Understanding the BASICS OF QSAR FOR APPLICATIONS IN PHARMACEUTICAL SCIENCES AND RISK ASSESSMENT

Understanding the BASICS OF QSAR FOR APPLICATIONS IN PHARMACEUTICAL SCIENCES AND RISK ASSESSMENT

KUNAL ROY
Department of Pharmaceutical Technology,
Jadavpur University, Kolkata, West Bengal, India

SUPRATIK KAR
Department of Pharmaceutical Technology,
Jadavpur University, Kolkata, West Bengal, India

RUDRA NARAYAN DAS
Department of Pharmaceutical Technology,
Jadavpur University, Kolkata, West Bengal, India

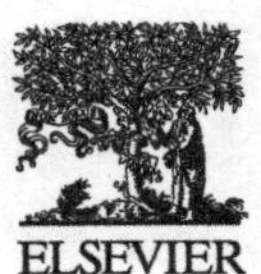

AMSTERDAM • BOSTON • HEIDELBERG • LONDON
NEW YORK • OXFORD • PARIS • SAN DIEGO
SAN FRANCISCO • SINGAPORE • SYDNEY • TOKYO
Academic Press is an imprint of Elsevier

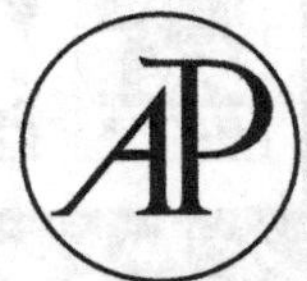

Academic Press is an imprint of Elsevier
32 Jamestown Road, London NW1 7BY, UK
525 B Street, Suite 1800, San Diego, CA 92101-4495, USA
225 Wyman Street, Waltham, MA 02451, USA
The Boulevard, Langford Lane, Kidlington, Oxford OX5 1GB, UK

ISBN: 978-0-12-801505-6

British Library Cataloguing-in-Publication Data
A catalogue record for this book is available from the British Library.

Library of Congress Cataloging-in-Publication Data
A catalog record for this book is available from the Library of Congress.

For Information on all Academic Press publications visit our website at http://store.elsevier.com/

Typeset by MPS Limited, Chennai, India
www.adi-mps.com

Printed and bound in the United States of America

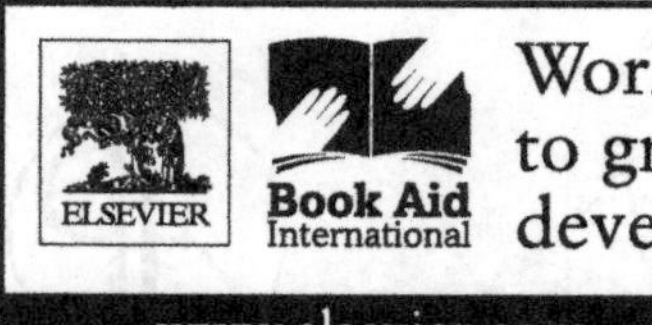

DEDICATION

In memory of Professor A. U. De

CONTENTS

FOREWORD

We are perhaps not far removed from the time when we shall be able to submit the bulk of chemical phenomena to calculation

Joseph-Louis Gay-Lussac, 1808

All of chemistry... would become a branch of mathematical analysis which, taking its constants from observation, would enable us to predict the character of any new compound...

Charles Babbage, 1838

Quantitative structure–activity relationships (QSARs) and quantitative structure–property relationships (QSPRs) have been part of scientific study for many years. As early as 1863, Cros [1] found that the toxicity of alcohols increased with decreasing aqueous solubility. Brown and Fraser [2] recognized in 1868 that "There can be no reasonable doubt but that a relation exists between the physiologic action of a substance and its chemical composition and constitution." Only a few years later, Mills [3] developed mathematical equations (almost certainly the very first QSPRs) to predict the melting and boiling points of several homologous series of chemicals as a function of their chain length.

By far the most widely quoted early work in QSAR is that of Overton [4] and Meyer [5], who independently observed in 1899 that the toxicity of simple organic chemicals to aquatic species increased with their partition coefficient. This discovery was most prescient, for the partitioning process is by far the most important factor controlling the biological activity of chemicals in living organisms.

Despite all this early activity, very little further progress was made in the field until the 1960s, when Corwin Hansch, the acknowledged "father" of QSAR, and his coworkers began to publish research showing that a range of biological activities could be modeled mathematically using simple physicochemical properties. Their first QSAR publication concerned the herbicidal effects of phenoxyacetic acids [6]; this seminal work was the touchstone for most of the thousands of QSAR publications that have followed in the 50+ years since then.

The multiple linear regression equation approach used by Hansch is still employed today for its simplicity and transparency. However, there is now also a plethora of other approaches to QSAR modeling, such as partial least squares, principal component analysis, artificial neural networks, regression trees and random forests, support vector machines, and comparative molecular field analysis (CoMFA), to name but a few. Of course, this is due in part to the huge increases in computing power and speed that we continue to see, as well as to the wide availability of databases and descriptors (physicochemical, quantum chemical, and structural properties that can be used in a QSAR to model the end point—biological or chemical—under consideration). Since 1999 in particular, there has been an almost exponential rise in the number of QSAR modeling papers published [7], driven in part by the increasing importance of QSAR in environmental and regulatory work.

There are regular conferences dedicated to QSAR, such as the European QSAR Symposia, started by MiloňTichý in Prague in 1973; the International Workshops on QSAR in Environmental and Health Sciences, started by Klaus Kaiser in Hamilton, Ontario, Canada, in 1983; and the Gordon Conferences on QSAR, first organized by Yvonne Martin in Rindge, New Hampshire, in 1975.

Despite all of this activity, very few books have been published specifically on QSAR. Therefore, this book by Roy, Kar, and Das, covering all aspects of QSAR modeling, is greatly to be welcomed. It will be useful to newcomers to QSAR, such as those having to cope with the requirements of the Registration, Evaluation, and Authorization of Chemicals (REACH) legislation, as well as to researchers and seasoned practitioners in pharmaceutical, agricultural, cosmetics, and environmental fields.

John C. Dearden
Emeritus Professor of Medicinal Chemistry,
School of Pharmacy and Biomolecular Sciences,
Liverpool John Moores University, Liverpool, UK

REFERENCES

[1] Cros AFA. Action de l'alcool amylique sur l'organisme (Action of amylalcohol on the organism). Thèse, Faculté de Médecine, Université de Strasbourg, Strasbourg, France; 1863.
[2] Brown AC, Fraser TR. On the connection between chemical constitution and physiological action; with special reference to the physiological action of the salts of the ammonium bases derived from Strychnia, Brucia, Thebaia, Codeia, Morphia, and Nicotia. Trans Roc Soc Edinburgh 1868;25:151–203.
[3] Mills EJ. On melting point and boiling point as related to composition. Phil Mag Ser 1884;5(17): 173–87.
[4] Overton E. Über die allgemeinenosmotischenEigenschaften der Zelle, ihrevermutlichenUrsachen und ihreBedeutungfür die Physiologie (On the general osmotic properties of the cell, their probable origin and their significance for physiology). Vierteljahrsschr Naturforsch Ges Zürich 1899;44: 88–135.
[5] Meyer H. ZurTheorie der Alkoholnarkose. ErsteMitteilung. WelcheEigenschaft der AnastheticabedingtihrenarkotischeWirkung? (On the theory of alcohol narcosis. Part 1. Which property of anaesthetics gives them their narcotic activity?) Naunyn-Schmiedebergs Arch Exp Pathol Pharmakol 1899;42:109–18.
[6] Hansch C, Maloney PP, Fujita T, Muir RM. Correlation of biological activity of phenoxyacetic acids with Hammett constants and partition coefficients. Nature 1962;194:178–80.
[7] Cherkasov A, Muratov E, Fourches D, Varnek A, Baskin I, Cronin MTD, et al. QSAR modeling: Where have you been? Where are you going to? J Med Chem 2014;57:4977–5010.

PREFACE

Quantitative structure–activity relationship (QSAR) modeling, originally evolved from physical organic chemistry, has seen wide application in the fields of medicinal chemistry (for lead optimization) and predictive toxicology (for risk assessment of chemicals). QSAR increases the probability of finding new drug candidates, thus avoiding the synthesis and biological screening of fewer potential molecules and saving time and money. It also helps in screening chemicals for target property or toxicity, thus helping in the prioritization of experimental testing and providing excellent statistical filtering tools. These techniques also have potential applications in other fields, such as materials science, nanoscience, and cosmetic technology for property and activity modeling and predictions. QSAR has now evolved as a well-recognized tool for application in chemistry when a biological activity or property or toxicity is the end point of the study for a series of chemicals of certain degree of structural similarity. The number of QSAR-related publications has grown very rapidly over the last two decades. However, the background knowledge about QSAR has remained confined mainly to researchers in the field and not been disseminated in general to students of and researchers into chemistry and the pharmaceutical sciences. There are many reference texts on advanced topics of QSAR, but there is no good resource covering the basic aspects of QSAR for the beginners in the field. In the present attempt, we have tried to incorporate all the necessary information so that readers may become acquainted with the various areas of the field, at least in a cursory manner.

Chapter 1 deals with the background knowledge and historical evolution of QSAR. Chapter 2 discusses chemical information and introduces the concept of descriptors. In the next chapter, classical QSAR, encompassing the Free–Wilson model, Fujita–Ban modification, the Hansch model, and the mixed approach, all of which have created the foundation of modern QSAR, are covered in detail. Chapter 4 deals with graph theory-based QSAR and topological descriptors. The use of computers in medicinal chemistry, computational chemistry, and related aspects are discussed in Chapter 5. The selected statistical methods used to develop linear and nonlinear QSARs are discussed in Chapter 6. The validation tools used for QSAR models are covered in Chapter 7. Chapter 8 discusses important 3D-QSAR models. Chapter 9 introduces some newer QSAR techniques. Other related (non-QSAR) techniques including docking and pharmacophore mapping used in drug design are dealt with in Chapter 10. Some examples of successful application of QSAR modeling in drug discovery are cited in Chapter 11. The last chapter discusses future avenues for further application of QSAR. We hope that the readers will get at least a bird's-eye view on different aspects of QSAR and related tools. Readers may consult the original references cited in the book for a more detailed discussion.

In this opportunity, we thank Professor C. Sengupta and Professor J. K. Gupta, Department of Pharmaceutical Technology, Jadavpur University, Kolkata, India, for giving us inspiration for writing this book. We must acknowledge the help and inspiration received from our respective family members during the development of the book. We are thankful to the publisher for releasing this book, which we hope will be of use to QSAR learners. We also thank Dr. Kristine Jones and Molly M. McLaughlin of Elsevier for their cooperation.

Kunal Roy
Supratik Kar
Rudra Narayan Das

CHAPTER 1

Background of QSAR and Historical Developments

Contents

Understanding the Basics of QSAR for Applications in Pharmaceutical Sciences and Risk Assessment.
ISBN: 978-0-12-801505-6, DOI: http://dx.doi.org/10.1016/B978-0-12-801505-6.00001-6

1.1 INTRODUCTION

Chemicals are essential components of human civilization. The applications of chemicals in the modern era span a wide range, from industrial to household environments. The esteemed goal of a chemist lies in the development of chemicals with the desired profile of their better behavioral manifestation; that is, activity/property. In cases of chemicals with pronounced biological activity or drugs, the chemist aims in enhancing the efficacy of the molecule while reducing any toxic effects exerted. Now, following the general axiom, development of a new chemical can be achieved either by designing a complete new entity or by modifying an existing one. In both cases, chemists need to possess sufficient knowledge regarding the nature of the chemical and its potential for interaction with the biological system. It is obvious that the biological activity (including toxicity) and property of any chemical (e.g., drugs, pharmaceuticals, and carcinogens) depend upon its interaction with the biological system concerned. Hence, the primary goal of a chemical designer lies in establishing a rational explanation of the mechanism of action of the chemical, which can lead to the derivation of a suitable theoretical basis and thus enabling the tailoring of its structure. Sometimes the lack of suitable explanation for a drug action limits the derivation of a hypothetical basis. In order to establish a proper theoretical basis for the action of chemicals, one would need to have a deep insight into the fundamental chemistry of the system that controls its physicochemical and structural behavior [1].

The biological activity elicited by chemicals is attributed by various interactions of the molecule at the critical reaction site in the biological system. The ligand molecule is recognized by a particular receptor followed by formation of a ligand–receptor complex involving different physicochemical forces. The complex then undergoes some conformational changes that lead to a series of events giving rise to the activity. The features possessed by a chemical entity get modified during its encounter with the biological system. Hence, elicitation of biological response is controlled by the way in which the chemical reacts at the active site of the biological system. In other words, the biological system plays a crucial role in determining the structural features of a chemical needed to elicit a desired response. Owing to the limited available space for this chapter, we shall not elaborate on this issue; instead, we would like to present a brief overview of the important steps and interactions involved at the biological reaction site when a chemical comes in contact with a biological system.

Before eliciting a desired response, drugs and other bioactive molecules are subjected to a complex path inside the biological system governed by their pharmacokinetic and pharmacodynamic behavior. Following administration, the drug molecules are subjected to the uncertainties arising from absorption, metabolism, excretion, and the *random walk* toward the critical reaction site, where it binds with a suitable receptor molecule. Figure 1.1 depicts different stages of pharmacokinetic movement of a drug

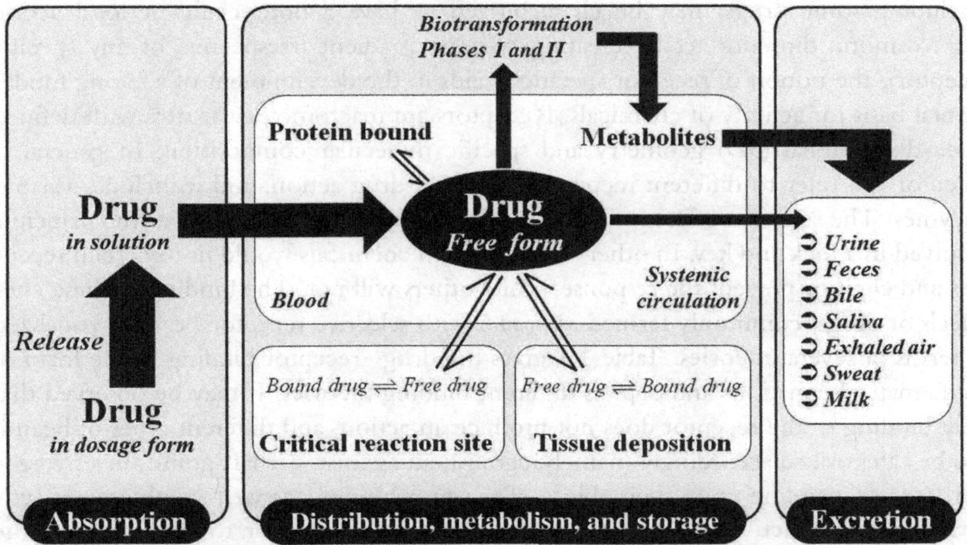

Figure 1.1 Different pharmacokinetic stages of bioactive ligands inside a living system.

inside the body. The random walk usually refers to the transportation of the drug molecule in various compartments, including the target site. The pharmacokinetic movements of the drug molecule, along with its pharmacodynamic properties, are regulated by a wide number of physical, chemical, and biological factors (e.g., partitioning behavior, solubility, pK_a value, ionization, interatomic distance, and stereochemical arrangement), and ultimately contribute to a considerable degree of complexity and uncertainty in some cases [2,3]. The drug molecules and other bioactive chemicals are considered to interact with macromolecular complexes present on the cellular surface or inside the cell to elicit a response. In the past, the response of several bioactive agents was considered to occur as a result of their interactions within a specific site of the living system. In the mid-1800s, Bernard [4] demonstrated that curare acts as a neuromuscular blocking agent by preventing the contraction of skeletal muscle following nerve stimulation, while its effect is lost when the muscle is subjected to direct stimulation. This study indicated the existence of chemical neurotransmission at the synapse between the nerve and muscle, and the curare was eliciting a localized response by cutting off the transmission. Later, Langley [5] provided further impetus to the concept of specific cellular component by showing the selective and potent action of parasympathomimetic agent pilocarpine which was selectively reversed by an atropine like compound. It was Ehrlich and Himmelweit [6] who introduced the term *receptor* or *receptive substance* in this realm and contemplated that an organic compound (which may be a drug) exerts its action via binding to specific receptive substances. Although some chemical agents (including some drugs) may be characterized to have a nonspecific or local action (e.g., osmotic diuretics act by creating osmotic gradient irrespective of any specific receptor), the notion of receptor specificity aids in the development of a strong fundamental basis for activity of chemicals. Receptors are macromolecular sites with defined three-dimensional (3D) geometry and specific molecular composition. In general, a receptor can refer to different recognition sites of drug action, and it includes various enzymes. The selective effects of drugs on receptors can be envisioned as the principle involved in a lock and key. In other words, certain chemicals would fit to certain receptors and elicit or prevent the response, while others will not. The binding of these chemicals or drugs, commonly termed as *ligands* with selective receptors, can be visualized in terms of several theories. Table 1.1 gives the drug–receptor binding in the form of mathematical equations and depicts different binding theories. It may be observed that only binding to the receptor does not produce an action, and different types of ligands can be categorized accordingly (namely, agonist, antagonist, partial agonist, inverse agonist, etc.), depending upon their ability of receptor binding, as well as subsequent activation (intrinsic activity). Apart from the affinity of a receptor toward a ligand, the number of receptors also plays an important function in a given tissue. Receptors are usually characterized by two types: (1) G-protein–coupled receptors and (2) ligand gated ion channels, while voltage-sensitive ion channels also act as receptors in some cases. The two major functions served by receptors include (1) specific ligand recognition and (2) transduction of the signal into a response; accordingly, receptors are possessed by a binding domain for ligand attachment and one effector domain to allow required conformational changes [3].

Now, the obvious question arises of how the ligand molecules bind with specific receptor sites. The answer lies in the chemical structure of the ligands. Biologically active ligands are characterized with various functional groups that are engaged in the formation of various types of chemical bonds like ionic bonds and hydrogen bonds, with the corresponding groups present in the receptor cavities. Various structural features (namely steric, geometric, and stereochemical) features of ligands also play a crucial role while interacting with a receptor. Apart from that, there are cases where the information of the receptor is not important since the ligand bypasses any receptor-mediated action. Examples of this include drugs altering solvent properties, drugs acting by physical or chemical means, and the antimetabolites that produce nonfunctional cellular components [3]. Hence, it is evident that in order to pursue a rational strategy for the design of a desired biologically active ligand, one would need to have sufficient knowledge regarding its interaction with the target receptor (if available) and other structural specificities. The predictive modeling studies aim in exploring all such potential attributes that affect the activity/property/toxicity of chemicals. In the following sections, we will present the impact of various types of physicochemical forces, as well as structural features of ligand molecules that enable them to

Table 1.1 An overview of different receptor-binding theories and classification of ligands

Mathematical expression for ligand binding

$[R] + [L] \rightleftharpoons [RL] \rightarrow$ Conformational changes $\rightarrow [R]$ + cellular effects

where R and L represent receptor and ligand (e.g., drug), respectively. The same relationship can also be used to designate the binding of a substrate to an enzyme and it takes the following form:

$[E] + [S] \rightleftharpoons [ES] \rightleftharpoons [E]$ + products

Here, the enzyme and the substrate are denoted by E and S, respectively.

The desired characteristics for receptor activation and categorization of ligands thereof

Affinity	Refers to the ability of a ligand to recognize and bind to a receptor. Also known as *potency of the ligand*.
Intrinsic activity	Refers to the ability of a ligand to activate a receptor. This involves induction of conformational changes in the receptor that leads to change in cellular process by the activating transmembrane transductional mechanism involving G-proteins or ion channel.
Agonist	Ligands possessing both affinity and maximal efficacy. Example: Morphine is a strong agonist of μ opioid receptor.
Competitive antagonists	Ligands possessing affinity but no intrinsic activity; that is, efficacy. Example: Naloxone is a competitive antagonist of μ opioid receptor.
Partial agonist	Ligands characterized by affinity and submaximal intrinsic activity. Example: Butorphanol is a partial agonist of μ opioid receptor.
Inverse agonist	Ligands characterized by affinity and negative intrinsic activity. Example: Dimethoxyethylcarbomethoxy-β-carboline is an inverse agonist to the benzodiazepine receptor.

Different Theories of Receptor Binding

Occupancy theory	Response is directly predicted by the number of agonist-bound receptors.
Rate theory	Intensity of the response depends on the ligand–receptor interaction per unit time.
Induced fit theory	The receptor adapts a conformational change as the ligand approaches toward it and results in effective binding.
Macromolecular perturbation theory	It combines rate and induced fit theory and considers the existence of two types of conformational changes. Here, the rate determines the ultimate presence of one of the conformers, and hence the response. Agonists produce response by initiating desired perturbation, while antagonists fail to do the same and do not yield a response.
Activation aggregation theory	It considers the receptors to belong in a dynamic equilibrium between active and inactive states. Agonists aid in shifting the equilibrium toward the active state and thereby eliciting response while antagonists cause prevention of the active state. The action of inverse agonists is explained by using this theory.

elicit different types of responses. Then we will give a sense of how quantitative predictive modeling analysis can be performed using all these information for the development of a rational theoretical basis of designing and developing novel chemical entities.

1.2 PHYSICOCHEMICAL ASPECTS OF BIOLOGICAL ACTIVITY OF DRUGS AND CHEMICALS

The kinetics (e.g., movement) and dynamics (e.g., mechanism of action of chemicals, including drugs, inside a biological system) are influenced by the physicochemical properties of drug molecules. Three important physicochemical properties implicated in drug action are hydrophobic, electronic, and steric features, which enable a biologically active ligand to interact with its target receptor [3]. The following section will give a brief account of these properties, whereas a more detailed discussion can be found in subsequent chapters of this book.

1.2.1 Hydrophobicity

The most fundamental criterion for eliciting a response by a bioactive ligand molecule involves its interaction with the biological system that comprises lipoid barriers. Lipids represent an inevitable constituent in all types of biological membranes, and hence the hydrophobicity of a bioactive ligand or drug molecule becomes important for its absorption from the site of administration and its distribution; that is, partitioning into different physiological compartments. Furthermore, the hydrophobic property is also crucial while interacting at the target site containing hydrophobic functionalities. However, the lipophilicity should be maintained at an optimum level in order to address two essential factors [namely, concentration of drug (or other bioactive chemical) in the extracellular fluid and its elimination from the body]. The *n*-octanol/water partition coefficient gives a suitable measure of the hydrophobic behavior of any chemical. However, features like the chromatographic retention constant R_M and log K' also give an account of the lipophilicity measure. The hydrophobic property of chemicals can also be theoretically computed for the whole molecule, as well as for molecular fragments.

1.2.2 Electronic effect

Drug interaction involves various electronic attributes for establishing bonding with the target site since the biological receptors may comprise amino acid species containing charged and polar functional groups. Various types of dispersion forces (charge transfer complex formation, ionic interaction, inductive effect, hydrogen bonding, polarization effect, acid–base catalytic property, etc.) characterize electronic features. Again, some of these parameters employ multiple mechanistic features.

1.2.3 Steric effect

Steric features are principally related to the 2D spatial arrangement of molecules. In order to satisfy the requirement of a specific spatial location in the receptor cavity (i.e., fitting to the receptor), suitable steric features are essential for bioactive molecules, including drugs. The steric influences include intramolecular contribution of substituents, molecular bulk, size, shape, spatial arrangement, and specific conformational attributes.

1.2.4 Forces and chemical bonding

The physicochemical characteristics of chemicals are governed by various types of forces and energies. Two principal forces that rule the behavior of chemicals are attractive and repulsive forces. Attractive forces attempt to keep the entities together and can be of the cohesive type (i.e., attraction of alike molecules) or the adhesive type (i.e., attraction of unlike molecules). On the other hand, repulsive forces keep molecules apart. These forces result from intramolecular and intermolecular bonding energies, which are governed by electron orbital interaction, and such forces must be in an energetically favorable balanced state in order to initiate a molecular interaction. Both the repulsion and attraction forces operate together when an interaction between molecules is instituted. With the gradual proximity of two atoms or molecules, attraction is established since the opposite charges and binding forces come closer than the similar charges and forces. In this case, the negatively charged electron cloud of the molecules plays a significant role in sustaining the equilibrium of forces between the participating molecules. However, bringing the molecules very close so that they overlap their outer cloud of charge would make them start pushing themselves apart. Hence, attractive forces aid in cohering, while repulsion tends to prevent the interpenetration and annihilation of molecules. The interaction between bioactive ligand molecule and the receptor involves different forms of attractive intermolecular forces to form bonding [7]. In the next section, we will present an account of these interactions (namely, van der Waals force, electrostatic force, hydrogen bonding, ion–dipole interaction, etc. [3,7,8]), which help in establishing a binding between ligand molecule and target cellular components followed by the expression of activity.

1.2.4.1 Covalent bond

The covalent bond implicates the strongest bond in the realm of ligand–receptor interactions. Such a bond is formed by the share of an electron from each of the two participating atoms. In case of drug-receptor interaction, the electrons are shared by atoms of the ligand and receptor molecule. The strength of covalent bonds varies from 50 to 150 kcal/mol. It has been observed that owing to the greater strength of the covalent bonds, ligands are irreversibly bound to the receptor when such bonding occurs. Hence, covalent bond formation usually leads to receptor inactivation or antagonism and normal biological action of drugs or endogenous substrate are not obtained in such cases since the dissociation of ligand becomes difficult. Such blockade of activity of a biological target due to covalent bond formation is found in many cases—namely, antagonism of the α-adrenoceptor by phenoxybenzamine through alkylation of an amino, sulfhydryl, or carboxyl group on the receptor, blockade of acetylcholinesterase receptor by organophosphates (dyflos, ecothiophate) by phosphorylation of an ester bond, etc.

1.2.4.2 Ionic bond

Ionic bonds are formed during attraction of two ions of opposite charge involving electrostatic force. Ionic bonds hold a strength varying between 5 and 10 kcal/mol in an aqueous environment. The strength of ionic bonds tends to decrease as two participating atoms are taken apart, and this decrease has been observed to be proportional to the squared distance between the atoms. Hence this decay with an increasing distance is slower than that of the dispersion forces (*vide infra*). There is an increased strength of ionic bond when a charged ligand or drug species approaches the target receptor. The strength of an ionic bond supports initial transient interaction between a ligand and a receptor, and it also allows dissociation of the bioactive ligand from receptor, unlike a covalent bond. A measure of electronegativity determines the propensity of an atom in forming ionic bonds. Atoms having a stronger electronegativity value than hydrogen, (i.e., a value more than 2.1 in Pauling scale), which include fluorine, chlorine, hydroxyl, sulfhydryl, and carboxyl, possess a stronger affinity toward electrons than groups like alkyl, which do not participate in such bonding.

Figure 1.2 shows a representation of covalent and ionic bond formation between functional groups of a hypothetical ligand molecule and a receptor surface.

1.2.4.3 Hydrogen bond

Hydrogen bonding refers to a weak bond formation between a hydrogen atom attached to a strong electronegative atom and another atom of higher electronegativity. Hence, the hydrogen atom, which is connected to a highly electronegative atom (e.g., oxygen, nitrogen, and sulfur) via a covalent bond develops a partial positive charge and gets attracted to another strong electronegative atom (e.g., oxygen, fluorine, nitrogen, and sulfur), which has developed a partial negative charge due to attraction between the electron cloud and its neighbor atom. Hence, it may be noted that hydrogen bond formation can take place within a single molecule, satisfying the presence of partially positive charged hydrogen and partially negatively charged heteroatoms, as well as between two different molecular species. The former case is considered intramolecular hydrogen bonding while it is intermolecular in the latter case. The molecules contributing hydrogen atom (i.e., hydrogen bond donors), as well as the other electronegative participant molecules (i.e., hydrogen bond acceptors), are characterized by a dipolar

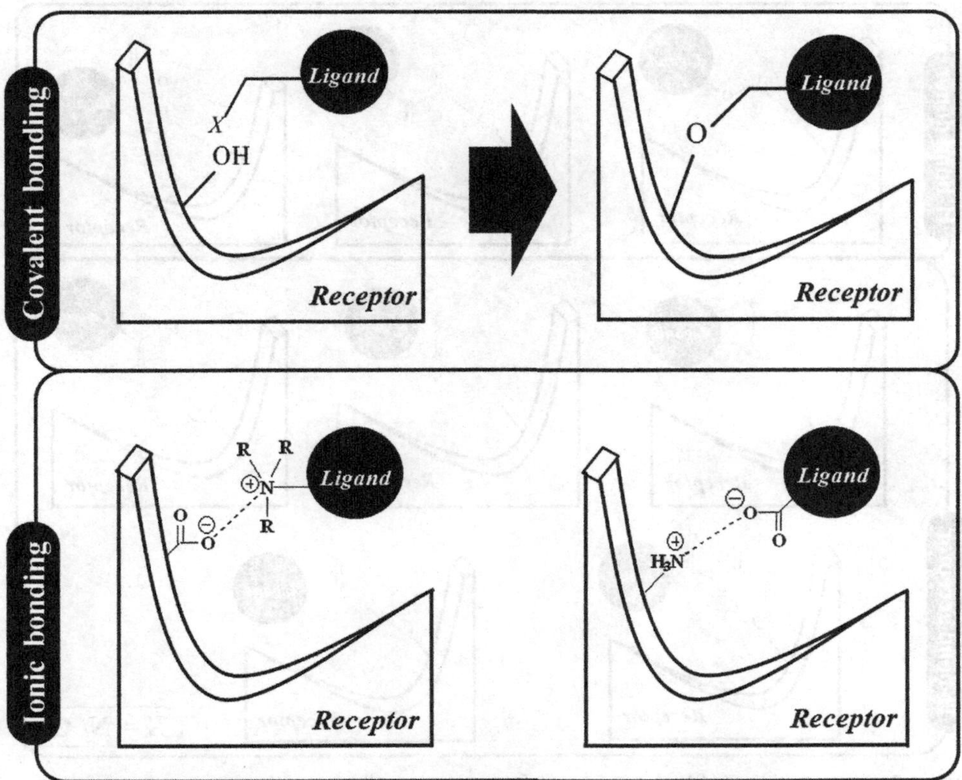

Figure 1.2 Formation of covalent and ionic bond between ligand and receptor.

nature. The simplest example probably would be the water molecule, which easily forms a hydrogen bond due to its behavior as an electron dipole. The strength of a single hydrogen bond usually varies from 2 to 5 kcal/mol. Hence, formation of single hydrogen bond is relatively weak and may not account for a ligand–receptor interaction by itself. However, a significant amount of bonding stability can be achieved when there is formation of multiple hydrogen bonds between two such systems and elicits a response. Because of the presence of amino acid residues in receptors containing both the hydrogen bond donor and acceptor functionalities, hydrogen bonding plays a crucial role in binding ligands like drug molecules possessing similar functionality and aids in the expression or suppression of the activity/property/toxicity. Figure 1.3 depicts different situations where an arbitrary ligand molecule develops a hydrogen bond with a receptor by acting as a hydrogen bond donor as well as an acceptor.

Hydrogen bonding plays a crucial role in the bonding and arrangement pattern of various molecular assemblies including complex protein structure. The bonding between a hydrogen bond donor and an acceptor atom is very selective and can be

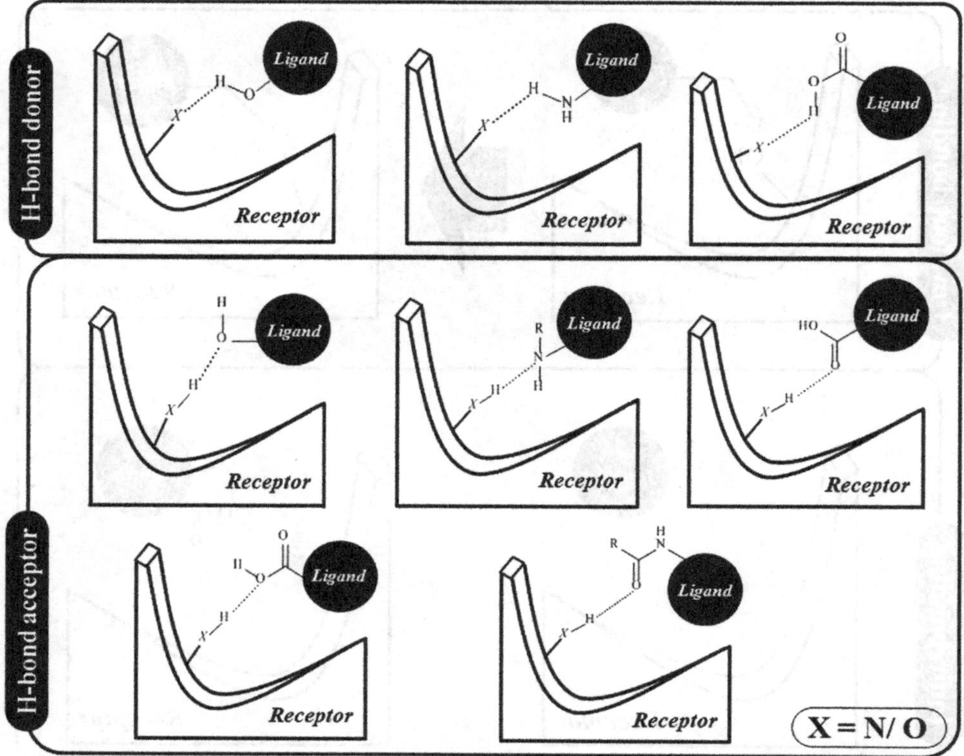

Figure 1.3 Representation of hydrogen bond formation by a ligand with receptor site.

defined in terms of specific distance and angle between them, as well as directionality. Various theoretical *ab initio* studies on the hydrogen-bonding pattern have shown the H-bond to be highly directional at the donor hydrogen atom. The binding selectivity of a receptor protein to a ligand is influenced by the directionality of the hydrogen-bonding groups on its surface. The H-bond formation is controlled by the orbital spatial distribution of the acceptor site, along with a dipolar orientation of the donor group. The tetrahedral hybridization of oxygen atom is justified by the angle of $R_1-H\cdots O$ which is approximately 180°, while for $R_2-O\cdots H$, it is 110°. Studies have shown that a decrease in the angle causes reduced stability [9].

1.2.4.4 Hydrophobic force

The hydrophobic interaction of molecules refers to an effect of dislikeness toward water, that is, insolubility in aqueous medium. Formation of such force is favored and accompanied with a change in entropy of the system. At rest, the water molecules remain in an orderly fashion characterized by reduced entropy of the system. This is characterized by the free Brownian movement of water molecule along all directions accompanied with the formation of favorable intermolecular hydrogen bonds. With the addition of chemicals possessing nonpolar groups, a constraint is applied on the water molecules limiting their free orientation. This unfavorable interaction is overcome by reducing contact of water molecule with the nonpolar interface, leading to the aggregation of the nonpolar chemical in an aqueous medium. Such a phenomenon triggers a favorable change of entropy that exceeds the enthalpy, giving a negative value for the free energy. The strength of such interaction is 0.37 kcal/mol per $-CH_2-$ group. Hence, we can see that molecules possessing long alkyl chains possess a higher value of hydrophobic force that may be stronger than ionic bonds or other such weak forces. Hydrophobic interaction may assist in binding a drug to its receptor, as well as stabilization of the protein structure.

1.2.4.5 van der Waals interaction

A van der Waals interaction is a relatively weak force ranging from 0.5 to 1 kcal/mol and is nonionic in nature. Neutral molecules containing electronegative atoms, like oxygen and nitrogen, have a tendency to draw the electron cloud toward itself through the covalent bond from its less electronegative neighbor atom. Such phenomenon institutes a dipolar nature into the molecule, creating a charge dispersion; that is, a partial positive ($\delta+$) as well as a partial negative ($\delta-$) charge inside the same molecule. A weak interaction force is established between opposite charges ($\delta+$ and $\delta-$) of two participating molecules when they are placed close to each other by aligning the positive end of one molecule close to the negative end of the other. Now, these forces can be classified based on the type of charge dispersion mechanism in participating molecules and the connection established thereof. Molecules enabling such partial charge distribution by itself because they have strong electronegative atoms are considered to establish a permanent dipole. Permanent dipole agents can persuade a dipolar nature in a neighbor molecule, which is known as *induced dipole*, and then interaction between the two is possible. If the connection occurs between two such permanent dipoles, the interaction becomes much like that of ionic fashion, although possessing much less strength. In this case, the force involved is recognized as a *Keesom force*. Whereas if a permanent dipole polarizes the electron cloud in its neighbor molecule, that is, induced dipole and establishes an interaction, the force is termed as a *Debye force*. One more such force, *London force* (induced dipole–induced dipole), acts between two neighboring neutral species (e.g., aliphatic hydrocarbon) by the induction of partial charge distribution. The London force explains the fluidity and cohesiveness of biological membranes under normal conditions. In short, a Keesom force is the weak attraction between dipole and dipole, a Debye force corresponds to a dipole-induced dipole interaction, and a London force is an induced dipole–induced dipole interaction caused by the induction of polarity in each other by nonpolar

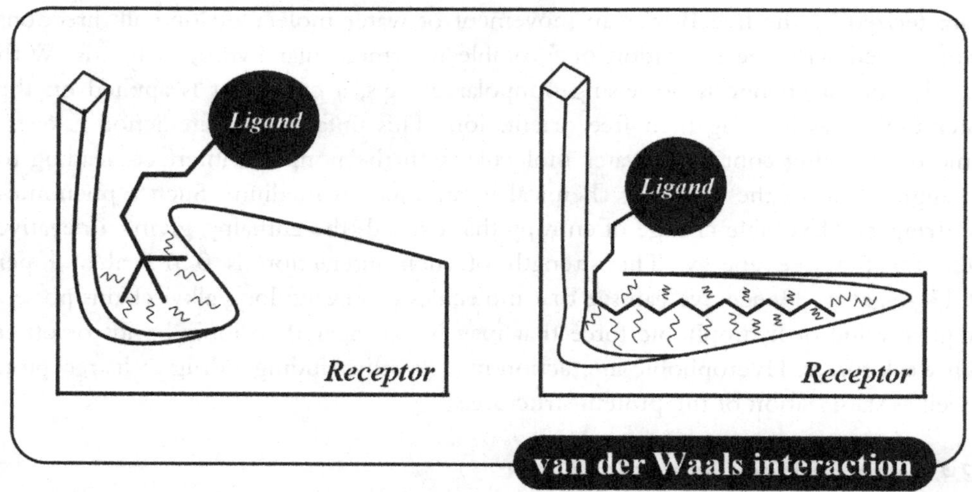

Figure 1.4 Establishment of van der Waals interaction at the receptor site by a suitable ligand.

molecules. The potential energy in all these three variants of the van der Waals force holds an inverse relation with the distance of separation raised to the sixth power. Figure 1.4 describes the establishment of a van der Waals interaction between a ligand molecule and a hypothetical receptor cavity and/or pocket. The representative formation of a dipole, as well as an induced dipole interaction, are shown in Figure 1.5.

1.2.4.6 Pi–pi (π–π) stacking interaction

The $\pi-\pi$ stacking interaction refers to a special type of noncovalent attractive force occurring between compounds possessing unsaturation; that is, pi (π) electrons. Such interactions, especially in the arene systems, play a significant role in the recognition process of a ligand molecule and its receptor. Although knowledge of the exact mechanism of pi–pi ($\pi-\pi$) stacking is incomplete, studies have revealed that pi orbitals of two molecules do not overlap like that of a conventional covalent bond. Simply expressed, two planar organic molecules, one of which is preferably aromatic and containing pi electrons, form a complex or stack by involving noncovalent-bonding forces. Formation of such stacked geometry between planar molecules enables minimization of the solvent-exposed surface area of the complex. Considering benzene as a representative model of the arene family, three stacked geometries (namely, parallel-displaced, T-shaped edge-to-face, and eclipsed face-to-face) can be identified as a result of the formation of a $\pi-\pi$ stacking interaction (Figure 1.6). Several researchers have attempted to hypothesize these patterns of interactions. One group of researchers hypothesizes that [10] the stacked pi–pi association can be attributed to an electrostatic type of interaction that controls the out-of-plane electron density between two aromatic molecules of

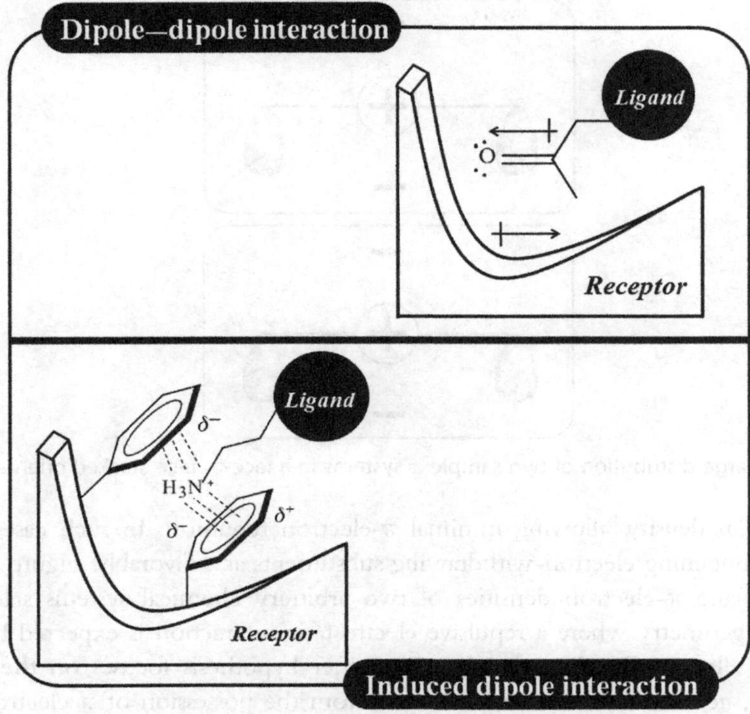

Figure 1.5 Depiction of dipolar and induced-dipolar interaction between a functional group of sample ligand and receptor surface.

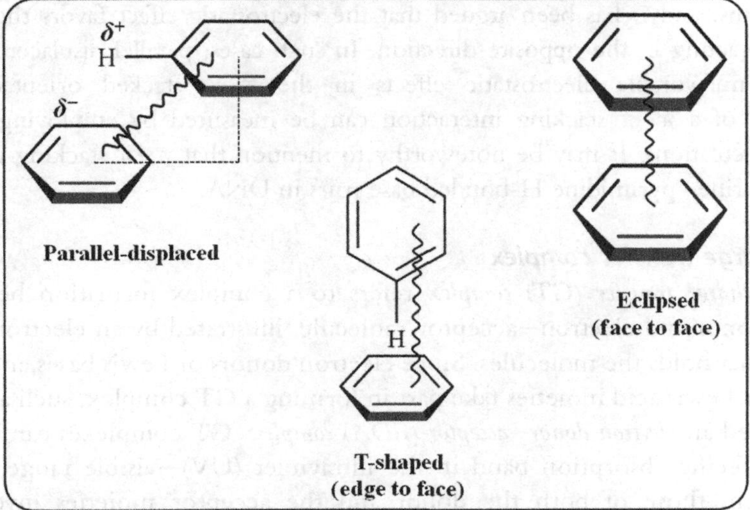

Figure 1.6 Representation of different π–π stacking geometries.

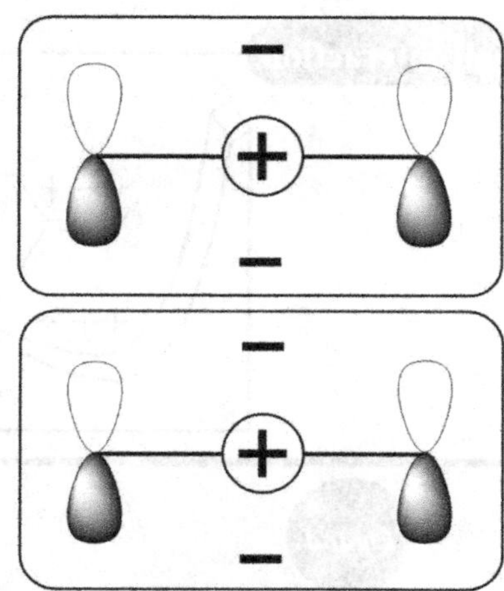

Figure 1.7 Charge distribution of two sample π systems in a face-to-face stacked orientation.

low π-electron density, allowing minimal π-electron repulsion. In such cases, an aromatic ring containing electron-withdrawing substituents acts favorably. Figure 1.7 shows the out-of-plane π-electron densities of two arbitrary chemical systems stacked in a face-to-face geometry where a repulsive electrostatic interaction is expected because of the negative charge. On the other hand, another hypothesis focuses on the mode of binding (i.e., geometry of the complex apart from the possession of π electron cloud), and it has been shown that the decrease in interaction energy of an aromatic system in a T-shaped complex is similar to saturated molecules [11]. A dispersion component has also been identified as the determinant factor in a $\pi-\pi$ stacked complex in large unsaturated systems, and it has been argued that the electrostatic effect favors the saturated complex by acting in the opposite direction. In such cases, parallel displacement minimizes the unfavorable electrostatic effects in the $\pi-\pi$ stacked orientation [11]. Occurrence of a $\pi-\pi$ stacking interaction can be measured by employing quantum chemical calculations. It may be noteworthy to mention that $\pi-\pi$ stacking interaction occurs in purine–pyrimidine H-bonded base pairs in DNA.

1.2.4.7 Charge transfer complex

The term *charge transfer (CT) complex* refers to a complex formation between an electron–donor and electron–acceptor molecule, illustrated by an electronic attraction force that holds the molecules. Since electron donors or Lewis bases and electron acceptors or Lewis acid moieties take part in forming a CT complex, such association is also termed an *electron donor–acceptor (EDA) complex*. CT complexes can be identified by a specific absorption band in the ultraviolet (UV)–visible range, which is separate from those of both the donor and the acceptor moieties involved. By employing a valence-bond formalism where each member represents an atom and the donor−atom pair (D−A) a diatomic like molecule, Mulliken and Person [12] proposed a diatomic wave function to characterize such complexes. The solved version of the equation can be represented as in Eq. (1.1):

$$h\nu_{C-T} = I_D - E_A + C \tag{1.1}$$

where I_D represents ionization energy of the donor, while E_A is the electron affinity of the acceptor for the C−T band $h\nu_{C-T}$. Here, C is a constant term. However, there are several other methods for the determination of CT complexes, including molecular orbital calculations. CT complexes are formed in biological systems, an example of which may be the stabilization of chemicals (drugs) that intercalate between the DNA bases. Example of some electron donor chemicals involved in CT complex formation includes diethyl ether, diethyl sulfide, methyl amines, *p*-chloranil, and benzene. while iodine, bromine, SO_2, BF_3, $AlCl_3$, and $TiCl_4$ are some representative acceptors in such complexes. Spectroscopic characterization of CT complexes of various drugs and pharmaceuticals are made to study the binding mechanism of drug-receptor. Figure 1.8, shows that the CT complex formation of drug sulfamethoxazole (antibacterial) and quinidine (antiarrhythmic agent) with two different benzoquinone derivates (namely, *p*-chloranil and dichlorodicyanobenzoquinone, respectively).

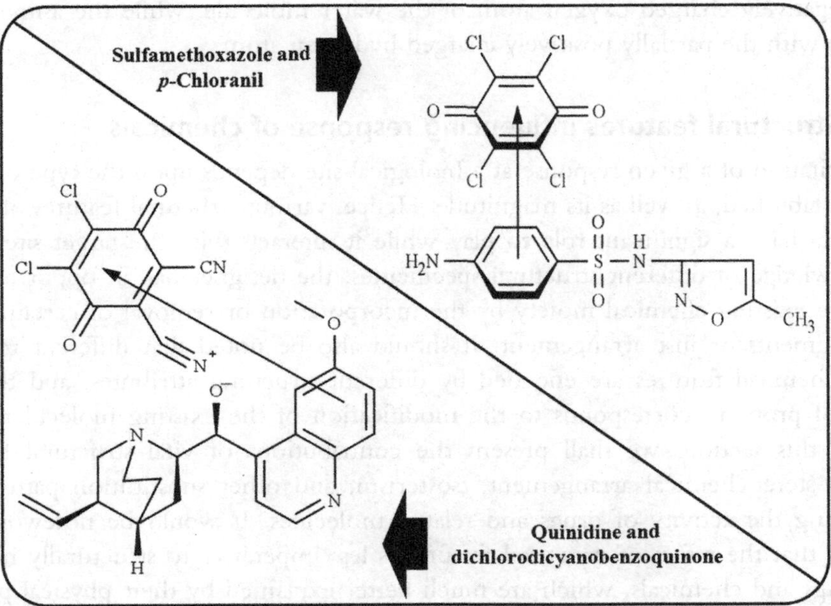

Figure 1.8 CT complex formation of sample drug molecules: sulfamethoxazole, *p*-chloranil, quinidine, and dichlorodicyanobenzoquinone.

1.2.4.8 Orbital-overlapping interaction

The pi electron orbital in a system sometimes creates a dipole–dipole force of attraction due to overlapping of the orbitals. Aromatic rings are special systems, and the π-orbital electron cloud imparts a partial negative charge above and below the ring while the equatorial hydrogen atoms remain positively charged. Hence, dipole–dipole interaction is possible between two aromatic rings due to the orbital-overlap phenomenon. It has been observed that the highest energy interaction in terms of intramolecular and intermolecular forces between two aromatic systems is supported by a near-perpendicular geometric alignment with respect to each other [13]. Such interaction provides stability to proteins containing aromatic amino acids. Aromatic stacking has an impact on the binding of drugs and other ligand molecules containing an aromatic system with receptor molecules. It may be noted that presence of atoms containing a lone electron pair, (e.g., oxygen and nitrogen on an aromatic ring) can influence such dipole–dipole bonding. Furthermore, such interaction is also affected by repulsive forces if the attractive interaction is changed.

1.2.4.9 Ion-dipole and ion-induced dipole interaction

Such interactions are shown in systems comprising of molecules (polar or nonpolar). Aqueous solubility of certain ionic crystalline systems is monitored by such forces because water behaves as a dipolar molecule. Here, the cationic part attracts the partially negatively charged oxygen atom of the water molecule, while the anionic part interacts with the partially positively charged hydrogen atom.

1.2.5 Structural features influencing response of chemicals

The elicitation of a given response at a biological site depends upon the type of interaction established, as well as its magnitude. Hence, various structural features of ligand molecules have a significant role to play while it interacts with the target site. From the knowledge of different structural specificities, the designer has an opportunity to tailor the existing chemical moiety by the incorporation or removal of certain structural fragments or just arrangement. It should also be noted that different required physicochemical features are encoded by different structural attributes, and the fine tuning of property corresponds to the modification of the existing molecular structure. In this section, we shall present the contributions of vital structural features (namely, stereochemical arrangement, isosterism, and other substitution patterns) in influencing the activity of drugs and related molecules. It would be noteworthy to mention that the effect of structural features is less imperative to structurally nonspecific drugs and chemicals, which are much better explained by their physical properties (e.g., action of general anesthetics, volatile insecticides, and antacids). In cases of structurally specific drugs, structural features contribute toward the affinity of the drug in binding to a receptor, as well as its ability to induce the desired conformational change (e.g., intrinsic activity).

1.2.5.1 Stereochemical features influencing drug activity

One of the fundamental properties of the biological system is chirality. Hence, the spatial arrangement of many drug molecules in 3D space plays a crucial role in optimal interaction with a stereospecific receptor site, thereby eliciting a response. Consideration of proper optical, geometric, and conformational specificity can enhance the drug activity to a very great extent. The use of only a single (active) enantiomer can also reduce the side effects arising from an inactive enantiomer. Apart from activity, stereospecificity offers selective metabolism, as well as membrane penetration of chemical agents. Diethylstilbestrol is characterized by better estrogenic activity in *trans*-isomeric form than the *cis*-form, and (−) epinephrine is more active than (+) epinephrine. The chair form of the piperidine ring with axial hydroxyl group in the compound 4-(4-hydroxypiperidino)-4′-fluorobutyrophenone provides the tranquilizing action. S-(−) propranolol has around 40 times more potency than its *R*-(+) form. The calcium channel blocker verapamil possesses varying stereoselectivity for vascular and cardiac tissues and it has been observed that *S*-verapamil shows both vasodialatory and cardio-depressant actions, while *R*-verapamil is majorly a vasodialator drug [7,14]. Figure 1.9 shows the mentioned stereochemical forms of the cited examples. In Figure 1.10, we have attempted to portray the stereochemical features influencing the binding of the epinephrine molecule to its receptor site. It may be observed that the less sympathomimetic potency of (+) epinephrine can be attributed to the stereochemical orientation of the hydroxyl group on the chiral carbon atom that hinders the formation of a third H-bond with the receptor site.

1.2.5.2 Isosterism features influencing drug activity

Sometimes bioactive chemicals suffer from unwanted side effects, physicochemical properties, bioavailability, and poor pharmacokinetic issues owing to the presence of undesirable functional groups. Isosterism provides a concept of replacing such groups or atoms with other groups (or atoms) having similar properties, thereby obtaining the desired response [14]. The notion of chemical isosterism was introduced by Langmuir [15] to depict similar physical behaviors among atoms, functional groups, radicals, and molecules. Langmuir's similarity considered atoms containing the same number of valence electrons. Later, Grimm [16] developed his hydride displacement law to consider similarity among groups possessing the same number of valence electrons but a different number of atoms. The hydride displacement depicts that the same number of valence electrons is maintained in the next group element in the periodic table when hydrogen atom is progressively added to the previous group element. Hence, OH, NH_2, and CH_3 groups represent isosters. Such groups were observed to depict

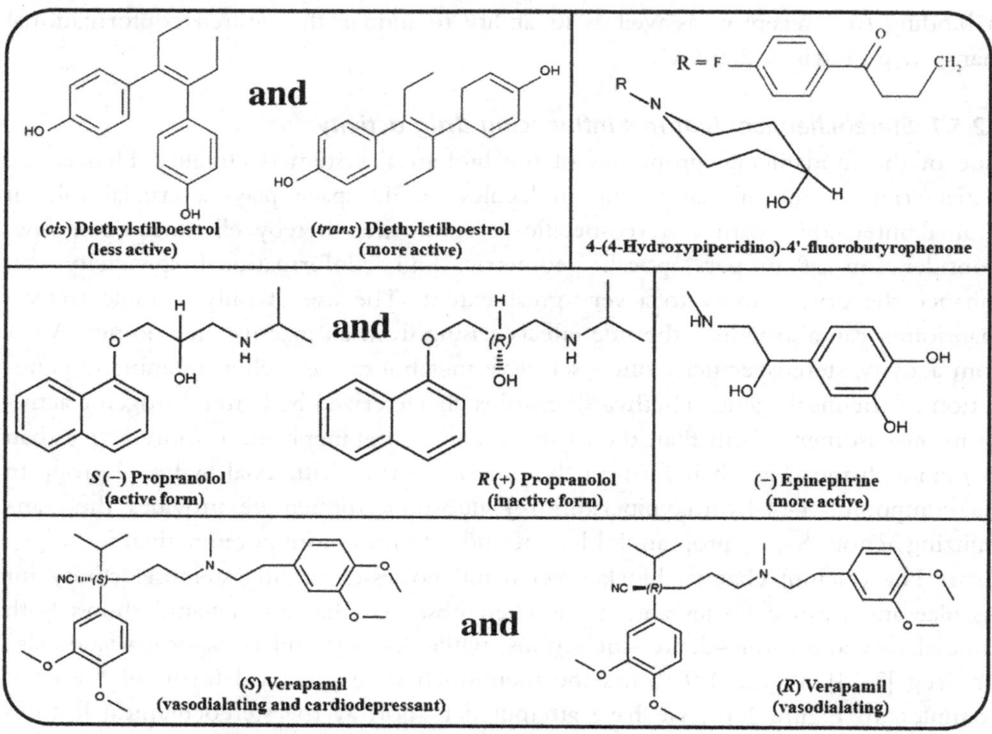

Figure 1.9 Examples showing stereospecific bioactive molecules and their less active analogs.

few similar properties; for instance, OH and NH_2 share similar hydrogen-bonding properties but do not share all inclusive identical properties with respect to parameters like electronegativity, polarizability, bond angle, size, and shape. The concept of isosterism was further extended to the entire molecule by Hinsberg [17] who introduced "ring equivalents," showing an exchange of groups in aromatic systems without causing significant change in the parent structure. Thiophene and pyridine can be represented as ring equivalents to benzene, considering that −CH=CH− in benzene is replaced by divalent sulfur (−S−) in thiophene and −CH= in benzene is replaced by trivalent nitrogen (−N=) to create pyridine. The antihistaminic property of tripelennamine is preserved when one of its benzene rings is replaced with thiophene to make methaphenilene. A concept called *bioisosterism* was employed to designate structurally related functional groups depicting similar biological properties. Later, bioisosters were designated as compounds or groups characterized by similar molecular shape, volume, electronic distribution, and physical properties. Bioisosteric replacements are made in molecules to obtain desired drug agents retaining the actual pharmacological action. Table 1.2 lists two classes of bioisosters: those according to Langmuir and Grimm's

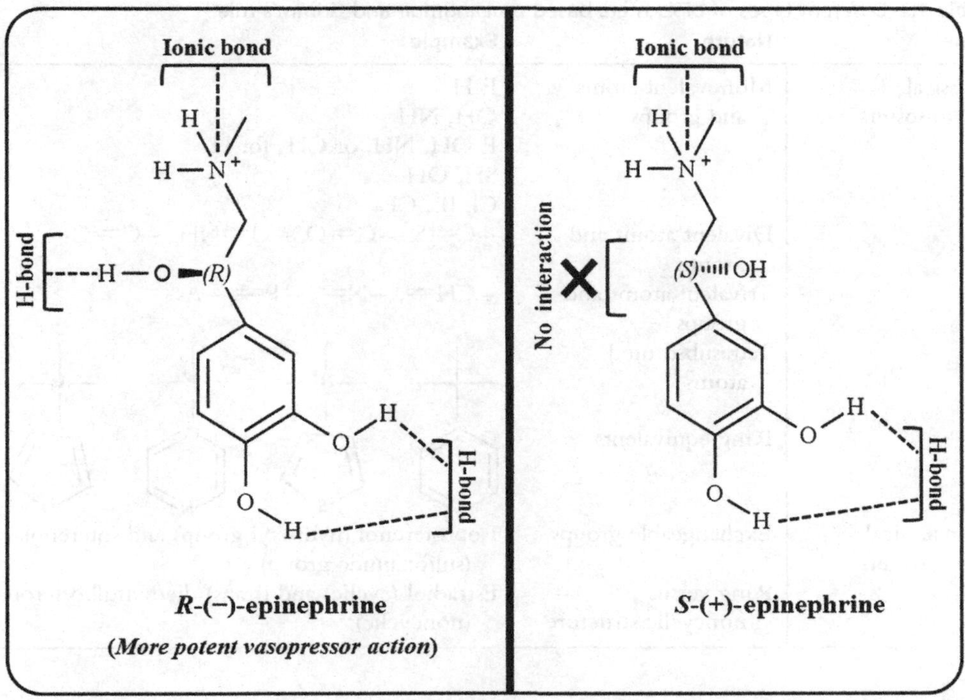

Figure 1.10 Representation of the potent binding of stereospecific (−)-epinephrine than its (+) form to the receptor site.

condition (classical bioisosters) and those avoiding the mentioned rules (nonclassical bioisosters). Replacement of a hydrogen atom in uracil by fluorine in 5-fluorouracil (antineoplastic agent) is an example of classical bioisosteric replacement. Another such example is the replacement of hydroxyl group of folic acid with amino to create aminopterin. Different bioisosteric forms of α-tocopherol have similar activity in terms of the scavenging of lipoperoxide and superoxide radicals. Replacement of the methyl sulfonamide group in soterenol (bronchodilator) with the hydroxyl group in isoproterenol maintains the similar activity and presents an example of nonclassical bioisosters. In this case, both groups preserve similar hydrogen-bonding potential with the receptor. Figure 1.11 shows the aforementioned examples of isosteric compounds.

1.2.5.3 Miscellaneous contribution of structural features

Incorporation of varying substituents in the same parent ring can result in drugs of different pharmacological classes. Incorporation of or change in a substituent in the same basic phenothiazine nucleus can yield antiparkinsonian (ethopropazine), antihistaminic (promethazine), and antipsychotic (chlorpromazine) drugs. Sometimes variation in the

Table 1.2 Different types of bioisosters based on Langmuir and Grimm's rule

Type	Nature	Example
Classical bioisosters	Monovalent atoms and groups	F, H OH, NH F, OH, NH, or CH_3 for H SH, OH Cl, Br, CF_3
	Divalent atoms and groups	–C=S, –C=O, –C=NH, –C=C–
	Trivalent atoms and groups	–CH=, –N=, –P=, –As=
	Tetrasubstituted atoms	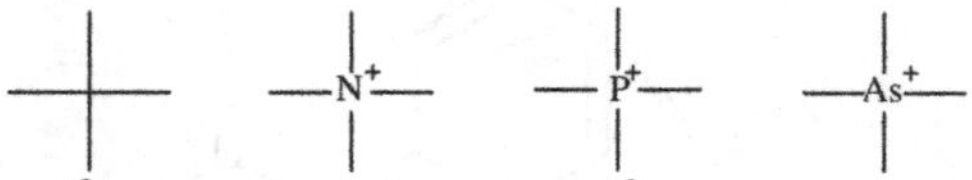 N^+ P^+ As^+
	Ring equivalents	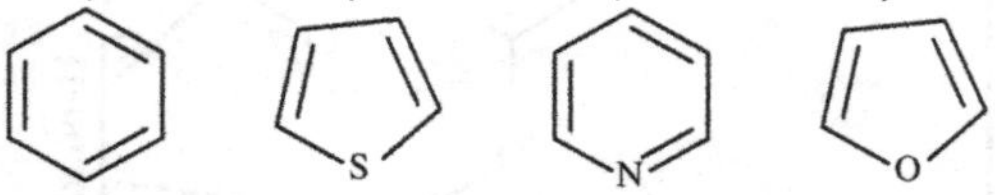 S N O
Nonclassical bioisosters	Exchangeable groups	Isoproterenol (hydroxyl group) and soterenol (sulfonamide group)
	Ring versus noncyclic structure	Estradiol (cyclic) and (trans) diethylstilbosterol (noncyclic)

structure can lead to the change in degree and kind of pharmacological effect. Replacing the methyl group of tolbutamide (a short-acting hypoglycemic) with chlorine gives chlorpropamide (a long-acting hypoglycemic). When the *N*-methyl substituent of epinephrine (a hypertensive agent) is replaced with the *N*-isopropyl group, the derived molecule isoproterenol shows hypotensive action. Presence of an additional methyl substituent sometimes causes change in activity. Addition of a methyl group at the nitrogen atom of morphine (analgesic) gives *N*-methyl morphine with muscle relaxant activity. *N*-methylation of nicotine (insecticidal action) gives *N*-methylnicotine with muscle relaxant action. Mydriatic action of atropine changes to muscle relaxant action on *N*-methylation. *Para*-aminobenzoic acid (PABA) shows a reversal of antibacterial activity of sulfanilamide when the carboxylic acid group of PABA is replaced with the sulfonamido substituent in sulfanilamide. The cited examples have been presented in Figure 1.12.

1.3 STRUCTURE–ACTIVITY RELATIONSHIP

1.3.1 Ideology

Chemistry has been an essential "central science" correlating and exploring different problems of scientific discipline [18]. Considering the large number of chemicals influencing our lives from the perspective of industrial application, laboratory research,

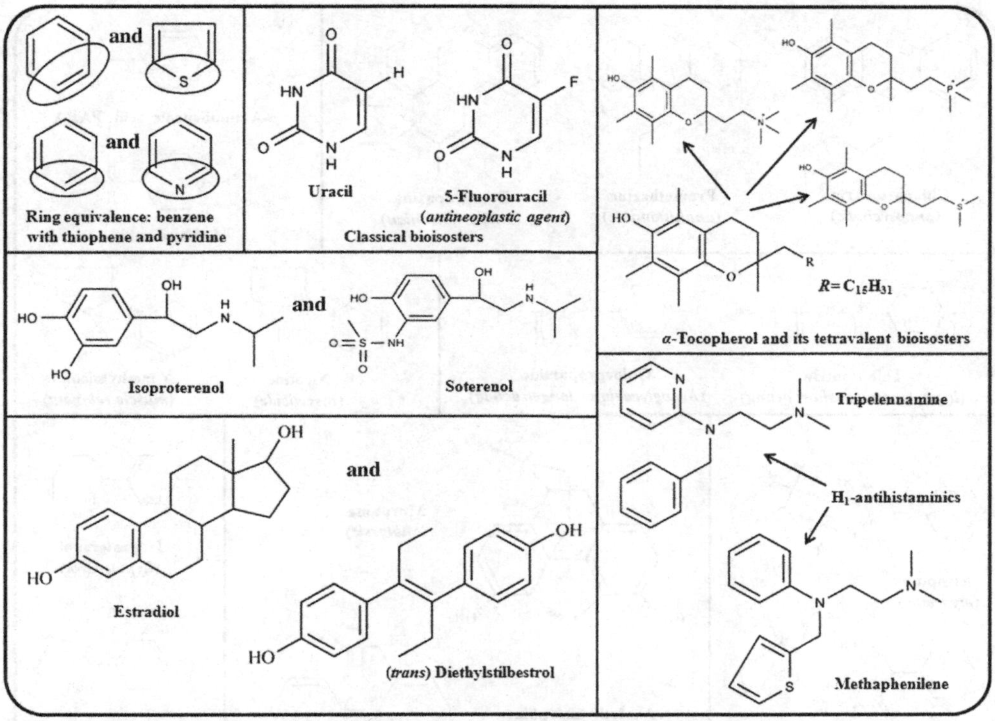

Figure 1.11 Examples showing various isosteric replacements in bioactive compounds.

and household consumption, it will be interesting to develop a basis that gives a suitable reason to explain the behavior of the chemicals. Once such basis is developed, it will also enable us modifying the behavior of those chemicals by incorporating reasonable structural changes. The structure–activity relationship (SAR) notion attempts to establish a relationship between various behavioral characteristics of chemical compounds (namely, activity/property/toxicity and chemical information derivable from chemical structures). Such process involves significant knowledge of chemistry and physics (defining the compounds), mathematics (allowing modeling analysis), and biology (giving reasons for the biological activity profile of chemicals) to develop a rational basis. In other words, the SAR study provides an option to construct a mathematical equation for a set of chemicals for their specific activity/property/toxicity behavior using information about their chemical structure. It may be noted that since we are talking about mathematical equations, it involves numbers or quantities. If the behavioral information of chemicals is expressed in qualitative terms, the study is named as qualitative SAR, while the presence of quantitative numbers representing activity of chemicals defines the process as a QSAR study [19]. However, both the qualitative and the quantitative studies are collectively termed as (Q)SAR.

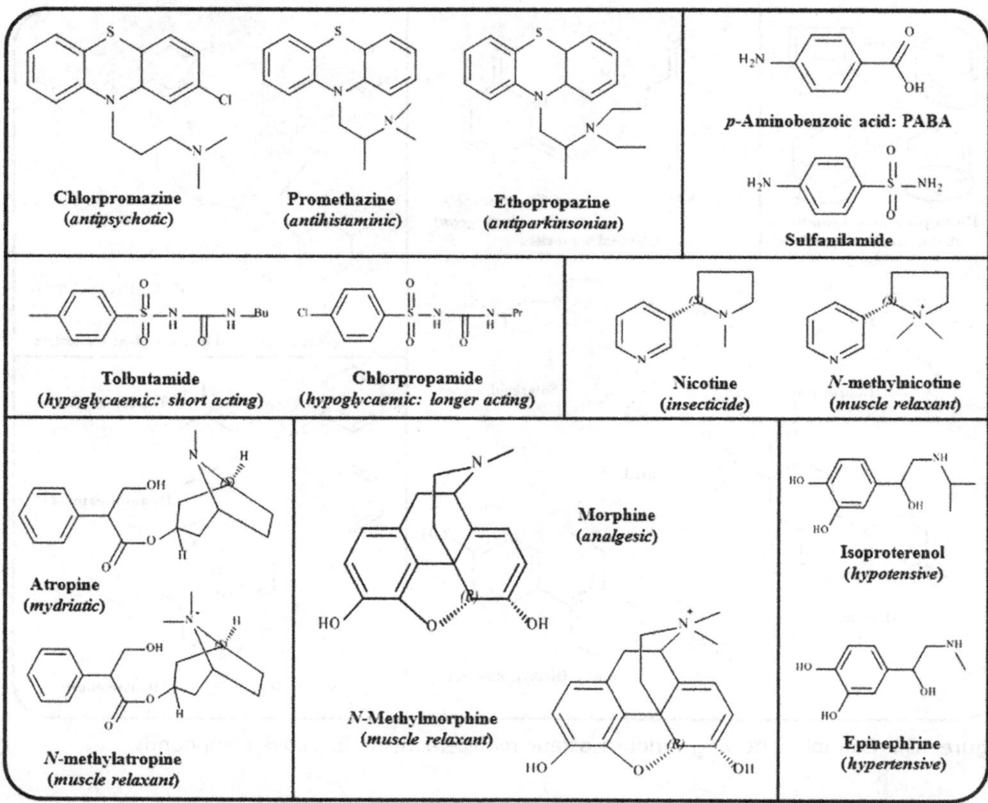

Figure 1.12 Example of drugs showing varying pharmacological activity due to changes in structural attributes.

The naming is also influenced by the end point modeled, and the process can be defined accordingly as QSAR/QSPR/QSTR considering that the response is activity, property, or toxicity. However, we shall use the term *QSAR* to designate all three of them throughout this chapter for convenience.

The central axiom of QSAR modeling lies in presenting the chemical response in terms of molecular attributes. These chemical features can represent theoretically determined parameters as well as experimental variables (namely, different types of physicochemical properties). Hence, it may be observed that any feature that contains significant and fundamental chemical information can be employed as predictor variables or descriptors. From the section "Historical Development of QSARs: A Journey of Knowledge Enrichment," later in this chapter, we will be able to know that the concept of computed descriptors came much later and the correlation models in the early days were developed using different physicochemical properties. Certainly, physicochemical properties like melting point, boiling point, and surface tension are characteristics for specific chemicals and contain relevant information in explaining the response of chemicals. Mathematically, the response of a chemical can be represented as the function of structural attributes and property [Eq. (1.2)]:

$$\text{Response} = f(\text{Chemical attributes, Property}) \tag{1.2}$$

Stated in a simpler way, a QSAR equation may be like the following expression [Eq. (1.3)]:

$$Y = a_0 + a_1X_1 + a_2X_2 + a_3X_3 + \cdots + a_nX_n \tag{1.3}$$

In this expression, Y is the response activity/property/toxicity being modeled, X_1, X_2, . . ., X_n are different structural features or physicochemical properties in the form of numerical quantities or descriptors, a_1, a_2, . . ., a_n are contributions of individual descriptors to the response, and a_0 is a constant.

It may also be noted that while various property parameters can be employed as predictor variables, they can also be used as the dependent or response variable during modeling of the property as an end point. Recent studies also show that even a response parameter (e.g., activity or toxicity) can be used as predictor variables in studies such as quantitative activity–activity relationship (QAAR) or quantitative toxicity–toxicity relationship (QTTR) modeling. Now, once a correlation equation is developed, the (Q)SAR formalism enables prediction of the response parameter (i.e., the activity/property or toxicity of untested or new chemical entities) that has not been used for developing the model. Furthermore, the (Q)SAR paradigm not only focuses on developing correlation models on chemicals, but also it emphasizes the modification of chemical structure to obtain the chemicals of interest with the desired response values. This fine-tuning of chemical structure is possible by suitably decoding the chemical information contained in chemical descriptors that gives a reasonable basis for the mechanism of action [19,20].

1.3.2 The components and principal steps involved

Simply speaking, the QSAR study aims at the quantification of chemical information and then the development of a logical mathematical relationship of the information with a response property or activity. Then the relationship can be employed to furnish the desired goal of the modeler; for example, enhancing the efficiency of an operation, reducing toxicity of hazardous chemicals, and improving pharmacological activity of drugs. Every step of predictive (Q)SAR modeling analysis uses different concepts of mathematics, and there is a large amount of quantitative data generated. It may be understood that here, mathematics provides an abstract ideological platform to encode the purpose of chemistry. The major goal is to encode the chemical information into suitable numbers, followed by the development of a mathematical relationship with the response such that the information can be used for prediction and molecular modification. The (Q)SAR modeling consists of quantitative data and suitable statistical tools. The quantitative data is obtained from chemicals in two forms: one is the response data, which may be quantitative or semiquantitative; and the other is the chemical information in the form of descriptors derived by processing the molecules. Various statistical tools are employed to derive a correlation equation between the response and the descriptors followed by judging the statistical reliability of the equation. Because of involvement of a large amount of data, computers are used to carry out the whole operation. Finally, the individual knowledge of the modeler aids the explanation of results based on the derived chemical information in the equation.

The four basic steps of QSAR study include (1) data preparation, (2) data processing, (3) data prediction and validation, and (4) data interpretation. The first step allows the modeler to arrange the data in a convenient and usable form. One needs to possess a set of chemicals with a response value (activity/property/toxicity) of interest. As long as a biological activity or toxicity is considered as the response property, two types of input data are possible: one being the dose required for a fixed response and the other being the response at a fixed dose. The examples of the former case may be EC_{50} (effective concentration in 50% population), IC_{50} (concentration required for 50% inhibition), and LD_{50} (the dose required to kill half the total population). As all these are determined in multiple assays at different dose or concentration levels, this kind of response (dose required for fixed response) is preferred as the dependent variable in a QSAR study. The response being fixed, it is the (required) dose or concentration of a series of compounds which is considered as the *Y*-variable [Eq. (1.3)]. In order to keep the wide range of response data over a smaller scale, a logarithmic transformation is usually applied that keeps the numbers closer. However, this is not the only reason. In cases while biological activity or toxicity is considered as the response, a dose–response curve gives a parabolic relationship (Figure 1.13), while the log

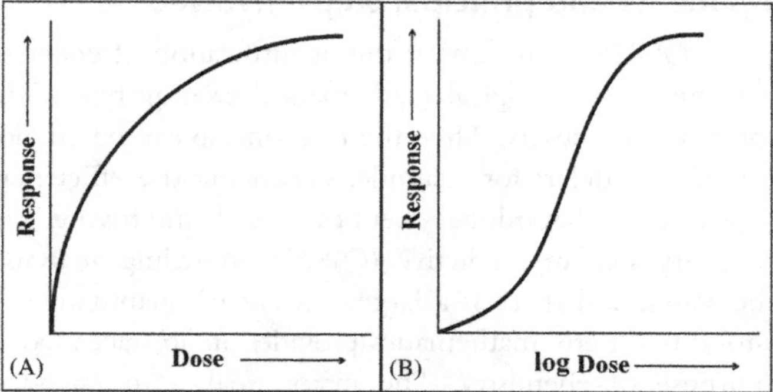

Figure 1.13 Representative (A) dose–response and (B) log dose–response curves of biologically active molecules.

dose−response curve gives a sigmoidal relationship, the middle portion of which is linear and easy to model. Note that the concentration term should be in a molar unit (M, mM, or μM). Also, note that a compound requiring a lower concentration (*C*) than another compound for the same response activity or toxicity is actually more active (or toxic), and thus the response activity or toxicity has an inverse relationship with concentration. For all practical purposes, log $1/C$ or −log *C* is used as the response or *Y*-variable in QSAR when the response property is an activity or toxicity. It is also desirable to have a data set with a span of at least 3−4 log units of the response property for which a QSAR model can be developed. All the compounds used in a particular model development are expected to have a same mechanism of action.

The predictor variables (i.e., descriptors) can be obtained from physicochemical experimentation on the chemicals or from theoretical computations. After the determination or computation of descriptors, a QSAR table is formed, which is a two-dimensional (2D) array of numbers with the columns representing descriptors and response and the compounds are depicted in successive rows. As QSAR is basically a statistical approach, in order to have sufficient reliability and robustness of the developed models, the number of observations must be much higher than the number of descriptors used in the final models. Usually a ratio of 5:1 (observations: descriptor) is used for this purpose. To have sufficient reliability of the developed statistical model, it is necessary to have a good number of observations (say, 50) based on which the model can be developed. Considering the presence of intercorrelated and redundant data, a pretreatment procedure is optionally used by the modeler in the data-processing step. For checking reliability of a QSAR model for prediction of the response property on a new set of data, an additional set of data may be required. Such new data often being unavailable, the original data set is divided into a training set and a test set. The division of the data set is one of the most crucial steps, and it may involve one of many chemometric operations (e.g., cluster analysis, Kennard stone, and sphere exclusion) aiming a rational division of the data set into a training and a test set. The training set chemicals are employed for model development, while the ability of the model to predict response value of the external chemicals is done using the test set. The developed models are subjected to extemporaneous statistical validation tests to establish their reliability. Once the model (or the developed equation) becomes acceptable, the diagnostic information encoded in the independent variables is unwrapped to explore the mechanism of action of the set of chemicals, and the design of a new set of chemicals with the desired response profile may also be possible [19,20]. In each step of the QSAR model development, several statistical operations are involved right from the generation of descriptors; that is, encoding of information to the pretreatment of data, division of the data set, development of model, and checking reliability and validation of the model. The basic workflow of (Q)SAR analysis, along with the principal components, are

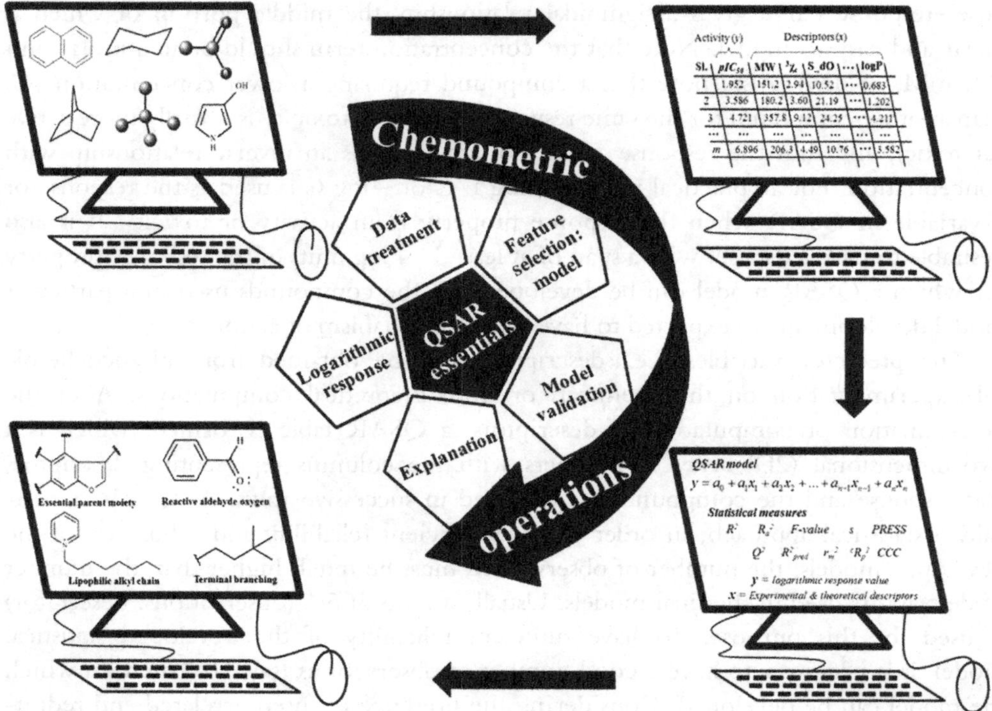

Figure 1.14 Depiction of the principal components of the (Q)SAR technique, along with the basic workflow involved.

depicted in Figure 1.14, while a more detailed schematic overview of a representative methodology is presented in Figure 1.15.

1.3.3 Naming of the components

The (Q)SAR formalism uses chemical information and correlates this with a behavior of the chemical (activity/property/toxicity) employing mathematical algorithms. Hence, different mathematical terminologies can define the process, and it will be useful to have an idea about the names employed to designate different components of such analysis. Since the developed equation is obtained by using an explicit mathematical algorithm, the components of the equation can be classified as the *Y*-variable and *X*-variables, where the dependent quantity or variable designates the *Y*-variable [i.e., the left side of an equation (usual convention)], while the *X*-variables denote independent variables [Eq. (1.3)]. Here, the dependent variable corresponds to the behavioral feature to be addressed, also termed the *response variable*, and it may be a biological (e.g., antimalarial, antiarrhythmic, and anti-HIV), physicochemical (e.g., aqueous solubility, octanol/water partition coefficient, and melting point), and toxicological (e.g., carcinogenicity, skin irritation,

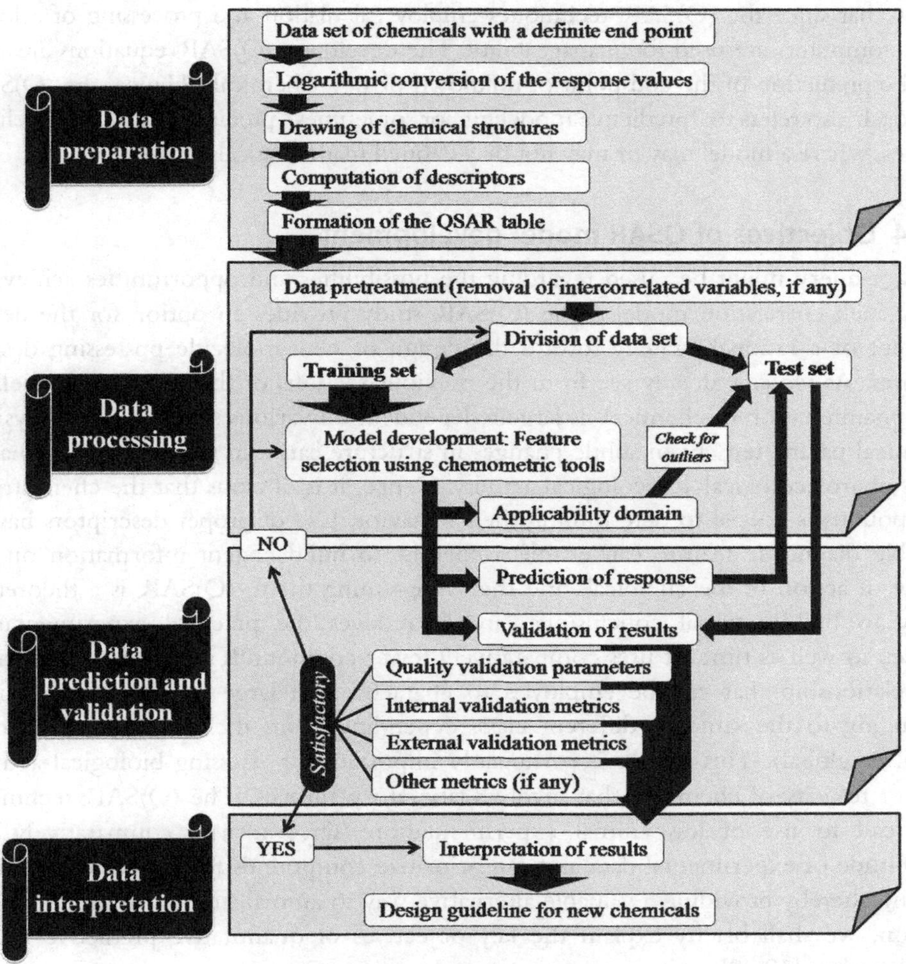

Figure 1.15 A schematic representation of the methodology employed in QSAR analysis.

genotoxicity, hepatotoxicity, toxicity toward ecological indicators like tetrahymena, daphnids, bacteria, and fungi) end point. The *Y*-variable can be qualitative or quantitative, while the *X*-variables are essentially independent quantitative entities defining the fundamental properties or features of the employed chemicals. These *X*-variables are also termed *descriptors* since they provide descriptive information of the chemicals, or predictor variables in (Q)SAR analysis. Various statistical operations are employed in the data treatment, model development, and model validation steps. Since such operations are designed on the basis of chemical platforms, dealing with the modeling of chemical data, they are also termed *chemometric tools*. Throughout this book, we shall gradually come to know that since the (Q)SAR techniques employ calculation and processing of a lot of data, computers are used for manageability. The developed (Q)SAR equations are used for the prediction of the end point of unknown or new chemicals. Hence, the (Q)SAR approach also refers to "predictive modeling" or sometimes "predictive *in silico* modeling" studies, where a model may or may not be a defined mathematical equation.

1.3.4 Objectives of QSAR model development

Now, a query might be raised regarding the possibilities and opportunities achievable using such correlation models. The (Q)SAR study provides an option for the development of a rational strategy toward the design of new molecule possessing desired features. As we can already see from the previous sections of this chapter, the behavioral manifestation of chemicals is largely dependent on various structural and physicochemical parameters. Even subtle changes in structure can lead to a significant change in its pharmacological/toxicological activity. Hence, it is obvious that the chemistry of compounds is crucial to determining their behavior. Use of proper descriptors having suitable diagnostic feature can enable a chemist to build cogent information on the mode of action of the chemicals and then fine-tuning them. (Q)SAR is a theoretical study to build rational conclusions, and it reduces the practical experimentation burden as well as time. It uses comparatively fewer compounds to build a mathematical relationship that can be employed to characterize a large number of chemicals belonging to the same or different class, depending upon the nature of the model (local or global). This feature is particularly important for assessing biological activity and/or toxicity of chemicals that involves laboratory animals. The (Q)SAR technique can lead to use of less animal experimentation (since it uses comparatively less magnitude of experimental data and can prioritize compounds for further experimentation), thereby providing a valuable alternative way to animal studies. In the following section, we shall briefly explain the key objectives of quantitative predictive model development [19,20].

1.3.4.1 Prediction of activity/property/toxicity

The primary purpose of a QSAR model is to predict the response value (activity/property/toxicity) of new chemicals. The prediction is done for the compounds that are not used to develop the model (test or validation set). Now the prediction for unknown compounds can be achieved by an extrapolation of data, and it is also obvious that in this method, there is a certain degree of uncertainty. In QSAR analysis, the training set chemicals are usually employed to define a chemical domain and any new, untested, or hypothetical compound lying within that domain can be predicted by a given QSAR equation. Thus, the QSAR study provides reasonably good support to a chemist in choosing molecules with desired properties before their synthesis.

1.3.4.2 Reduction and replacement of experimental (laboratory) animals

Biological analysis involves animal studies at the preclinical stage of development of drugs. The use of animals in biological and toxicological experimentation of drugs and other industrial chemicals is objectionable because it shows cruelty to the living animals. However, lack of proper safety data of such essential chemicals can also lead to disastrous outcomes. In 1959, Russell and Burch [21] introduced the "3R" concept (namely, replacement, reduction, and refinement), with the aim of improving the treatment of animals toward scientific procedures. Replacement refers to substitution for sentient living higher animals, while reduction confers employment of less number of animals to generate information of a given amount and precision in a study. Refinement corresponds to the decrease of severity inhuman methodology applied to the animals still to be used for experiment. Some recognized organizations working for animal welfare, namely, Fund for the Replacement of Animals in Medicinal Experiments (FRAME) [22], People for the Ethical Treatment of Animals (PETA) [23], etc. propose the use of alternative methods of experimentation to reduce the employment of *in vivo* animal models. QSAR provides a rational alternative path to reduce the animal experimentation by choosing the selected desirable compounds. The use of an animal model also creates ethical obligations while assessing hazardous potential of chemicals and in this regard QSAR analysis is supported and purported as a valid alternative tool by various international organizations, including the European Commission's European Centre for the Validation of Alternative Methods (ECVAM) [24], the Council for International Organizations of Medical Sciences [25], the European Union's Registration, Evaluation and Authorization of Chemicals (REACH) regulations [26], Office of Toxic Substances of the U.S. Environmental Protection Agency (EPA) [27], Agency for Toxic Substances and Disease Registry (ATSDR) [28], and the Organisation for Economic Co-operation and Development (OECD) [29].

1.3.4.3 Virtual screening of library data

(Q)SAR studies enable screening of chemical library comprising a large number of compounds. The mathematical information derived from a (Q)SAR analysis can be employed as filter criteria to screen the molecules of interest. Virtual screening can be performed employing the information of ligands (i.e., ligand-based), as well as the receptor structure (i.e., structure-based). (Q)SAR methodology can be employed to perform ligand-based searches for desired chemicals. Two aspects of such operation can be identified; namely, searching for the compounds having similar structural features, as in the developed model; and second, screening of chemical databases of known response (e.g., anticancer database) to predict and check the response value using the model. There are several chemical libraries available containing a large number of compounds; namely, ZINC, DUD benchmark, PubChem, ChemBank,

ChEMBL, DrugBank, Interbioscreen, FDA database, Maybridge, and ChemSpider, which are widely employed by the (Q)SAR practitioners [30].

1.3.4.4 Diagnosis of mechanism

Interpretation of the mechanism involved in a process is one of most interesting and challenging task of QSAR models. The quality of descriptors employed plays a significant role in explaining the mechanism of a process. In the case of biological and toxicological end points, knowledge of the specific biological (or toxicological) process is also important. The variables obtained in a QSAR model can be used to establish a link between the mechanism involved and the factors affecting it and thereby providing a guideline in designing molecules possessing desired properties. For example, chemicals acting via narcosis have been observed to be well predicted by lipophilicity measure log *P* [31]. Here, partitioning of the chemical accounts for its accumulation in the lipid layer and therefore acts as the prerequisite for the mechanism involved. The same logic of lipophilicity is also applicable for anesthetic action of chemicals. Note that QSAR is originally a ligand-based approach; however, it can also use the information derived from receptor-based approaches. A combination of both approaches has a better promise in finding out novel drug candidates.

1.3.4.5 Classification of data

Sometimes the quantitative response data to certain biological and/or toxicological end points are scarce. The reason of this can be attributed to difficulty in executing experiments on such end points. Relatively new or less explored research areas are supplied with insufficient biological (or toxicological) data. In some cases, the data points comprise a mixture of quantitative and qualitative information. QSAR provides an option for performing a classification analysis (like discriminant analysis) to such response values and thereby categorizing the compounds into different semiquantitative categories like "highly active," "moderately active," "active" and "inactive," or "toxic" and "nontoxic." Discriminant analysis enables the use of the same descriptors which are employed in normal regression-based QSAR analysis, and allows categorization of the data. During toxicological screening of chemical libraries, a classification model is useful for prioritization of chemicals by eliminating the toxic ones.

1.3.4.6 Optimization of leads

Drug discovery projects are costly, as well as time-consuming research involving a risk of failures. Only therapeutic activity seems to be an insufficient characteristic of a candidate molecule to succeed as a drug, and many of the candidates get failed at the preclinical developmental stage owing to poor pharmacokinetic issues. QSAR can provide a rational guidance for the design of new compounds obtained from a chemical data screening project. Apart from the selective end-point ones, the big chemical libraries

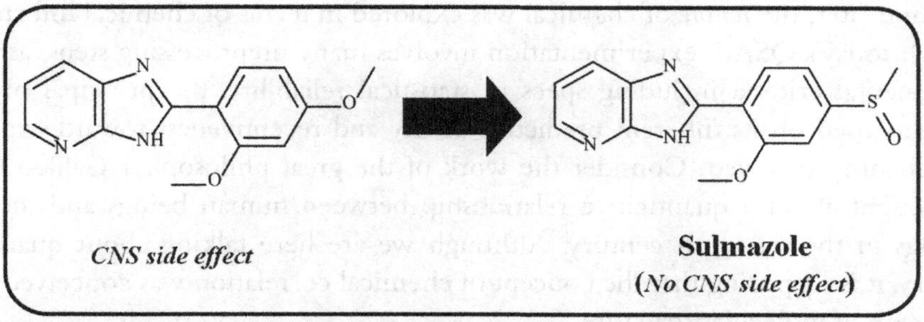

Figure 1.16 Example showing the structural refinement of a candidate molecule, resulting in a more suitable drug called sulmazole.

usually comprise molecules corresponding to varying pharmacological classes. Following screening of the library, specific QSAR models can be applied to fine-tune the structure of the selected lead molecules toward a particular activity profile.

1.3.4.7 Refinement of synthetic targets

Design of synthetic drug molecules can be fine-tuned by using the knowledge of existing/developed QSAR models. Hansch [32] showed the implementation of the concept of lipophilicity during the design of the drug sulmazole. Following the development of the concept of QSAR, a good number of studies were conducted using log P as a free-energy variable during the early days. A significant amount of study on anesthetic action of chemicals showed the lipophilicity to be an important modulator of activity of such compounds and it appeared that compounds bearing log P value of 2 or thereabouts can penetrate the central nervous system (CNS). It was reported that a potent cardiotonic agent, the 2,4-dimethoxy analogue of sulmazole depicted CNS side effects termed *bright vision* in patients during the clinical trial stage. The log P of the compound was 2.59, causing the molecule to penetrate the CNS of the trial patients. Then replacement of the 4-methoxy group with 4-S(O)CH_3 led to the development of sulmazole molecule (Figure 1.16) possessing log P value of 1.17 and bearing no such CNS side effects.

1.4 HISTORICAL DEVELOPMENT OF QSARS: A JOURNEY OF KNOWLEDGE ENRICHMENT

The development of the QSAR methodology was not a sudden discovery; rather, it has been a gradual evolution of an ideology. The ideology came as a resultant combination of core concepts of chemistry and mathematics, which was later extrapolated to other interdisciplinary branches of natural sciences. In the distant past, the notion came from the approach of correlating behavior of chemical compounds with their nature; and later, the *nature* of chemical was explored in terms of chemical information. Although today's QSAR experimentation involves many preprocessing steps, as well as developmental criteria including specs of statistical reliability, the principal objective remains focused on its inherent predictive ability and receptiveness toward explaining the mechanism involved. Consider the work of the great philosopher Galileo Galilei, who thought about a quantitative relationship between human beings and their surroundings in the sixteenth century. Although we are here talking about quantitative chemistry, it is surprising that the concept of chemical correlation was conceived before any concept of molecular structure.

The development of fundamentals of molecular structures can be attributed to the decisive contribution of Kekule, Couper, and Crum-Brown during the period of 1858–1870. However, it was Blake who noted similar action elicited by salts of isomorphous bases in 1841 [33]. Ten years later, Horsford and Baird [34] observed a relationship between the taste of compounds and their composition and a few years after, in 1854, Pelikan [35] noted that chemical composition influences the toxic effect of compounds. In 1858, Borodin came to the realization that a toxicological property is closely related to the chemical makeup of compounds [36]. A similar type of behavior on the organisms was observed to be elicited by chemicals possessing same elements or taking part in similar chemical reaction. In 1863, Cros [37] observed a relationship between aqueous solubility and toxicity of primary alcohols. Hence, it may be observed that the early notion of QSAR modeling is associated with the field of toxicology. By this time, Mendeleev observed a relationship among elements using their atomic weight and developed periodic table of elements [20]. The use of atomic weight to develop the "rule of eight" by Mendeleev can be visualized as one of the oldest approach of using a "parameter" in a relationship study involving chemistry. The first proposition for the existence of a mathematical relationship between chemical structure and activity was inevitably done by Crum-Brown and Fraser in 1868 [38] by showing physiological activity (φ) as a mathematical function of chemical constitution (C) [Eq. (1.4)]. It may be observed that the term *chemical constitution* merely represented elemental composition at that period of time since the concepts of molecular structure was not established. They showed that a series of strychnine derivatives possessing muscle paralytic activity similar to curare can be prepared by varying the quaternary substituent.

$$\phi = f(C) \tag{1.4}$$

In 1869, Richardson [39] observed the molecular weight of primary alcohol proportionately controlling their narcotic effect. Reynolds in 1877 carried out another preliminary study and reported an effect of chemical constitution on physiological activity of chemicals. Some years later, in 1893, Richet [40] imparted further confidence to the proposition of Crum-Brown and Fraser by showing that the toxicity of ether, alcohol, and ketones is inversely affected by their solubility measure. At the turn of the century, Meyer [41], Overton [42], and Baum [43] added further light to Eq. (1.4) by employing the olive oil/water partition coefficient to correlate potencies of narcotic substances. Overton performed an extended research in this perspective and observed a systemic increase in narcotic potency in tadpoles when the chain length in groups was increased, and concluded the partitioning of the compounds into lipid cells to be responsible for such action. Furthermore, while experimenting with morphine, he observed varying toxic effects to human and tadpoles and assumed a difference in protein structure in both the organism responsible for complex formation. Further essence to the research was added by Traube in 1904 [44], who observed narcosis to be linearly related with the surface tension of the chemicals and later, in 1912, Seidell [45] considered both the partition coefficient and solubility measure to establish such correlation. Additional impetus to this line of thinking was instituted in 1939 by Ferguson [46], who fused the concept of thermodynamics with narcosis and partition coefficient and stated that the relative saturation of the substance in the applied phase is related to narcotic activity. At the beginning of the 1940s, Albert et al. [47] and Bell and Roblin [48] explored the influence of ionization of bases and weak acids toward their bacteriostatic activity. It may be noted that at that point of time, pioneering research was going on in the field of physical organic chemistry to derive the impact of substituents of organic compounds toward the behavior of chemicals. The decisive study by Hammett [49] on relative reaction rate of *meta*- and *para*-substituted benzoic acid derivatives led to the development of the famous electronic substituent constant Hammett sigma (σ), as shown in Eqs. (1.5) and (1.6).

$$\log(k_X/k_H) = \rho \cdot \sigma_X \tag{1.5}$$

Or,

$$\log(K_X/K_H) = \rho \cdot \sigma_X \tag{1.6}$$

where k_H and k_X are the respective rate constant terms, K_H and K_X are respective equilibrium constant terms for the unsubstituted and substituted benzoic acid derivatives, ρ is the reaction constant, and σ_X is the Hammett electronic constant of the substituent X. It was the first linear free energy related (LFER) model established in the realm of QSAR since the ionization constant terms used to describe σ can be related to the free energy equation [Eq. (1.7)], where G is the Gibbs free energy change, R is ideal gas constant, and T is temperature (in Kelvin):

$$\Delta G^0 = -RT \ln K \tag{1.7}$$

Extensive research on this aspect evolved a "sigma–rho" formalism at that time. Later, Taft [50] introduced the first steric parameter E_S and by employing LFER analysis on the rates of base- and acid-catalyzed hydrolysis of aliphatic esters and separated the polar, steric, and resonance effects. In the beginning of the 1960s, Corwin Hansch, also known as the "Father of modern QSAR," provided further momentum to QSAR research by using Hammett constants and hydrophobicity parameters to develop correlation models on plant growth regulators [51]. A relative hydrophobicity measure of the substituent parameter (π) was introduced. Later, the famous linear Hansch equation was developed by Hansch and Fujita [52] by combining hydrophobic constant terms with the Hammett sigma (σ). The principal equation is presented in Eq. (1.8), while it may be noted that this form of the equation has been modified and extended many times, including development of its parabolic form:

$$\log 1/C = k_1\pi + k_2\sigma + k_3E_s + k_4 \quad (1.8)$$

where k_1, k_2, and k_3 are the coefficient terms, while k_4 presents a constant. At the same time, another significant approach of QSAR modeling was instituted by Free and Wilson [53] on a congeneric series of compounds. In this approach, biological activity is expressed as the summed contribution of parent moiety and each structural features present. The Free—Wilson approach may be defined in Eq. (1.9), where μ is the contribution of the parent moiety and a_i is the contribution of individual structural features, x_i is a variable that depicts the presence ($x_i = 1$) or absence ($x_i = 0$) of a specific structural feature:

$$BA = \sum a_i x_i + \mu \quad (1.9)$$

The limitations of this equation was addressed by Fujita and Ban [54], who developed a similar equation just by using logarithmic activity to bring the activity term in same level with other free energy terminologies.

Hence, it is evident that the journey of QSAR started with the concept of obtaining a correlation of the activity of chemicals with the chemical composition, which gradually led to the exploration of the chemistry of compounds. Following some basic assumptions at the initial stage, researchers came up with mathematical equations bearing thermodynamic relations which can be considered as chemical property. As the time progressed, independent parameters in the QSAR equation were also modified and structural measures (namely, substituent constant, occurrence of substituent, etc.) came into light. Now, it should be noted that along with different approaches and algorithms, the pathway of QSAR has been paved by the discovery and development of various independent variables commonly known as *descriptors*. At the mid-twentieth century, the research and knowledge in chemical structure was increasing, and scientists were trying to find a way to create numerical representation of structures. Chemical graph theory, although an old concept, became an inevitable tool for this quantification of chemical structures, and in 1947, the first theoretically derived descriptors (the Wiener index [55] and Platt index [56]) were reported. The use of structurally derived theoretical descriptors bought a new wave of research in the QSAR paradigm. The concept of graph theory and chemical topology was significantly exploited in the 1970s–1980s for addressing various QSAR problems. The minimum topological difference (MTD) method of Simon [57] and Hall and Kier's molecular connectivity [58] can be cited in this regard, although it is beyond the scope of this chapter to mention all notable contributions of different researchers at that time all over the world. Throughout this time, the QSAR studies were principally one-dimensional (1D) and two-dimensional (2D). In the late 1980s, molecular features were characterized based on their alignment in space. Interaction energy between a molecule and probes in 3D space known as the *molecular interaction field (MIF)* were used to determine the chemical feature of molecules. This field of study was pioneered by Goodford, with his GRID method [59], and Cramer et al. [60] with his comparative molecular field analysis (CoMFA) formalisms. Some other methods and descriptors based on MIF include comparative molecular similarity indices analysis (CoMSIA), G-WHIM descriptors, Compass method, Voronoi field analysis, GRIND descriptors, and VolSurf approach. Following the three-dimensional (3D)-QSAR formalisms, other higher dimensional approaches involving receptor–ligand interaction, as well as some newer techniques such as hologram-based QSAR (HQSAR), binary QSAR, and inverse QSAR have evolved. It is not surprising to say that new concepts in the QSAR paradigm as well as modification of the existing ones are still taking place. Figure 1.17 shows a chronological list of significant events that lead to the discovery and development of QSAR techniques.

1.5 APPLICATIONS OF QSAR

Different kinds of chemicals influence a large part of human endeavor spanning from laboratory experiments to industrial processes, including household applications. The chemical attributes facilitate designing of better analogues by the optimization of the desired response and/or reduction of hazardous outcome, if any. (Q)SAR presents an ideology of developing a mathematical correlation between response and information of the employed objects (i.e., chemicals) here. Hence, any suitable response elicited by chemicals can be modeled to develop a theoretical basis for that process. Considering a vast area of functional chemicals (e.g., pharmaceuticals, agrochemicals, flavor, perfumeries, analytical reagents, solvents, and household chemicals), the domain of application of QSAR techniques will also be significantly large, and practically, it will be difficult to mention all processes where QSAR can be of great importance. We already know that from a global point of view of the modeling nature of response data, the area of application of QSAR analysis can be visualized in terms of modeling different biological activity, property, and toxicity end points. Table 1.3 gives a representative list of different end points employed in the QSAR modeling paradigm. With respect to the nature of purposes addressed by chemicals, we can divide the application areas into the chemicals of health benefits, the chemicals responsible for

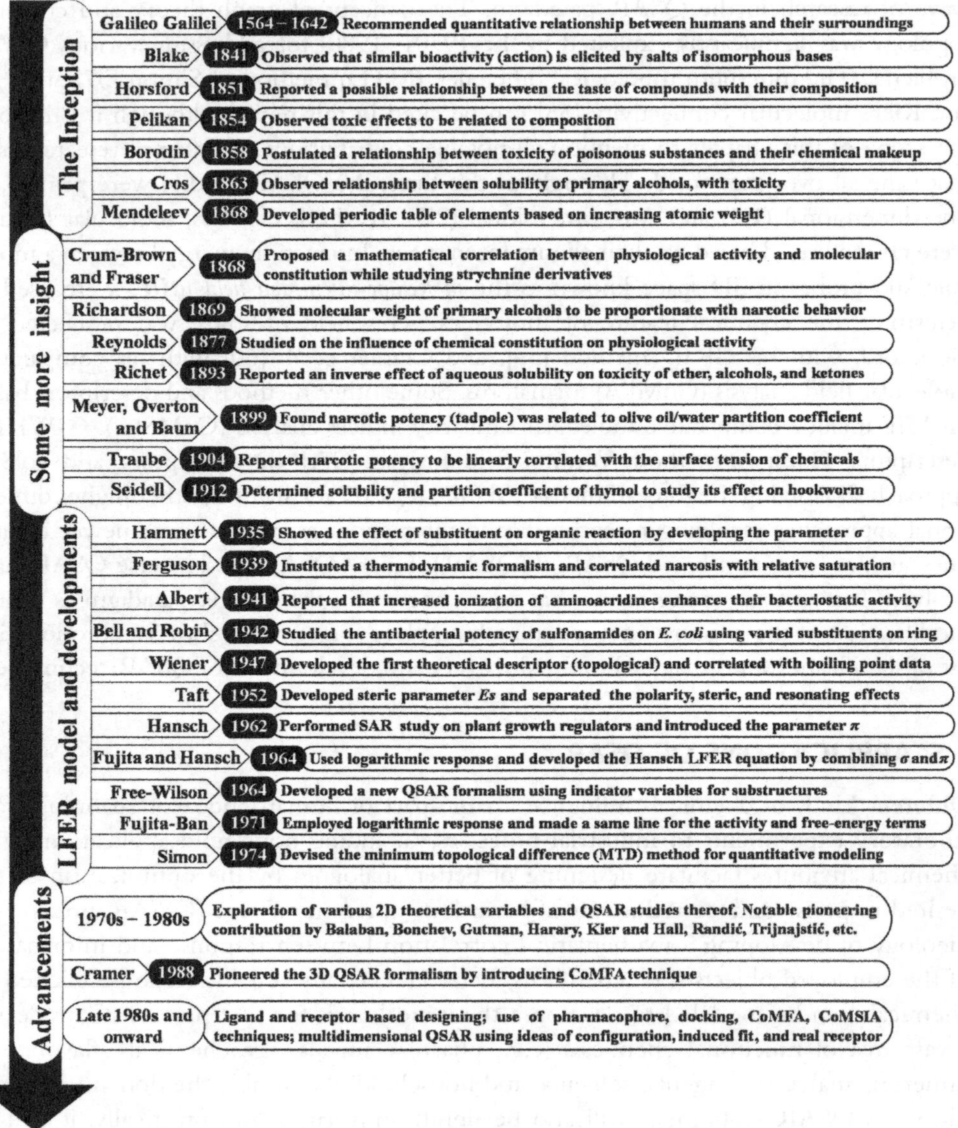

Figure 1.17 A look at the historical journey of predictive (Q)SAR model development.

environmental hazard, and the chemicals responsible for the industrial/laboratory process (Figure 1.18).

The chemicals of health benefits include all different types of drugs and pharmaceuticals and some food ingredients that are widely subjected to (Q)SAR modeling

Table 1.3 Various end points employed in predictive modeling analysis using (Q)SAR technique

Nature of end point	Representative examples
Activity	Antimalarial, antipsychotic, antioxidant, antiarrhythmic, antianginal, antihypertensive, anti-HIV, antidiuretic, antibacterial, anticholinergic, antiadrenergic, antihistaminic, antianxiety, antiepileptic, antiparkinsonian, antidepressant, analgesic, antipyretic, antiemetic, hypoglycemic, etc.
Property	Melting point, boiling point, vapor pressure, glass transition temperature, adsorption, rate of reaction, octanol/water partition coefficient, water solubility, molar refractivity, chromatographic retention data, biodegradation, hydrolysis, atmospheric oxidation, bioaccumulation, critical micelle concentration of surfactants, odor threshold of flavors, etc.
Toxicity	Acute fish toxicity, long-term aquatic toxicity, acute oral toxicity, acute inhalation toxicity, acute dermal toxicity, skin irritation/corrosion, eye irritation/corrosion, skin sensitization, toxicity due to repeated dose, genotoxicity, reproductive toxicity, developmental toxicity, carcinogenicity, organ toxicity, e.g., hepatotoxicity, cardiotoxicity, and nephrotoxicity, toxicity toward ecotoxicological indicator organisms, namely, algae (*Scenedesmus, Selenastrum*, etc.), daphnids, *Tetrahymena*, bacteria (*Vibrio, Escherichia*, etc.), yeast (*Saccharomyces*), etc.

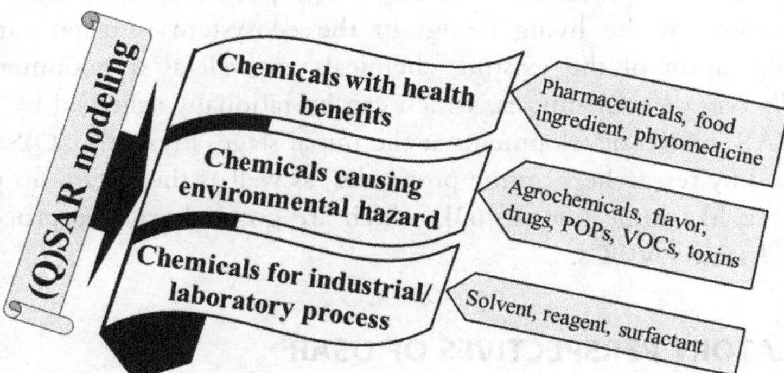

Figure 1.18 Three broad application areas of (Q)SAR modeling.

for the optimization of their potency, receptor specificity, and improved pharmacokinetic profile, while reduction toxicity is also desired. The study of (Q)SAR has also led to the development of some drugs molecules (e.g., norfloxacin, ketoconazole, danazole, griseofulvin, and amlodipine). Any chemicals coming in contact with the environment can pose risks to the ecosystem by exerting unwanted hazardous outcomes. Hence, quantitative structure–toxicity (QSTR) relationship studies (i.e., QSTR modeling) have many applications in modeling hazardous profile of chemicals. The chemicals of interest include various persistent organic pollutants (POPs), volatile organic compounds (VOCs), different aldehyde containing flavor and fragrance materials, toxins, and toxic xenobiotic. Such modeling analysis also aids in filling of data gaps and prioritization of chemicals before their synthesis. Furthermore, the (Q)SAR technique allows environmental monitoring by modeling the biodegradation and bioaccumulation of chemicals. It may be noted here that the chemicals with biological activity; namely, drugs and pharmaceuticals also pose an ecotoxicological threat, as they are also released in the environment via wastewater or as metabolic products, and (Q)SAR modeling is also employed for their safety assessment. Physiologically based pharmacokinetic (PBPK) modeling can be employed for modeling chemicals like VOCs using physicochemical (log *P*), as well as biochemical parameters (Michaelis constant K_m, maximal velocity V_{max}, hepatic clearance, etc.). The third important aspect for the application of (Q)SAR is diagnosing the attributes of process chemicals in order to maximize the efficiency of an operation. These include modeling of specific features like critical micelle concentration of surfactants, odor threshold of odorants, thermal degradation data, data on oxidation of metal by chemicals, analytical data like chromatographic retention time, and modeling of tribochemical property. Fine-tuning of the structure of all such process chemicals can improve the performance of a given industrial operation. Considering the environmental and health hazard issues caused by chemicals of different sources, guidelines have been built toward the development of "sustainable" [61] and "green" chemicals [62] so that the existence of the living beings in the ecosystem is taken care of. This involves modification of the existing chemicals, as well as development of novel *environmentally benevolent* chemicals, which can be rationally achieved by performing suitable (Q)SAR model developments at the initial stage. Presently, (Q)SAR modeling is practiced by researchers on the properties, as well as the hazardous potential of novel chemicals like ionic liquids [63], which are good alternative process solvents replacing the harmful VOCs.

1.6 REGULATORY PERSPECTIVES OF QSAR

Considering the widespread existing body of research, applications, and immense possibilities, predictive modeling studies employing the QSAR technique is practiced by various regulatory authorities throughout the world. The regulatory agencies aid in the assessment of risk and hazardous potential posed by chemicals employed in industries, laboratories, and used by consumers. The regulatory monitoring of chemicals includes several aspects, which can be summarized as follows [64]:

1. Assessment of chemical hazard: It involves identification of hazard as well as dose–response characterization, including the classification and labeling of chemicals
2. Assessment of exposure

3. Assessment of hazard and exposure
4. Identification of persistent, bioaccumulative, and toxic (PBT), as well as very persistent and very bioaccumulative (vPvB) chemicals

(Q)SAR studies can assist in achieving the goals of regulatory assessment by allowing chemical prioritization, filling of data gaps, as well as replacement of extensive animal experimentation. It may be observed that modeling of categorical data (if present) plays an important role here since the toxicological data can be categorized into several groups, thereby identifying different levels of hazard (e.g., high, moderate, and low). Because of the rational designing algorithm coupled with the option for hazardous assessment of chemicals, different international authorities (namely, ECVAM, US-EPA, ATSDR as mentioned earlier) provide their consent for employing such predictive modeling analysis as a reliable tool for toxicological evaluation. In 2006, European Commission enacted the REACH regulations to perform systematic evaluation of new as well as existing chemicals (imported or produced).

Following the recommendations taken in a workshop, the OECD published a guideline document for the validation of (Q)SAR models in 2007. This document prescribes a set of five seminal principles to be followed by the OECD member countries for (Q)SAR model development and validation. Gradually, with the progress of time, research, and development on (Q)SAR have become more intense, and presently many countries have developed their own guidelines for (Q)SAR modeling analysis. Considering a huge number of chemicals prevailing in the environment, different (Q)SAR databases on hazardous assessment of chemicals are available online (both open access and commercial). Different countries have also developed various (Q)SAR expert systems on potentially toxic and hazardous chemicals. Expert systems are computational applications that provide a subject-matter expertise to nonexperts by employing suitable logical reasoning. In the realm of (Q)SAR, these are trusted systems, prepared and maintained by professional people, containing models on different toxicological end points. Following the input of a query molecule (drug, etc.), the structure is parsed by the expert program and then toxicity prediction/comparison/categorization is made with respect to the available knowledge-base on that system. Table 1.4 offers a list of representative (Q)SAR expert systems principally allowing assessment of chemical hazards.

1.7 OVERVIEW AND CONCLUSION

Chemistry is one of the fundamental natural sciences affecting a wide variety of processes. Needless to say, we are controlled by a multitude of chemical processes from birth to death. How different chemicals act differently (and even the same chemical elicits varying responses in different circumstances) is a matter of deep interest among the scientists. With the technological developments, it has been a prime focus

Table 1.4 A representative overview of various (Q)SAR expert systems used for the assessment of chemical hazards

Expert system	Short description (with web link)
Open-source systems (Freely accessible)	
QSAR TOOLBOX (OECD)	It allows grouping of chemicals into categories and data filling in ecotoxicity end points and facilitates mechanistic comparison while assessing hazard of chemicals. Web site: http://www.qsartoolbox.org/
Lazar	Lazar stands for "lazy SAR." It involves *k*-nearest-neighbor technique for the prediction of chemical end points and develops local QSAR model for each compound to be predicted. The predicted end points include fish toxicity, carcinogenicity (mouse, hamster, rat), mutagenicity, and repeated dose toxicity. It employs mining of end point–related substructure. Web site: http://lazar.in-silico.de/predict
Toxtree	It uses the decision tree approach for categorization and prediction of toxicity. It incorporates Cramer classification scheme, Kroes TTC decision tree, Verhaar scheme for aquatic modes of action, rulebases for skin and eye irritation and corrosion, Benigni–Bossa rulebase for mutagenicity and carcinogenicity, structural alerts for Michael acceptors, etc. It was developed by Ideaconsult Ltd (Sofia, Bulgaria). Web site: http://ihcp.jrc.ec.europa.eu/our_labs/eurl-ecvam/laboratories-research/predictive_toxicology/qsar_tools/toxtree
VEGA	It combines QSAR and read across tools. It allows modeling of skin sensitization, mutagenicity, bioconcentration factor, toxicity toward fathead minnow, carcinogenicity, developmental toxicity, and log *P*. Web site: http://www.vega-qsar.eu/
DEMETRA	DEMETRA is a project of the European Commission and stands for "Development of Environmental Modules for Evaluation of Toxicity of pesticide Residues in Agriculture." Five toxicity end points involving four organisms can be modeled, namely, *Oncorhynchus mykiss*, *Daphnia magna*, *Colinus virginianus*, and *Apis melifera* employing linear and nonlinear techniques for classification as well as prediction. Web site: http://www.demetra-tox.net/
EPI Suite™	It is the abbreviated form of "Estimation Program Interface Suite" and is a product of the Office of Pollution Prevention Toxics and Syracuse Research Corporation (SRC), US-EPA. It performs prediction of physical/chemical property and environmental fate. Web site: http://www.epa.gov/opptintr/exposure/pubs/episuite.htm
TEST	TEST stands for Toxicity Estimation Software Tool. It performs testing of acute toxicity. The end points include toxicity toward daphnia, tetrahymena, rat, ames mutagenicity, bioaccumulation factor, and developmental toxicity. TEST is a product of the US-EPA. Web site: http://www.epa.gov/nrmrl/std/qsar/qsar.html

(*Continued*)

Table 1.4 (Continued)

Expert system	**Short description (with web link)**
OncoLogic™	It assesses the likelihood of causal of cancer by organic compounds as well as polymers, metals, and fibers. A product of the US-EPA. Web site: http://www.epa.gov/oppt/sf/pubs/oncologic.htm
Commercial systems (Paid systems)	
Derek Nexus	It is a knowledge-based toxicity expert system developed by Lhasa Limited. It allows modeling carcinogenicity, mutagenicity, genotoxicity, skin sensitization, teratogenicity, irritation, respiratory sensitization, reproductive toxicity. Web site: http://www.lhasalimited.org/products/derek-nexus.htm
HazardExpert	The first computer-based toxicity prediction expert system of CompuDrug Chemistry Ltd. Toxicity end points include irritation, neurotoxicity, immunotoxicity, teratogenicity, mutagenicity, and carcinogenicity, and prediction is done on the basis of toxic fragments accompanied by expert judgment and fuzzy logic. Web site: http://www.compudrug.com/hazardexpertpro
The BfR Decision Support System (DSS)	It is employed for determining skin/eye irritation/corrosion potential of chemicals leading to classification and labeling. It considers physicochemical properties like log *P*, surface tension, and melting point during prediction. The system employs two approaches for toxicity prediction namely exclusion rule for those chemicals not possessing certain hazard by the use of physicochemical cutoff values, and inclusion rule for chemicals with specific toxicological potency using structural alerts. It was formerly developed by the Bundesinstitut für gesundheitlichen Verbraucherschutz und Veterinärmedizin (German Institute for Consumer Health Protection and Veterinary Medicine) and is now with the Bundesinstitut für Risikobewertung (Federal Institute for Risk Assessment). Web site: http://www.tandfonline.com/doi/pdf/10.1080/10629360701304014
TOPKAT	It is one of the earliest systems. Hansch QSAR equation is derived from the substructural fragments producing toxicity. The end points include carcinogenicity, mutagenicity, acute lethal toxicity, and skin sensitization. Web site: http://www.sciencedirect.com/science/article/pii/0027510794901252
MCASE and CASE Ultra	The prediction in MCASE (MultiCASE) is done using fragments comprising of all linear atom and bond chains within a preset range of bond numbers in the training set. CASE Ultra is the end-user application of MCASE. Toxicity end points include genotoxicity, mutagenicity, carcinogenicity, cardiotoxicity, and hepatotoxicity. Web site: http://www.multicase.com/

(*Continued*)

Table 1.4 (Continued)

Expert system	Short description (with web link)
Leadscope	The modelable end points include genetic Toxicity, carcinogenicity, reproductive toxicity, developmental toxicity, neurotoxicity, adverse hepatobiliary effects, adverse urinary tract effects, and adverse cardiological effects. Web site: http://www.leadscope.com/
TerraQSAR™	It uses a probabilistic neural network (PNN) method on the basis of conditional average estimation. The toxicity end points include skin irritation, toxicity toward daphnia, fathead minnow, fish, rat, and mouse. Web site: http://www.terrabase-inc.com/
ACD/Percepta	It performs prediction of pharmacokinetic profile (ADME-Tox). It allows a single interface for analysis and interpretation of ADME, physicochemical property, and toxicological data. A product of the ACD/Labs. Web site: http://www.acdlabs.com/products/percepta/physchem_adme_tox/
MolCode Toolbox	It allows prediction of physicochemical and biological properties, ADME-Tox, ecological pathways/ecotoxicity, and adverse drug effect. A product of the MolCode. Web site: http://www.molcode.com/
TIMES	It stands for "TIssue MEtabolism Simulator" and is a product of the Laboratory of Mathematical Chemistry (LMC), Bourgas University, Bulgaria. It is used for the prediction of toxicity of chemicals as a matter of their metabolic activation; produces metabolic map from biotransformation and abiotic reaction library by employing heuristic algorithm; used for assessing skin sensitization, mutagenicity, chromosomal aberrations, and micronucleus formation due to metabolites of chemicals. Web site: http://oasis-lmc.org/products/software/times.aspx
CATALOGIC	It is used for assessing environment fate and ecotoxicity, namely, abiotic and biotic degradation, bioaccumulation, acute aquatic toxicity, etc. A product of LMC, Bourgas University, Bulgaria. Web site: http://oasis-lmc.org/products/software/catalogic.aspx

of the scientists to search for the suitable explanation of a scientific process and thereby defining it logically. Quantification of chemistry and incorporation of mathematical algorithms in chemical sciences allows the development of a logical basis to define a chemistry-activity/property/toxicity correlation. The aftermath of chemical interactions producing the pharmacological effects of chemicals can be understood from such analysis. Although it sounds simple, such correlation analysis can be amplified in a very broad way to solve complex problems spanning from prediction of drug action in human body to the assessment of environmental hazard produced by chemicals.

The concept being same, the purpose of application can be varied. It should be remembered that no QSAR analysis can do more than suggesting molecules for synthesis and testing. The only way to determine a molecule's activity (or toxicity) is through experiments. QSAR analyses can save needless synthesis and biological evaluation of less potential compounds.

As the time has passed, development of predictive (Q)SAR modeling has traversed a long path, and presently is accepted, defined and described by the regulatory agencies. Various new methodologies for data treatment, processing, modeling and validation are emerging nowadays. However, the aim of a modeler should be maintaining unambiguity and reproducibility in selecting data points, defining descriptors, choosing the transparent modeling method, performing suitable validation, and finally providing an explanation of the results that define the process with an apt logic. It may be noted that the explanation of the results depends on the descriptors present in the model (equation) and hence care should be exercised while selecting appropriate descriptors as predictor variables from the available ones or defining a novel one. The success of (Q)SAR modeling lies in establishing a rational basis for chemical action such that the designer can incorporate desirable modification to an existing process; otherwise, it will merely be a "black-box" correlation analysis obtained as a consequence of a series of abstract mathematical algorithms.

REFERENCES

[1] Hansch C, Leo A, Hoekman DH. Exploring QSAR: structure activity relations in chemistry and biology. Washington, DC: Am Chem Soc; 1995.

[2] Ramsden CA. (volume editor), Quantitative drug design, vol. 4 of comprehensive medicinal chemistry. The rational design, mechanistic study; therapeutic application of chemical compounds. Hansch C, Sammes PG, Taylor JB, editors. Oxford: Pergamon Press; 1990.

[3] Daniels TC, Jorgensen EC. Physicochemical properties in relation to biological action. In: Doerge RF, editor. Wilson and Gisvold's textbook of organic medicinal and pharmaceutical chemistry. 8th ed. Philadelphia, PA: J.B. Lippincott Co; 1982.

[4] Leake CD. A historical account of pharmacology to the twentieth century. Springfield, IL: Charles C Thomas; 1975.

[5] Langley JN. On the reaction of cells and of nerve-endings to certain poisons, chiefly as regards the reaction of striated muscle to nicotine and to curari. J Physiol 1905;33:374–413.

[6] Ehrlich P. In: Himmelweit F, editor. Collected papers of Paul Ehrlich, vol. 3. London: Pergamon Press; 1957.

[7] Sinko PJ, editor. Martin's physical pharmacy and pharmaceutical sciences. 6th ed. Baltimore, MD: Lippincott Williams & Wilkins; 2011.

[8] Maher TA, Johnson DA. Receptors and drug action. In: Williams DA, Lemke TL, editors. Foye's principles of medicinal chemistry. Philadelphia, PA: Lippincott Williams & Wilkins; 2002. pp. 86–99.

[9] Kolář M, Jiří H, Hobza P. The strength and directionality of a halogen bond are co-determined by the magnitude and size of the σ-hole. Phys Chem Chem Phys 2014;16:9987–96.

[10] Hunter CA. Arene–arene interactions: electrostatic or charge transfer? Angew Chem Int Ed Engl 1993;32:1584–6.

[11] Grimme S. Do special noncovalent $\pi-\pi$ stacking interactions really exist? Angew Chem Int Ed Engl 2008;47:3430–4.

[12] Mulliken RS, Person WB. Molecular complexes. New York, NY: Wiley; 1969.

[13] Serrano L, Bycroft M, Fersht A. Aromatic–aromatic interactions and protein stability: investigation by double-mutant cycles. J Mol Biol 1991;218:465–75.

[14] Knittel JJ, Zavod RM. Drug design and relationship of functional groups to pharmacologic activity. In: Williams DA, Lemke TL, editors. Foye's principles of medicinal chemistry. Philadelphia, PA: Lippincott Williams & Wilkins; 2002. pp. 37–67.

[15] Langmuir I. The arrangement of electrons in atoms and molecules. J Am Chem Soc 1919;41: 868–934.

[16] Grimm HG. Structure and size of the non-metallic hydrides. Z Elekrochemie 1925;31:474–80.

[17] Hinsberg O. The sulfur atom. J Prakt Chem 1916;93:302–11.

[18] Balaban AT, Klein DJ. Is chemistry "the central science"? How are different sciences related? Co-citations, reductionism, emergence, and posets. Scientometrics 2006;69:615–37.

[19] Todeschini R, Consonni V, Gramatica P. Chemometrics in QSAR. In: Brown S, Tauler R, Walczak R, editors. Comprehensive chemometrics, vol. 4. Oxford: Elsevier; 2009. pp. 129–72.

[20] Tute MS. History and objectives of quantitative drug design. In: Hansch C, Sammes PG, Taylor JB, editors. Comprehensive medicinal chemistry, vol. 4. Oxford: Pergamon Press; 1990. pp. 1–31.

[21] Russell WMS, Burch RL. The principles of humane experimental technique. London: Methuen; 1959<http://altweb.jhsph.edu/pubs/books/humane_exp/het-toc>; [accessed 12.08.14].

[22] Fund for the Replacement of Animals in Medicinal Experiments (FRAME). <http://www.frame.org.uk/>; [accessed 12.08.14].

[23] People for the Ethical Treatment of Animals (PETA). Alternatives to animal testing. <http://www.peta.org/issues/animals-used-for-experimentation/alternatives-animal-testing/>; [accessed 12.08.14].

[24] Zuang V, Hartung T. Making validated alternatives available—the strategies and work of the European Centre for the Validation of Alternative Methods (ECVAM). Altern Anim Test Exp 2005;11:15–26.

[25] International Guiding Principles for Biomedical Research Involving Animals. Council for international organizations of medical sciences (CIOMS). <http://cioms.ch/publications/guidelines/1985_texts_of_guidelines.htm>; 1985 [accessed 12.08.14].

[26] Hengstler JG, Foth H, Kahl R, Kramer P-J, Lilienblum W, Schulz T, et al. The REACH concept and its impact on toxicological sciences. Toxicology 2006;220:232–9.

[27] Auer CM, Nabholz JV, Baetcke KP. Mode of action and the assessment of chemical hazards in the presence of limited data: use of structure–activity relationships (SAR) under TSCA, Section 5. Environ Health Perspect 1990;87:183–97.

[28] El-Masri HA, Mumtaz MM, Choudhary G, Cibulas W, De Rosa CT. Application of computational toxicology methods at the agency for toxic substances and disease registry. Int J Hyg Environ Health 2002;205:63–9.

[29] OECD environment health and safety publications series on testing and assessment No. 69 Guidance document on the validation of (quantitative) structure–activity relationship [(Q)SAR] models. <http://www.oecd.org/officialdocuments/publicdisplaydocumentpdf/?cote=env/jm/mono(2007)2&doclanguage=en>; 2007 [accessed 12.08.14].

[30] Sotriffer C, editor. Virtual screening, principles, challenges, and practical guidelines. Weinheim, Germany: Wiley-VCH Verlag GmBH & Co. KGaA; 2011.

[31] Albert A, Rubbo SD, Goldacre RJ, Davey ME, Stone JD. The influence of chemical constitution on antibacterial activity. Part II: a general survey of the acridine series. Br J Exp Pathol 1945; 26:160–92.

[32] Hansch C. On the state of QSAR. Drug Inf J 1984;18:115–22.

[33] Charton M, Philip S. Magee: a life in QSAR. J Comput Aided Mol Des 2008;22:335–7.

[34] Horsford E.N. In: Baird S.P., editor. Proceedings of the American association for the advancement of science fourth meeting. New Haven, CT; 1851. pp. 216–222.

[35] Pelikan EV (1854) Opyt prilozheniya sovremennykh fizilo-khimischeskikh issledovanii k ucheniyu o yadakh (Experience with the application of modern physiochemical concepts to the study of poisons). St. Petersburg; Toksikologiya tsianistykh metallov. (The toxicology of cyanides of metals). St. Petersburg, 1855.
[36] Borodin A. Ob analogii myshiakovoi kislotys fosforoyu v khimischeskom i toksicheskov otnosheniyakh (Concerning the analogy between arsenic and phosphoric acids in chemical and toxicological respects). Dissertation, St. Petersburg, 1858.
[37] Cros. Action de l'alcohol amylique sur l'organisme" at the Faculty of Medicine. University of Strasbourg, Strasbourg, France, 1863 (January 9).
[38] Crum-Brown A, Fraser TR. On the connection between chemical constitution and physiological action. Part I. On the physiological action of the salts of the ammonium bases, derived from strychnine, brucia, thebaia, codeia, morphia, and nicotia. J Anat Physiol 1868;2:224–42.
[39] Richardson BJ. Physiological research on alcohols. Med Times Gazzette 1869;2:703–6.
[40] Richet C. On the relationship between the toxicity and the physical properties of substances. Compt Rendus Seances Soc Biol 1893;9:775–6.
[41] Meyer H. Zur Theorie der Alkoholnarkose: 1. Welche Eigenschaft der Anästhetica bedingt ihre narkotische Wirkung? Arch Exp Pathol Pharmakol 1899;42:109–18.
[42] Overton E. Ueber die allgemeinen osmotischen Eigenschaften der Zelle, ihre vermutlichen Ursachen und ihre Bedeutung fur die Physiologie. Vierteljahrsschr Naturforsch Ges Zurich 1899; 44:88–114.
[43] Baum F. Zur Theorie der Alkoholnarkose. Arch Exp Pathol Pharmakol 1899;42:119–37.
[44] Traube J. Theorie der Osmose and Narkose. Pflüg Arch Physiol 1904;105:541–58.
[45] Seidell A. A new bromine method for the determination of thymol, salicylates, and similar compounds. Am Chem J 1912;47:508–26.
[46] Ferguson J. The use of chemical potentials as indices of toxicity. Proc R Soc London Ser B 1939; 127:387–403.
[47] Albert A, Rubbo SD, Goldacre R. Correlation of basicity and antiseptic action in an acridine series. Nature 1941;147:332–3.
[48] Bell PH, Roblin Jr RO. Chemotherapy. VII. A Theory of the relation of structure to activity of sulfanilamide-type compounds. J Am Chem Soc 1942;64:2905–17.
[49] Hammett LP. Some relations between reaction rates and equilibrium constants. Chem Rev 1935;17:125–36.
[50] Taft Jr RW. Linear free-energy relationships from rates of esterification and hydrolysis of aliphatic and ortho-substituted benzoate esters. J Am Chem Soc 1952;74:2729–32.
[51] Hansch C, Maloney PP, Fujita T, Muir RM. Correlation of biological activity of phenoxyacetic acids with Hammett substituent constants and partition coefficients. Nature 1962;194:178–80.
[52] Hansch C, Fujita T. ρ–σ–π analysis. A method for the correlation of biological activity and chemical structure. J Am Chem Soc 1964;86:1616–26.
[53] Free SM, Wilson JW. A mathematical contribution to structure–activity studies. J Med Chem 1964;7:395–9.
[54] Fujita T, Ban T. Structure–activity relation. 3. Structure–activity study of phenethylamines as substrates of biosynthetic enzymes of sympathetic transmitters. J Med Chem 1971;14:148–52.
[55] Wiener H. Structural determination of paraffin boiling points. J Am Chem Soc 1947;69:17–20.
[56] Platt JR. Influence of neighbor bonds on additive bond properties in paraffins. J Chem Phys 1947; 15:419–20.
[57] Simon Z. Specific interactions. Intermolecular forces, steric requirements, and molecular size. Angew Chem Int Ed Engl 1974;13:719–27.
[58] Hall LH, Kier LB. Structure–activity studies using valence molecular connectivity. J Pharm Sci 1977;66:642–4.
[59] Goodford PJ. A computational procedure for determining energetically favorable binding sites on biologically important macromolecules. J Med Chem 1985;28:849–57.

[60] Cramer III RD, Patterson DE, Bunce JD. Comparative Molecular Field Analysis (CoMFA). 1. Effect of shape on binding of steroids to carrier proteins. J Am Chem Soc 1988;110:5959–67.
[61] Proceedings of the OECD workshop on sustainable chemistry. Part 1: ENV/JM/MONO(99)19/PART1, 15–17 October, 1998. <http://www.oecd.org/officialdocuments/publicdisplaydocumentpdf/?doclanguage=en&cote=env/jm/mono(99)19/PART1>; [accessed 12.08.14].
[62] Anastas PT, Warner JC. Green chemistry: theory and practice. Oxford: Oxford University Press; 1998.
[63] Das RN, Roy K. Advances in QSPR/QSTR models of ionic liquids for the design of greener solvents of the future. Mol Divers 2013;17:151–96.
[64] Worth AP. The role of QSAR methodology in the regulatory assessment of chemicals. In: Puzyn T, Leszczynski J, Cronin MTD, editors. Recent advances in QSAR studies methods and applications. The Netherlands: Springer; 2010. pp. 367–82.

CHAPTER 2

Chemical Information and Descriptors

Contents

Understanding the Basics of QSAR for Applications in Pharmaceutical Sciences and Risk Assessment.
ISBN: 978-0-12-801505-6, DOI: http://dx.doi.org/10.1016/B978-0-12-801505-6.00002-8

2.1 INTRODUCTION

The quantitative structure–activity relationship (QSAR) technique, being directly related to the molecular structures of chemicals, can explain the effects exerted by the chemicals in relation to their structures and properties. Any significant search for the required chemical information of molecules for a particular end point can provide a strong tool for the predictive assessment of the response of existing untested as well as new chemicals [1]. QSAR is a simple mathematical model that can correlate chemistry with the properties (physicochemical/biological/toxicological) of molecules using various computationally or experimentally derived quantitative parameters known as *descriptors*. These descriptors are correlated with the response variable using a variety of chemometric tools in order to obtain a meaningful QSAR model. The developed models provide a significant insight regarding the essential structural requisites of the molecules, thus enabling us to identify the features contributing to the biological activity/property/toxicity of the studied molecules [2].

2.2 CONCEPT OF DESCRIPTORS

Molecular descriptors are terms that characterize specific information about a studied molecule. They are the "numerical values associated with the chemical constitution for correlation of chemical structure with various physical properties, chemical reactivity, or biological activity" [3,4]. In other words, the modeled response (activity/property/toxicity of query molecules) is represented as a function of quantitative values of structural features or properties that are termed as descriptors for a QSAR model. Cheminformatics methods depend on the generation of chemical reference spaces into which new chemical entities are predictable by the developed QSAR model. The definition of chemical spaces significantly depends on the use of computational descriptors of studied molecular structure, physical or chemical properties, or specific features.

$$\text{Response(activity/property/toxicity)} = f(\text{Information in form of chemical structure or property}) = f(\text{Descriptors})$$

The type of descriptors used and the extent to which they can encode the structural features of the molecules that are correlated to the response are critical determinants of the quality of any QSAR model. The descriptors may be physicochemical (hydrophobic, steric, or electronic), structural (based on frequency of occurrence of

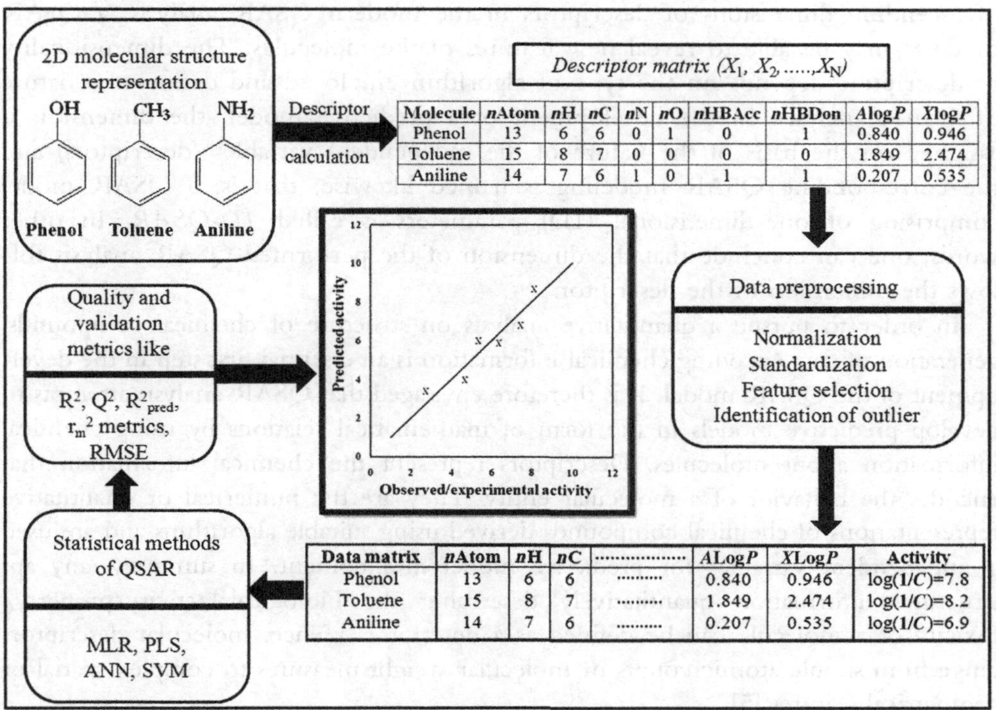

Figure 2.1 How chemical structure is used to calculate descriptors and QSAR model development.

a substructure), topological, electronic (based on molecular orbital calculations), geometric (based on a molecular surface area calculation), or simple indicator parameters (dummy variables). A schematic overview is presented in Figure 2.1 in order to show the steps how a chemical structure is used to calculate descriptors and used in QSAR model development.

A dimension in the QSAR analysis acts as the constraint that controls the nature of the analysis. The term *dimension* in predictive model development is roughly associated with the complexity of the modeling technique that directly signifies the degree of descriptors. The dimension of an object can be mathematically attributed to the minimum number of coordinates needed for specifying a particular point in it [1]. The addition of dimension to a specific geometric object assists in identifying it in a different way by adding more information. Thus, it is clear that dimension is an intrinsic property of an object and does not depend on the space of the object [1]. The addition of new dimensions to the QSAR technique helps in deriving structural information at a higher level of analysis. With the use of ascending dimensions of descriptors in the modern QSAR analysis, a QSAR modeler may be able to reveal new features of the molecules. The dimensionality of descriptors depends on the type of algorithm employed and defines the nature of QSAR analysis. In the development of a predictive model, the dimension is assigned on the basis of the nature of the independent variables (descriptors) and the corresponding QSAR modeling is named likewise; that is, a QSAR model comprising of one-dimensional (1D) parameters is called *1D-QSAR*. In other words, one can conclude that the dimension of the performed QSAR analysis follows the dimension of the descriptor.

In order to pursue a quantitative analysis on structure of chemical compounds, generation of data encoding chemical information is an essential first step in the development of the QSAR model. It is therefore envisaged that QSAR analysis attempts to develop predictive models in the form of mathematical relations by using chemical information about molecules. Descriptors represent the chemical information that encodes the behavior of a molecular entity. They are the numerical or quantitative representations of chemical compounds derived using suitable algorithms and are used as independent variables for predictive model development. In summary, any apt structural information quantitatively describing the biological activity/property/toxicity of a molecule can be defined as a descriptor. Hence, molecular descriptors range from simple atomic counts or molecular weight measures to complex spatial or geometrical features [5].

One can describe a single molecule in many ways. It is possible to compute thousands of numerical descriptors for a given chemical. Many of these descriptors are very closely related to each other and even capture the same information at times. Thus, the selection of relevant descriptors is a well-known problem, and it requires a lot of experience for the QSAR modeler to select the appropriate ones for the model development [6]. In addition, one has to take into account the nature of the chemical structure being considered. A set of descriptors may efficiently encode the chemical information perfectly for the small molecules, but the same set of descriptors may not be able to encode the required features for polymers, protein structures, and inorganic molecules. Thus, not only the calculation but also the selection of suitable descriptors requires a lot of knowledge and experience in QSAR model development.

Counts of types of atoms or bonds can be considered as constitutional descriptors that only consider atom and bond labels of the compound. Topological descriptors take into account connectivity and labeled graph theory [7]. An advantage of these descriptors is that they do not require exhaustive three-dimensional (3D) coordinate generation and conformational analysis. On the contrary, geometric and 3D descriptors require a 3D structure as input, and therefore the analysis needs to be extensive in order to get the output. Geometrical descriptors are those that describe the molecular shape that is a key factor in ligand–receptor interactions and is an important approach to virtual screening. A variety of descriptors have been invented to characterize molecular shape. Apart from the numerical descriptors, other helpful descriptors are called *fingerprint descriptors.* Conventionally, these descriptors are symbolized in the form of bit strings. In case of inorganic materials, traditional small molecule descriptors are not at all useful. In recent times, a number of periodic table–derived descriptors for inorganic materials, which are very similar to constitutional descriptors, are proving to be helpful [8,9].

This discussion has focused on various facets of descriptors that make them useful in developing QSAR models. It is interesting to point out that the efficacy of a descriptor can rely heavily on the problem being considered. More precisely, certain end points may need to take into account exact molecular features. The best possible features that make a descriptor ideal for the construction of a QSAR model are summarized here:

1. A descriptor must be correlated with the structural features for a specific end point and show negligible correlation with other descriptors.
2. A descriptor should be applicable to a broad class of compounds.
3. A descriptor that can be calculated rapidly and does not depend on experimental properties can be considered more suitable than one that is computationally exhaustive and relies heavily on experimental results.
4. A descriptor should generate dissimilar values for structurally different molecules, even if the structural differences are small. This means that the descriptor should show minimal degeneracy. In addition to degeneracy, a descriptor should be continuous. It signifies that small structural changes should lead to small changes in the value of the descriptor.
5. It is always important that the descriptor has some form of physical interpretability to encode the query features of the studied molecules.
6. Another significant aspect is the ability to map descriptor values back to the structure for visualization purposes [10]. These visualizations are sensible only when descriptor values can be associated to structural features.

Different features of ideal descriptors are summarized in a graphical way in Figure 2.2.

Figure 2.3 illustrates an outline of the types of descriptors and the form of molecular structure required to calculate them. Here, the representation is very general and focuses only on small molecule descriptors. In the following section, various molecular descriptors are discussed for different chemical entities, not just only for small organic molecules.

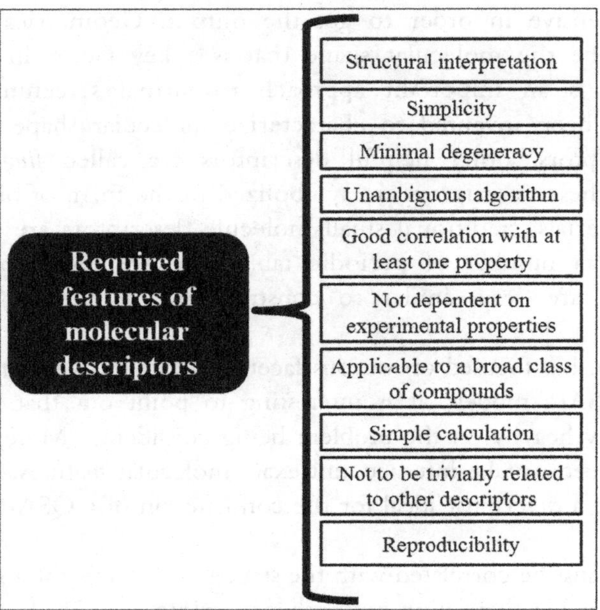

Figure 2.2 Ideal features of descriptors for the development of the QSAR model.

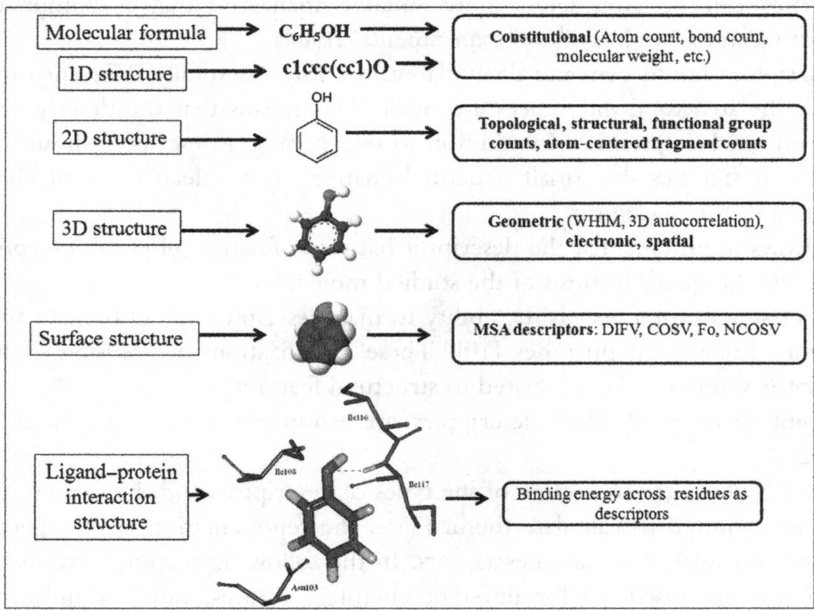

Figure 2.3 An outline of the types of descriptors can be calculated from the different forms of molecular structure.

2.3 TYPE OF DESCRIPTORS

Descriptors can be classified in multiple ways. In general, there are several types of descriptors like structure explicit descriptors (topological), structure implicit (hydrophobicity and electronic), and cryptic descriptors (quantum chemical). It is interesting to point out that the majority of QSAR researchers prefer to classify the types of descriptors in respect to their dimensions. Considering this aspect, Table 2.1 gives a useful illustration of largely used molecular descriptors based on dimensions [5].

In a broader perspective, descriptors (specifically, physicochemical descriptors) can be classified into two major groups: (1) substituent constants and (2) whole molecular descriptors.

2.3.1 Substituent constants

QSAR grew out of physical organic chemistry based on studies to show how differential reaction rates of chemical reactions depend on the differences in molecular structure. Characterization of these differences in structure, which are due to functional group substitutions into a fixed core structure, led to the development of substituent constants [11]. The substituent constants may encode the electronic, hydrophobic, and steric aspects of a series of compounds by which QSAR models can be generated. Substituent constants are basically physicochemical descriptors that are designed on

Table 2.1 Commonly used molecular descriptors based on different dimensions

Dimension of descriptors	Parameters
0D descriptors	Constitutional indices, molecular property, atom, and bond count.
1D descriptors	Fragment counts, fingerprints.
2D descriptors	Topological, structural, physicochemical parameters including thermodynamic descriptors.
3D descriptors	Electronic, spatial parameters, MSA parameters, MFA parameters, RSA parameters.
4D descriptors	Volsurf, GRID, Raptor, etc. derived descriptors.
5D descriptors	These descriptors consider induced-fit parameters and aim to establish a ligand-based virtual or pseudoreceptor model. These can be explained as 4D-QSAR + explicit representation of different induced-fit models. Example: flexible-protein docking.
6D descriptors	These are derived using the representation of various solvation circumstances along with the information obtained from 5D descriptors. They can be explained as 5D-QSAR + simultaneous consideration of different solvation models. Example: Quasar.
7D descriptors	They comprise real receptor or target-based receptor model data.

the basis of factors, which govern the physicochemical properties of chemical entities. Due to changes in physicochemical properties, absorption, distribution, and transport of chemical entities may be changed.

2.3.2 Whole molecular descriptors

Advancement of structural representation and exploitation of chemical structures have led to the generation of novel methods for representing entire molecular structures. Many of the whole molecule descriptors are expansions of the substituent constant approach, but many of them are also derived from entirely new approaches or from experiments. There are now many commercial molecular modeling programs that can produce descriptors from the whole molecule. Some examples of most commonly used whole molecule descriptors in the QSAR study include the octanol–water partition coefficient, acidic dissociation constant (pK_a), and van der Waals volume (Vw).

2.4 DESCRIPTORS COMMONLY USED IN QSAR STUDIES

Most commonly used descriptors in the QSAR studies are elaborately described in the following sections.

2.4.1 Physicochemical descriptors

These descriptors are derived from the results of some physicochemical experimental findings, and they have connections with the physicochemical properties of the molecules.

2.4.1.1 Hydrophobic parameters

2.4.1.1.1 Partition coefficient (log *P*)

The relative affinity of a drug molecule for an aqueous or lipid medium is important for the drug's activity because absorption, transport, and excretion depend on partitioning phenomena [12,13]. The most widely used molecular descriptor to encode this property is the logarithm of the partition coefficient, *P*, between *n*-octanol and water:

$$P = [C]_{\text{octanol}}/[C]_{\text{aqueous}} \tag{2.1}$$

In Eq. (2.1–2.3), $[C]_{\text{octanol}}$ is the concentration of a solute in the lipid phase (*n*-octanol) and $[C]_{\text{aqueous}}$ is the concentration of the solute in the aqueous phase. Compounds for which $P > 1$ are lipophilic or hydrophobic, and compounds for which $P < 1$ are hydrophilic. Lipophilicity represents the affinity of a molecule or a moiety for a lipophilic environment. It is commonly measured by its distribution behavior in a biphasic system, either liquid–liquid or solid–liquid. In addition, log *P* values can also be computed based on atomic/fragmental contributions and various correction factors, and several such algorithms like $C\log P$, $A\log P$, $A\log P98$, $M\log P$, and $X\log P$ are available.

One of the important methods for calculating $\log P$ from the molecular structure is substituent additivity based on fragmental and atomic contributions, with consideration of surface area, molecular properties, and solvatochromic parameters [14]. In this method, after summing fragment constants for the molecule in query, any necessary correction factors for intramolecular interactions between the fragments, such as electronic, steric, or hydrogen-bonding effects, are added. This fragment addition method developed by Hansch et al. [14] is widely used in recent times. Here, the $\log P$ of a compound is computed by summing the contributions for the fragments and then applying a number of correction factors as needed:

$$\log P = \sum_i a_i f_i + \sum_j b_j f_j \tag{2.2}$$

where f_i are fragment constants and f_j are correction factors. The contribution for each fragment f_i multiplied by the occurrence of that fragment (a_i) is added cumulatively. This sum is then corrected for a number of factors according to the solvent theory. Each correction factor has an associated value, f_j, and this is multiplied by the number of instances of the correction in the structure, b_j. Correction factors include those due to molecular flexibility, branching, polar fragment interaction factors, *ortho* effects, and aromatic interactions [14].

2.4.1.1.2 Hydrophobic substituent constant (π)

Hydrophobicity [12,13] is the association of nonpolar groups or molecules in an aqueous environment, which arises from the tendency of water to exclude nonpolar molecules. The hydrophobicity of the compounds in the series can be represented on a relative scale with the hydrophobic substituent constant π. The value for the substituent X is defined as follows:

$$\pi_X = \log P_X - \log P_H \tag{2.3}$$

In Eq. (2.3), P_X is the partition coefficient of the derivative and P_H is the partition coefficient of the parent compound. The variable π_X expresses the variation in lipophilicity, which results when the substituent X replaces H in RH. For example, the value of the chloro substituent π_{Cl} is the difference between the partition coefficient values of chlorobenzene and benzene. As another example, one may note that the $\log P$ values for benzene and benzamide are 2.13 and 0.64, respectively. Since benzene is the parent compound, the substituent constant for $CONH_2$ is -1.49 (Figure 2.4).

A positive value of π indicates that the substituent is more hydrophobic than hydrogen, and a negative value indicates that the substituent is less hydrophobic. The π value

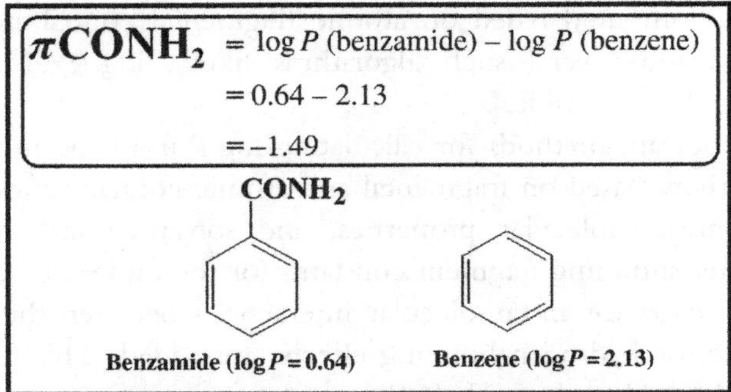

Figure 2.4 Sample calculation of the hydrophobic substituent constant for $CONH_2$ group.

is a characteristic for an individual substituent and can be used to calculate how the partition coefficient of a drug would be affected by adding that particular substituent.

2.4.1.1.3 Hydrophobic fragmental constant (f, f')

The hydrophobic fragmental constant of a substituent or molecular fragment represents the lipophilicity contribution of that molecular fragment [12–14].

2.4.1.2 Electronic parameters

Electronic substituent constants were developed as a direct result of an empirical observation made from certain chemical systems that substituents have the same relative effects on the rates of reaction equilibria, regardless of which reaction was being studied [13,15].

2.4.1.2.1 Acid dissociation constant

An important whole molecular parameter defining electronic nature of the tested molecules is the acid dissociation constant [5], which can be explained by the following equation:

$$K_a = \frac{[A^-][H^+]}{[HA]} \tag{2.4}$$

where A^- is the conjugate base of acid HA and H^+ is the proton. The negative logarithmic function (pK_a) is used for modeling purposes and can be defined as $pK_a = -\log_{10} K_a$. It is usually determined using the famous Henderson–Hasselbalch equation:

$$pK_a = pH - \log\frac{[A^-]}{[HA]} \tag{2.5}$$

where pH is the negative logarithmic concentration of H^+ ion; that is, $pH = -\log[H^+]$.

2.4.1.2.2 Hammett constant

Hammett proposed the electronic substituent constant from the rate constants of ionization reaction of *meta*- and *para*-substituted benzoic acid derivatives:

$$\log\frac{k}{k_0} = \rho\sigma \tag{2.6}$$

In Eq. (2.6), the slope ρ is a proportionality reaction constant pertaining to a given equilibrium that relates the effect of substituents on that equilibrium to the effect on the benzoic acid equilibrium. The parameter σ describes the electronic properties of aromatic substituents; that is, electron withdrawing or donating power. The constant k_0 refers to the rate constant for the unsubstituted compound, while k refers to that of a *meta*- or *para*-substituted congener. The substituent constant, σ, reflects the intrinsic polar effect of a given substituent relative to hydrogen. This effect is independent of the reaction.

One of the limitations of the Hammett constant is that it does not hold for *ortho* substituents. This characteristic is known as the *ortho effect*. Taft and Newman [16] proposed a quantitative measure for separating the inductive influence of a substituent from its steric effect. The substituent constant σ^* is based on the rates of acid- and base-catalyzed hydrolysis of esters of the form $X{-}CH_2{-}COOR$:

$$\sigma^* = (1/2.48)[\log(k/k_0)_{BASE} - \log(k/k_0)_{ACID}] \tag{2.7}$$

where X = H for k_0. Taft argued that σ^* should measure only the inductive influence of a substituent.

There are several other variants of electronic substituent constants. For example, σ^- may be used instead of σ_p when cross-conjugation with an electron-withdrawing substituent occurs. Similar to the σ^- constants for electron-withdrawing groups, there is another variant σ^+, which can be used for groups that release electron density via resonance. The *meta*-substituted systems are employed to find out the appropriate reaction constant ρ, and these, in turn, may be used to find the normalized substituent constant, σ^0, for *para* substituents. The σ^0 values indicate that electron donor groups such as $-N(CH_3)_2$, $-NH_2$, and $-OCH_3$ have much less influence in *p*-substituted phenylacetic acid systems than in the corresponding *para*-substituted benzoic acids. This helps to prove that cross-conjugation is a significant component of the Hammett constants for such substituents.

Efforts were made to include inductive and resonance components in the general quantitation for the electronic effects, which can be shown as follows:

$$\sigma_p = \sigma_I + \sigma_R \tag{2.8}$$

$$\sigma_m = \sigma_I + \alpha\sigma_R \tag{2.9}$$

In Eqs. (2.8) and (2.9), σ_I is the field/inductive component, which is a scaled version of Taft's σ^* parameter; α is the transmission effect; and σ_R is the resonance component.

2.4.1.3 Steric parameters

In a homologous series of compounds, different biological activities for the compounds are often related to the size of the substituents [13,16,17]. Bulky substituents can interfere with the intermolecular reactions, which lead to the drug's activity. The quantitative encoding of the steric aspect of the drug structure can be accomplished by a series of steric substituent constants.

2.4.1.3.1 Taft steric constant

The first steric parameter to be quantified and used in QSAR studies was Taft's steric (E_S) constant [16,17], which was proposed as a measure of steric effects that a substituent X exerts on the acid-catalyzed hydrolytic rate of esters of substituted acetic acids XCOOR. The basic assumption is that the effect of X on acid hydrolysis is purely steric, as the reaction constant ρ for acid hydrolysis of substituted esters is close to zero. It was a modification to the Hammett constant equation. While the Hammett equation accounts for how field, inductive, and resonance effects influence the reaction rates, the Taft equation describes the steric effects of a substituent. E_S is defined as

$$E_S = \log(k_x)_A - \log(k_{CH3})_A = \log(k_x/k_{CH3})_A \tag{2.10}$$

where k_x and k_{CH3} are the rate constants for the substituted (substituent is X) and unsubstituted ($X = CH_3$) esters or acids, respectively; and the subscript A denotes hydrolysis in acid solution. The bulkier is the substituent, the more negative are the E_S constant values.

2.4.1.3.2 Charton's steric parameter (ν) and van der Waals radius

Charton found that Taft's steric (E_S) constant is linearly dependent on the van der Waals radius of the substituent, which led to the development of Charton's steric parameter (υ_X) [18]. Taft also pointed out that E_S varies parallel to the atom group radius. Charton's steric parameter can be defined as

$$\upsilon_X = r_X - r_H = r_X - 1.20 \tag{2.11}$$

where r_X and r_H are the minimum van der Waals radii of the substituent and hydrogen, respectively.

Charton's steric parameter is related to the van der Waals radius of any symmetrical substituent or to the minimum width of unsymmetrical ones. To overcome the problem of asymmetrical substituents, Verloop introduced the STERIMOL set of five parameters, which is explained in a later section of this chapter [13,16].

2.4.1.3.3 Effective Charton's steric parameter (υ_{ef})

Taft developed his steric effect constants based on the assumption that rates of esterification of carboxylic acids with alcohols and of acid-catalyzed hydrolysis of carboxylate esters were structurally reliant on steric effects. This assumption was supported by the work of Charton, who showed that the Taft E_S values for H, a no conformational dependence (NCD) group, and for CH_3, CCl_3, CBr_3, and CF_3, minimal conformational dependence (MCD) groups, were well correlated by Eq. (2.12):

$$E_{S,X} = a_1 r_{v,min,X} + a_0 \tag{2.12}$$

where *min* denotes minimum radius. Effective values, υ_{ef}, of the steric parameter for some intermediate conformational dependence (ICD) groups have been obtained by means of a two-step procedure:

1. The log k_X values, which are available for NCD and MCD groups, are correlated with Eq. (2.13):

$$\log(k_X)_A = s\nu_{min,X} + h \tag{2.13}$$

2. The s and h values obtained from this correlation are used to calculate the values of υ_{eff} from Eq. (2.14):

$$\nu_{eff,X} = \frac{\log(k_X)_A - h}{s} \tag{2.14}$$

The values of υ_{eff} for some frequently occurring substituents are given in Table 2.2.

2.4.1.3.4 STERIMOL parameters

In an attempt to go beyond the Taft parameter, which was designed for simple homogenous organic reactions, Verloop [19] designed a multiparametric method for characterizing the steric features of the substituents in more complex biological systems. Verloop [19] developed the STERIMOL parameters, which are a set of five descriptors (L, $B1$, $B2$, $B3$, and $B4$), to describe the shape of a substituent. L is the length of the substituent along the axis of the bond between the first atom of the substituent and the parent molecule. The width parameters $B1-B4$ are all orthogonal to L and form angles of 90° to each other. The large number of parameters required to define each substituent and the large number of compounds necessary to incorporate all the parameters in a QSAR resulted in pruning of the descriptors to L, $B1$, and $B5$, with $B1$ as the smallest and $B5$ the largest width parameter, which does not have any directional relationship to L [19]. Verloop STERIMOL parameters for the carboxylic acid group in *para*-hydroxy benzoic acid are presented in Figure 2.5.

Table 2.2 υ_{ef} **values for common substituents**

Groups	υ_{ef}	Groups	υ_{ef}
CH_3	0.52	CH_3CHOH	0.50
CH_2CH_3	0.56	C_2H_5CHOH	0.71
$CH_2CH_2CH_3$	0.68	C_6H_5CHOH	0.69
$CH_2CH_2CH_2CH_3$	0.68	CH_2NH_2	0.54
$C_6H_5(CH_2)_3$	0.70	CH_3CHNH_2	0.58
CH_2F	0.62	$C_2H_5CHNH_2$	0.89
CH_2Cl	0.60	H	0
CH_2Br	0.64	F	0.27
CH_2I	0.67	Cl	0.55
CHF_2	0.68	Br	0.65
$CHCl_2$	0.81	I	0.78
$CHBr_2$	0.89	OH	0.32
CHI_2	0.97	NH_2	0.35
CF_3	0.90	SH	0.60
CCl_3	1.38	CH_3OCH_2	0.63
CBr_3	1.56	$CH_3CH_2OCH_2$	0.61
CI_3	1.79	$CH_3OCH_2CH_2$	0.89
CH_2CH_2Cl	0.97	CH_2OH	0.53
CH_2CH_2Br	0.92	CH_2CH_2OH	0.77
CH_2CH_2I	0.93	$C_3H_7OCH_2$	0.65

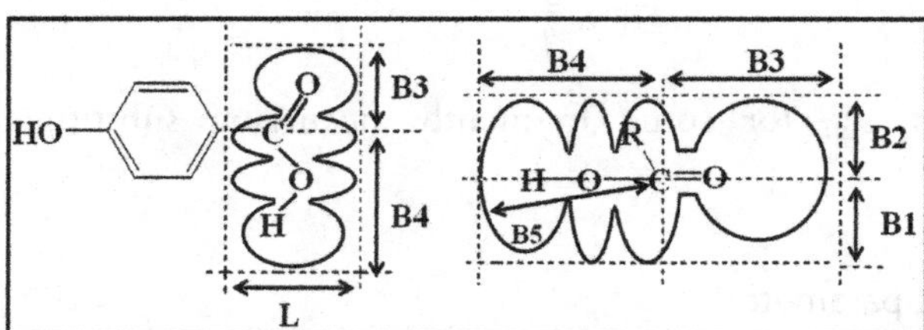

Figure 2.5 Verloop STERIMOL parameters for the carboxylic acid group of *para*-hydroxy benzoic acid.

2.4.1.3.5 Molar refractivity

The molar refractivity (MR) [13,16] is the molar volume corrected by the refractive index. It represents the size and polarizability of a fragment or a molecule. In an atom-based approach, each atom of the molecule is assigned to a particular class, with additive contributions to the total value of MR:

$$MR = \left[\frac{(n^2 - 1)}{(n^2 + 2)}\right]\left(\frac{MW}{d}\right) \tag{2.15}$$

In Eq. (2.15), n is the refractive index, MW is the molecular weight, and d is the density of the compound.

2.4.1.3.6 Parachor

An important whole molecular parameter defining the steric nature is parachor, which can be derived by the following equation:

$$PA = \gamma^{1/4} \cdot \frac{MW}{\rho_L - \rho_V} \tag{2.16}$$

where γ is the surface tension of the liquid, MW is the molecular weight, and ρ_L and ρ_V are the densities of the liquid and vapor states, respectively. Parachor depends on molecule volume [5].

We have enlisted here some of the most commonly used substituent constant parameters for a representative list of common aromatic substituents (Table 2.3).

2.4.2 Topological descriptors

Topological descriptors are calculated based on the graphical representation of the molecules and thus neither require estimation of any physicochemical parameters nor need the rigorous calculations involved in the estimation of the quantum chemical descriptors. The structure representation of the molecule depends on its topology, which indicates the position of the individual atoms and the bonded connections between them. Topological indices are computed by applying a specific algorithm using information obtained from the hydrogen-suppressed graph; that is, the number of elements defining it and their connectivity information [20]. The graph theoretic determination of the molecular structure involves the covalently bonded compounds, considering atoms as the vertices and bonds as the edges. Various topological indices constitute a major portion of the development of successful and predictive QSAR models. Computation of such parameters is very fast and efficient, as they require only hydrogen-suppressed 2D-structural information of the molecule under consideration [21,22]. Their simplicity and easy calculability make them useful for studying large databases of compounds.

In Table 2.4, we list the most commonly used topological descriptors [5,20–38] along with their formal mathematical definitions. The topological descriptors are discussed more thoroughly in Chapter 4 due to their immense application in QSAR model development.

2.4.3 Structural descriptors

Structural parameters [5] are classified and described in Table 2.5.

2.4.4 Indicator variables

Indicator variables have been employed in QSAR models due to their simplicity. Substructure descriptors can be easily employed as indicator variables. Two sets of

Table 2.3 Representative list of substituent constant parameters for common aromatic substituents

Substituent	π	MR	σ_m	σ_p	*L*	*B1*	*B2*	*B3*	*B4*	*B5*
H	0.00	0.103	0.00	0.00	2.06	1.00	1.00	1.00	1.00	1.00
CH_3	0.56	0.565	−0.07	−0.17	3.00	1.52	2.04	1.90	1.90	2.04
CH_2CH_3	1.02	1.030	−0.07	−0.15	4.11	1.52	2.97	1.90	1.90	3.17
CH_2OH	−1.03	0.719	0.00	0.00	3.97	1.52	2.70	1.90	1.90	2.70
CH_2CN	−0.57	1.011	0.16	0.01	3.99	1.52	4.12	1.90	1.90	4.12
CH_2Cl	0.17	1.049	0.11	0.12	3.89	1.52	3.46	1.90	1.90	3.46
CH_2Br	0.79	1.339	0.12	0.14	4.09	1.52	3.75	1.95	1.95	3.75
CH_2I	1.50	1.886	0.10	0.11	4.36	1.52	4.15	2.15	2.15	4.15
$CH_2C_6H_5$	2.01	3.001	−0.08	−0.09	3.63	1.52	6.02	3.11	3.11	6.02
$CH(CH_3)_2$	1.53	1.496	−0.07	−0.15	4.11	2.04	2.76	3.16	3.16	3.17
n-C_3H_7	1.55	1.496	−0.07	−0.13	5.05	1.52	3.49	1.90	1.90	3.49
n-C_4H_9	2.13	1.969	−0.08	−0.16	6.17	1.52	4.42	1.90	1.90	4.54
C_5H_{11}	2.67	2.426	−0.08	−0.16	7.11	1.52	4.94	1.90	1.90	4.94
C_6H_5	1.96	2.536	0.06	−0.01	6.28	1.70	1.70	3.11	3.11	3.11
$COCH_3$	−0.55	1.118	0.38	0.50	4.06	1.90	1.90	2.36	2.93	3.13
$CONH_2$	−1.49	0.981	0.28	0.36	4.06	1.60	1.60	2.42	3.07	3.07
COC_6H_5	1.05	3.033	0.34	0.43	4.57	2.36	5.98	3.11	3.11	5.98
OH	−0.67	0.285	0.12	−0.37	2.74	1.35	1.93	1.35	1.35	1.93
$OCOCH_3$	−0.64	1.247	0.39	0.31	4.87	1.35	3.68	1.90	1.90	3.68
OCH_3	−0.02	0.787	0.12	−0.27	3.98	1.35	2.87	1.90	1.90	3.07
OCH_2CH_3	0.38	1.247	0.10	−0.24	4.92	1.35	3.36	1.35	1.90	3.36
OC_3H_7	0.85	1.706	0.10	−0.25	6.05	1.35	4.30	1.90	1.90	4.42
OC_4H_9	1.55	2.166	0.10	−0.32	6.99	1.35	4.79	1.90	1.90	4.79
OC_6H_5	2.08	2.768	0.25	−0.03	4.51	1.35	5.89	3.11	3.11	5.89
CH_2OCH_3	−0.78	1.207	0.02	0.03	4.91	1.52	2.88	1.90	1.90	3.41
CHO	−0.65	0.688	0.35	0.42	3.53	1.60	1.60	2.00	2.36	2.36
COOH	−0.32	0.693	0.37	0.45	3.91	1.60	1.60	2.36	2.66	2.66
CN	−0.57	0.633	0.56	0.66	4.23	1.60	1.60	1.60	1.60	1.60
CF_3	0.88	0.502	0.43	0.54	3.30	1.98	2.61	2.44	2.44	2.61
F	0.14	0.092	0.34	0.06	2.65	1.35	1.35	1.35	1.35	1.35
Cl	0.71	0.603	0.37	0.23	3.52	1.80	1.80	1.80	1.80	1.80
Br	0.86	0.888	0.39	0.23	3.83	1.95	1.95	1.95	1.95	1.95
I	1.12	1.394	0.35	0.18	4.23	2.15	2.15	2.15	2.15	2.15
NO	−1.20	0.520	0.62	0.91	3.44	1.70	2.44	1.70	1.70	2.44
NO_2	−0.28	0.736	0.71	0.78	3.44	1.70	1.70	2.44	2.44	2.44
NH_2	−1.23	0.542	−0.16	−0.66	2.93	1.50	1.50	1.84	1.84	1.97
$N(CH_3)_2$	0.18	1.555	−0.15	−0.83	3.53	1.50	2.56	2.80	2.80	3.08
$NHCH_3$	−0.47	1.033	−0.30	−0.84	3.53	1.50	3.08	1.90	1.90	3.08
NHC_6H_5	1.37	3.004	−0.12	−0.40	4.53	1.50	5.95	3.11	3.11	5.95
$N{=}NC_6H_5$	1.69	3.131	0.32	0.39	8.43	1.70	1.70	1.92	4.31	4.31
SH	0.39	0.922	0.25	0.15	3.47	1.70	2.33	1.70	1.70	2.33
SCH_3	0.61	1.382	0.15	0.00	4.30	1.70	3.26	1.90	1.90	3.26
SO_2CH_3	−1.63	1.349	0.60	0.72	4.37	2.11	3.15	2.67	2.67	3.15
SO_2NH_2	−1.82	1.228	0.46	0.57	3.82	2.11	3.07	2.67	2.67	3.07

Table 2.4 A representative overview of topological descriptors used in QSAR model development

Name	Mathematical definition	Additional information
Wiener index (W)	$W = \frac{1}{2}\sum_{i=1}^{N}\sum_{j=1}^{N}\delta_{ij}$ where N is the number of vertices or atoms and δ_{ij} is the distance matrix of the shortest possible path between vertices i and j.	Sum contribution of all connecting bonds in a molecular graph.
Zagreb group indices	$\text{Zagreb} = \sum_i \delta_i^2$ where δ_i is the valency of vertex atom i.	Principally depends on vertex adjacency.
Balaban J index	$J = \frac{M}{\mu+1}\sum_{\text{all edges}}(\delta_i\delta_j)^{-0.5}$ where M is the number of edges, μ represents cyclomatic number, and δ_i (or δ_j) can be defined as: $\delta_i = \sum_{j=1}\delta_{ij}$	Acyclic graph is pruned toward its center in order to obtain the sequences of numbers.
Randic branching index (χ)	$\chi = \sum_{\text{all edges}}(\delta_i\delta_j)^{-0.5}$ where δ_i and δ_j represent the number of other nonhydrogen atoms bonded to atoms (vertices) i and j, respectively, forming an edge ij.	Basic connectivity parameter based on which, various higher order graph connectivities are established.
Molecular connectivity index	${}^m\chi_t = \sum_{j=1}^{n_m} {}^mS_j$ where n_m represents the number of t type subgraphs of order m. The term ${}^mS_j$ may be defined as follows: ${}^mS_j = \prod_{i=1}^{m+1}(\delta_i)_j^{-0.5}$ and δ_i for the ith atom may be defined as $\delta_i = \sigma_i - h_i$, where σ_i is the number of valence electrons in σ orbital of the ith atom and h_i represents the number of hydrogen atoms attached to vertex i.	The δ_i represents the number of skeletal neighbors, whereas the valence delta value explicitly considers the hybridization states of each atom. In cases of saturated carbon systems, that is, alkanes, $\delta_i^v = \delta_i$.

(Continued)

Table 2.4 (Continued)

Name	Mathematical definition	Additional information
Valence molecular connectivity index	$^m\chi_t^{vv} = \sum_{j=1}^{n_m} {}^mS_j^{vv}$ Here, the corresponding term δ^v is defined as $\delta_i^v = \frac{(Z_i^v - h)}{Z - Z_i^v - 1}$, where Z and Z^v are the atomic number and the total number of valence electron respectively for the ith vertex.	
Bond/edge connectivity indices	$\in = \sum_{l=1}^{p_2} [\delta(e_i)\delta(e_j)]_l^{-0.5}$ where $\delta(e)$ corresponds to edge degree and is summed (l) over all the p_2 adjacent edges.	This index coincides with Randic connectivity parameter in case of line graph where number of edges equals number of connections.
Extended bond/edge connectivity indices	$^m\in_t = \sum_s \prod_i [\delta(e_i)]_s^{-0.5}$ where m represents the order of the index, t is the type of fragment, and $\delta(e_i)$ is the degree of the edge e_i.	They characterize a generalization of the edge connectivity index. The subscript t denotes the subgraph type is represented as follows. ch: chain or ring; pc: path-cluster; c: cluster; p: path
Kappa shape indices	$^1\kappa = 2\frac{^1P_{max}\,^1P_{min}}{(^1P_i})^2;\ ^2\kappa = 2\frac{^2P_{max}\,^2P_{min}}{(^2P_i})^2;\ ^3\kappa = 4\frac{^3P_{max}\,^3P_{min}}{(^3P_i})^2$ where the numbers of one, two, and three path lengths are denoted by ^1P_i, ^2P_i, and ^3P_i respectively. Furthermore, the maximum and minimum path lengths of a specific type may be represented in terms of the number of atoms (A) and thus the corresponding Kappa shape indices can be defined as follows: $^1P_{max} = (A(A-1))/2;\ ^1P_{min} = (A-1)$ $^1\kappa = \frac{A(A-1)^2}{(^1P_i)^2};\ ^2\kappa = \frac{(A-1)(A-2)^2}{(^2P_i)^2};\ ^3\kappa = \frac{(A-1)(A-3)^2}{(^3P_i)^2}$ for odd value of A and $^3\kappa = \frac{(A-2)^2(A-3)}{(^3P_i)^2}$ for even value of A.	Also known as the Kier's shape indices. Here, the shape of a molecule is defined in terms of number of atoms and their bonding pattern. The index Kappa 1 ($^1\kappa$) shows the degree of complexity, Kappa 2 ($^2\kappa$) defines the degree of linearity or "star-likeness," while Kappa 3 ($^3\kappa$) represents the branching degree at the molecular center.

Kappa modified (alpha) shape indices	The Kappa indices are modified by using an α term which is defined as $\alpha_x = \frac{r_x}{r_{Csp^3}} - 1,$ where r_x and r_{Csp3} are the covalent radii of desired atom and sp^3 hybridized carbon atom, respectively. The corresponding alpha-modified Kappa shape indices are defined here: $^1\kappa_\alpha = \frac{(A+\alpha)(A+\alpha-1)^2}{(^1P_i+\alpha)^2}$; $^2\kappa_\alpha = \frac{(A+\alpha-1)(A+\alpha-2)^2}{(^2P_i+\alpha)^2}$; $^3\kappa_\alpha = \frac{(A+\alpha-1)(A+\alpha-3)^2}{(^3P_i+\alpha)^2}$ for odd A values and $^3\kappa_\alpha = \frac{(A+\alpha-2)^2(A+\alpha-3)}{(^3P_i+\alpha)^2}$ for even A values.	The basic Kappa shape indices consider equivalency of all atoms, which is avoided here by comparing the atomic radius of individual atoms with C_{sp3} carbon.
E-state index	$S_i = I_i + \Delta I_i$ where I_i is an intrinsic state parameter and ΔI_i is the perturbation factor. Both the terms are defined as $I_i = \frac{[2/N]^2\delta^v + 1}{\delta}$ and $\Delta I_i = \sum_{j \neq i} \frac{(I_i - I_j)}{r_{ij}^2}$ where N is the principal quantum number and r_{ij} being the topological distance between atoms *i* and *j*.	Within the electrotopological state atom index, the intrinsic state part denotes the possible partitioning influence of nonsigma (σ) electrons along the path of the chosen atom, whereas the perturbation factor corresponds to an electronegative gradient.
Flexibility index (Kier and Hall's)	$\Phi = \frac{(^1\kappa_\alpha {}^2\kappa_\alpha)}{A}$ where A is the number of vertices and $^1\kappa_\alpha$ and $^2\kappa_\alpha$ are the modified Kappa shape indices of the one and two paths respectively.	This index was derived to provide a direct interpretation of degree of linearity, presence of cycles and branching of the studied structural moiety.

(*Continued*)

Table 2.4 (Continued)

Name	Mathematical definition	Additional information
Information theoretic indices	$I = N\log_2 N - \sum_{i=1}^{n} N_i \log_2 N_i$ where the number of elements present in the ith set is represented by N_i and the number of different sets of elements are denoted by n.	In order to measure the information content in bits, base-2 logarithmic value has been used to define this index.
Extended topochemical atom (ETA) indices	Definitions of some basic ETA indices are given here: $\alpha = \frac{Z - Z^v}{Z^v} \cdot \frac{1}{PN - 1}, \quad \beta = \Sigma x\sigma + \Sigma y\pi + \delta, \quad \gamma_i = \frac{\alpha_i}{\beta_i},$ $[\eta]_i = \sum_{j \neq i} \left[\frac{\gamma_i \gamma_j}{r_{ij}^2}\right]^{0.5}, \quad \varepsilon = -\alpha + 0.3 \times Z^v, \quad \psi = \frac{\alpha}{\varepsilon}$ where α is the core count, β is the valence electron mobile (VEM) count, γ is the VEM vertex count, η is an atom level index, ε is an electronegativity count, and ψ is a measure of hydrogen-bonding propensity parameter. Z and Z^v are the respective atomic number and valence electron number; PN corresponds to periodic number; σ and π are the representation of sigma and pi bond respectively with their contributions being x and y; δ gives a measure of the resonating lone pair electron in an aromatic system; r_{ij} is the topological distance between two atoms.	The ETA indices were introduced as a refinement of different topologically arrived unique (TAU) scheme indices. All the ETA indices are available under two headings: (a) the basic (first generation) ETA indices and (b) the more novel ETA indices. The ETA indices are thoroughly discussed in Chapter 4.
Subgraph count index	It is the number of subgraphs of a given type and order. Subgraph count index is classified from zero order to third order (SC_0, SC_1, SC_2, SC_3). It is notable that third-order subgraphs are divided into three types on the basis of path, cluster, and ring (SC_3_P, SC_3_C, SC_3_CH). Subgraph count index are thoroughly discussed in Chapter 4.	

Table 2.5 Structural parameters used in the development of QSAR models

Parameter	Explanation
Chiral centers	It counts the number of chiral centers (R or S) in a molecule.
Molecular weight (MW)	It is the simple molecular weight of a chemical entity.
Rotatable bonds (Rotlbonds)	This descriptor counts the number of bonds in the molecule having rotations that are considered to be meaningful for molecular mechanics. All terminal H atoms are ignored.
Hbond donor	It counts the number of groups or moieties capable of donating hydrogen bonds.
Hbond acceptor	This descriptor calculates the number of hydrogen-bond acceptors present in the molecule.

compounds, whose only difference is that a substructure exists in one set but not the other, can be studied as an entire set when using an indicator variable. This creates a model that simultaneously utilizes all other independent variables and then combines the models via the indicator variable. The major limitation of this variable is that this approach should be used only when the two sets of compounds are identical in every respect, except for the substructure being coded with the indicator variable. It can be considered as the extension of a structure-based descriptor.

2.4.5 Thermodynamic descriptors

The most commonly used thermodynamic descriptors in QSAR models are described in Table 2.6 [5].

Table 2.6 Thermodynamic parameters used in the development of QSAR models

Descriptor	Description
*A*log*P*	Log of the partition coefficient using Ghose and Crippen's method
*A*log*P*98	The *A*log*P*98 descriptor is an implementation of the atom-type-based *A*log*P* method
*A*logp_atypes	The 120 atom types defined in the calculation of *A*log*P*98 are available as descriptors. Each *A*log*P*98 atom-type value represents the number of atoms of that type in the molecule.
Fh2o	Desolvation free energy for water derived from a hydration shell model developed by Hopfinger
Foct	Desolvation free energy for octanol derived from a hydration shell model developed by Hopfinger
Hf	Heat of formation

2.4.6 Electronic parameters

Electronic descriptors [5] are used to describe electronic aspects of both the whole molecule and particular regions, such as atoms, bonds, and molecular fragments. Electronic charges in the molecule are the driving force of electrostatic interactions, and it is well known that local electron densities or charges play a fundamental role in many chemical reactions and physicochemical properties. The electronic descriptors are summarized in Table 2.7.

Table 2.7 Electronic parameters used in the development of QSAR models

Parameter	Explanation
Sum of atomic polarizabilities	It is the summation of atomic polarizabilities (A_i). The polarizabilities are calculated as follows: $P_a = \sum_i A_i$
Dipole moment (Dipole)	This 3D descriptor represents the strength and orientation behavior of a molecule in an electrostatic field. Both the magnitude and the components (X, Y, and Z) of the dipole moment are calculated. It is determined by using partial atomic charges and atomic coordinates.
Highest occupied molecular orbital (HOMO) energy	This is the highest energy level in the molecule that contains electrons. It governs molecular reactivity and properties. When a molecule acts as a Lewis base (an electron-pair donor) in bond formation, the electrons are supplied from this orbital. It measures the nucleophilicity of a molecule.
Lowest unoccupied molecular orbital (LUMO) energy	This is the lowest energy level in the molecule that contains no electrons. It is also important in governing molecular reactivity and properties. When a molecule acts as a Lewis acid (an electron-pair acceptor) in bond formation, incoming electron pairs are received in this orbital. It measures the electrophilicity of a molecule.
Superdelocalizability (S_r)	This is an index of reactivity in aromatic hydrocarbons, represented as follows: $S_r = 2\sum_{j=1}^{m}\left(\frac{c_{jr}^2}{e_j}\right)$ S_r = superdelocalizability at position r, e_j = bonding energy coefficient in jth molecular orbital (eigenvalue), c = molecular orbital coefficient at position r in the HOMO, m = index of the HOMO. The index is based on the idea that early interaction of the molecular orbitals of two reactants may be regarded as a mutual perturbation, so that the relative energies of the two orbitals change together and maintain a similar degree of overlap as the reactants approach one another.

2.4.7 Quantum chemical descriptors

2.4.7.1 Mulliken atomic charges

Charges (e.g., Mulliken atomic charges) computed from structures optimized at different levels of theory may be used as descriptors. Energy minimization may be carried out at different levels of theory: (i) the semiempirical AM1 (or PM3) method, (ii) the Hartree–Fock method at the HF/3-21G(d) level, (iii) Hartree–Fock method at the HF/6-31G(d) level, (iv) B3LYP/6-31 + G(d,p), (v) B3LYP/6-311 + G(2d,p), and (vi) MP2/6-311 + G(2d,p). The output from each level may be used as the input for the next level for energy minimization [39].

2.4.7.2 Quantum topological molecular similarity indices

Quantum topological molecular similarity (QTMS) descriptors focus on bond critical points (BCPs), which occur when the gradient of the electron density, ρ vanishes ($\nabla\rho = 0$) at some point between two bonded nuclei. The electron density at a BCP, denoted by ρ_b, can be related to bond order via an exponential relationship. Seven types of descriptors (ρ, $\nabla^2\rho$, λ, ε, K, G, and equilibrium bond lengths) can be calculated for each of the bonds connecting the adjacent common atoms [40,41]. For the molecules sharing a common skeleton, properties are calculated at each BCP formed by the common atoms. At a BCP, the Hessian of ρ has two negative eigenvalues ($\lambda_1 < \lambda_2 < 0$) and one positive value ($\lambda_3 > 0$). The eigenvalues express local curvature of ρ in a point: negative eigenvalues are curvatures perpendicular to the bond, while the positive eigenvalue measures the curvature along the bond [42,43]. If the positive eigenvalue λ_3 dominates, electron density is accumulated along the bond path toward the nuclei. The descriptor λ_3 gives a measure the σ character of a bond, while the summation of values of $\lambda_1 + \lambda_2$ measure the degree of π character. The Laplacian, denoted by $\nabla^2\rho$, refers to the sum of eigenvalues and is a measure of how much ρ is concentrated ($\nabla^2\rho < 0$) or depleted ($\nabla^2\rho > 0$) in a point. Another descriptor in this series is the ellipticity of a bond, which also measures the degree of π character of a bond together with the susceptibility of the ring bonds to rupture and is defined as, $\varepsilon = \lambda_1/\lambda_2 - 1$. In the QTMS bond descriptor vector, there are two more components: the kinetic energy density $K(r)$ and a more classical kinetic energy $G(r)$. In addition, the equilibrium bond length (R_e) has also been used as one of the descriptors, along with other QTMS descriptors. It has been reported that the BCP descriptors have been successful at translating the predicted electronic effects of orbital theories into observable consequences of variation in bond electron densities [44,45].

2.4.8 Spatial parameters

They comprise a series of descriptors calculated based on the spatial arrangement of the molecules and the surface occupied by the molecules [5].

2.4.8.1 RadofGyration

Radius of gyration (RadofGyration) is a measure of the size of an object, a surface, or an ensemble of points. It is calculated as the root mean square distance of the objects' parts from either its center of gravity or an axis [5]. This can be calculated as per Eq. (2.17):

$$\text{RadofGyration} = \sqrt{\left[\sum \frac{(x_i^2 + y_i^2 + z_i^2)}{N}\right]} \tag{2.17}$$

where N is the number of atoms and x, y, z are the atomic coordinates relative to the center of mass.

2.4.8.2 Jurs descriptors

These descriptors combine shape and electronic information to characterize molecules. These descriptors are calculated by mapping atomic partial charges on solvent-accessible surface areas of individual atoms [46]. The various descriptors included in this category are listed in Table 2.8.

Table 2.8 List of Jurs descriptors used in QSAR model development

Category of descriptors	Definition/Remarks
Partial negative surface area (PNSA1)	Sum of the solvent-accessible surface areas (SASAs) of all negatively charged atoms.
Partial positive surface area (PPSA1)	Sum of the SASAs of all positively charged atoms.
Total charge-weighted negative surface area (PNSA2)	Partial negative SASA multiplied by the total negative charge.
Total charge-weighted positive surface area (PPSA2)	Partial positive SASA multiplied by the total positive charge.
Atomic charge-weighted negative surface area (PNSA3)	Sum of the products of atomic SASAs and partial charges over all negatively charged atoms.
Atomic charge-weighted positive surface area (PPSA3)	Sum of the products of atomic SASAs and partial charges over all positively charged atoms.
Difference in charged partial surface area (DPSA1)	Partial positive SASA minus the partial negative SASA.
Difference in total charge-weighted surface area (DPSA2)	Total charge-weighted positive SASA minus the total charge-weighted negative SASA.
Difference in atomic charge-weighted surface area (DPSA3)	Atomic charge weighted positive SASA minus the atomic charge weighted negative SASA.
Fractional charged partial negative surface areas (FNSA1, FNSA2, FNSA3)	They are obtained by multiplication of PNSA1, PNSA2, and PNSA3 descriptors with SASA and then dividing the fraction by 1,000, respectively.

(Continued)

Table 2.8 (Continued)

Category of descriptors	Definition/Remarks
Fractional charged partial positive surface areas (FPSA1, FPSA2, FPSA3)	They are obtained by multiplication of PPSA1, PPSA2, and PPSA3 descriptors with SASA and then dividing the fraction by 1,000, respectively.
Surface-weighted charged partial negative surface areas (WNSA1, WNSA2, WNSA3)	They are obtained by multiplication of PNSA1, PNSA2, and PNSA3 descriptors with SASA and then dividing the fraction by 1,000, respectively.
Surface-weighted charged partial positive surface areas (WPSA1, WPSA2, WPSA3)	They are obtained by multiplication of PPSA1, PPSA2, and PPSA3 descriptors with SASA and then dividing the fraction by 1,000, respectively.
Relative negative charge (RNCG)	Partial charge of the most negative atom divided by the total negative charge.
Relative positive charge (RPCG)	Partial charge of the most positive atom divided by the total positive charge.
Relative negative charge surface area (RNCS)	SASA of the most negative atom divided by the relative negative charge.
Relative positive charge surface area (RPCS)	SASA of the most positive atom divided by the relative positive charge.
Total hydrophobic surface area (TASA)	Sum of SASAs of atoms with absolute value of partial charges less than 0.2.
Total polar surface area (TPSA)	Sum of SASAs of atoms with absolute value of partial charges greater than or equal to 0.2
Relative hydrophobic surface area (RASA)	TASA divided by the total molecular SASA.
Relative polar surface area (RPSA)	TPSA divided by the total molecular SASA.

2.4.8.3 Shadow indices

These indices help to characterize the shape of the molecules. These are calculated by projecting the molecular surface on three mutually perpendicular planes; that is, *XY*, *YZ*, and *XZ*. These descriptors depend not only on conformation, but also on the orientation of molecules. Molecules are rotated to align principal moments of inertia with *X*-, *Y*-, and *Z*-axes [47]. The various descriptors included in this category are listed in Table 2.9. Projections and embedding rectangles of query molecule in the three principal planes for shadow indices are presented in Figure 2.6.

2.4.8.4 Molecular surface area

Molecular surface area is a 3D descriptor that describes the van der Waals area of a molecule. It measures the extent to which a molecule exposes itself to the external environment. It is related to binding, transport, and solubility [5].

Table 2.9 List of shadow descriptors used in QSAR model development

Mode of calculation	Descriptors	Description
Areas of molecular shadows	Shadow-*XY*	Area of the molecular shadow in the *XY* plane (*Sxy*)
	Shadow-*XZ*	Area of the molecular shadow in the *XZ* plane (*Sxz*)
	Shadow-*YZ*	Area of the molecular shadow in the *YZ* plane (*Syz*)
Fractional areas of molecular shadows	Shadow-*XY*fr	Fraction of the area of molecular shadow in the *XY* plane over the area of enclosing rectangle (*Sxy,f*)
	Shadow-*XZ*fr	Fraction of the area of molecular shadow in the *XZ* plane over the area of enclosing rectangle (*Sxz,f*)
	Shadow-*YZ*fr	Fraction of the area of molecular shadow in the *YZ* plane over the area of enclosing rectangle (*Syz,f*)
Extents of molecular shadows	Shadow-*X*length	Length of molecule in the *X* dimension (*Lx*)
	Shadow-*Y*length	Length of molecule in the *Y* dimension (*Ly*)
	Shadow-*Y*length	Length of molecule in the *Z* dimension (*Lz*)
	Shadow-nu	Ratio of largest to smallest dimension

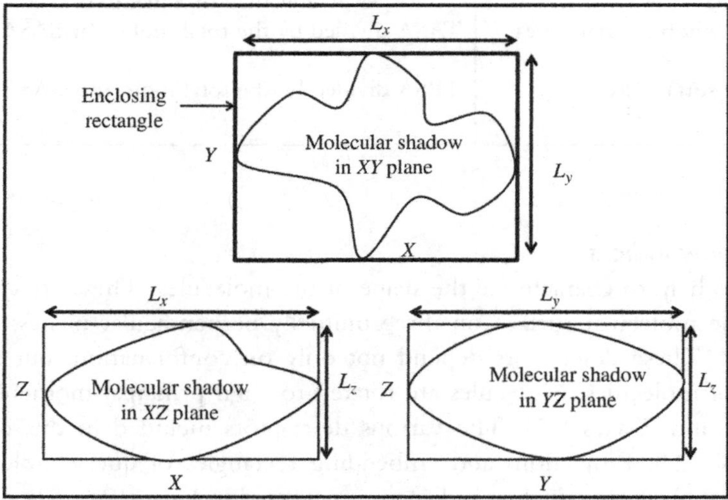

Figure 2.6 Projections and embedding rectangles of a query molecule in the three principal planes for shadow indices.

2.4.8.5 Density

The 3D descriptor known as density is the ratio of molecular weight to molecular volume. This descriptor represents the type of atoms and how tightly they are packed in a molecule. It is related to transport and melt behavior [5].

2.4.8.6 Principal moment of inertia

The moments of inertia are calculated for a series of straight lines through the center of mass. These are associated with the principal axes of the ellipsoid [48]. If all three moments are equal, the molecule is considered to be a symmetrical top.

2.4.8.7 Molecular volume

This 3D descriptor known as molecular volume is the volume inside the contact surface [5]. It is related to binding and transport.

2.4.9 Information indices

In this approach, molecules are viewed as structures that can be partitioned into subsets of elements that are in some sense equivalent. The concept of equivalence depends on the particular descriptor. For a partition of a set of N elements into k subsets, each consisting of N_k elements [49–51]:

$$\text{Equivalence class} = 1, 2, \ldots, k$$

The number of elements in each $N_1\ N_2 \ldots N_k$ and N is mathematically represented as

$$N = N_1 + N_2 + N_3 + \cdots + N_k \tag{2.18}$$

For a given partition P, the following relationship is obtained:

$$P = N(N_1, N_2, N_3, \ldots, N_k) \tag{2.19}$$

A probability distribution can be associated with the partition and may be represented as

$$p_i = \frac{N_i}{N_V} \tag{2.20}$$

where p_i is the probability for a randomly chosen element to belong to class i. This degree of uncertainty also can be expressed by the entropy as follows:

$$H_i = -\text{lb}\ p_i \tag{2.21}$$

where H_i is the entropy and lb is the base-2 logarithm. Then the mean entropy of such a probability distribution can be defined as

$$H = -\sum_{i=1}^{k} p_i\ \text{lb}\ p_i \tag{2.22}$$

This parameter can be considered as a measure of the mean quantity of information contained in each structure element (in bits per element) [49].

2.4.9.1 Information of atomic composition index

Here, equivalence classes of the atoms in a molecule are formed by considering their atomic numbers. Two types of information of atomic composition (IAC) descriptors are IAC-mean and IAC-total. The partition of atoms then yields the descriptor IAC-mean as the mean quantity of information H (as defined previously). The descriptor IAC-total is defined as

$$\text{IAC-total} = N \times \text{IAC-mean} \tag{2.23}$$

where N is the number of atoms in the molecule.

2.4.9.2 Information indices based on the A-matrix

The concept is based on partitioning elements of the A-matrix according to two basic modes:

1. The *equality* mode: The matrix elements are considered as equivalent if their values are equal.
2. The *magnitude* mode: This mode assumes that each matrix element is an equivalence class unto itself whose cardinality (number of elements) is equal to the magnitude of the matrix element.

The two information indices in this category are:

1. *Total vertex adjacency/equality (V_ADJ_equ)*: Here, the A-matrix (N-by-N) consists of zeros and 1s, so the partitioning consists of two classes. If C_k represents the number of matrix elements for each class k in the A-matrix, the vertex adjacency/equality will be defined as

$$V\_ADJ\_equ = -N^2 \sum_k \frac{C_k}{N^2} \operatorname{lb} \frac{C_k}{N^2} \tag{2.24}$$

2. *Total vertex adjacency/magnitude (V_ADJ_mag)*: The magnitude descriptor uses the actual A-matrix values a_{ij}, unlike the equality values used for the populations of each class in the A-matrix. Here, the nonzero elements are not included in the expression of *V_ADJ_mag*:

$$V\_ADJ\_mag = -N^2 \sum_{a_{ij} \neq o} \frac{a_{ij}}{n^2} \operatorname{lb} \frac{a_{ij}}{N^2} \tag{2.25}$$

2.4.9.3 Information indices based on the D-matrix

The information indices based on the D-matrix are similar descriptors like the vertex adjacency indices, but the difference is that the distance matrix is used instead of the adjacency matrix. Two types of indices based on this matrix are:

1. Vertex distance/equality (V_DIST_equ)
2. Vertex distance/magnitude (V_DIST_mag)

2.4.9.4 Information indices based on the E-matrix and the ED-matrix

The information indices based on the *E*-matrix and *ED*-matrix are descriptors based on the edge adjacency and the edge distance matrices. The indices based on these matrices are:

1. Edge adjacency/equality (E_ADJ_equ)
2. Edge adjacency/magnitude (E_ADJ_mag)
3. Edge distance/equality (E_DIST_equ)
4. Edge distance/magnitude (E_DIST_mag)

2.4.9.5 Multigraph information content indices (IC, BIC, CIC, SIC)

For multigraph information content, an *unordered* sequence of *ordered* pairs is assigned to each vertex *v*, termed as a *coordinate*, as follows:

$$\{(m_1, n_1), (m_2, n_2), \ldots, (m_k, n_k)\}$$

where *k* is the valence of the vertex [with one ordered pair (m_j, n_j) per each neighboring vertex, v_j], and for every $j = 1, \ldots, k$, n_j is the valence of v_j and the bond between *v* and v_j is of order m_j.

The coordinates are assigned to vertices, and the partition of vertices is constructed in the usual way, in which two vertices are considered equivalent if their coordinates are the same as unordered *k*-tuples; that is, the repetitions of ordered pairs are not ignored, as they would be if we treated the *k*-tuples purely as sets.

After the partition, the index is termed as information content (IC). The different classes of IC are as follows [49–51]:

1. Bonding information content (BIC): This index corresponds to the number of bonds counting bond orders, defined as

$$\text{BIC} = \text{IC}/\text{lb} \tag{2.26}$$

2. Structural information content (SIC): This index refers to the number of vertices, defined as

$$\text{SIC} = \text{IC}/\text{lb} \tag{2.27}$$

3. Complementary information content (CIC): This index measures the deviation of IC from its maximum possible value, corresponding to a partition into classes containing one element each. The definitions of IC_{max} and CIC are derived as follows:

$$\text{IC}_{\text{max}} = -N_X(1/N) \times \text{lb}(1/N) = \text{lb}(N) \tag{2.28}$$

$$\text{CIC} = \text{lb}(N) - IC \tag{2.29}$$

2.4.10 Molecular shape analysis descriptors

Different types of molecular shape analysis (MSA) descriptors [5] are summarized in Table 2.10.

Table 2.10 MSA descriptors

Parameter	Explanation
Difference volume (DIFFV)	It is the difference between the volume of the individual molecule and the volume of the shape reference compound.
Common overlap steric volume (COSV)	This is the common volume between each individual molecule and the reference molecule. It is the measurement of similarity of steric shape between analogs to reference compound.
Common overlap volume ratio (Fo)	It is obtained from the ratio of common overlap steric volume to the volume of the individual molecule.
Noncommon overlap steric volume (NCOSV)	It is the volume of the individual molecule and the common overlap steric volume.
Root mean square to shape reference (ShapeRMS)	This is the root mean square deviation between the individual molecule and the shape reference compound.

2.4.11 Molecular field analysis parameters

The molecular field analysis (MFA) [52] formalism calculates probe interaction energies on a rectangular grid around a bundle of active molecules. The surface is generated from a *shape field*. The atomic coordinates of the contributing models are used to compute field values on each point of a 3D-grid. MFA evaluates the energy between a probe (H^+ and CH_3) and a molecular model at a series of points defined by a rectangular grid. The fields of molecules are represented using grids in MFA, and each energy value associated with an MFA grid point can serve as input for the calculation of a QSAR.

2.4.12 Receptor surface analysis parameters

The energies of interaction between the receptor surface model and each molecular model can be used as descriptors for generating QSARs [52]. The surface points that organize as triangle meshes in the construction of the receptor surface analysis (RSA) store these properties as associated scalar values. Receptor surface models provide compact, quantitative descriptors that capture 3D information of interaction energies in terms of steric and electrostatic fields at each surface point.

QSAR has become more attractive for researchers with the development of new and advanced software tools, which have allowed them to determine and understand how molecular structure is responsible for a compound's activity/property/toxicity. Table 2.11 gives a representative list of various software tools used to generate descriptors from molecular structures.

Table 2.11 List of software tools for computation of molecular descriptors

Software	Web link
4D FAP	http://www.ra.cs.uni-tuebingen.de/software/4DFAP/welcome_e.html
ADAPT	http://research.chem.psu.edu/pcjgroup/adapt.html
ADMET Predictor	http://www.simulations-plus.com/Products.aspx?grpID=1&cID=11&pID=13
ADRIANA.Code	http://www.molecular-networks.com/products/adrianacode
Alchemy 2000	http://www.chemistry-software.com/modelling/10235.htm
ALMOND	http://www.moldiscovery.com/soft_almond.php
BlueDesc	http://www.ra.cs.uni-tuebingen.de/software/bluedesc/welcome_e.html
CAChe	http://www.cache.fujitsu.com/cache/index.shtml
Cerius^2	http://accelrys.com/
ChemEnlightenTM	http://www.tripos.com/sciTech/inSilicoDisc/media/LITCTR/CHEMENLI.PDF
CODESSA PRO	http://www.codessa-pro.com/index.htm
Discovery Studio	http://accelrys.com/
DRAGON	http://www.talete.mi.it/products/dragon_description.htm
GRID	http://www.moldiscovery.com/soft_grid.php
JChem	http://www.chemaxon.com/jchem/intro/index.html
JOELib	http://www.ra.cs.uni-tuebingen.de/software/joelib/index.html
ISIDA	http://infochim.u-strasbg.fr/spip.php?rubrique53
MOE	http://www.chemcomp.com/software.htm
MOLCONN-Z	http://www.edusoft-lc.com/molconn/
MOLGEN-QSPR	http://www.molgen.de/?src=documents/molgenqspr.html
OAK	http://www.ra.cs.uni-tuebingen.de/software/OAKernels/welcome_e.html
OASIS QSAR	http://toolbox.oasis-lmc.org/
OpenBabel	http://openbabel.org/
PaDEL-Descriptor	http://padel.nus.edu.sg/software/padeldescriptor/
Pentacle	http://www.moldiscovery.com/soft_pentacle.php
PowerMV	http://nisla05.niss.org/PowerMV/?q= PowerMV/
PreADMET	http://preadmet.bmdrc.org/index.php?option=com_content&view=frontpage&Itemid=1
QSARModel	http://www.molcode.com/
QuaSAR	http://www.chemcomp.com/feature/qsar.htm
RDKit	http://www.rdkit.org/
SciQSAR	http://www.scimatics.com/jsp/qsar/QSARIS.jsp
Sarchitect	http://www.strandls.com/sarchitect/index.html
SYBYL-X	http://tripos.com/index.php?family=modules,SimplePage&page=SYBYL-X
Tsar™	http://www.accelrys.com/products/tsar/tsar.html
Unscrambler X	http://www.camo.com/rt/Products/Unscrambler/unscrambler.html
V-Life MDS	http://www.vlifesciences.com/products/VLifeMDS/Product_VLifeMDS.php

2.5 OVERVIEW AND CONCLUSION

The selection of suitable descriptors from a large pool of diverse classes of descriptors plays a major role in the development of acceptable and robust predictive QSAR models. To some extent, this depends upon the end point to be modeled. The experience of the QSAR researcher also helps in choosing suitable descriptors. An important aspect is to choose the relevant descriptors considering the problem at hand. Again, one must consider, before developing QSAR models, how the descriptors have been calculated and whether calculations can be reproduced. Lower-dimensional parameters like zero-dimensional (0D), 1D, or 2D are easily computable and are used alone or in combination with other higher-dimensional descriptors for successful model development. But due to the complexity of the endpoint and advancement of QSAR studies, as well as the requirements of mechanistic interpretation of the activity/property/toxicity of chemicals, the use of higher-dimensional parameters is increasing every day.

REFERENCES

[1] Katritzky AR, Fara DC, Petrukhin RO, Tatham DB, Maran U, Lomaka A, et al. The present utility and future potential for medicinal chemistry of QSAR/QSPR with whole molecule descriptors. Curr Top Med Chem 2002;2:1333–56.

[2] Guha R, Willighagen EA. Survey of quantitative descriptions of molecular structure. Curr Top Med Chem 2012;12(18):1946–56.

[3] van de Waterbeemd H, Carter RE, Grassy G, Kubinyi H, Martin YC, Tute MS, et al. Glossary of terms used in computational drug design (IUPAC recommendations 1997). Ann Rep Med Chem 1998;33:397–409.

[4] Randic M. On characterization of chemical structure. J Chem Inf Comput Sci 1997;37:672–87.

[5] Todeschini R, Consonni V. Handbook of molecular descriptors. Weinheim, Germany: Wiley-VCH; 2000.

[6] Kohavi R, John G. Wrappers for feature subset selection. Artif Intell 1997;97:273–324.

[7] Dehmer M, Varmuza K, Borgert S, Emmert-Streib F. On entropy-based molecular descriptors: statistical analysis of real and synthetic chemical structures. J Chem Inf Model 2009;49:1655–63.

[8] Willems T, Rycroft C, Kazi M, Meza J, Haranczyk M. Algorithms and tools for high-throughput geometry-based analysis of crystalline porous materials. Microporous Mesoporous Mater 2012;149 (1):134–41.

[9] Mackay A. Descriptors for complex inorganic structures. Croat Chem Acta 1984;57:725–36.

[10] Segall M, Champness E, Obrezanova O, Leeding C. Beyond profiling: using ADMET models to guide decisions. Chem Biodivers 2009;6(11):2144–51.

[11] Livingstone DJ. The characterization of chemical structures using molecular properties. A survey. J Chem Inf Comput Sci 2000;40:195–209.

[12] Taylor PJ. In: Hansch C, Sammes PG, Taylor JB, editors. Comprehensive medicinal chemistry. vol. 4. Quantitative drug design. The rational design, mechanistic study and therapeutic applications of chemical compounds. Oxford: Pergamon Press; 1991. pp. 241–94.

[13] Rekker R. In the hydrophobic fragmental constant. Amsterdam, the Netherlands: Elsevier; 1977.

[14] Hansch C, Leo A, Hoekman D. In exploring QSAR vol. 2: hydrophobic, electronic and steric constants. Washington, DC: ACS; 1995.

[15] Selassie CD, Mekapati SB, Verma RP. QSAR: then and now. Curr Top Med Chem 2002;2(12): 1357–79.

[16] Taft RW. In: Newman MS, editor. Steric effects in organic chemistry. New York, NY: John Wiley & Sons; 1956. p. 556.
[17] Hansch C, Leo A. Substituent constants for correlation analysis in chemistry and biology. New York, NY: Wiley; 1979.
[18] Charton M. Steric effects. IV. E1 and E2 eliminations. J Am Chem Soc 1975;97:6159–61.
[19] Verloop A. The STERIMOL approach to drug design. New York, NY: Marcel Dekker; 1987.
[20] García-Domenech R, Gálvez J, de Julián-Ortiz JV, Pogliani L. Some new trends in chemical graph theory. Chem Rev 2008;108:1127–69.
[21] Broto P, Moreau G, Vandycke C. Molecular structure: perception, autocorrelation descriptor and SAR studies. System of atomic contributions for the calculation of the *n*-octanol/water partition coefficients. Eur J Med Chem Chim Ther 1984;19:71–8.
[22] Wold S, Geladi P, Esbensen K, Ohman J. Multiway principal components and PLS analysis. J Chemom 1987;1:41–56.
[23] Estrada E, Ivanciuc O, Gutman I, Gutierreza A, Rodríguez L. Extended wiener indices. A new set of descriptors for quantitative structure–property studies. New J Chem 1998;22:819–23.
[24] Balaban AT. Chemical graphs. Theor Chim Acta 1979;53(4):355–75.
[25] Bonchev D, Balaban AT, Mekenyan O. Generalization of the graph center concept and derived topological centric indexes. J Chem Inf Comput Sci 1980;20:106–13.
[26] Wiener H. Structural determination of paraffin boiling points. J Am Chem Soc 1947;69:17–20.
[27] Randic M. Characterization of molecular branching. J Am Chem Soc 1975;97:6609–15.
[28] Balaban AT. Distance connectivity index. Chem Phys Lett 1982;89:399–404.
[29] Kier LB, Hall LH. Derivation and significance of valence molecular connectivity. J Pharm Sci 1981; 70(6):583–90.
[30] Hall LH, Kier LB. The electrotopological state: an atom index for QSAR. Quant Struct-Act Relat 1991;10:43–51.
[31] Hall LH, Kier LB. The E-state as the basis for molecular structure space definition and structure similarity. J Chem Inf Comput Sci 2000;30:784–91.
[32] Bonchev D, Trinajstić N. Overall molecular descriptors. 3. Overall Zagreb indices. SAR QSAR Environ Res 2001;12(1–2):213–35.
[33] Kier LB. In: Rouvray DH, editor. Computational chemical graph theory. New York, NY: Nova Science Publishers; 1990. pp. 152–74.
[34] Kier LB. A shape index from molecular graphs. Quant Struct-Act Relat 1985;4(3):109–16.
[35] Kier LB. Shape indexes of orders one and three from molecular graphs. Quant Struct-Act Relat 1986;5(1):1–7.
[36] Estrada E. Spectral moments of the edge adjacency matrix in molecular graphs. 1. Definition and applications to the prediction of physical properties of alkanes. J Chem Inf Comput Sci 1996;36:844–9.
[37] Roy K, Das RN. On Extended Topochemical Atom (ETA) indices for QSPR studies. In: Castro EA, Hagi AK, editors. Advanced methods and applications in chemoinformatics: research progress and new applications. Hershey, PA: IGI Global; 2011. pp. 380–411.
[38] Roy K, Ghosh G. Introduction of Extended Topochemical Atom (ETA) indices in the Valence Electron Mobile (VEM) environment as tools for QSAR/QSPR studies. Internet Electron J Mol Des 2003;2(9):599–620.
[39] Mitra I, Roy K, Saha A. QSAR of anti-lipid peroxidative activity of substituted benzodioxoles using chemometric tools. J Comput Chem 2009;30(16):2712–22.
[40] Roy K, Popelier PLA. Predictive QSPR modeling of acidic dissociation constant (pK_a) of phenols in different solvents. J Phys Org Chem 2009;22(3):186–96.
[41] Roy K, Popelier PLA. Exploring predictive QSAR models using Quantum Topological Molecular Similarity (QTMS) descriptors for toxicity of nitroaromatics to *Saccharomyces cerevisiae*. QSAR Comb Sci 2008;27(8):1006–12.
[42] Popelier PLA. Quantum molecular similarity. 1. BCP space. J Phys Chem A 1999;103(15): 2883–90.
[43] Bader RFW, Preston HJT. The kinetic energy of molecular charge distributions and molecular stability. Int J Quantum Chem 1969;3(3):327–47.

[44] Howard ST, Lamarche O. Description of covalent bond orders using the charge density topology. J Phys Org Chem 2003;16(2):133–41.
[45] Bader RFW, Slee TS, Cremer D, Kraka E. Description of conjugation and hyperconjugation in terms of electron distributions. J Am Chem Soc 1983;105(15):5061–8.
[46] Rohrbaugh RH, Jurs PC. Description of molecular shape applied in studies of structure/activity and structure/property relationships. Anal Chim Acta 1987;199:99–109.
[47] Stanton DT, Jurs PC. Development and use of charged partial surface area structural descriptors in computer-assisted quantitative structure–property relationship studies. Anal Chem 1990;62: 2323–9.
[48] Hill TL. Introduction to statistical thermodynamics. Reading, MA: Addison-Wesley; 1960.
[49] Bonchev D. In: Bawden DD, editor. Information theoretic indices for characterization of chemical structures. Chemometrics series, vol. 5. New York, NY: Research Studies Press Ltd.; 1983.
[50] Bonchev D, Mekenyan O, Trinajstic N. Isomer discrimination by topological information approach. J Comput Chem 1981;2(2):127–48.
[51] Katritzky AR, Gordeeva EV. Traditional topological indices vs. electronic, geometrical, and combined molecular descriptors in QSAR/QSPR research. J Chem Inf Comput Sci 1993;33(6):835–57.
[52] Hopfinger AJ, Tokarsi JS. In: Charifson PS, editor. Practical applications of computer-aided drug design. New York, NY: Marcel Dekker; 1997. pp. 105–64.

CHAPTER 3

Classical QSAR

Contents

3.1 INTRODUCTION

Quantitative structure–activity relationship (QSAR) is basically a lead optimization process seeking the most active compounds of a series, thus systematically minimizing the expense, delay, and manpower requirements. It tries to maximally utilize the information obtained from a relatively small series of data for which biological experimental data are available. In classical QSAR (which formed the foundation of QSAR science), model development is possible with the physicochemical properties of the training molecules in linear free-energy-related (LFER) models, or simply based on the sum of contributions of different substituents to the biological activity without requiring estimation of any physicochemical properties of the molecule or computation of any descriptors from the molecular structure (mathematical models). Several prerequisites are necessary for model development in classical QSAR [1]: (i) the compounds to be studied should be closely related congeners, thereby increasing the probability of having the same mechanism of action; (ii) the biological activity data to be used in modeling should be accurate and measured under uniform conditions; and (iii) the activity parameter must be intrinsically additive. For statistical reliability of

Understanding the Basics of QSAR for Applications in Pharmaceutical Sciences and Risk Assessment.
ISBN: 978-0-12-801505-6, DOI: http://dx.doi.org/10.1016/B978-0-12-801505-6.00003-X

such models, it is desirable to have a high ratio of the number of observations to the number of unknown terms in the linear equations.

3.2 THE FREE–WILSON MODEL

3.2.1 The concept

The Free–Wilson model (also known as the *de novo* model) is an additive mathematical model developed by Free and Wilson in 1964 [2]. This is based on the measurement of contributions of different substituents at specified positions of a congeneric series of compounds to the biological activity (e.g., EC_{50}, IC_{50}, or percent inhibition). Note that in the original Free–Wilson model, logarithmic transformation of the biological activity was not used. In their original paper [2], Free and Wilson used the biological activities of 10 tetracycline antibiotics and the analgesic activities of 29 indanamines for model development. Later, in 1965, Purcell [3] used this method for developing a model for butyrylcholineasterase inhibitory potency of alkyl-substituted 3-carbamoylpiperidines. Based on the developed model, the activity of 26 new congeners was predicted. In 1969, these predictions were found to be quantitative when one of these predicted derivatives was actually synthesized and experimentally tested, showing the experimental IC_{50} value to be in good agreement with the predicted value [4]. This was the first reported successful prediction of the biological activity of compounds with the Free–Wilson model.

3.2.2 The methodology

The development of the Free–Wilson model has some prerequisites [5] for characteristics of the input data:

1. The data set should be a congeneric series with substituents at specified positions.
2. There should be at least two positions of substitutions.
3. A particular substituent should occur at least twice at a specified position of the data set to avoid creating error from measurement of the response activity of a compound.

There are other prerequisites for the selection of the data set, some of which are valid for classical QSAR analysis (and many other types of analysis) as well:

1. In addition to understanding the basic type of data that is being used (type of experiment, unit, etc.), one should be aware of its quantitative nature, reproducibility, and reliability.
2. The biological activity of all the compounds under consideration has been measured under the same conditions.
3. The congeners used for model development should be very similar to ensure that they have the same mechanism of action for all compounds.

4. The substituent group additivity contributions to the selected response must be intrinsically additive.
5. It is desirable to have a high ratio of the number of observations to the number of unknowns in the linear equations, which allows a maximum degree of freedom and higher statistical significance.
6. If necessary, some compounds may be omitted from the data set due to outlier behavior (showing a large difference between the observed and calculated values), which may be because of the presence of groups with nonadditive contributions.
7. Precautions should be taken when selecting the data to avoid ill-conditioned matrices.
8. The biological activity data should be of the equiresponse type. If that is not the case, the data should be adjusted to obtain this effect.

The basic formalism of the model tries to develop a relationship like this:

$$\text{Biological activity(equiresponse)} = \sum G_i X_i + \mu \tag{3.1}$$

In Eq. (3.1), G_i is the contribution of a particular group i, while X_i takes a value of 1 when the group is present and 0 otherwise. The constant μ is the contribution of the parent moiety (i.e., the scaffold without considering the substituents). The basic assumption of the Free–Wilson model is that the contribution of a particular group in a specified position of the congeneric series of compounds is the same in all such compounds, without considering the cross-interaction terms. The Free–Wilson model also considers a hypothesis that the substituents at each position must obey a "symmetry equation" stating that the net contributions of all the substituents occurring at a particular position equal zero. This constraint helps to achieve unique solutions for the substituent constants.

3.2.3 Example of Free–Wilson model development

As an example, we cite here the work of Smithfield and Purcell [1] on using the Free–Wilson model for the hypoglycemic activity of substituted piperidinesulfamylsemicarbazides. This analysis had two purposes: ranking the group contributions to the biological activity and estimating the hypoglycemic activity of analogs that were not screened experimentally.

Note that Table 3.1 contains 24 piperidinesulfamylsemicarbazides, out of which 12 compounds (shown by the shaded rows) have no experimental hypoglycemic activity values. Thus, these 12 compounds cannot be used for model development, as experimental activity values are used as input (in addition to the structural features in the form of descriptors) for QSAR model development. Again, among the compounds with experimental activity values, compounds **8** and **24** contain substituents that occur only once in the reduced data set (as indicated by the bold faces). Thus, these

Table 3.1 Hypoglycemic activity (maximum percent fall in blood glucose at a dose level of 100 mg/kg) of substituted sulfamyl semicarbazides

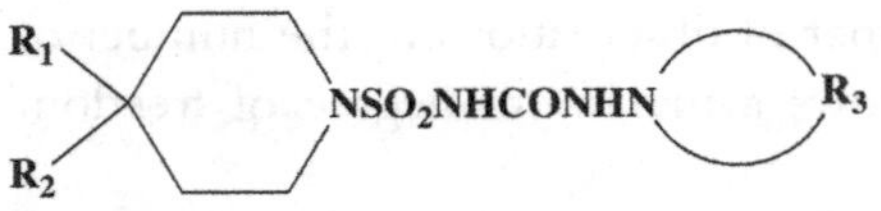

Sl. No.	R¹	R²	R³	Observed activity	Calculated activity[a]
1	H	H	$(CH_2)_5$	14.8 ± 7.0	14.9
2	H	H	$(CH_2)_6$	11.1 ± 1.9	14.0
3	H	CH_3	$(CH_2)_5$	26.1 ± 2.6	27.3
4	H	CH_3	$(CH_2)_6$	33.9 ± 1.5	26.4
5	H	C_2H_5	$(CH_2)_5$	N/A	27.3
6	H	C_2H_5	$(CH_2)_6$	N/A	26.3
7	H	OCH_3	$(CH_2)_5$	N/A	N/A
8	**H**	**OCH_3**	**$(CH_2)_6$**	**24.8 ± 3.1**	N/A
9	CH_3	CH_3	$(CH_2)_5$	39.1 ± 2.8	40.0
10	CH_3	CH_3	$(CH_2)_6$	34.9 ± 3.3	38.8
11	CH_3	C_2H_5	$(CH_2)_5$	N/A	39.6
12	CH_3	C_2H_5	$(CH_2)_6$	42.0 ± 3.3	38.7
13	CH_3	OCH_3	$(CH_2)_5$	N/A	N/A
14	CH_3	OCH_3	$(CH_2)_6$	N/A	N/A
15	C_2H_5	C_2H_5	$(CH_2)_5$	N/A	40.0
16	C_2H_5	C_2H_5	$(CH_2)_6$	34.4 ± 2.8	36.5
17	C_2H_5	OCH_3	$(CH_2)_5$	N/A	N/A
18	C_2H_5	OCH_3	$(CH_2)_6$	N/A	N/A
19	OCH_3	OCH_3	$(CH_2)_5$	N/A	N/A
20	OCH_3	OCH_3	$(CH_2)_6$	N/A	N/A
21	$(CH_2)_2$	$(CH_2)_2$	$(CH_2)_5$	35.6 ± 2.4	33.6
22	$(CH_2)_2$	$(CH_2)_2$	$(CH_2)_6$	30.8 ± 3.7	32.7
23	$(CH_2)_{2.5}$	$(CH_2)_{2.5}$	$(CH_2)_5$	N/A	N/A
24	**$(CH_2)_{2.5}$**	**$(CH_2)_{2.5}$**	**$(CH_2)_6$**	**25.0 ± 3.7**	N/A

[a]Based on contribution values in Table 3.3.
The shaded rows represent compounds without experimental activity values.
The bold rows represent compounds with experimental activity and a unique substituent that was not present in other compounds with experimental activity values.

compounds need to be removed from the analysis; otherwise, they would lead to perfect quantitative fits for contributions of such groups, yielding misleading statistical tests. This means that we can use 10 compounds only for model development. Although the number of compounds considered here is very limited, this example may be used for learning purposes. Based on Eq. (3.1), we can write the following 10 equations for compounds 1, 2, 3, 4, 9, 10, 12, 16, 21, and 22, respectively:

$$[H]R^1 + [H]R^2 + [(CH_2)_5]R^3 + \mu = 14.8 \quad (3.2)$$

$$[H]R^1 + [H]R^2 + [(CH_2)_6]R^3 + \mu = 11.1 \quad (3.3)$$

$$[H]R^1 + [CH_3]R^2 + [(CH_2)_5]R^3 + \mu = 26.1 \quad (3.4)$$

$$[H]R^1 + [CH_3]R^2 + [(CH_2)_6]R^3 + \mu = 33.9 \quad (3.5)$$

$$[CH_3]R^1 + [CH_3]R^2 + [(CH_2)_5]R^3 + \mu = 39.1 \quad (3.6)$$

$$[CH_3]R^1 + [CH_3]R^2 + [(CH_2)_6]R^3 + \mu = 34.9 \quad (3.7)$$

$$[CH_3]R^1 + [C_2H_5]R^2 + [(CH_2)_5]R^3 + \mu = 42.0 \quad (3.8)$$

$$[C_2H_5]R^1 + [C_2H_5]R^2 + [(CH_2)_6]R^3 + \mu = 34.4 \quad (3.9)$$

$$[(CH_2)_2]R^1 + [(CH_2)_2]R^2 + [(CH_2)_5]R^3 + \mu = 35.6 \quad (3.10)$$

$$[(CH_2)_2]R^1 + [(CH_2)_2]R^2 + [(CH_2)_6]R^3 + \mu = 30.8 \quad (3.11)$$

In these equations, $[H]R^1$ indicates contribution of the H atom at the R^1 position, $[CH_3]R^1$ indicates the contribution of the CH_3 group at the R^1 position, etc. Note that in this example, the biological activity is not in the log scale, although in modern QSAR, logarithmic transformation of biological activity is essential. From Eqs. (3.2)–(3.11), we seek to derive the contributions of different substituents (like H, CH_3, and C_2H_5) at different positions like R^1, R^2, and R^3. Hence, the unknown quantities here are $[H]R^1$, $[H]R^2$, $[CH_3]R^1$, etc. One can see that in these 10 equations, there are 10 unknowns (without considering μ, which is a constant that can be obtained from the values of other unknowns determined from the regression analysis), leading to an algebraic solution, which is undesirable. The quality of the model is heavily dependent on the quality of biological activity data, which would have some inherent error values due to experimental errors or biological variation. Thus, it is always desirable to use a larger number of samples to avoid the impact of erroneous data from a particular sample and to obtain an average picture for all the molecules. This is why the quality of a QSAR model is always judged in terms of statistical tests. In the present preliminary example, we have 10 data points with 10 unknowns, which is not suitable for a statistical model development.

If we carefully observe the data set, R^1 and R^2 substituent positions may be considered equivalent. This means that a compound containing H at R^1 and CH_3 at R^2 will be no different from the congener with CH_3 at R^1 and H at R^2, provided that the R^3 position is substituted for a particular group in both cases. Thus, the variable $[H]R^1$ is the same as $[H]R^2$, etc. Instead of considering R^1 and R^2 positions separately, we can define a new position as R^1, R^2, thus reducing the number of unknowns by 4.

We can rewrite Eqs. (3.2)–(3.11) as follows:

$$2[H]R^1,R^2 + [(CH_2)_5]R^3 + \mu = 14.8 \tag{3.12}$$

$$2[H]R^1,R^2 + [(CH_2)_6]R^3 + \mu = 11.1 \tag{3.13}$$

$$[H]R^1,R^2 + [CH_3]R^1,R^2 + [(CH_2)_5]R^3 + \mu = 26.1 \tag{3.14}$$

$$[H]R^1,R^2 + [CH_3]R^1,R^2 + [(CH_2)_6]R^3 + \mu = 33.9 \tag{3.15}$$

$$2[CH_3]R^1,R^2 + [(CH_2)_5]R^3 + \mu = 39.1 \tag{3.16}$$

$$2[CH_3]R^1,R^2 + [(CH_2)_6]R^3 + \mu = 34.9 \tag{3.17}$$

$$[CH_3]R^1,R^2 + [C_2H_5]R^1,R^2 + [(CH_2)_5]R^3 + \mu = 42.0 \tag{3.18}$$

$$2[C_2H_5]R^1,R^2 + [(CH_2)_6]R^3 + \mu = 34.4 \tag{3.19}$$

$$2[(CH_2)_2]R^1,R^2 + [(CH_2)_5]R^3 + \mu = 35.6 \tag{3.20}$$

$$2[(CH_2)_2]R^1,R^2 + [(CH_2)_6]R^3 + \mu = 30.8 \tag{3.21}$$

Therefore, we now have 10 equations with 6 unknowns, leading to a better situation. The number of unknowns may further be reduced to 4 by the use of the following two symmetry equations:

$$6[H]R^1,R^2 + 7[CH_3]R^1,R^2 + 3[C_2H_5]R^1,R^2 + 4[(CH_2)_2]R^1,R^2 = 0 \tag{3.22}$$

$$4[(CH_2)_5]R^3 + 6[(CH_2)_6]R^3 = 0 \tag{3.23}$$

Equations (3.22) and (3.23) may be used to eliminate two variables. Theoretically, any one of the variables present in a particular equation may be eliminated, but practically it would be wise to eliminate the variable with lowest coefficients, thus requiring fewer changes in the elimination process. Based on this concept, $[C_2H_5]R^1, R^2$ was selected for elimination in Eq. (3.22) and $[(CH_2)_5]R^3$ in Eq. (3.23):

$$[C_2H_5]R^1, R^2 = -2[H]R^1, R^2 - 2.33[CH_3]R^1, R^2 - 1.33[(CH_2)_2]R^1, R^2 \quad (3.24)$$

$$[(CH_2)_5]R^3 = -1.5[(CH_2)_6]R^3 \quad (3.25)$$

These values of the unknowns to be eliminated may be incorporated into Eqs. (3.12)–(3.21), thus reducing the number of unknowns to 4. A matrix notation of the problem can be seen in Table 3.2. Note that the matrix entries are just the coefficient values of individual unknowns in Eqs. (3.12)–(3.21) after elimination of the two unknowns $[C_2H_5]R^1$, R^2 and $[(CH_2)_5]R^3$.

A multiple linear regression analysis may be applied on the matrix given in Table 3.2 (see Chapter 6). The regression results directly give the values of $[H]R^1$, R^2, $[CH_3]R^1, R^2$, $[(CH_2)]R^1, R^2$, and $[(CH_2)_6]R^3$, while the values of $[(C_2H_5)]R^1$, R^2 and $[(CH_2)_6]R^3$ can be obtained from Eqs. (3.24) and (3.25). The value of μ can be obtained from any of Eqs. (3.2)–(3.11). The calculated contributions of the substituent groups and the parent moiety are given in Table 3.3.

Table 3.3 shows that a hydrogen substitution at the R^1 and R^2 positions (unsubstituted positions) decreases the activity, while the CH_3 and C_2H_5 groups have a more beneficial role than tetramethylene substituents in the same positions. Again, at the R^3 position, $(CH_2)_5$ has a positive contribution (preferred), while $(CH_2)_6$ at the same

Table 3.2 A matrix representation of the data set in Table 3.1

Sl. No.	Substituents at R^1, R^2			Substituent at R^3	Biological activity
	H	CH_3	$(CH_2)_2$	$(CH_2)_6$	
1	2	0	0	−1.5	14.8
2	2	0	0	1	11.1
3	1	1	0	−1.5	26.1
4	1	1	0	1	33.9
9	0	2	0	−1.5	39.1
10	0	2	0	1	34.9
12	−2	−1.33	−1.33	1	42
16	−4	−4.33	−2.66	1	34.4
21	0	0	2	−1.5	35.6
22	0	0	2	1	30.8

Table 3.3 Calculated group contribution values from the Free–Wilson analysis

Substituent position	Group	Calculated value of contribution
R^1, R^2	CH_3	4.36
R^1, R^2	C_2H_5	4.26
R^1, R^2	$(CH_2)_2$	1.29
R^1, R^2	H	−8.07
R^3	$(CH_2)_5$	0.56
R^3	$(CH_2)_6$	−0.37
μ	Parent structure	30.5

position is not preferred. Based on these group contributions, one can calculate the hypoglycemic activities of compounds appearing in Table 3.1. Note that there is good agreement between the observed and calculated activity values. The activity can also be predicted for the compounds without any experimental hypoglycemic activity values (5, 6, 11, and 15), but not for compounds 7, 13, 14, or 17–20 containing a substituent (OCH_3 at R^1 or R^2) not present in the modeling set; thus, the corresponding group contribution cannot be determined. The activity of compound 5 can be calculated as

$$\text{Biological activity (compound 5)} = [\text{H}]R^1 + [C_2H_5]R^2 + [(CH_2)_6]R^3 + \mu \quad (3.26)$$

Again, the activity of compound 15 can be calculated as

$$\text{Biological activity (compound 15)} = [C_2H_5]R^1 + [C_2H_5]R^2 + [(CH_2)_5]R^3 + \mu \quad (3.27)$$

Prediction of the activity of untested molecules is one of the uses of QSAR models. However, note that the Free–Wilson model cannot be used to predict compounds with groups not appearing in the training molecules (compounds 8 and 24 in the present example). This is one of the shortcomings of the Free–Wilson model. However, its advantage is that it does not require the computation of any descriptors. The presence or absence of a group at a particular position (an indicator variable with a 1 or 0 value, respectively) may be used as a descriptor for model development. It may give a quick idea about the contributions of the groups appearing as the data set to the response activity.

3.3 THE FUJITA–BAN MODEL

3.3.1 The concept

The Fujita–Ban model is basically a modification [6] of the original Free–Wilson model. It has two differences from the Free–Wilson model. First, in the Free–Wilson model, [H] is considered as a substituent to the parent moiety, and its contribution to the activity must be considered along with the application of symmetry equations. In the Fujita–Ban method, the activity contribution of a substituent relative to that of [H] at each position is considered, obviating the requirement of symmetry equations and simplifying calculations. Second, in the Free–Wilson model, the constant term signifies the contribution of the parent moiety, while in the Fujita–Ban model, it is the value of the unsubstituted compound itself. Third, the log of activity is considered as the response in the Fujita–Ban model, as it is an additive free energy related parameter (*vide infra*).

3.3.2 The methodology

The Fujita–Ban model is based on the following expression:

$$\log A = \sum G_i X_i + \log A_0 \tag{3.28}$$

In Eq. (3.28), $\log A$ is the activity of the substituted compound, while $\log A_0$ is the activity of the unsubstituted compound. G_i is the contribution of the ith substituent to the activity relative to [H], and X_i is a binary variable having a value of 1 or 0 according to the presence or absence of the ith substituent.

As an example, we will cite here the exercise reported by Fujita and Ban in their original paper [6]. They considered the substrate action of phenylethylamine derivatives on dopamine-β-hydroxylase.

Based on the presence and absence of substitutions in the phenylethylamine structure, the X values (0 or 1) for different groups may be entered in the QSAR table as descriptors (as given in Table 3.4), and then this may be subjected to the development of a multiple linear regression equation patterned after the generalized expression shown in Eq. (3.28). The values of the regression coefficients give an indication about the contribution of a particular group to the activity relative to [H] (Table 3.5). Thus, a *p*-hydroxy substituent increases activity of phenylethylamine while a *p*-methoxy substituent decreases the activity. In fact, all other groups present in the data set (*m*-OH, *m*-OCH_3, α-CH_3, *N*-CH_3, and *m*′-OCH_3) reduce the activity of phenylethylamine, as suggested by Eq. (3.28) (Table 3.5). Note that any QSAR equation is a statistical model, and its acceptability is always checked with different statistical measures. All QSAR equations are not statistically acceptable and hence not reliable. Thus, a series of tests are required before one can believe the interpretations of a QSAR model (as detailed in Chapters 6 and 7). Not only that, each term (i.e., the contribution of a particular group in the case of the Fujita–Ban model) in the QSAR equation can be checked for

Table 3.4 The substrate action (log *A*) of phenylethylamine derivatives on dopamine-β-hydroxylase

H_2N

Sl. No.	Compound	Occurrence of groups								log *A*	
		X(*p*-OH)	X(*p*-OCH_3)	X(*m*-OH)	X(*m*-OCH_3)	X(α-CH_3)	X(*N*-CH_3)	X(*m'*-OCH_3)	X[a](OH:OCH_3)	Obs.	Calc.[a]
1	Phenylethylamine	0	0	0	0	0	0	0	0	1.80	1.87
2	4-hydroxy	1	0	0	0	0	0	0	0	2.00	2.02
3	3-hydroxy	0	0	1	0	0	0	0	0	1.89	1.93
4	4-methoxy	0	1	0	0	0	0	0	0	0.48	0.54
5	4-hydroxy, *N*-methyl	1	0	0	0	0	1	0	0	1.40	1.37
6	4-hydroxy-α-methyl	1	0	0	0	1	0	0	0	1.81	1.68
7	3-hydroxy-α-methyl	0	0	1	0	1	0	0	0	1.70	1.59
8	3,4-dihydroxy	1	0	1	0	0	0	0	0	1.97	2.08
9	4-hydroxy-3-methoxy	1	0	0	1	0	0	0	1	1.85	1.52
10	3-hydroxy-4-methoxy	0	1	1	0	0	0	0	1	0.30	0.27
11	3,4-dimethoxy	0	1	0	1	0	0	0	0	0.30	0.36
12	3,4-dihydroxy-*N*-methyl	1	0	1	0	0	1	0	0	1.40	1.43
13	3,4-dihydroxy-α-methyl	1	0	1	0	1	0	0	0	1.76	1.73
14	4-hydroxy-3-methoxy-α-methyl	1	0	0	1	1	0	0	1	0.90	1.17
15	4-hydroxy-3,5-dimethoxy	1	0	0	1	0	0	1	1	1.45	1.54
16	3,4,5-trimethoxy	0	1	0	1	0	0	1	0	0.48	0.39

[a]Calculated from Eq. (3.30).

statistical significance, and if it is found unacceptable at a particular probability level, may be discarded. Similarly, a new term may be added to the existing QSAR equation if the incoming term is found statistically significant and capable of increasing the quality of the previous equation. With this objective, Fujita and

Table 3.5 Computed group contributions from the Fujita–Ban analysis

Group	Contribution to the Activity	
	Equation (3.28)	**Equation (3.30)**
p-OH	0.054	0.147
p-OCH_3	−1.345	−1.334
m-OH	−0.012	0.054
m-OCH_3	−0.376	−0.180
α-CH_3	−0.305	−0.343
N-CH_3	−0.555	−0.649
m′-OCH_3	−0.080	0.026
OH:OCH_3	–	−0.326
Phenylethylamine	1.906	1.875

Ban used a few interaction terms considering the possible interaction among substituents on the benzene ring in order to derive a relationship like the following:

$$\log A = \sum G_i X_i + \sum G^* X^* + c \tag{3.29}$$

The terms superscripted with * in Eq. (3.29) correspond to the interaction terms among different substituents (e.g., OH and OH, and OH and OCH_3). Now, based on the statistical significance, Fujita and Ban found the interaction between OH and OCH_3 as an important contributor and obtained the following general expression for this set of compounds:

$$\log A = \sum G_i X_i + X^*(\mathrm{OH{:}OCH_3})G^*(\mathrm{OH{:}OCH_3}) + c \tag{3.30}$$

The statistical quality of the model derived from Eq. (3.30) was better than the previous model obtained from Eq. (3.28). From the contributions of different groups to the activity as found from this model, the interaction between OH and OCH_3 has a negative impact on the activity. Fujita and Ban hypothesized that when OH and OCH_3 are vicinally placed, the activity may reduce due to the formation of an intramolecular hydrogen bond or the steric hindrance presented by the methoxy group. Again, the interaction between two vicinal OH groups was not found to be important, which Fujita and Ban hypothesized to be because the interaction of each OH group with the receptor site was stronger than the intramolecular H bond formation. Again, the difference of the contribution values of *p*-OH and *p*-OCH_3 was thought to be due to H bond formation with the enzyme (in the case of *p*-OH), in addition to hydrophobic and steric effects. This example helps us to understand how QSAR may be useful in mechanistic interpretation of the activity.

3.4 THE LFER MODEL

3.4.1 The concept

The Hansch approach (also known as the *LFER approach*) is basically a property-based QSAR method that considers correlation of the biological response with hydrophobic, electronic, and steric properties. This approach is very general, as any kind of drug–receptor interactions are caused by factors that can be broadly categorized into any one or more of these three properties. One may be able to use this approach to explore the relative contributions of different properties to the response activity and role of each factor in the biological mechanism. This approach is applicable for closely related congeners and a given biological activity. The Hansch model is based on the following postulates:

1. The drug molecules reach the receptor site via a "random walk" process (described in Section 3.4.2).
2. The drug molecules bind with the receptor, forming a complex.
3. The drug–receptor complex undergoes a chemical reaction or conformational changes for the desired activity.
4. The drugs in a congeneric series should have the same mechanism of action.

3.4.2 Genesis

The biological system offers a very reactive environment to the drugs [5]. After a drug is introduced to a biological system, it must find its target before any pharmacological action takes place. Before reaching the target, the administered drug takes part in many processes like absorption, distribution, metabolism, and sometimes elimination, allowing only a fraction of the administered drug to reach its target. The true effectiveness of a drug also depends on its selectivity, as it should not bind with some non-target sites. The reaction of a drug with its target forms the basis of the theory of LFER models. Partition coefficient of a drug is a significant determinant of the transport process of the drug to its target.

The first LFER approach was introduced by Hammett [7] for the hydrolysis rates of benzoic acid derivatives in either of the following expressions:

$$\log(K_X/K_H) = \rho\sigma \tag{3.31}$$

or

$$\log(k_X/k_H) = \rho\sigma \tag{3.32}$$

In Eqs. (3.31) and (3.32), K_X and K_H are the equilibrium constants for the reactions of substituted and unsubstituted benzoic acids, respectively; k_X and k_H are corresponding rate constants; ρ is a constant that depends on the type and conditions of the reaction, as well as the nature of compounds; σ is a constant denoting electronic contribution of the substituent depending on its nature and position. Equation (3.31) may be rewritten as

$$\log K_X = \rho\sigma + \log K_H \tag{3.33}$$

Equation (3.32) may be similarly rewritten. Equation (3.33) suggests a linear relationship between the substituent constant σ and the logarithm of reactivity of the compound (K_X). Although the Hammett equation was originally suggested for chemical reactions, the same logic can also be applied to "reactions" of drugs with the receptor in a biological system.

Gibbs free energy is related to the equilibrium constant of a reaction through the following expression:

$$\Delta G^{\text{o}} = -RT \ln K \tag{3.34}$$

where ΔG^{o} is the change in Gibbs free energy, R is the ideal gas constant, T is the absolute temperature, and K is the equilibrium constant of the reaction. This explains why the Hammett equation (as well as its expanded form of the Hansch equation) is considered as an LFER approach.

Considering the importance of the partition coefficient in the drug's transport to the ultimate site of action, Hansch et al. [8] considered additional physicochemical parameters for inclusion in the Hammett LFER model. Patterned after Hammett σ, Hansch and Fujita [9] introduced another substituent constant π in the following manner:

$$\pi_X = \log(P_X/P_H) \tag{3.35}$$

In Eq. (3.35), π_X is the hydrophobic substituent constant of substituent X (its contribution to the molecular hydrophobicity), and P_X and P_H are (n-octanol—water) partition coefficients of substituted and unsubstituted compounds.

An oversimplified picture of biological action of a drug may be hypothesized as shown in Figure 3.1 [9].

The first step in this process is the random walk process, in which the drug molecule makes its way from the dilute solution in the extracellular phase to the intracellular site of action. This process is primarily governed by the partition coefficient of the

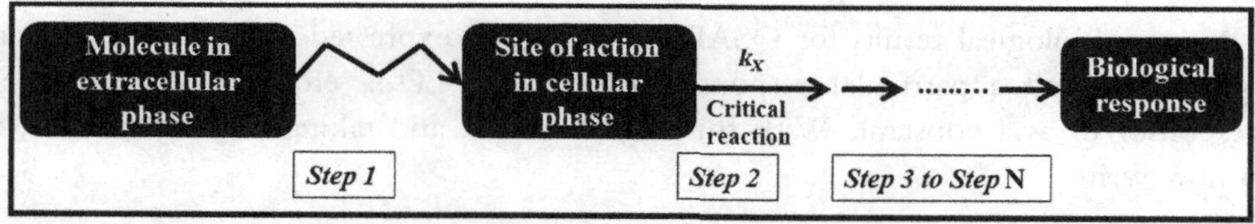

Figure 3.1 An oversimplified picture of the biological action of a drug.

drug. Among the series of events playing at the critical reaction site, there would be one rate controlling the reaction. This may be formulated in the following expression:

$$\text{Rate of biological reaction} = \mathrm{d(response)}/\mathrm{d}t = ACk_X \tag{3.36}$$

In Eq. (3.36), A is the probability of the drug molecule reaching the site of action in a given time interval, C is the extracellular molar concentration of the drug, and k_X is the rate or equilibrium constant for the critical step. The parameter AC is the effective concentration at the critical reaction site. It is assumed that a relatively large number of active sites are available, so this may be considered constant during the test interval. The parameters A and k_X will be important determinants of the effectiveness of individual member of a series of compounds in this steady-state model. The parameter A depends heavily on the partition coefficient P of the congener. Instead of P, Hansch used the previously defined LFER term π, which is a measure of the relative free energy change that results in moving a derivative from one phase to another. The A molecule would have to make many partitions between aqueous phases and a variety of different membranes, making the process more complex than simple partitioning because there will be many adsorption–desorption steps accompanying this at solid surfaces. It can be expected that the relative polarity of the molecules will play a role here parallel to that played in the partitioning process. The molecule with the minimum sum of the free energy changes for the many boundary crossings of the two types will be the one with the ideal lipohydrophilic character (π_0); any increase or decrease from π_0 will result in a slower rate of movement of the molecule in the partitioning-diffusion process by which the site of action is attained. It has long been known that as one increases the partition coefficient of a biologically active function, activity often rises, but after a certain point, it falls off and eventually reaches zero. Thus, there is abundant evidence to indicate that there is often an optimum partition coefficient (or value of π in a group of derivatives) for a biologically active series. Hansch and Fujita [9] hypothesized a normal distribution of biological activity with respect to log P or π, other factors being constant, and expressed A as the following relation:

$$A = f(\pi) = a \cdot \mathrm{e}^{-(\pi-\pi_0)^2/b} \tag{3.37}$$

In Eq. (3.37), a and b are constants. Substituting A into Eq. (3.36), one gets

$$\mathrm{d(response)}/\mathrm{d}t = a \cdot \mathrm{e}^{-(\pi-\pi_0)^2/b} Ck_X \tag{3.38}$$

As most biological results for QSAR modeling are expressed as the concentration required to elicit a particular response (IC_{50}, EC_{50}, LD_{50}, etc.), we can consider d(response)/dt as a constant. With this consideration, and taking the logarithm, we can now write

$$\log 1/C = -k\pi^2 + k'\pi\pi_0 - k''\pi_0^2 + \log k_X + k''' \tag{3.39}$$

The terms k, $k^{/}$, $k^{//}$, and $k^{///}$ are constants in Eq. (3.39). Again, log k_X in this equation may be eliminated using the Hammett equation in the following manner:

$$\log 1/C = -k\pi^2 + k^{/}\pi\pi_0 - k^{//}\pi_0^2 + \rho\sigma + k^{////} \tag{3.40}$$

where $k^{////}$ is a new constant. Note that log k_H is a constant by definition.

In Eq. (3.40), π_0 is the ideal value for a substituent such that the sum of the many free energy changes in the penetration process is minimal. Since both π_0 and ρ are constants for a given type of parent molecule in a particular biological system, Eq. (3.40) reduces to

$$\log 1/C = k_1\pi - k_2\pi^2 + k_3\sigma + k_4 \tag{3.41}$$

The parameters k_1, k_2, k_3, and k_4 are constant values in Eq. (3.41).

Depending on a particular series of biologically active compounds, all the terms mentioned in Eq. (3.41) may not be present, or some additional terms may be inserted.

In the case of nonspecific toxicity or narcosis, where an equilibrium between the drug outside the cell and that within the cell is established very rapidly, as considered in the classical works of Meyer and Overton and Ferguson, π_0 is very large in comparison to π and the contribution of the electronic effect (σ) is very small; thus, Eq. (3.41) reduces to

$$\log 1/C = a\pi + b \tag{3.42}$$

where a and b are two new constants.

In cases where π is close to π_0 (e.g., the carcinogenic activity of the dimethylaminoazobenzenes), Eq. (3.41) takes the following form:

$$\log 1/C = a\pi - b\pi^2 + c \tag{3.43}$$

Note that the values of the constants a, b, and c are found from the multiple linear regression exercise and will obviously be different from those of the constants of Eq. (3.42).

It may be possible that π could have no importance in determining the in vitro activity of a series of compounds. In such cases, Eq. (3.41) takes the form of the Hammett equation:

$$\log 1/C = a\sigma + b \tag{3.44}$$

When π_0 is larger than π and when σ is significant (e.g., local anesthetic action on guinea pigs), Eq. (3.41) reduces to

$$\log 1/C = a\pi + b\sigma + c \tag{3.45}$$

In some cases, additional parameters may be required to be incorporated in the Hansch model. For example, when a steric E_s is important, Eq. (3.41) may take the following form:

$$\log 1/C = k_1\pi - k_2\pi^2 + k_3\sigma + k_4E_s + k_5 \tag{3.46}$$

Equation (3.46) may be considered as the generalized expression of the Hansch model as it shows hydrophobic, electronic, and steric terms. For a particular data set, different variants of these terms (e.g., chromatographic parameter $\log k_0$ for hydrophobicity, pK_a for electronic effect, and van der Waals volume for steric effect) may be important; and it is the task of the QSAR modeler to select appropriate descriptors using feature selection tools. All descriptors appearing in the final model should have statistically significant regression coefficients; otherwise, such terms should be omitted.

In selecting the physicochemical parameters to be used in the QSAR models, one should check the possibility of intercorrelation among various pairs of substituent constants. Craig [10] studied such interdependence and prepared useful diagrams for the proper combination of substituent constants in a particular model. Remember that experimentally determined and theoretically computed physicochemical properties are only approximation of the factors involved in the biological processes. One may also try to use in the final model other kinds of descriptors, like topological or substructural ones, in addition to the physicochemical property-based descriptors as mentioned previously. This flexibility of modification by the incorporation or deletion of physicochemical or other parameters to describe a particular biological response more adequately is an important advantage of the LFER approach. This approach is also known as the *extrathermodynamic approach*, as the terms used in the model are applied in biological systems that are different from those (chemical systems) in which they were originally determined. Certain compounds (observations) may be omitted from the analysis due to reasons like steric restriction, high chemical reactivity, susceptibility to metabolic transformation, or unavailability of reliable substituent constant values. In cases where limited data points with experimental activity values are available, and thus meaningful statistical model development is not possible, it may be beneficial to adopt a rational method for guidance in selecting the most promising successive compounds for synthesis. Topliss [11] suggested nonmathematical operational schemes for analog synthesis based on the assumptions of Hansch analysis.

3.4.3 An example

In this section, we cite an example of Hansch analysis from the work of Kutter and Hansch [12]. The monoamine oxidase (MAO) inhibitory activity (pIC_{50} or the negative logarithm of the molar concentration necessary to inhibit 50% of the enzyme) of 18 *N*-(phenoxyethyl)cyclopropylamines was considered for the analysis. The substituent constants of the *meta* and *para* substituents on the phenyl ring (π as the hydrophobicity contribution, σ as the electronic contribution, and E_s as the steric contribution) obtained from the phenoxyacetic acid system were considered for the analysis and sum of the contributions of all *meta* and *para* substituents for a particular property (hydrophobic, electronic, or steric; $\Sigma\pi$, $\Sigma\sigma$, or ΣE_s) were considered as descriptors. Table 3.6 gives the data set along with the descriptor values, while Table 3.7 gives the substituent constant values of the substituents occurring in Table 3.6.

Note that in Hansch analysis, one can use a compound containing a substituent occurring only once in the data set. This is unlike the Free–Wilson model, where the descriptor values used in the former analysis are in a continuous scale. Similarly, from the developed Hansch model, one can predict the activity of a compound containing substituents not occurring in the modeling set.

Table 3.6 MAO (Rat liver) inhibitory activity of *N*-(phenoxyethy1)cyclopropylamines

Sl. No.	Substituent (*X*)	Descriptors			Log 1/IC$_{50}$	
		$\Sigma\pi$	$\Sigma\sigma$	ΣE_s	Obs.	Calc.[a]
1	4-Br	1.02	0.23	2.48	6.64	6.45
2	3,4-Cl_2	1.46	0.60	1.51	6.30	6.50
3	3-NO_2	0.11	0.71	−0.04	5.76	5.44
4	3-CF_3	1.07	0.42	0.08	4.98	5.17
5	4-CH_3	0.52	−0.17	2.48	5.69	5.69
6	3,5-Cl_2	1.52	0.74	0.54	5.68	6.09
7	3-Cl-4-CH_3	1.28	0.20	1.51	5.75	5.78
8	3-Br	0.94	0.39	1.32	5.64	5.93
9	3-CH_3-4-Cl	1.21	0.16	1.24	6.06	5.52
10	4-Cl	0.76	0.37	1.51	5.82	6.00
11	4-OCH_3	−0.04	−0.27	2.48	5.46	5.43
12	3,4-$(CH_3)_2$	1.03	−0.24	1.24	4.71	4.81
13	3,5-$(CH_3)_2$	1.02	−0.14	0.00	4.85	4.14
14	3-CH_3	0.51	−0.07	1.24	4.78	5.02
15	4-Cl-3,5-$(CH_3)_2$	1.72	0.09	0.00	4.70	4.65
16	3,4,5-$(CH_3)_3$	1.54	−0.31	0.00	3.54	3.93
17	4-N=NC_6H_5	1.71	0.64	2.48	7.56	7.26
18	4-NH_2	−1.63	−0.66	2.48	4.40	4.52

[a]From Eq. (3.47).

Table 3.7 Substituent constants from the phenoxyacetic acid system

Substituent	π_m	π_p	σ_m	σ_p	E_{s-m}	E_{s-p}
H	0.00	0.00	0.00	0.00	1.24	0.00
Br	0.94	1.02	0.39	0.23	0.08	0.00
Cl	0.76	0.70	0.37	0.23	0.27	0.00
NO_2	0.11	–	0.71	–	−1.28	0.00
CF_3	1.08	–	0.42	–	−1.16	0.00
CH_3	0.51	0.52	−0.07	−0.17	0.00	0.00
OCH_3	–	−0.05	–	−0.27	–	0.00
$N{=}NC_6H_5$	–	1.71	–	0.64	–	0.00
NH_2	–	−1.63	–	−0.66	–	0.00

A different combination of the descriptors may be tested to generate different models, and a comparative study can be made for their statistical quality (see Chapters 6 and 7). One of the models thus obtained may be

$$\log 1/IC_{50} = 4.226 + 0.154\sum\pi + 1.716\sum\sigma + 0.674\sum E_s \tag{3.47}$$

Equation (3.47) suggests that hydrophobic (i.e., a positive value of π denotes a more hydrophobic substituent than H) and electron-withdrawing (i.e., a positive value of σ indicates a more electron-withdrawing substituent than H) substituents increase MAO inhibitory activity. The interpretation of the E_s term is less obvious, as it also contains a resonance effect. Table 3.6 gives the calculated activity values according to Eq. (3.47).

3.4.4 Applications

The Hansch approach has been very successful in QSAR studies of drugs and other biologically active chemicals. Many successful applications of this approach have been reported in the literature [13]. By approximating the physicochemical properties with measured or theoretical values, one may be able to use this method as a measure to determine the relative importance and role of each factor in the biological mechanism. However, this approach is applicable only to closely related congeners sharing a common mechanism of action.

3.5 KUBINYI'S BILINEAR MODEL

Although linear relationships exist between the biological activity and hydrophobic character for a large number of homologous compounds, as shown in Eq. (3.48), this cannot go on infinitely. A cutoff point is reached in each homologous series: the biological activity increases with increasing lipophilicity, reaches a maximum, and then decreases with further increase of hydrophobic character:

$$\log 1/C = a \log P + b \tag{3.48}$$

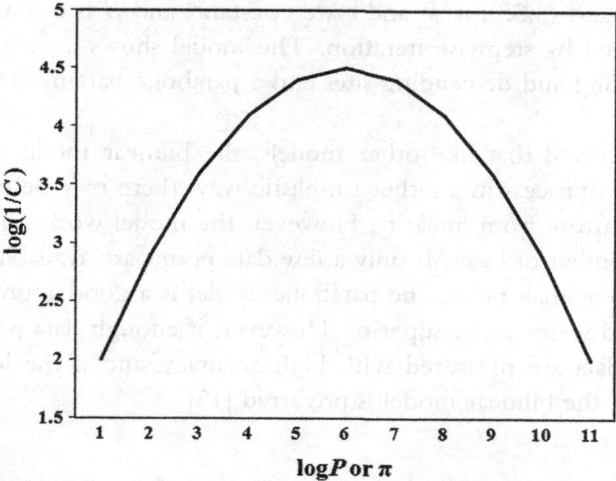

Figure 3.2 A parabolic relationship of the biological activity with logP (or π).

Fujita and Hansch [9] proposed a parabolic model to denote the dependence of biological activity on hydrophobic character on the basis of a random walk process (Figure 3.2). On their way from the outer phase, where the drug is administered, to their receptor sites, the drug molecules have to penetrate a number of lipophilic and hydrophilic barriers. While hydrophilic molecules tend to remain in the aqueous phases and lipophilic molecules tend to go into the lipid (membrane) phases, molecules with an optimal hydrophilic–lipophilic balance will have the best chance to penetrate all barriers and reach the receptor sites. A quadratic dependence on log P (or π) is usually interpreted as indicating the importance of transport, while a linear dependence is considered to imply that hydrophobic bonding plays an important role in the expression of biological activity. Also note that the octanol–water partition coefficient reflects more than simple hydrophobic bonding (i.e., hydrogen bonding and van der Waals interactions):

$$\log 1/C = a \log P - b(\log P)^2 + c \tag{3.49}$$

$$\log 1/C = a\pi - b\pi^2 + c \tag{3.50}$$

Apart from the parabolic model, there are several other nonlinear models correlating biological activity with hydrophobicity, among which the bilinear approach of McFarland [14] is most interesting. The original bilinear model was modified by Kubinyi [15], and its two variants are shown here:

$$\log 1/C = a \log P - b \log(\beta \cdot P + 1) + c \tag{3.51}$$

$$\log 1/C = a\pi - b \log(\beta \cdot 10^{\pi} + 1) + c \tag{3.52}$$

In Eqs. (3.51) and (3.52), a, b, and c are constants and β is a nonlinear term that must be determined by stepwise iteration. The model shows an unsymmetric curve with linear ascending and descending sites and a parabolic part in the region of optimal lipophilicity.

It can be conceived that like other models, the bilinear model is an attempt to simulate a complex process in a rather simplistic way; there may be other factors that could cause a departure from linearity. However, the model works in a nearly perfect way for a large number of cases. If only a few data points are available, or if the log P values vary within a small range, the parabolic model is a good approximation of the bilinear model and seems to be superior. However, if enough data points are present, if the biological data are measured with high accuracy, and if the log P values vary over a wide range, the bilinear model is preferred [15].

3.6 THE MIXED APPROACH

The Free–Wilson model is a mathematical approach for the quantitative description of structure–activity relationships. The Fujita–Ban modification is a linear transformation of the classical Free–Wilson model. The Fujita–Ban model is characterized by a number of advantages [16] over the classical Free–Wilson model: (i) no transformation of the structural matrix and no symmetry equations are necessary; (ii) all group contributions are based on an arbitrarily chosen reference compound, preferably the unsubstituted compound; (iii) the constant term, which is the theoretically predicted activity value of the reference compound, and the values of the group contributions are not markedly influenced by the addition or elimination of a compound; (iv) the problem of linear dependence (the singularity problem) sometimes can be circumvented by preparing a contracted matrix; and (v) if the unsubstituted compound is chosen as the reference compound, the group contributions are numerically equivalent to Hansch-derived group contributions. Therefore, the Hansch approach and the Fujita–Ban model can be combined into a mixed approach. If, for one definite region of the molecule, a Hansch correlation can be obtained for the substituents, while substituents in another position of the molecule must be treated by Free–Wilson analysis (using indicator variables for the presence or absence of substituents at particular positions), the Fujita–Ban model and the Hansch approach can be combined into a mixed approach [16]:

$$\log 1/C = k_1\pi + k_2\sigma + \sum G_iX_i + c \tag{3.53}$$

In Eq. (3.53), $k_1\pi + k_2\sigma$ is the Hansch part for the substituents Y_j, ΣG_iX_i is the (modified) Free–Wilson part for the substituents X_i (with G_i being the corresponding group contributions), and c is the theoretically predicted activity value of the unsubstituted parent compound ($X = Y = H$) or of an arbitrarily chosen reference compound. Taking all these facts into consideration, the Fujita–Ban model is considered the most suitable approach for the calculation of *de novo* group contributions.

3.7 OVERVIEW AND CONCLUSIONS

The classical QSAR approaches dominated the domain of theoretical modeling in medicinal chemistry in the 1970s and 1980s. The Hansch modeling approach is still useful today due to its fundamental nature. However, it is more appropriate for application to a congeneric series of compounds with a particular mechanism of action. With the introduction of more sophisticated 3D and higher-order QSARs coupled with receptor-based approaches, and in order to deal with molecular series of greater structural diversity, the use of classical QSAR has declined nowadays to some extent. However, these methods will continue to contribute to the understanding of the basic principles of QSAR studies.

REFERENCES

[1] Smithfield WR, Purcell WP. Application of regression analysis to hypoglycemic activities of 12 piperidinesulfamylsemicarbazides and activity predictions for 12 analogs. J Pharm Sci 1967;56(5): 577–9.

[2] Free SM, Wilson JW. A mathematical contribution to structure–activity studies. J Med Chem 1964;7(4): 395–9.

[3] Purcell WP. Cholinesterase inhibitory prognoses of thirty-six alkyl substituted 3-carbamoylpiperidines. Biochim Biophys Acta 1965;105:201–4.

[4] Beasley JG, Purcell WP. An example of successful prediction of cholinesterase inhibitory potency from regression analysis. Biochim Biophys Acta 1969;178:175–6.

[5] Purcell WP, Bass GE, Clayton JM. Strategy of drug design: a guide to biological activity. New York, NY: John Wiley & Sons; 1973.

[6] Fujita T, Ban T. Structure–activity study of phenethylamines as substrates of biosynthetic enzymes of sympathetic transmitters. J Med Chem 1971;14(2):148–52.

[7] Hammett LP. Some relations between reaction rates and equilibrium constants. Chem Rev 1935; 17:125–36.

[8] Hansch C, Muir RM, Fujita T, Maloney PP, Geiger F, Streich M. The correlation of biological activity of plant growth regulators and chloromycetin derivatives with Hammett constants and partition coefficients. J Am Chem Soc 1963;85:2817–24.

[9] Hansch C, Fujita T. ρ–σ–π Analysis. A method for the correlation of biological activity and chemical structure. J Am Chem Soc 1964;86:1616–26.

[10] Craig PN. Interdependence between physical parameters and selection of substituent groups for correlation studies. J Med Chem 1971;14:680–4.

[11] Topliss J. Utilization of operational schemes for analog synthesis in drug design. J Med Chem 1972;15:1006–11.

[12] Kutter E, Hansch C. Steric parameters in drug design. Monoamine oxidase inhibitors and antihistamines. J Med Chem 1969;12:647–52.

[13] Kubinyi H. QSAR: Hansch analysis and related approaches. In: Mannhold R, Krogsgaard-Larsen P, Timmerman H, editors. Methods and principles in medicinal chemistry. Weinheim, Germany: VCH; 1993.
[14] McFarland JW. Parabolic relation between drug potency and hydrophobicity. J Med Chem 1970; 13:1192–6.
[15] Kubinyi H. Quantitative structure–activity relationships. 7. The bilinear model, a new model for nonlinear dependence of biological activity on hydrophobic character. J Med Chem 1977;20: 625–9.
[16] Kubinyi H, Kehrhahn OH. Quantitative structure–activity relationships. 3. A comparison of different Free–Wilson Models. J Med Chem 1976;19:1040–9.

CHAPTER 4

Topological QSAR

Contents

4.1 INTRODUCTION

Science provides a systematic path of study for solving natural problems using logical observations and deriving the explanations thereof. The knowledge from a study is built through the logical nourishment of its basic components defining different facets of fundamental understanding. The quantitative study of chemistry involves basic and fundamental components that allow its coherence with mathematics and thereby solving the problems of nature. Descriptors being one such very essential component allow interaction between chemistry and mathematics toward the development of theoretical basis for predictive mathematical models.

Before going into the details of topological descriptors, we would like to provide a brief discussion on the impact and role of dimension in chemistry. Representation of chemical structure plays a major part in chemistry, involving different patterns of description of atoms and bonds. Dimension, in mathematical terms, is recognized

Understanding the Basics of QSAR for Applications in Pharmaceutical Sciences and Risk Assessment.
ISBN: 978-0-12-801505-6, DOI: http://dx.doi.org/10.1016/B978-0-12-801505-6.00004-1

as the number of coordinates used to locate an object or point in it. Although any subjects observed in nature have three dimensions, scientists have developed hypotheses on lower as well as higher dimensions than three with the aim of solving specific problems. The journey of the quantitative structure–activity relationship (QSAR) paradigm has been associated with a gradually increasing dimensional perspective that has led to the evolution of various predictor variables or descriptors corresponding to different levels of dimension. Topology is one such concept that addresses the two-dimensional (2D) geometry of the molecules under investigation.

4.2 TOPOLOGY: A METHOD OF CHEMICAL STRUCTURE REPRESENTATION

Representation of chemical structure has been of great interest to chemists. In chemistry, molecular representation refers to the symbolic way of presenting a chemical moiety using a specific format coupled with definite rules [1]. Chemical representation provides a rational way of studying molecules by providing a pattern of coded information. Readers should understand that different types of representation of chemicals are made based on a theoretical basis to achieve specific needs and hence the amount of information regarding the chemical structure held up by the "symbolic" representation depends on the type of representation used. An example may be the chemical formula of a compound, which provides an easy way of expressing the type and number (which is usually subscripted) of atoms in a molecule. The formula C_6H_6 easily codes the presence of six carbon and six hydrogen atoms together in a molecule. However, the chemical/molecular formula is one of the most primitive forms of chemical structure representation and does not account for the arrangement of atoms. One of the major objectives of a QSAR modeler is to extract quantitative information from chemical structures, and different chemical representation mechanisms aid this perspective by enlightening different dimensional features. Molecular formula is essentially a zero dimensional (0D) feature since it deals only with the composition, not the arrangement of molecules. Other parameters of this kind are atomic weight, mass, charge, and count of number of atoms. When the fragments of a molecule are used for molecular representation (e.g., substructural fragment or functional groups), it adds another dimension to the process and depicts the type of substitution or fragments present and they are considered in the one-dimensional (1D) group. Next comes 2D representation of molecules and the information derived thereof. 2D representation considers the type of atoms, their numbers, and their connection pattern with each other, hence providing a more detailed color to the picture. Topological descriptors are 2D features of chemical compounds derived using a suitable algorithm. Likewise, there are higher dimensions than 2D, and several features are derived at each level of dimension. However, considering the scope of this chapter (topological features), we shall restrict our discussion principally to 2D, with some discussion of the relationship between 2D and 3D features.

4.3 GRAPHS AND MATRICES: PLATFORMS FOR THE TOPOLOGICAL PARADIGM

4.3.1 Graph theory and chemical graphs

Evolution of the graph theoretic formalism has been one of the best developments in the field of quantitative chemistry. The topological concept is purely based on the graphical representation of molecular structure. Graphs essentially stem from mathematics and refer to the collection of a set of objects in a plane and the binary relationship held therein [2]. Mathematics is an abstract branch of natural science where concepts from other branches are brought under rational algorithmic expression. The inclusion of graph theory in chemistry has given rise to a novel concept of representing chemical structures using mathematical formalism. Hence, chemical graphs are used to characterize the interaction between chemical objects; for example, atoms, bonds, and molecules. The two basic elements in the context of chemical graph theory are vertex and edge, which depict the connected structure of chemical compounds. Atoms are represented by vertices, while different types of bond are designated by edges. Hence, chemical graphs provide a way of representing the chemical structures using a 2D perspective. Figure 4.1 depicts a hydrogen-suppressed (or depleted) chemical graph of *n*-butane comprising vertices (carbon atom) and edges (sigma bond). Since the formalism is entirely 2D, there is no such restriction of providing specific bond length or angle, but it aptly describes the bonded connections present among different type of atoms. Although carbon atoms are represented as dots or points in a graph theoretical representation, heteroatoms are denoted by their symbols.

It may be noted that the practice of graph theory to address practical problems was introduced long ago. Leonhard Euler [3] was the first to use graph theory, and he provided an ingenious solution to the Königsberg seven bridges problem in 1736. Kirchhoff [4] employed a graphical notion for the study of electrical circuits. Sylvester [5] is considered to be the first to use the term *graph* in the literature from a contemporary chemical background and also introduced the term *chemicograph*. William Cullen [6] was the first to use the term *affinity diagram* and introduced the idea of a chemical graph. From a concept of gravitational attraction, William Higgins [7] was the next to depict the connection between atoms by employing chemical graphs. It should be noted here that at that time, concepts of chemical bonds and spatial arrangement of molecules were not established. It was at the beginning of the

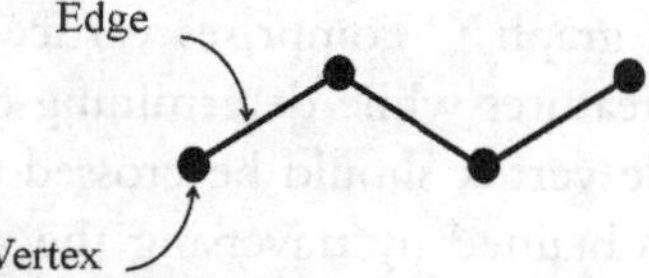

Figure 4.1 Hydrogen-depleted chemical graph of *n*-butane.

nineteenth century when Dalton [8] and Wollaston [9] devised the concept of arranging molecules in a 3D plane, and Dalton used ball-and-stick models to identify molecules. Dalton, in his ball-and-stick models, used circles (tiny hard spheres) to designate atoms, while the force of holding was denoted using sticks. In the mid-nineteenth century, further momentum was gained in the study using the concept of tetrahedral carbon atoms by Kekulé [10], van't Hoff [11], and Le Bel [12]. In 1861, Loschmidt [13] used graphical representation to denote organic molecules, where he used small circles to denote H-atoms and large circles for carbon atoms. The development of theories regarding chemical bonding and structural elucidation was accompanied by the graph theoretical presentation. Cayley [14] used alkane tree graphs for enumerating alkane isomers known as *kenograms.* Following the bare beginning of the journey, the actual and vivid usage of graph theory with respect to the chemical structures started in the mid-twentieth century. The need was to enumerate various chemical isomers obtained from the field of synthetic chemistry. Henze and Blair [15] incorporated corrections into Cayley's assumptions. The mathematical formulation of the chemical graph theory was created by Pólya and Read [16]. Graph theory has been extensively cultivated by scientists and researchers since then, and topological descriptors were the fruitful output serving the QSAR fraternity. It will be beyond the scope of this chapter to discuss all the discoveries in the graph theoretic and topological paradigm in detail. However, the authors would like to mention the names of some of the great pioneers who took the simple graphical representation to the topological QSAR formalism still used widely by researchers: Alexandru T. Balaban, Danail D. Bonchev, Dennis H. Rouvray, Douglas J. Klein, Frank Harary, Harry P. Schultz, Haruo Hosoya, Ivan Gutman, Lemont B. Kier, Lowell H. Hall, Milan Randić, and Nenad Trinajstić.

In other, simpler words, chemical structures were represented by scientists as connected lines. Vertices or atoms were joined by edges or bonds. It may be noted that the concept of graphs are utilized to serve a wide number of purposes, including canonical coding, constitutional symmetry perception, reaction graph, synthon graph, and optimal planning graph. In the literature, various kinds of terminologies regarding chemical graphs are available. Figure 4.2 shows a representative list of some of the commonly used phrases related to graph theoretic chemistry, along with their meanings. In this chapter, we shall focus on the graphs used on the topological perspective of chemical compounds. These are termed as *hydrogen-depleted* or *hydrogen-suppressed* graphs, and the hydrogen atoms attached to carbon are not shown in the connected molecule. Hence, a chemical graph G comprises vertices V, and edges E connecting those vertices. Two essential features while determining distance or path between any two vertices are that no single vertex should be crossed more than once and a minimum topological distance is obtained by traversing the shortest path among vertices. These two facts are illustrated in Figure 4.3.

Graph theoretic terminologies

Term	Definition
Cyclic graph	Begins and ends on a same vertex consisting of at least one walk such that each vertex is visited once.
Isomorphic graph	One-to-one matching of the vertices and edges of one graph to that of a second graph.
Homeomorphic graph	Similar graphs obtained by further dividing one's edges with vertices.
Connected graph	A graph where all pairs of vertices are joined by path.
Pseudograph	Presence of multiple edges and loops between pairs of vertices. May contain multiple bonds and lone electron pairs.
Vertex	The points, that is chemical atoms joining edges in a molecular graph.
Edge	The bond joining two vertices in a molecular graph.
Tree	A graph without cycle that is having two distinct terminals.
Chain	Connected acyclic graph (analogous).
Star	A tree with maximum possible number of terminals with the existing number of vertices and edges.
Arc	An edge with assigned direction; graphs are called oriented graphs.
Walk	The alternating sequence of vertices and edges. Starting as well as ending is commenced with vertex.
Path	A walk with no vertex repeating for more than single occurrence.
Elongation	Longest distance in a graph.
Loop	Edges from a vertex to itself defining a self-connection.
Rooted tree	A tree containing a dissimilar vertex.
Subgraph	Obtained by eliminating vertices and edges of a molecular graph without removal of the endpoints of an unremoved edge.
Spanning tree	A tree where all vertices are connected with arc.
Terminal	The end vertex in molecular graph.
Cyclomatic number	Number of independent cycles present.
Order of a graph	The number of vertices present in a connected molecular graph.
Vertex degree	The number of edges connected to a vertex in a molecular graph.
Regular graph	A molecular graph where all vertex degrees are equal.
Topological distance	The number of edges joining two vertices in the shortest path.
Adjacent vertices	The vertices joined by a single edge.
Adjacent edges	The edges having a common vertex.

Figure 4.2 Various terminologies commonly employed in graph theoretic chemistry.

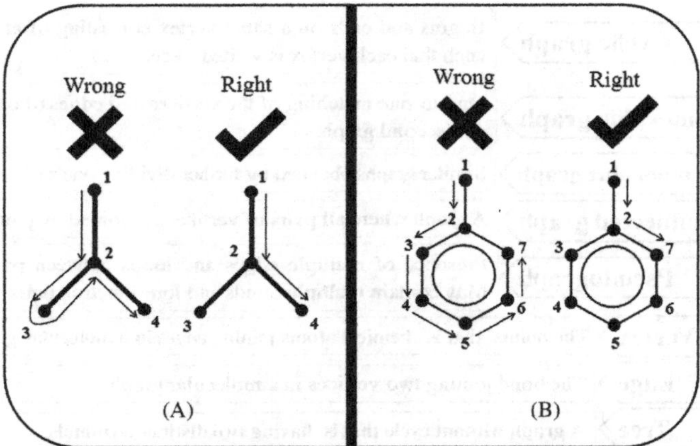

Figure 4.3 (A) The correct way of traversing path in isobutane molecule. (B) Determining minimum topological distance between vertices 1 and 7 in toluene.

4.3.2 Matrix: aiding the numerical presentation of graph theory

Matrix plays a crucial role in graph theoretical chemistry in deriving quantitative topological information. *Matrices* are arrays of numbers or some other mathematical objects that are utilized to get desired information. In graph theoretic chemistry, matrices are treated with operators to derive topological indices. Hence, a matrix acts as a suitable and convenient device for the numerical codification of chemical graphs. Different types of matrices are used in relation to the chemical graph theory, and they are associated with algebraic operators.

In order to derive a matrix from a chemical structure, one needs to follow some basic steps. This includes drawing of the hydrogen-depleted graph followed by numbering and then formation of a 2D-graphical matrix by gradual removal of adjacent vertices or edges of the given H-suppressed graph and using them one by one as matrix elements following a rule. Once the matrix is completed, then replacing the graphical elements with a numerical value yields the desired matrix of interest. This matrix is further treated to derive descriptors. Different kinds of rules give rise to different matrices from a same molecular graph. In Figure 4.4, we have attempted to show a pictorial representation of this operation; that is, how to derive a matrix from a chemical structure. We have used a distance-based rule (namely, distance between two vertices) to derive the distance matrix for the chemical isopentane. Bold bonds depict the derived distances, while narrow bonds represent the edges (or the vertices) removed. Finally, conversion of the graph distances into numbers gives the final required matrix.

Again, it will be beyond the scope of this chapter to present a great deal of information about different matrices, and we would like to limit the discussion to some of the commonly used ones so that novices are familiar with the formalism of basic matrices in relation to the chemical graphs. Detailed information on matrices related

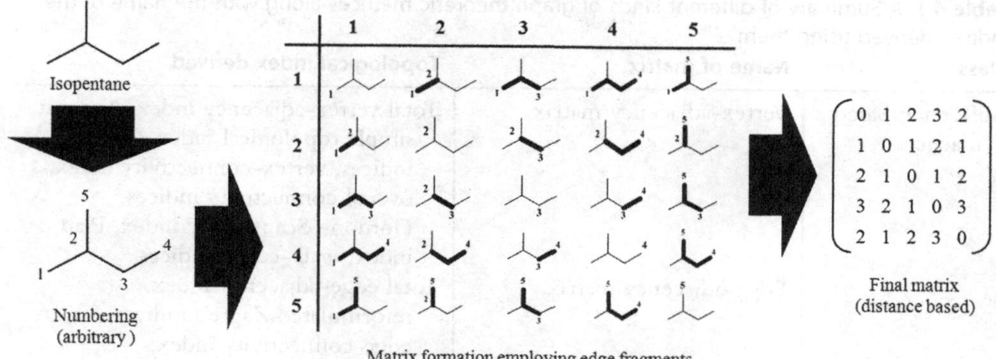

Figure 4.4 Schematic diagram showing the formation of a matrix from a sample chemical structure (isopentane).

to chemical graphs can be found in the literature [17–19]. Table 4.1 gives a list of different matrices used in connection to chemical graphs.

The next section discusses some representative matrices. One point to be noted here is that the vertices or the edges in a connected molecular graph are numbered in order to get a matrix representation. These numbers are completely arbitrary, and one should just follow the method of deriving the matrix entries since for a whole molecule, the final topological parameter gives the same value regardless of numbering pattern (thus, these indices are termed *topological invariants*).

a. Adjacency matrix

The term *adjacency matrix* refers to a square symmetric matrix showing the adjacencies between vertices (V) or edges (E) in chemical graphs. The adjacency matrix can be framed to vertices, as well as to edges giving two different matrices.

i. Vertex-adjacency matrix: Mallion [20] used this term in relation to chemical graph theory. For a connected molecular graph G, the vertex-adjacency matrix with $V \times V$ dimension can be defined as

$$\begin{aligned}[A_v(G)]_{ij} &= 1 \quad \text{when } i \neq j \text{ and } e_{ij} \in E(G), \text{ i.e., vertices } i \text{ and } j \text{ are adjacent} \\ &= 0 \quad \text{when } i = j \text{ and } e_{ij} \notin E(G)\end{aligned} \tag{4.1}$$

where e_{ij} is the edge defined by the vertices i and j and $E(G)$ is the set of edges present in the connected molecular graph G (Boxes 4.1 and 4.2).

ii. Edge-adjacency matrix: The edge-adjacency matrix of a connected graph G can be defined as

$$\begin{aligned}[A_e(G)]_{ij} &= 1 \quad \text{when } e_{ij} \in E(G); \text{ i.e., edges } i \text{ and } j \text{ are adjacent} \\ &= 0 \quad \text{when } e_{ij} \notin E(G)\end{aligned} \tag{4.2}$$

Table 4.1 A Summary of different kinds of graph theoretic matrices along with the name of the indices derived using them

Class	Name of matrix	Topological index derived
Adjacency-based matrices	Vertex-adjacency matrix	Total vertex-adjacency index, Narumi simple topological index, Zagreb indices, vertex-connectivity index, overall connectivity indices, Gordon–Scantlebury index, Platt index, walk-count indices
	Edge-adjacency matrix	Total edge-adjacency index, reformulated Zagreb indices, edge-connectivity index, reformulated Gordon–Scantebury index, reformulated Platt index
	Augmented vertex-adjacency matrix	Variable Zagreb indices, variable vertex-connectivity index
	Edge-weighted edge-adjacency matrix	Edge-connectivity index
	Vertex-connectivity matrix	Connectivity identification (ID) number
	Edge-connectivity matrix	Edge-connectivity index
	Zagreb matrix	Zagreb index
	Augmented vertex-degree matrix	Complexity index of Randić and Plavšić connectivity indices
	Laplacian matrix	Mohar indices, Wiener index of trees, *quasi*-Wiener index, spanning-tree density, reciprocal spanning-tree density
Distance-based matrices	Vertex-distance matrix	Wiener index, multiplicative Wiener index, Balaban index, distance-sum index
	Vertex-distance-path matrix	Hyper-Wiener index
	Reciprocal vertex-distance-path matrix	Hyper-Harary indices
	Vertex-distance-complement matrix	Includes the Wiener index, complement hyper-Wiener index, and the complement Balaban index
	Augmented vertex-distance matrix	Variable Wiener index, variable hyper-Wiener index, variable Balaban index
	Complementary vertex-distance matrix	Wiener-like molecular descriptors
	Detour matrix	Detour index
	Detour-path matrix	Hyper-detour index
	Detour-complement matrix	Detour-complement index
	Vertex-Harary matrix	Vertex-Harary index, hyper-Harary index, Harary–Balaban index
	Distance-degree matrices	Distance-degree descriptors
	Resistance-distance matrix	Kirchhoff index

(*Continued*)

Table 4.1 (Continued)

Class	Name of matrix	Topological index derived
Other matrices	Adjacency-plus-distance matrices	Edge-Schultz index
	Distance-sum-connectivity matrix	Weighted identification number
	Wiener matrices	Wiener index
	Reverse-Wiener matrix	Reverse-Wiener index, reverse-distance sum
	Reverse-detour matrix	Reverse-detour index
	Szeged matrices	Szeged index
	Hosoya matrices	*Z*-index, Hosoya index
	All-path matrix	All-path Wiener index
	Expanded vertex-distance matrix	Expanded distance indices, expanded square distance indices

BOX 4.1 Vertex-Adjacency Matrix Elements of Sample Chemicals

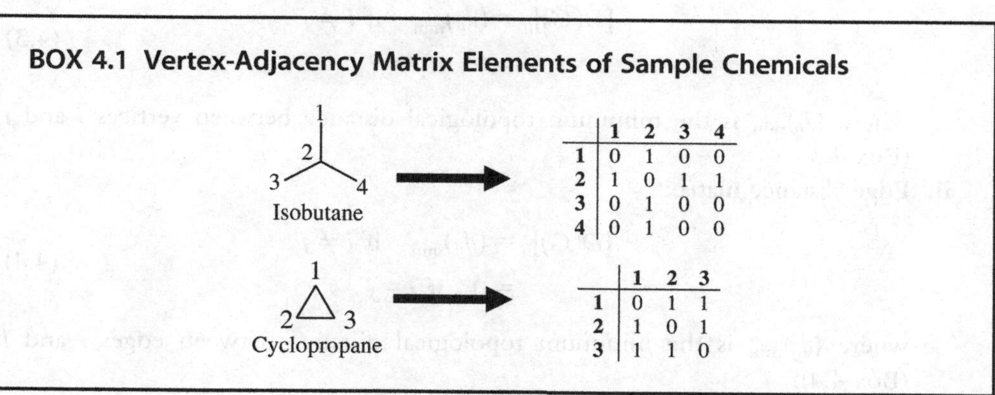

	1	2	3	4
1	0	1	0	0
2	1	0	1	1
3	0	1	0	0
4	0	1	0	0

	1	2	3
1	0	1	1
2	1	0	1
3	1	1	0

BOX 4.2 Edge-Adjacency Matrix Elements of Sample Chemicals

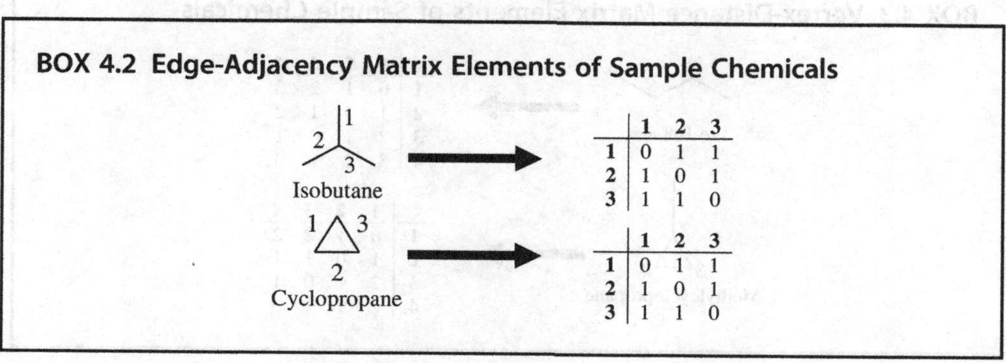

	1	2	3
1	0	1	1
2	1	0	1
3	1	1	0

	1	2	3
1	0	1	1
2	1	0	1
3	1	1	0

It may be observed that the diagonal elements of an adjacency matrix give zero value. Furthermore, it is also interesting to note that a vertex-adjacency matrix is distinctive in determining a specific type of graph, whereas an edge-adjacency matrix may not be so in cases of nonisomorphic graphs (e.g., same matrix elements for isobutane and cyclopropane).

b. Distance matrix

The distance matrix works on the assumption of distances between objects in the shortest way. When one has to compute the distance between two vertices (or edges), there might be different ways to do so; however, the objective here is to find the connection path that travels the minimum distance through a connected molecular graph (G). Such distance is called *minimum topological distance*, and the shortest distance between two vertices in a graph is also known as the *geodesic distance* [2]. Like the adjacency matrix, distance matrix can also be applicable to vertices, as does the edge-distance matrix, discussed later.

i. Vertex-distance matrix: It can be defined as

$$\begin{aligned}[D(G)]_{ij} &= (d_{ij})_{\min} \quad \text{if } i \neq j \\ &= 0 \quad \text{if } i = j\end{aligned} \tag{4.3}$$

where $(d_{ij})_{\min}$ is the minimum topological distance between vertices i and j (Box 4.3).

ii. Edge-distance matrix:

$$\begin{aligned}[D(G)]_{ij} &= (d_{ij})_{\min} \quad \text{if } i \neq j \\ &= 0 \quad \text{if } i = j\end{aligned} \tag{4.4}$$

where $(d_{ij})_{\min}$ is the minimum topological distance between edges i and j (Box 4.4).

BOX 4.3 Vertex-Distance Matrix Elements of Sample Chemicals

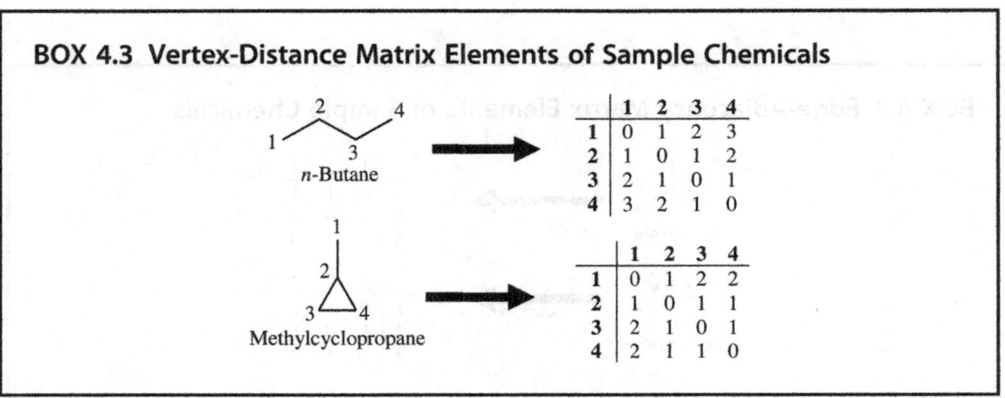

	1	2	3	4
1	0	1	2	3
2	1	0	1	2
3	2	1	0	1
4	3	2	1	0

	1	2	3	4
1	0	1	2	2
2	1	0	1	1
3	2	1	0	1
4	2	1	1	0

Therefore, it is evident that a matrix can be computed for the arbitrarily assigned vertices, as well as for the edges for a same molecular graph. However, in order to keep the text simple, we shall be dealing with vertex-derived matrices only in the definitions that will be discussed later.

c. Distance-complement matrix

It can be defined as follows:

$$[D_c(G)]_{ij} = V - [D(G)]_{ij} \quad \text{if } i \neq j$$
$$= 0 \quad \text{if } i = j \tag{4.5}$$

where V is the number of vertices present in the connected molecular graph G (Box 4.5).

BOX 4.4 Edge-Distance Matrix Elements of Sample Chemicals

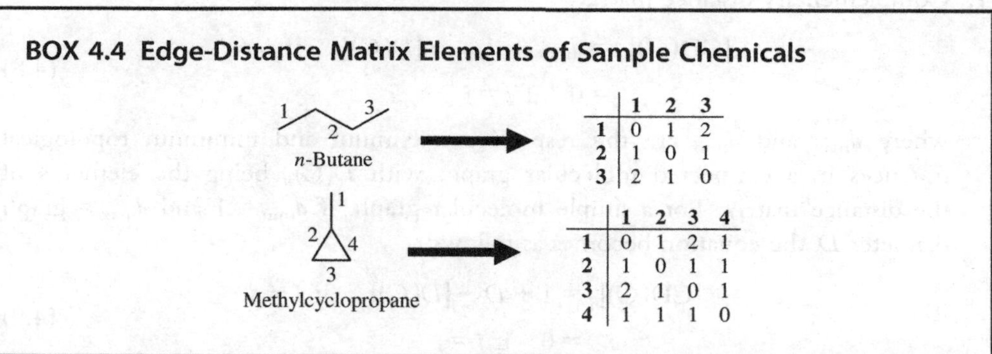

	1	2	3
1	0	1	2
2	1	0	1
3	2	1	0

	1	2	3	4
1	0	1	2	1
2	1	0	1	1
3	2	1	0	1
4	1	1	1	0

BOX 4.5 Distance-Complement Matrix Elements of Sample Chemicals

5
2
4
1
3
Isopentane

	1	2	3	4	5
1	0	4	3	2	3
2	4	0	4	3	4
3	3	4	0	4	3
4	2	3	4	0	2
5	3	4	3	2	0

1
6
2
5
3
4
Benzene

	1	2	3	4	5	6
1	0	5	4	3	4	5
2	5	0	5	4	3	4
3	4	5	0	5	4	3
4	3	4	5	0	5	4
5	4	3	4	5	0	5
6	5	4	3	4	5	0

d. Reciprocal distance matrix

It may be defined as follows:

$$[RD(G)]_{ij} = 1/[D(G)]_{ij} \quad \text{if } i \neq j \\ = 0 \quad \text{if } i = j \tag{4.6}$$

where $[D(G)]_{ij}$ is the topological graph distance between vertices i and j. This matrix is also termed the *Harary matrix* (or *vertex-Harary matrix*) (Box 4.6).

e. Reciprocal distance-complement matrix

$$[RD_c(G)]_{ij} = 1/[D_c(G)]_{ij} \quad \text{if } i \neq j \\ = 0 \quad \text{if } i = j \tag{4.7}$$

where $D_c(G)_{ij}$ is the distance-complement matrix formed by vertices i and j in a connected graph (Box 4.7).

f. Complementary distance matrix

$$[CD(G)]_{ij} = d_{max} + d_{min} - [D(G)]_{ij} \quad \text{if } i \neq j \\ = 0 \quad \text{if } i = j \tag{4.8}$$

where d_{max} and d_{min} are the respective maximum and minimum topological distances in a connected molecular graph, with $D(G)_{ij}$ being the elements of the distance matrix. For a simple molecular graph, if $d_{min} = 1$ and d_{max} = graph diameter D, the equation becomes as follows:

$$[CD(G)]_{ij} = 1 + D - [D(G)]_{ij} \quad \text{if } i \neq j \\ = 0 \quad \text{if } i = j \tag{4.9}$$

where, graph diameter D corresponds to the longest geodesic distance between any two vertices i and j (Box 4.8).

BOX 4.6 Reciprocal Distance Matrix Elements of Sample Chemicals

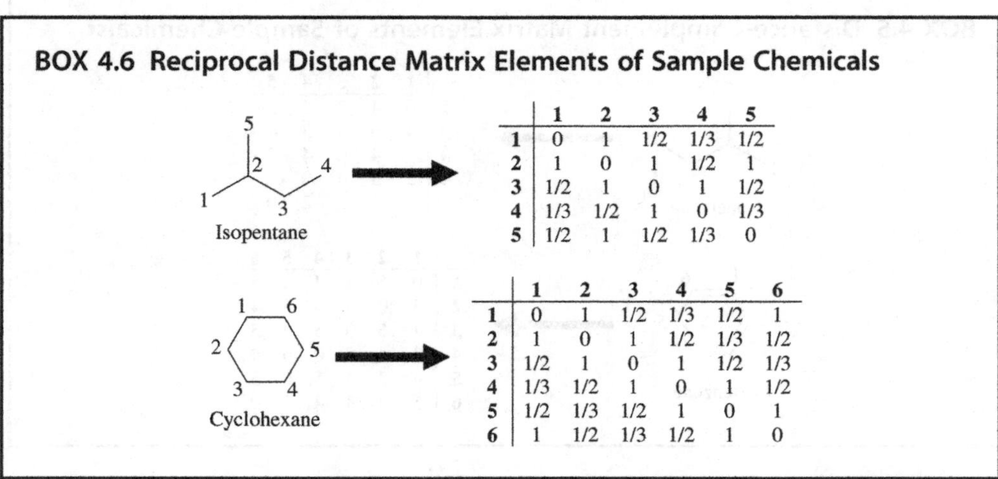

	1	2	3	4	5
1	0	1	1/2	1/3	1/2
2	1	0	1	1/2	1
3	1/2	1	0	1	1/2
4	1/3	1/2	1	0	1/3
5	1/2	1	1/2	1/3	0

	1	2	3	4	5	6
1	0	1	1/2	1/3	1/2	1
2	1	0	1	1/2	1/3	1/2
3	1/2	1	0	1	1/2	1/3
4	1/3	1/2	1	0	1	1/2
5	1/2	1/3	1/2	1	0	1
6	1	1/2	1/3	1/2	1	0

A reciprocal version of the complementary distance matrix can be generated using a similar method as discussed previously.

g. Distance-path matrix

$$[D_p(G)]_{ij} = [D(G)]_{ij}([D(G)]_{ij} + 1)/2 \quad \text{if } i \neq j$$
$$= 0 \quad \text{if } i = j \tag{4.10}$$

where $D(G)_{ij}$ is the element of the distance matrix formed between vertices i and j. The parameter $D_p(G)_{ij}$ considers all the internal paths possible between vertices i and j (Box 4.9).

BOX 4.7 Reciprocal Distance-Complement Matrix Elements of Sample Chemicals

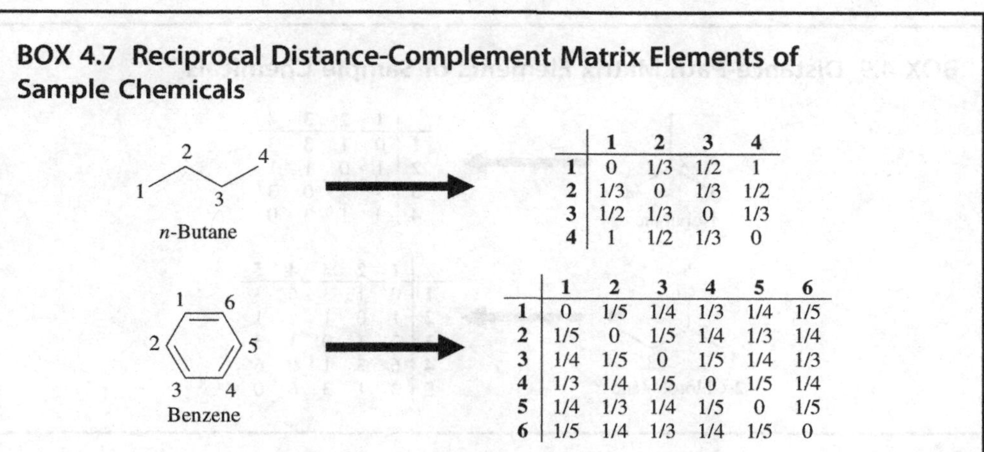

	1	2	3	4
1	0	1/3	1/2	1
2	1/3	0	1/3	1/2
3	1/2	1/3	0	1/3
4	1	1/2	1/3	0

	1	2	3	4	5	6
1	0	1/5	1/4	1/3	1/4	1/5
2	1/5	0	1/5	1/4	1/3	1/4
3	1/4	1/5	0	1/5	1/4	1/3
4	1/3	1/4	1/5	0	1/5	1/4
5	1/4	1/3	1/4	1/5	0	1/5
6	1/5	1/4	1/3	1/4	1/5	0

BOX 4.8 Complementary Distance Matrix Elements of Sample Chemicals

n-Butane

	1	2	3	4
1	0	3	2	1
2	3	0	3	2
3	2	3	0	3
4	1	2	3	0

Methylcyclopropane

	1	2	3	4
1	0	2	1	1
2	2	0	2	2
3	1	2	0	2
4	1	2	2	0

h. Detour matrix

$$[\Delta(G)]_{ij} = \max[l(p_{ij})] \quad \text{if } i \neq j \\ = 0 \quad \text{if } i = j \tag{4.11}$$

where p_{ij} is the path, $l(p_{ij})$ refers to the length of the path, and $\max[l(p_{ij})]$ corresponds to the longest path between vertices i and j. Usually the longest distance in a graph is termed *elongation* and the length is called the *detour distance.* The longest path connected by vertices i and j is also known as the *detour-path* (Box 4.10).

A detour-complement matrix can be obtained by applying a similar operation, as in the case of distance-complement matrix.

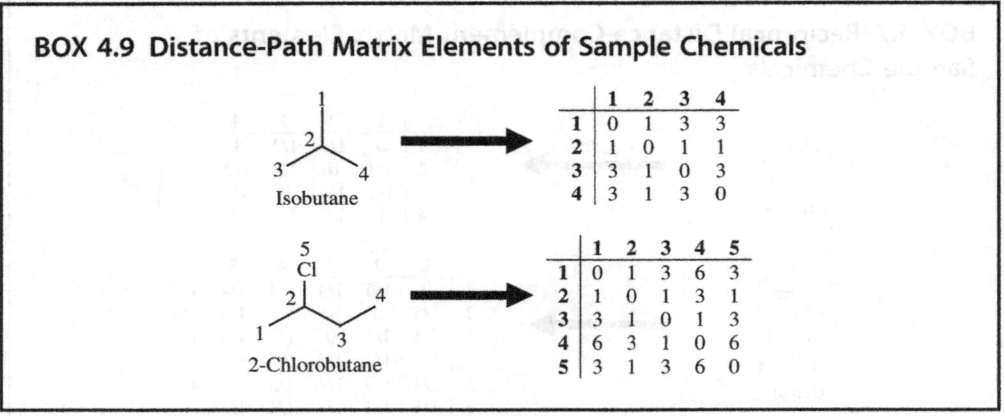

BOX 4.9 Distance-Path Matrix Elements of Sample Chemicals

	1	2	3	4
1	0	1	3	3
2	1	0	1	1
3	3	1	0	3
4	3	1	3	0

	1	2	3	4	5
1	0	1	3	6	3
2	1	0	1	3	1
3	3	1	0	1	3
4	6	3	1	0	6
5	3	1	3	6	0

BOX 4.10 Detour Matrix Elements of Sample Chemicals

Isopentane

	1	2	3	4	5
1	0	1	2	3	2
2	1	0	1	2	1
3	2	1	0	1	2
4	3	2	1	0	3
5	2	1	2	3	0

Mehtylcyclobutane

	1	2	3	4	5
1	0	3	2	3	1
2	3	0	3	2	4
3	2	3	0	3	3
4	3	2	3	0	4
5	1	4	3	4	0

i. Reverse detour matrix

$$[R\,\Delta(G)]_{ij} = d_{\max} - [\Delta(G)]_{ij} \quad \text{if } i \neq j$$
$$= 0 \quad \text{if } i = j \tag{4.12}$$

where $d_{\max}$ is the longest detour distance in a connected molecular graph (Box 4.11).

j. Detour-distance matrix

Such a matrix contains information about both the distance and the detour matrices.

$$[\Delta - D]_{ij} = [\Delta(G)]_{ij} \quad \text{if } i < j$$
$$= [D(G)]_{ij} \quad \text{if } i > j \tag{4.13}$$
$$= 0 \quad \text{if } i = j$$

where $\Delta(G)_{ij}$ and $D(G)_{ij}$ present the elements of detour and distance matrices, respectively. This represents that the elements of the matrix in the upper half (triangle, above diagonal) are those of the detour matrix, and the lower half (triangle) corresponds to the distance matrix (Box 4.12).

k. Laplacian matrix

$$[L]_{ij} = \deg_i \quad \text{if } i = j$$
$$= -1 \quad \text{if } i \text{ and } j \text{ are adjacent} \tag{4.14}$$
$$= 0 \quad \text{if } e_{ij} \notin E(G)$$

where $\deg_i$ corresponds to the degree of the ith vertex (atom). A vertex degree matrix (Δ) using the element $\deg_i$ can be defined as follows:

$$[\Delta] = \begin{cases} \deg(i) & \text{if } i = j \\ 0 & \text{otherwise} \end{cases} \tag{4.15}$$

BOX 4.11 Reverse Detour Matrix Elements of Sample Chemicals

Isopentane

	1	2	3	4	5
1	0	2	1	0	1
2	2	0	2	1	2
3	1	2	0	2	1
4	0	1	2	0	0
5	1	2	1	0	0

Mehtylcyclobutane

	1	2	3	4	5
1	0	1	2	1	3
2	1	0	1	2	0
3	2	1	0	1	1
4	1	2	1	0	0
5	3	0	1	0	0

BOX 4.12 Detour-Distance Matrix Elements of Sample Chemicals

Isopentane

	1	2	3	4	5
1	0	1	2	3	2
2	1	0	1	2	1
3	2	1	0	1	2
4	3	2	1	0	3
5	2	1	2	3	0

Mehtylcyclobutane

	1	2	3	4	5
1	0	3	2	3	1
2	1	0	3	2	4
3	2	1	0	3	3
4	1	2	1	0	4
5	1	2	3	2	0

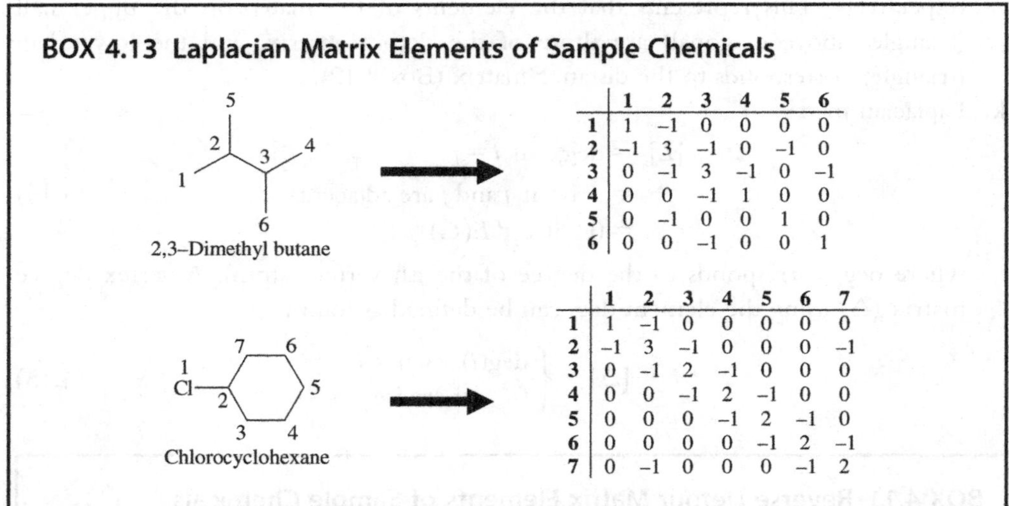

BOX 4.13 Laplacian Matrix Elements of Sample Chemicals

	1	2	3	4	5	6
1	1	−1	0	0	0	0
2	−1	3	−1	0	−1	0
3	0	−1	3	−1	0	−1
4	0	0	−1	1	0	0
5	0	−1	0	0	1	0
6	0	0	−1	0	0	1

	1	2	3	4	5	6	7
1	1	−1	0	0	0	0	0
2	−1	3	−1	0	0	0	−1
3	0	−1	2	−1	0	0	0
4	0	0	−1	2	−1	0	0
5	0	0	0	−1	2	−1	0
6	0	0	0	0	−1	2	−1
7	0	−1	0	0	0	−1	2

where Δ is a diagonal matrix. It can be noted that the Laplacian matrix is sometimes also termed the *Kirchhoff matrix*, owing to its contribution to the matrix-tree theorem and to electrical network graphs of Kirchhoff (Box 4.13).

1. Resistance distance matrix

$$[\Omega(G)]_{ij} = \omega_{ij} \quad \text{if } i \neq j$$
$$= 0 \quad \text{if } i = j \qquad (4.16)$$

Here, ω_{ij} represents the resistance distance between vertices i and j in the connected molecular graph G. This matrix has been developed based on the concept

BOX 4.14 Resistance Distance Matrix Elements of a Sample Chemical

3 4
2 1
Cyclobutane

	1	2	3	4
1	0	3/4	1	3/4
2	3/4	0	3/4	1
3	1	3/4	0	3/4
4	3/4	1	3/4	0

BOX 4.15 Szeged Matrix Elements of a Sample Chemical

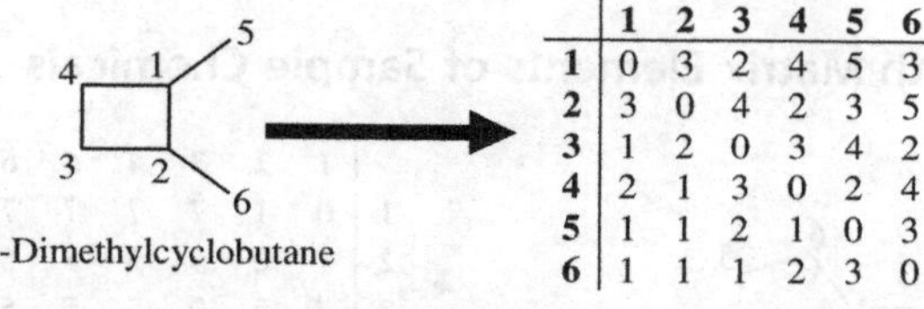

	1	2	3	4	5	6
1	0	3	2	4	5	3
2	3	0	4	2	3	5
3	1	2	0	3	4	2
4	2	1	3	0	2	4
5	1	1	2	1	0	3
6	1	1	1	2	3	0

of resistive electrical network, where graph vertices correspond to unit resistors, and the resistance distance is presented by the graph theoretical distance. The value of $[\Omega]_{ij}$ equals the sum of resistances along vertices i and j for an acyclic system, while for a cyclic system, Kirchhoff's laws are advised (Box 4.14).

The construction of a resistance distance matrix involves several steps: namely, formation of Laplacian matrix, assumption of an auxiliary matrix (all elements are unity), followed by summation and matrix inverse operations, as described in the literature [17].

m. Szeged matrix

$$[\mathrm{Sz}]_{ij} = n_{ij} \quad \text{if } i \neq j \\ = 0 \quad \text{if } i = j \tag{4.17}$$

where the number of vertices closer to i is represented by n_{ij} (Box 4.15).

n. Cluj matrix

$$[\mathrm{CJ}_u(G)]_{ij} = N_{i,p(ij)} \quad \text{if } i \neq j \\ = 0 \quad \text{if } i = j \tag{4.18}$$

where $N_{i,p(ij)}$ is the number of vertices lying closer to i after the removal of any internal vertices that corresponds to path $p(i,j)$ (Box 4.16).

BOX 4.16 Cluj Matrix Elements of a Sample Chemical

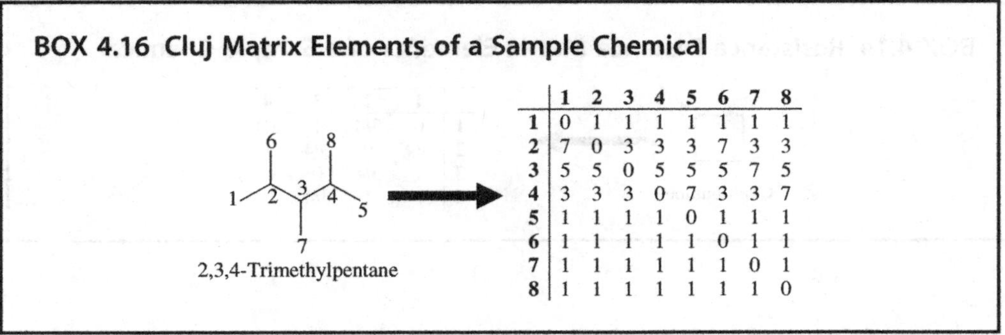

	1	2	3	4	5	6	7	8
1	0	1	1	1	1	1	1	1
2	7	0	3	3	3	7	3	3
3	5	5	0	5	5	5	7	5
4	3	3	3	0	7	3	3	7
5	1	1	1	1	0	1	1	1
6	1	1	1	1	1	0	1	1
7	1	1	1	1	1	1	0	1
8	1	1	1	1	1	1	1	0

BOX 4.17 All Path Matrix Elements of Sample Chemicals

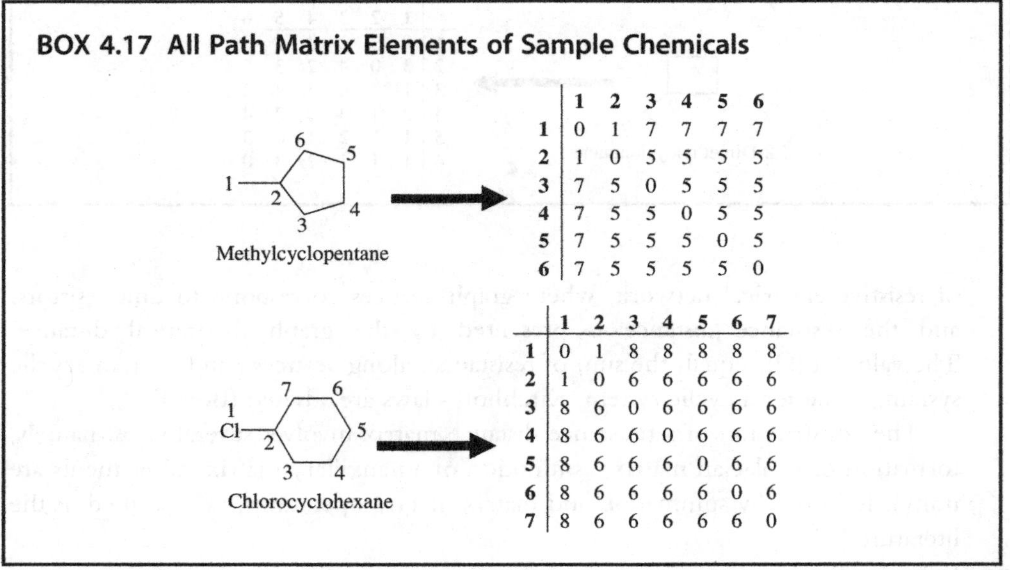

	1	2	3	4	5	6
1	0	1	7	7	7	7
2	1	0	5	5	5	5
3	7	5	0	5	5	5
4	7	5	5	0	5	5
5	7	5	5	5	0	5
6	7	5	5	5	5	0

	1	2	3	4	5	6	7
1	0	1	8	8	8	8	8
2	1	0	6	6	6	6	6
3	8	6	0	6	6	6	6
4	8	6	6	0	6	6	6
5	8	6	6	6	0	6	6
6	8	6	6	6	6	0	6
7	8	6	6	6	6	6	0

o. All path matrix

$$[\mathrm{AP}]_{ij} = \sum |p(i,j)| \quad \text{if } i \neq j \\ = 0 \quad \text{if } i = j \tag{4.19}$$

where the path length between vertices i and j is denoted by $|p(i, j)|$. The elements of this matrix give the value of all path counts possible between vertices i and j. This matrix gives a measure of total path count in a graph theoretic problem. It is quite obvious from the definition that for an acyclic graph, this matrix will be identical to that of a vertex-based distance matrix (Box 4.17).

4.4 TOPOLOGICAL INDICES

4.4.1 The context and formalism

In order to develop mathematical correlation for a set of samples, one needs to have two important components: a dependent variable and a set of independent variables. The central axiom of QSAR lies in establishing a correlation between chemical responses, as dependent variables, and descriptors, as independent features. Since QSAR analysis attempts to establish a chemical relationship, these independent variables are the numbers that are either experimentally derived properties or theoretically computed features. Topological indices are theoretically derived chemical features used for developing predictive correlation models, thereby exploring the responsible chemical information.

Topology is originally a mathematical concept, and the term has a relationship to "rubber sheet geometry." This means that the surface of a topological object behaves as an elastic rubber, and it can retain its property after being subjected to various force operations like twisting, bending, and pulling. but not tearing. The chemical structure representation that gives information regarding the number of elements and their connectivity is considered as the topological representation, and any independent variable derived thereof can be broadly defined as the topological indices. We have already mentioned that chemical graphs form the representational basis for topological indices. Topological indices represent the graphical properties that are conserved by graph theoretic isomorphism, meaning that the properties with identical values for isomorphic graphs are being preserved. Since the topological indices are derived from 2D-graph theoretic presentation, they are assumed to reflect changes made with respect to 2D-graphical features. In other words, the topological indices portray changes in size, shape, branching, symmetry, and cyclicity of a molecular structure. From the viewpoint of chemical encoding, topological indices comprise two major classes [21]:

1. Topostructural indices: They focus on adjacency and distance (graph theoretic) among atoms.
2. Topochemical indices: Along with topology, they consider specific chemical information like atom identity, state of hybridization, and number of core or valence electron.

In this text, we are using the term *topological index* to refer to both of them; that is, topostructural and topochemical indices. Classification can also be made with respect to the complexity and enrichment obtained with the historical development of such parameters. The topological indices have come across a long way since the time of their introduction. Research on the development of topological indices has been directed toward incorporating more complex information in newer parameters and overcoming loopholes in the older ones. A torrential amount of research on this matter has led to the development of several thousand topological indices to date.

It is beyond the scope of this chapter to enlighten all such indices developed hitherto. Instead, we would like to present some basic and mostly used parameters so that the reader can have an idea how such indices are defined from the basis of simple 2D graphs.

Topological indices play an essential as well as a memorable role concerning QSAR descriptors since they are the first theoretically defined predictor variables used in predictive modeling analysis. Following the emergence of chemical graph theory, scientists came up with the idea of (initially) applying algebraic operators on the graph matrix in order to get rational numbers to be used as independent variables in QSAR analysis. There was a growing interest in considering the number of carbon atoms of hydrocarbons as graph–theoretical invariant. It was Kopp [22] who attempted to determine specific volumes and densities of molecules by summing atoms or vertices (that later became known) of different kinds. In 1947, Wiener [23] and Platt [24] were the first to come up with graph theoretical indices for modeling the boiling point of hydrocarbons. Following this inception, a good amount of research was done on this topic in the 1960s and 1970s, giving rise to a number of descriptors [25–29]. It is beyond the scope of this discussion to furnish elaborate details on all the different topological indices, and hence omission of any specific index should be considered unintentional. Definitions of some basic topological indices, with suitable examples, are given in the next sections.

4.4.2 Wiener, Platt, Hosoya, Zagreb, and Balaban indices

4.4.2.1 Wiener index (W)

The Wiener index gives an additive measure of the connections or bonds present in a molecular graph. It can be defined as follows [23]:

$$W = \frac{1}{2}\sum_{i=1}^{N}\sum_{j=1}^{N}\delta_{ij} \tag{4.20}$$

where N is the number of vertices or nonhydrogen atoms and δ_{ij} is the distance of the shortest possible path between vertices i and j. It was first reported as having the ability to develop predictive models on the boiling point of paraffin hydrocarbons. The Wiener index can be computed from the distance matrix of a graph employing a Wiener operator. The formula can be rewritten as

$$W = W_i(D) = \frac{1}{2}\sum_{i=1}^{N}\sum_{j=1}^{N}\delta_{ij} = \sum_{k=1}^{D}{}^{k}f\cdot k \tag{4.21}$$

where W_i is the Wiener operator, D is the maximum topological distance in the molecular graph, and ${}^{k}f$ is the number of distances in the graph having kth order.

It might be noted that since the Wiener index deals with a symmetric matrix, the elements of the matrix above and below the diagonal contains the same elements, which is nullified by multiplying by 1/2 (Box 4.18).

From these examples, it may be observed that the Wiener index can be obtained by performing individual summation of the row elements of the matrix, followed by summation of all the row values and then dividing by 2.

4.4.2.2 Platt number (F)

The Platt number is obtained from an addition operation on the edge-adjacency matrix of a molecular graph. It is also known as the *total-edge-adjacency index* (A_E). This number [24] can be defined as

$$F = \sum_{i=1}^{B} \sum_{j=1}^{B} [E]_{ij} \tag{4.22}$$

where B is the number of bonds or edges and E represents an edge. John Platt reported this topological parameter while studying the influence of neighbor bonds on additive bond properties of paraffin hydrocarbons (Box 4.19).

4.4.2.3 Hosoya index (Z)

The Hosoya index can be defined as [30]

$$Z = \sum_{k=0}^{n/2} a(G, k) \tag{4.23}$$

where n is the number of vertices in the molecular graph G and $a(G, k)$ refers to the number of ways of choosing k edges of the graph such that no two of them are adjacent. In other words, it corresponds to the number of k matchings in the molecular graph. The phrase $a(G, k)$ is also called the *nonadjacent number.* For a given chemical graph, $a(G, 0) = 1$.

The Hosoya Z index reflects molecular size, branching, and ring closure of an analyzed chemical structure (Box 4.20).

4.4.2.4 Zagreb index

The Zagreb index is a topological index defined and described on the basis of the vertex degree of atoms in the molecular graph [31]:

$$\text{Zagreb} = \sum_{i=1}^{N} \delta_i^2 \tag{4.24}$$

where δ_i corresponds to the vertex degree of the ith vertex for a molecular graph comprising N number of vertices. The Zagreb index is related to molecular branching for an isomeric series of compounds (Box 4.21).

BOX 4.18 Wiener Index Computation for Sample Molecules

Molecule:

Isopentane (2-methylbutane)

Matrix elements:

	1	2	3	4	5	Σ
1	0	1	2	3	2	8
2	1	0	1	2	1	5
3	2	1	0	1	2	6
4	3	2	1	0	3	9
5	2	1	2	3	0	8
					Σ	36

$W = 36/2 = 18$

Computation of the index:

$$W = \frac{1}{2} \times \left\{ \begin{array}{l} (0+1+2+3+2)+(1+0+1+2+1) \\ +(2+1+0+1+2)+(3+2+1+0+3) \\ +(2+1+2+3+0) \end{array} \right\}$$

$$= \frac{1}{2} \times 36 = 18$$

Molecule:

Phenol

Matrix elements:

	1	2	3	4	5	6	7	Σ
1	0	1	2	3	4	3	2	15
2	1	0	1	2	3	2	1	10
3	2	1	0	1	2	3	2	11
4	3	2	1	0	1	2	3	12
5	4	3	2	1	0	1	2	13
6	3	2	3	2	1	0	1	12
7	2	1	2	3	2	1	0	11
							Σ	84

$W = 84/2 = 42$

Computation of the index:

$$W = \frac{1}{2} \times \left\{ \begin{array}{l} (0+1+2+3+4+3+2)+(1+0+1+2+3+2+1) \\ +(2+1+0+1+2+3+2)+(3+2+1+0+1+2+3) \\ +(4+3+2+1+0+1+2)+(3+2+3+2+1+0+1) \\ (2+1+2+3+2+1+0) \end{array} \right\}$$

$$= \frac{1}{2} \times 84 = 42$$

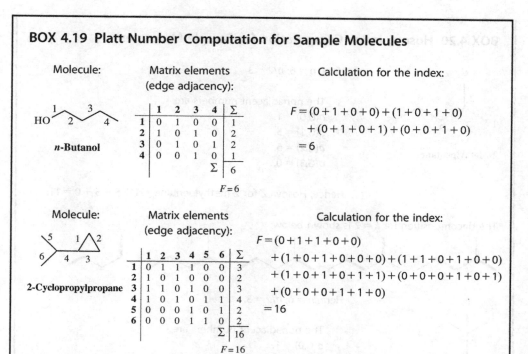

BOX 4.19 Platt Number Computation for Sample Molecules

Molecule: Matrix elements (edge adjacency): Calculation for the index:

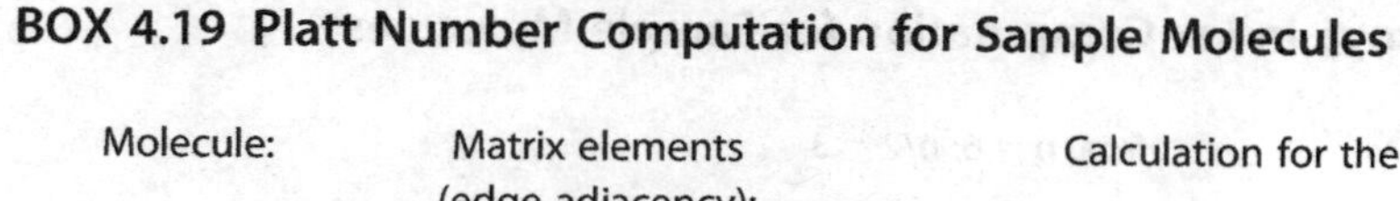

	1	2	3	4	Σ
1	0	1	0	0	1
2	1	0	1	0	2
3	0	1	0	1	2
4	0	0	1	0	1
				Σ	6

$F=6$

$$F=(0+1+0+0)+(1+0+1+0)+(0+1+0+1)+(0+0+1+0)=6$$

Molecule: Matrix elements (edge adjacency): Calculation for the index:

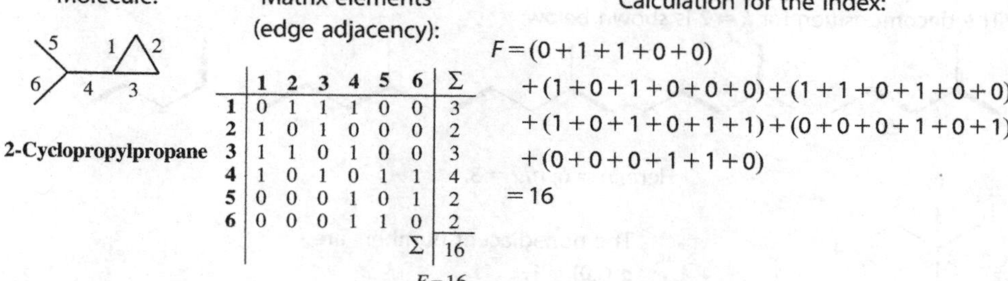

	1	2	3	4	5	6	Σ
1	0	1	1	1	0	0	3
2	1	0	1	0	0	0	2
3	1	1	0	1	0	0	3
4	1	0	1	0	1	1	4
5	0	0	0	1	0	1	2
6	0	0	0	1	1	0	2
						Σ	16

$F=16$

$$F=(0+1+1+0+0)+(1+0+1+0+0+0)+(1+1+0+1+0+0)+(1+0+1+0+1+1)+(0+0+0+1+0+1)+(0+0+0+1+1+0)=16$$

4.4.2.5 Balaban index (J)

The Balaban index can be defined as follows [32]:

$$J=\frac{M}{\mu+1}\sum_{\text{all edges}}(\delta_i\delta_j)^{-0.5} \tag{4.25}$$

where M is the number of edges, μ represents cyclomatic number, δ_i and δ_j represent vertex-distance degrees of the adjacent vertices, and δ_i can be defined as $\delta_i=\sum_{j=1}^{A}\delta_{ij}$, where A is the number of vertices. This index can be computed from the distance matrix of the molecular graph (Box 4.22).

4.4.3 Molecular connectivity indices

Connectivity indices present one of the major developments in the realm of topological indices and are widely employed for modeling purposes. These are computed using the vertex degree of atoms in the H-suppressed molecular graph. Molecular connectivity indices are presented by the Greek alphabet χ (chi).

BOX 4.20 Hosoya Index Computation for Sample Molecules

2-Methylpentane

Here, $n = 6$; $n/2 = 3$

The nonadjacent numbers are:
$a(G,0) = 1.$
$a(G,1) = 5.$
$a(G,2) = 5.$
$a(G,3) = 0.$

Hence, Hosoya Z for 2-methylpentane $= 1 + 5 + 5 + 0 = 11$.

The decomposition for $k = 2$ is shown below:

2,2-Dimethylbutane

Here, $n = 6$; $n/2 = 3$.

The nonadjacent numbers are:
$a(G,0) = 1.$
$a(G,1) = 6.$
$a(G,2) = 3.$
$a(G,3) = 0.$

Hence, Hosoya Z for 2,2-dimethylbutane $= 1 + 6 + 3 + 0 = 10$.

The decomposition for $k = 2$ is:

4.4.3.1 Randić connectivity index

The Randić connectivity index, also known as the *connectivity index* or *branching index*, was the first proposed connectivity index. It can be defined as [33]

$$\chi_R = {}^1\chi = \sum_{i=1}^{n-1} \sum_{j=i+1}^{n} a_{ij} \cdot (\delta_i \cdot \delta_j)^{-0.5} \tag{4.26}$$

where n is the total number of vertices in the molecular graph, a_{ij} represents the adjacency matrix elements, and δ_i and δ_j are the vertex degree; that is, the number of other vertices attached to vertex i and j, respectively. The term $(\delta_i \cdot \delta_j)^{-0.5}$ applies to each pair of adjacent vertices or edges of the first order and is called *edge connectivity*.

BOX 4.21 Zagreb Index Computation for Sample Molecules

2,3,4-Trimethyl pentane

Vertex	1	2	3	4	5	6	7	8
δ_i	1	3	3	3	1	1	1	1

$$\text{Zagreb} = 1^2 + 3^2 + 3^2 + 3^2 + 1^2 + 1^2 + 1^2 + 1^2 = 32$$

Acetyl salicylic acid (aspirin)

Vertex	1	2	3	4	5	6	7	8	9	10	11	12	13
δ_i	3	3	2	2	2	2	1	3	1	2	3	1	1

$$\text{Zagreb} = 3^2 + 3^2 + 2^2 + 2^2 + 2^2 + 2^2 + 1^2 + 3^2 + 1^2 + 2^2 + 3^2 + 1^2 + 1^2 = 60$$

However, it can be extended to more than two adjacent vertices as well. The Randić connectivity index principally accounts for branching in a molecular graph (Box 4.23).

4.4.3.2 Kier and Hall's connectivity index

Following Randić's index, Kier and Hall developed a general formalism and provided a more detailed insight to compute zeroth- as well as higher-order connectivity indices. These are called *molecular connectivity* or *Kier and Hall connectivity indices* [26,34]. The equations to calculate zeroth-, first-, and second-order connectivity indices, along with the generalized expression for higher-order indices, are furnished here:

$$^0\chi = \sum_{i=1}^{n} \delta_i^{-0.5} \tag{4.27}$$

$$^1\chi = \sum_{b=1}^{B} (\delta_i \cdot \delta_j)_b^{-0.5} \tag{4.28}$$

$$^2\chi = \sum_{k=1}^{^2P} (\delta_i \cdot \delta_l \cdot \delta_j)_k^{-0.5} \tag{4.29}$$

$$^m\chi_t = \sum_{k=1}^{K} \left(\prod_{i=1}^{n} \delta_i \right)_k^{-0.5} \tag{4.30}$$

BOX 4.22 Balaban Index Computation for Sample Molecules

Molecule:

5, 4, 3, 2, 1, 6

2,3-Dimethyl butane

Matrix representation:

	1	2	3	4	5	6	Σ
1	0	1	2	3	2	3	11
2	1	0	1	2	1	2	7
3	2	1	0	1	2	1	7
4	3	2	1	0	3	2	11
5	2	1	2	3	0	3	11
6	3	2	1	2	3	0	11

Computation of the index:

Here,
$M = 5$, $\mu = 0$.

$$J = 5 \times \left\{ \begin{array}{l} (\delta_1 \cdot \delta_2)^{-0.5} + (\delta_2 \cdot \delta_5)^{-0.5} + (\delta_2 \cdot \delta_3)^{-0.5} \\ + (\delta_3 \cdot \delta_4)^{-0.5} + (\delta_3 \cdot \delta_6)^{-0.5} \end{array} \right\}$$

$$= 5 \times \left\{ \begin{array}{l} (11 \times 7)^{-0.5} + (7 \times 11)^{-0.5} + (7 \times 7)^{-0.5} \\ + (7 \times 11)^{-0.5} + (7 \times 11)^{-0.5} \end{array} \right\} = 2.9934$$

Molecule:

1, 2, 3, 4, 5, 6

Methyl cyclopentane

Matrix representation:

	1	2	3	4	5	6	Σ
1	0	1	2	3	3	2	11
2	1	0	1	2	2	1	7
3	2	1	0	1	2	2	8
4	3	2	1	0	1	2	9
5	3	2	2	1	0	1	9
6	2	1	2	2	1	0	8

Computation of the index:

Here,
$M = 6$, $\mu = 1$.

$$J = \tfrac{6}{2} \times \left\{ \begin{array}{l} (\delta_1 \cdot \delta_2)^{-0.5} + (\delta_2 \cdot \delta_3)^{-0.5} + (\delta_2 \cdot \delta_6)^{-0.5} + (\delta_3 \cdot \delta_4)^{-0.5} \\ + (\delta_4 \cdot \delta_5)^{-0.5} + (\delta_5 \cdot \delta_6)^{-0.5} \end{array} \right\}$$

$$= 3 \times \left\{ \begin{array}{l} (11 \times 7)^{-0.5} + (7 \times 8)^{-0.5} + (7 \times 8)^{-0.5} + (8 \times 9)^{-0.5} \\ + (9 \times 9)^{-0.5} + (9 \times 8)^{-0.5} \end{array} \right\}$$

$$= 2.1841$$

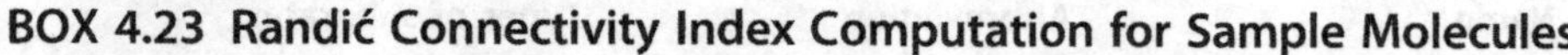

BOX 4.23 Randić Connectivity Index Computation for Sample Molecules

2,5-Dimethylhexane

Atom	1	2	3	4	5	6	7	8
δ	1	3	2	2	3	1	1	1

For 1st order,

$$\begin{aligned}{}^{1}\chi &= (\delta_1 \cdot \delta_2)^{-0.5} + (\delta_2 \cdot \delta_3)^{-0.5} + (\delta_3 \cdot \delta_4)^{-0.5} + (\delta_4 \cdot \delta_5)^{-0.5} \\ &\quad + (\delta_5 \cdot \delta_6)^{-0.5} + (\delta_2 \cdot \delta_7)^{-0.5} + (\delta_5 \cdot \delta_8)^{-0.5} \\ &= (1 \times 3)^{-0.5} + (3 \times 2)^{-0.5} + (2 \times 2)^{-0.5} + (2 \times 3)^{-0.5} + (3 \times 1)^{-0.5} \\ &\quad + (3 \times 1)^{-0.5} + (3 \times 1)^{-0.5} \\ &= 3.6258\end{aligned}$$

2-Cyclohexylopropane

Atom	1	2	3	4	5	6	7	8	9
δ	1	3	1	3	2	2	2	2	2

For 1st order,

$$\begin{aligned}{}^{1}\chi &= (\delta_1 \cdot \delta_2)^{-0.5} + (\delta_2 \cdot \delta_3)^{-0.5} + (\delta_2 \cdot \delta_4)^{-0.5} + (\delta_4 \cdot \delta_5)^{-0.5} + (\delta_5 \cdot \delta_6)^{-0.5} \\ &\quad + (\delta_6 \cdot \delta_7)^{-0.5} + (\delta_7 \cdot \delta_8)^{-0.5} + (\delta_8 \cdot \delta_9)^{-0.5} + (\delta_4 \cdot \delta_9)^{-0.5} \\ &= (1 \times 3)^{-0.5} + (3 \times 1)^{-0.5} + (3 \times 3)^{-0.5} + (3 \times 2)^{-0.5} + (2 \times 2)^{-0.5} \\ &\quad + (2 \times 2)^{-0.5} + (2 \times 2)^{-0.5} + (2 \times 2)^{-0.5} + (3 \times 2)^{-0.5} \\ &= 4.3045\end{aligned}$$

In these equations, k runs over the mth-order subgraphs comprising n vertices and B edges. The term ${}^{2}P$ refers to a path length of two. K corresponds to the total number of mth-order subgraphs present in the system. The product is considered for the simple vertex degree δ for all the vertices, while the subscript t in the equation of higher-order indices (Eq. (4.29)) corresponds to the type of molecular subgraph. The subgraph types, along with their subscript notation used for Kier and Hall connectivity indices, are presented in Table 4.2. It should be noted that the Kier and Hall connectivity index of the first order is actually the Randić connectivity index.

In order to account for the effects of multiple bonds and heteroatoms in a molecular graph, Kier and Hall incorporated a valence vertex degree (δ^{v}) formalism, which considers the effect of valence shell electrons of an atom. Hence, another

Table 4.2 Various types of subgraphical fragments used to define connectivity indices

Name	Abbreviation or subscript	Types of subgraph
Path	p	
Cluster	c	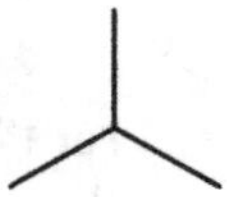
Path-cluster	pc	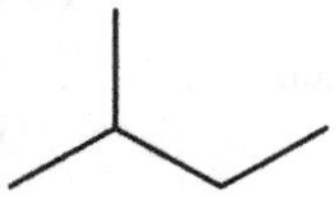
Chain (ring)	ch	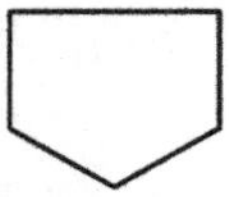

set of similar valence connectivity indices can be defined just by replacing δ with δ^v in Eqs. (4.26–4.29), as follows:

$$ {}^{0}\chi^{v} = \sum_{i=1}^{n} (\delta_i^{v})^{-0.5} \tag{4.31}$$

$$ {}^{1}\chi^{v} = \sum_{b=1}^{B} (\delta_i^{v} \cdot \delta_j^{v})_b^{-0.5} \tag{4.32}$$

$$ {}^{2}\chi^{v} = \sum_{k=1}^{2p} (\delta_i^{v} \cdot \delta_l^{v} \cdot \delta_j^{v})_k^{-0.5} \tag{4.33}$$

$$ {}^{m}\chi_t^{v} = \sum_{k=1}^{K} \left(\prod_{i=1}^{n} \delta_i^{v} \right)_k^{-0.5} \tag{4.34}$$

In these equations, all other terms have the same meaning as before except δ^v. The valence vertex degree of an atom may be defined in the following manner:

$$ \delta_i^{v} = \frac{Z_i^{v} - H}{Z_i - Z_i^{v} - 1} \tag{4.35}$$

where the total number of electrons and the number of electrons present in the valence shell of atom i are presented by the terms Z_i and Z_i^v, respectively; and H denotes the number of hydrogen atoms directly attached to the atom under investigation. The δ^v and ${}^1\chi^v$ values of some sample atoms attached to a carbon atom having $\delta^v = 3$

Table 4.3 δ^v and ${}^1\chi^v$ values of representative atoms attached to a carbon atom having δ^v value = 3

Sl. No.	Atom/Group	Z	Z^v	H	δ^v	${}^1\chi^v$
1	H	1	1	1	$\delta^v(\mathrm{H}) = 0$	${}^1\chi_v(\mathrm{H}) = 0$
2	$-CH_3$	6	4	3	$\delta^v(\mathrm{CH_3}) = \frac{(4-3)}{(6-4-1)} = 1$	${}^1\chi_v(\mathrm{CH_3}) = \frac{1}{\sqrt{(3\times 1)}} = 0.57735$
3	$-CH_2-$	6	4	2	$\delta^v(\mathrm{CH_2}) = \frac{(4-2)}{(6-4-1)} = 2$	${}^1\chi_v(\mathrm{CH_2}) = \frac{1}{\sqrt{(3\times 2)}} = 0.40824$
4	$-NH_2$	7	5	2	$\delta^v(\mathrm{NH_2}) = \frac{(5-2)}{(7-5-1)} = 3$	${}^1\chi_v(\mathrm{NH_2}) = \frac{1}{\sqrt{(3\times 3)}} = 0.33333$
5	$-OH$	8	6	1	$\delta^v(\mathrm{OH}) = \frac{(6-1)}{(8-6-1)} = 5$	${}^1\chi_v(\mathrm{OH}) = \frac{1}{\sqrt{(3\times 5)}} = 0.25819$
6	$=O$	8	6	0	$\delta^v(\mathrm{O}) = \frac{(6-0)}{(8-6-1)} = 6$	${}^1\chi_v(\mathrm{O}) = \frac{1}{\sqrt{(3\times 6)}} = 0.23570$

(e.g., >CH– or –CH=) are listed in Table 4.3. Hence, valence chi indices provide a measure to separate alkenes or alkynes from alkanes composed of the same number of carbon atoms.

Furthermore, Kier and Hall [34] postulated that the addition of the cardinal numbers obtained from δ^v and δ gives a measure of volume of a bonding atom ($\delta^v + \delta$), while their subtraction denotes electronegativity ($\delta^v - \delta$) (Box 4.24).

4.4.4 Kappa shape indices

Kappa shape indices are also known as *Kier shape parameters* [35] and designated by the Greek alphabet κ. The two components that define the Kappa parameters are the number of vertices and the number of desired path lengths of the molecular graph. The Kappa shape parameters for first-, second-, and third-order path lengths can be defined as follows:

$$ {}^1\kappa = 2\times\frac{{}^1P_{max}\times {}^1P_{min}}{({}^1P)^2} = \frac{A\times(A-1)^2}{({}^1P)^2} \tag{4.36}$$

$$ {}^2\kappa = 2\times\frac{{}^2P_{max}\times {}^2P_{min}}{({}^2P)^2} = \frac{(A-1)\times(A-2)^2}{({}^2P)^2} \tag{4.37}$$

$$ \begin{aligned} {}^3\kappa &= 4\times\frac{{}^3P_{max}\times {}^3P_{min}}{({}^3P)^2} = \frac{(A-3)\times(A-2)^2}{({}^3P)^2} \quad \text{for even values of } A\ (A>3) \\ &= \frac{(A-1)\times(A-3)^2}{({}^3P)^2} \quad \text{for odd values of } A\ (A>3) \end{aligned} \tag{4.38}$$

BOX 4.24 Kier and Hall's Connectivity Index Computation for Sample Molecules

2-Methyl-2-butene

Atom	Z	Z^v	H	δ_i	δ_i^v
1	6	4	3	1	$(4-3)/(6-4-1)=1$
2	6	4	0	3	$(4-0)/(6-4-1)=4$
3	6	4	1	2	$(4-1)/(6-4-1)=3$
4	6	4	3	1	$(4-3)/(6-4-1)=1$
5	6	4	3	1	$(4-3)/(6-4-1)=1$

Connectivity indices:

$${}^0\chi = (\delta_1)^{-0.5} + (\delta_2)^{-0.5} + (\delta_3)^{-0.5} + (\delta_4)^{-0.5} + (\delta_5)^{-0.5} = \frac{1}{\sqrt{1}} + \frac{1}{\sqrt{3}} + \frac{1}{\sqrt{2}} + \frac{1}{\sqrt{1}} + \frac{1}{\sqrt{1}} = 4.28446$$

$${}^1\chi = (\delta_1 \cdot \delta_2)^{-0.5} + (\delta_2 \cdot \delta_3)^{-0.5} + (\delta_3 \cdot \delta_4)^{-0.5} + (\delta_2 \cdot \delta_5)^{-0.5} = \frac{1}{\sqrt{(1\times 3)}} + \frac{1}{\sqrt{(3\times 2)}} + \frac{1}{\sqrt{(2\times 1)}} + \frac{1}{\sqrt{(3\times 1)}} = 2.27006$$

$${}^2\chi = (\delta_1 \cdot \delta_2 \cdot \delta_3)^{-0.5} + (\delta_2 \cdot \delta_3 \cdot \delta_4)^{-0.5} + (\delta_1 \cdot \delta_2 \cdot \delta_5)^{-0.5} + (\delta_5 \cdot \delta_2 \cdot \delta_3)^{-0.5} = \frac{1}{\sqrt{(1\times 3\times 2)}} + \frac{1}{\sqrt{(3\times 2\times 1)}} + \frac{1}{\sqrt{(1\times 3\times 1)}} + \frac{1}{\sqrt{(1\times 3\times 2)}} = 1.80210$$

$${}^3\chi_p = (\delta_1 \cdot \delta_2 \cdot \delta_3 \cdot \delta_4)^{-0.5} + (\delta_5 \cdot \delta_2 \cdot \delta_3 \cdot \delta_4)^{-0.5} = \frac{1}{\sqrt{(1\times 3\times 2\times 1)}} + \frac{1}{\sqrt{(1\times 3\times 2\times 1)}} = 0.81650$$

$${}^3\chi_c = (\delta_1 \cdot \delta_2 \cdot \delta_3 \cdot \delta_5)^{-0.5} = \frac{1}{\sqrt{(1\times 3\times 2\times 1)}} = 0.40825$$

$${}^4\chi_{pc} = (\delta_1 \cdot \delta_2 \cdot \delta_3 \cdot \delta_4 \cdot \delta_5)^{-0.5} = \frac{1}{\sqrt{(1\times 3\times 2\times 1\times 1)}} = 0.40825$$

Valence connectivity indices:

$${}^0\chi^v = (\delta_1^v)^{-0.5} + (\delta_2^v)^{-0.5} + (\delta_3^v)^{-0.5} + (\delta_4^v)^{-0.5} + (\delta_5^v)^{-0.5} = \frac{1}{\sqrt{1}} + \frac{1}{\sqrt{4}} + \frac{1}{\sqrt{3}} + \frac{1}{\sqrt{1}} + \frac{1}{\sqrt{1}} = 4.07735$$

$${}^1\chi^v = (\delta_1^v \cdot \delta_2^v)^{-0.5} + (\delta_2^v \cdot \delta_3^v)^{-0.5} + (\delta_3^v \cdot \delta_4^v)^{-0.5} + (\delta_2^v \cdot \delta_5^v)^{-0.5} = \frac{1}{\sqrt{(1\times 4)}} + \frac{1}{\sqrt{(4\times 3)}} + \frac{1}{\sqrt{(3\times 1)}} + \frac{1}{\sqrt{(4\times 1)}} = 1.86603$$

$${}^2\chi^v = (\delta_1^v \cdot \delta_2^v \cdot \delta_3^v)^{-0.5} + (\delta_2^v \cdot \delta_3^v \cdot \delta_4^v)^{-0.5} + (\delta_1^v \cdot \delta_2^v \cdot \delta_5^v)^{-0.5} + (\delta_5^v \cdot \delta_2^v \cdot \delta_3^v)^{-0.5} = \frac{1}{\sqrt{(1\times 4\times 3)}} + \frac{1}{\sqrt{(4\times 3\times 1)}} + \frac{1}{\sqrt{(1\times 4\times 1)}} + \frac{1}{\sqrt{(1\times 4\times 3)}} = 1.36603$$

$${}^3\chi_p^v = (\delta_1^v \cdot \delta_2^v \cdot \delta_3^v \cdot \delta_4^v)^{-0.5} + (\delta_5^v \cdot \delta_2^v \cdot \delta_3^v \cdot \delta_4^v)^{-0.5} = \frac{1}{\sqrt{(1\times 4\times 3\times 1)}} + \frac{1}{\sqrt{(1\times 4\times 3\times 1)}} = 0.57735$$

$${}^3\chi_c^v = (\delta_1^v \cdot \delta_2^v \cdot \delta_3^v \cdot \delta_5^v)^{-0.5} = \frac{1}{\sqrt{(1\times 4\times 3\times 1)}} = 0.28868$$

$${}^4\chi_{pc}^v = (\delta_1^v \cdot \delta_2^v \cdot \delta_3^v \cdot \delta_4^v \cdot \delta_5^v)^{-0.5} = \frac{1}{\sqrt{(1\times 4\times 3\times 1\times 1)}} = 0.28868$$

(Continued)

BOX 4.24 Kier and Hall's Connectivity Index Computation for Sample Molecules—cont'd

${}^2\chi$ and ${}^2\chi^v$ fragments:

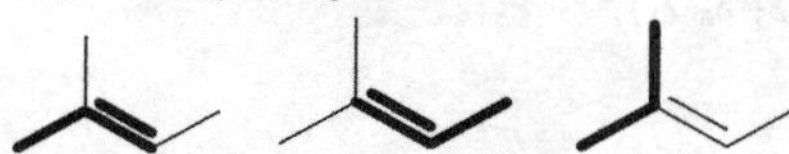

${}^3\chi_p$ and ${}^3\chi_p^v$ fragments:

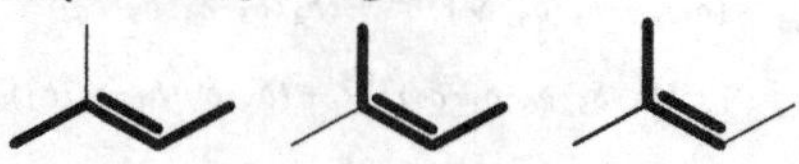

2-Chloro-3-hydroxypyridine

Atom	Z	Z^v	H	δ_i	δ_i^v
1	7	5	0	2	$(5-0)/(7-5-1)=5$
2	6	4	0	3	$(4-0)/(6-4-1)=4$
3	6	4	0	3	$(4-0)/(6-4-1)=4$
4	6	4	1	2	$(4-1)/(6-4-1)=3$
5	6	4	1	2	$(4-1)/(6-4-1)=3$
6	6	4	1	2	$(4-1)/(6-4-1)=3$
7	8	6	1	1	$(6-1)/(8-6-1)=5$
8	17	7	0	1	$(7-0)/(17-7-1)=7/9$

Connectivity indices:

$$
\begin{aligned}
{}^0\chi &= (\delta_1)^{-0.5}+(\delta_2)^{-0.5}+(\delta_3)^{-0.5}+(\delta_4)^{-0.5}+(\delta_5)^{-0.5}+(\delta_6)^{-0.5}+(\delta_7)^{-0.5}+(\delta_8)^{-0.5}\\
&= \tfrac{1}{\sqrt{2}}+\tfrac{1}{\sqrt{3}}+\tfrac{1}{\sqrt{3}}+\tfrac{1}{\sqrt{2}}+\tfrac{1}{\sqrt{2}}+\tfrac{1}{\sqrt{2}}+\tfrac{1}{\sqrt{1}}+\tfrac{1}{\sqrt{1}}=5.98313
\end{aligned}
$$

$$
\begin{aligned}
{}^1\chi &= (\delta_1\cdot\delta_2)^{-0.5}+(\delta_2\cdot\delta_3)^{-0.5}+(\delta_3\cdot\delta_4)^{-0.5}+(\delta_4\cdot\delta_5)^{-0.5}+(\delta_5\cdot\delta_6)^{-0.5}+(\delta_6\cdot\delta_1)^{-0.5}\\
&\quad+(\delta_2\cdot\delta_8)^{-0.5}+(\delta_3\cdot\delta_7)^{-0.5}\\
&= \frac{1}{\sqrt{(2\times3)}}+\frac{1}{\sqrt{(3\times3)}}+\frac{1}{\sqrt{(3\times2)}}+\frac{1}{\sqrt{(2\times2)}}+\frac{1}{\sqrt{(2\times2)}}+\frac{1}{\sqrt{(2\times2)}}\\
&\quad+\frac{1}{\sqrt{(3\times1)}}+\frac{1}{\sqrt{(3\times1)}}=3.80453
\end{aligned}
$$

$$
\begin{aligned}
{}^2\chi &= (\delta_1\cdot\delta_2\cdot\delta_3)^{-0.5}+(\delta_2\cdot\delta_3\cdot\delta_4)^{-0.5}+(\delta_3\cdot\delta_4\cdot\delta_5)^{-0.5}+(\delta_4\cdot\delta_5\cdot\delta_6)^{-0.5}+(\delta_5\cdot\delta_6\cdot\delta_1)^{-0.5}\\
&\quad+(\delta_6\cdot\delta_1\cdot\delta_2)^{-0.5}+(\delta_1\cdot\delta_2\cdot\delta_8)^{-0.5}+(\delta_3\cdot\delta_2\cdot\delta_8)^{-0.5}+(\delta_2\cdot\delta_3\cdot\delta_7)^{-0.5}+(\delta_4\cdot\delta_3\cdot\delta_7)^{-0.5}\\
&= \frac{1}{\sqrt{(2\times3\times3)}}+\frac{1}{\sqrt{(3\times3\times2)}}+\frac{1}{\sqrt{(3\times2\times2)}}+\frac{1}{\sqrt{(2\times2\times2)}}+\frac{1}{\sqrt{(2\times2\times2)}}+\frac{1}{\sqrt{(2\times2\times3)}}\\
&\quad+\frac{1}{\sqrt{0(2\times3\times1)}}+\frac{1}{\sqrt{(3\times3\times1)}}+\frac{1}{\sqrt{(3\times3\times1)}}+\frac{1}{\sqrt{(2\times3\times1)}}=3.23902
\end{aligned}
$$

$$
\begin{aligned}
{}^3\chi_p &= (\delta_1\cdot\delta_2\cdot\delta_3\cdot\delta_4)^{-0.5}+(\delta_2\cdot\delta_3\cdot\delta_4\cdot\delta_5)^{-0.5}+(\delta_3\cdot\delta_4\cdot\delta_5\cdot\delta_6)^{-0.5}+(\delta_4\cdot\delta_5\cdot\delta_6\cdot\delta_1)^{-0.5}\\
&\quad+(\delta_5\cdot\delta_6\cdot\delta_1\cdot\delta_2)^{-0.5}+(\delta_6\cdot\delta_1\cdot\delta_2\cdot\delta_3)^{-0.5}+(\delta_6\cdot\delta_1\cdot\delta_2\cdot\delta_8)^{-0.5}+(\delta_1\cdot\delta_2\cdot\delta_3\cdot\delta_7)^{-0.5}\\
&\quad+(\delta_7\cdot\delta_3\cdot\delta_2\cdot\delta_8)^{-0.5}+(\delta_7\cdot\delta_3\cdot\delta_4\cdot\delta_5)^{-0.5}+(\delta_4\cdot\delta_3\cdot\delta_2\cdot\delta_8)^{-0.5}\\
&= \frac{1}{\sqrt{(2\times3\times3\times2)}}+\frac{1}{\sqrt{(3\times3\times2\times2)}}+\frac{1}{\sqrt{(3\times2\times2\times2)}}+\frac{1}{\sqrt{(2\times2\times2\times2)}}\\
&\quad+\frac{1}{\sqrt{(2\times2\times2\times3)}}+\frac{1}{\sqrt{(2\times2\times3\times3)}}+\frac{1}{\sqrt{(2\times2\times3\times1)}}\\
&\quad+\frac{1}{\sqrt{(2\times3\times3\times1)}}+\frac{1}{\sqrt{(1\times3\times3\times1)}}+\frac{1}{\sqrt{(1\times3\times2\times2)}}\\
&\quad+\frac{1}{\sqrt{(2\times3\times3\times1)}}=2.54034
\end{aligned}
$$

(*Continued*)

BOX 4.24 Kier and Hall's Connectivity Index Computation for Sample Molecules—cont'd

$$^3\chi_c = (\delta_1\cdot\delta_2\cdot\delta_3\cdot\delta_8)^{-0.5} + (\delta_2\cdot\delta_3\cdot\delta_4\cdot\delta_7)^{-0.5} = \frac{1}{\sqrt{(2\times3\times3\times1)}} + \frac{1}{\sqrt{(3\times3\times2\times1)}} = 0.47140$$

$$\begin{aligned}^4\chi_p &= (\delta_1\cdot\delta_2\cdot\delta_3\cdot\delta_4\cdot\delta_5)^{-0.5} + (\delta_2\cdot\delta_3\cdot\delta_4\cdot\delta_5\cdot\delta_6)^{-0.5} + (\delta_3\cdot\delta_4\cdot\delta_5\cdot\delta_6\cdot\delta_1)^{-0.5}\\ &\quad + (\delta_4\cdot\delta_5\cdot\delta_6\cdot\delta_1\cdot\delta_2)^{-0.5} + (\delta_5\cdot\delta_6\cdot\delta_1\cdot\delta_2\cdot\delta_3)^{-0.5}\\ &\quad + (\delta_5\cdot\delta_6\cdot\delta_1\cdot\delta_2\cdot\delta_8)^{-0.5}\\ &\quad + (\delta_6\cdot\delta_1\cdot\delta_2\cdot\delta_3\cdot\delta_4)^{-0.5}\\ &\quad + (\delta_6\cdot\delta_1\cdot\delta_2\cdot\delta_3\cdot\delta_7)^{-0.5} + (\delta_8\cdot\delta_2\cdot\delta_3\cdot\delta_4\cdot\delta_5)^{-0.5}\\ &\quad + (\delta_7\cdot\delta_3\cdot\delta_4\cdot\delta_5\cdot\delta_6)^{-0.5}\\ &= \frac{1}{\sqrt{(2\times3\times3\times2\times2)}} + \frac{1}{\sqrt{(3\times3\times2\times2\times2)}} + \frac{1}{\sqrt{(3\times2\times2\times2\times2)}}\\ &\quad + \frac{1}{\sqrt{(2\times2\times2\times2\times3)}} + \frac{1}{\sqrt{(2\times2\times2\times3\times3)}} + \frac{1}{\sqrt{(2\times2\times2\times3\times1)}}\\ &\quad + \frac{1}{\sqrt{(2\times2\times3\times3\times2)}} + \frac{1}{\sqrt{(2\times2\times3\times3\times1)}} + \frac{1}{\sqrt{(1\times3\times3\times2\times2)}}\\ &\quad + \frac{1}{\sqrt{(1\times3\times2\times2\times2)}} = 1.50166\end{aligned}$$

$$\begin{aligned}^4\chi_{pc} &= (\delta_6\cdot\delta_1\cdot\delta_2\cdot\delta_3\cdot\delta_8)^{-0.5} + (\delta_1\cdot\delta_2\cdot\delta_3\cdot\delta_4\cdot\delta_7)^{-0.5} + (\delta_1\cdot\delta_2\cdot\delta_3\cdot\delta_4\cdot\delta_8)^{-0.5}\\ &\quad + (\delta_2\cdot\delta_3\cdot\delta_4\cdot\delta_5\cdot\delta_7)^{-0.5} + (\delta_4\cdot\delta_3\cdot\delta_2\cdot\delta_8\cdot\delta_7)^{-0.5} + (\delta_1\cdot\delta_2\cdot\delta_3\cdot\delta_7\cdot\delta_8)^{-0.5}\\ &= \frac{1}{\sqrt{(2\times2\times3\times3\times1)}} + \frac{1}{\sqrt{(2\times3\times3\times2\times1)}} + \frac{1}{\sqrt{(2\times3\times3\times2\times1)}}\\ &\quad + \frac{1}{\sqrt{(3\times3\times2\times2\times1)}} + \frac{1}{\sqrt{(2\times3\times3\times1\times1)}} + \frac{1}{\sqrt{(2\times3\times3\times1\times1)}} = 1.13807\end{aligned}$$

Valence connectivity indices:

By using similar sub-structural divisions like that of normal connectivity indices and just by replacing δ with δ^v the following results can be obtained:

$$^0\chi_v = (5)^{-0.5} + (4)^{-0.5} + (4)^{-0.5} + (3)^{-0.5} + (3)^{-0.5} + (3)^{-0.5} + (5)^{-0.5} + (7/9)^{-0.5} = 4.76037$$

$$\begin{aligned}^1\chi_v &= (5\times4)^{-0.5} + (4\times4)^{-0.5} + (4\times3)^{-0.5} + (3\times3)^{-0.5} + (3\times3)^{-0.5} + (3\times5)^{-0.5}\\ &\quad + (4\times7/9)^{-0.5} + (4\times5)^{-0.5} = 2.47770\end{aligned}$$

$$\begin{aligned}^2\chi_v &= (5\times4\times4)^{-0.5} + (4\times4\times3)^{-0.5} + (4\times3\times3)^{-0.5} + (3\times3\times3)^{-0.5}\\ &\quad + (3\times3\times5)^{-0.5} + (3\times5\times4)^{-0.5}\\ &\quad + (5\times4\times7/9)^{-0.5} + (4\times4\times7/9)^{-0.5}\\ &\quad + (4\times4\times5)^{-0.5} + (3\times4\times5)^{-0.5} = 1.67135\end{aligned}$$

$$\begin{aligned}^3\chi_p^v &= (5\times4\times4\times3)^{-0.5} + (4\times4\times3\times3)^{-0.5} + (4\times3\times3\times3)^{-0.5} + (3\times3\times3\times5)^{-0.5}\\ &\quad + (3\times3\times5\times4)^{-0.5} + (3\times5\times4\times4)^{-0.5} + (3\times5\times4\times7/9)^{-0.5} + (5\times4\times4\times5)^{-0.5}\\ &\quad + (5\times4\times4\times7/9)^{-0.5} + (5\times4\times3\times3)^{-0.5} + (3\times4\times4\times7/9)^{-0.5} = 1.03062\end{aligned}$$

$$^3\chi_c^v = (5\times4\times4\times7/9)^{-0.5} + (4\times4\times3\times5)^{-0.5} = 0.191323$$

(Continued)

BOX 4.24 Kier and Hall's Connectivity Index Computation for Sample Molecules—cont'd

$$^4\chi_p^v = (5\times4\times4\times3\times3)^{-0.5} + (4\times4\times3\times3\times3)^{-0.5} + (4\times3\times3\times3\times5)^{-0.5}$$
$$+ (3\times3\times3\times5\times4)^{-0.5} + (3\times3\times5\times4\times4)^{-0.5} + (3\times3\times5\times4\times7/9)^{-0.5}$$
$$+ (3\times5\times4\times4\times3)^{-0.5} + (3\times5\times4\times4\times5)^{-0.5}$$
$$+ (7/9\times4\times4\times3\times3)^{-0.5} + (5\times4\times3\times3\times3)^{-0.5} = 0.49689$$

$$^4\chi_{pc}^v = (3\times5\times4\times4\times7/9)^{-0.5} + (5\times4\times4\times3\times5)^{-0.5} + (5\times4\times4\times3\times7/9)^{-0.5}$$
$$+ (4\times4\times3\times3\times5)^{-0.5} + (3\times4\times4\times7/9\times5)^{-0.5} + (5\times4\times4\times5\times7/9)^{-0.5}$$
$$= 0.3424$$

We restrict this example up to fourth order. However, fifth and sixth order connections for the compound 2-chloro-3-hydroxypyridine can also be explored by using the same concept of graph division.

$^2\chi$ & $^2\chi^v$ fragments:

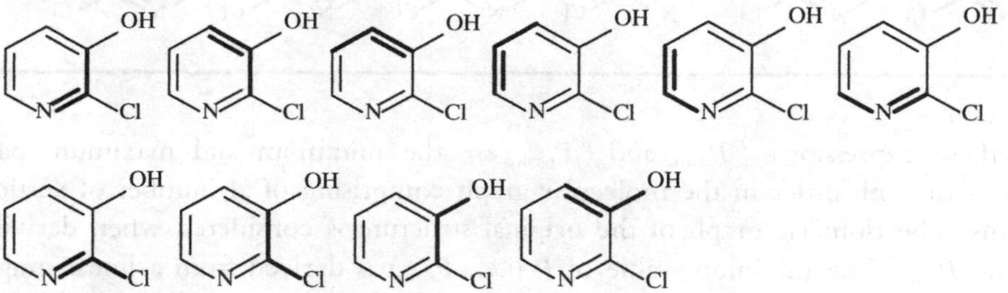

$^3\chi_p$ & $^3\chi_p^v$ fragments:

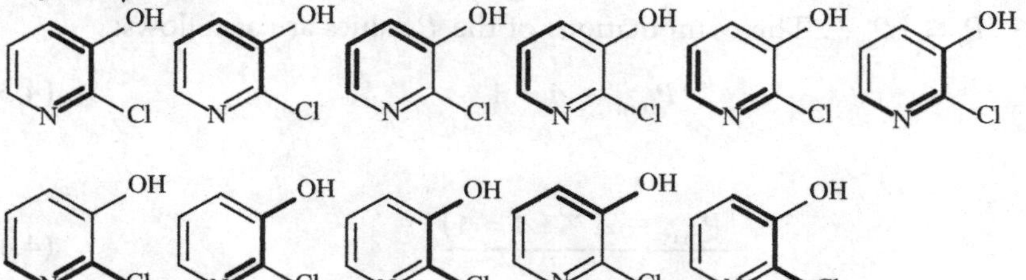

$^3\chi_c$ & $^3\chi_c^v$ fragments:

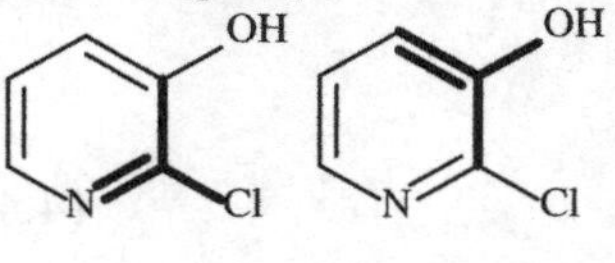

(*Continued*)

BOX 4.24 Kier and Hall's Connectivity Index Computation for Sample Molecules—cont'd

$^4\chi_p$ & $^4\chi_p^v$ fragments:

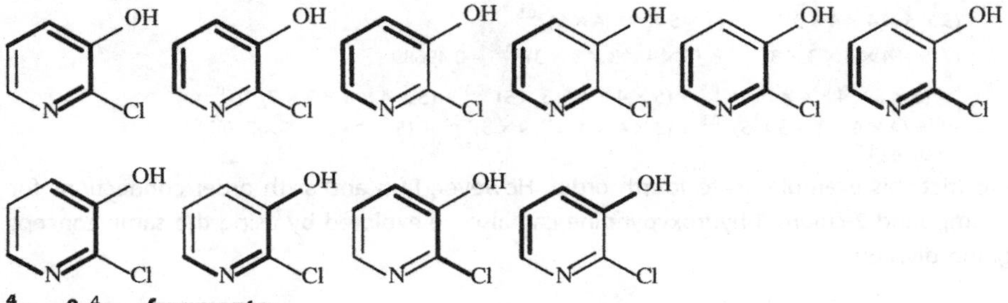

$^4\chi_{pc}$ & $^4\chi_{pc}^v$ fragments:

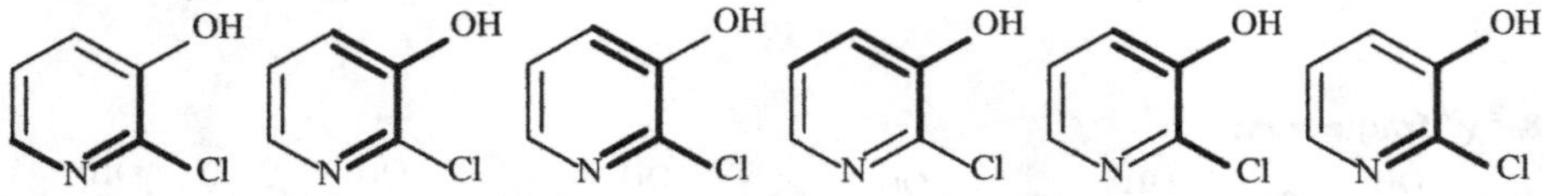

In these expressions, $^mP_{\min}$ and $^mP_{\max}$ are the minimum and maximum path counts of the mth order in the molecular graph comprising of A number of vertices or atoms. The isomeric graph of the original structure is considered when deriving $P_{\min}$ and $P_{\max}$. The minimum value of P (i.e., $P_{\min}$) is derived from a linear graph, while $P_{\max}$ is derived considering the original graph where all vertices are bonded to each other. For the ith molecule, the following relationship is held up by $P_{\min}$ and $P_{\max}$: $^mP_{min} \leq {}^mP_i \leq {}^mP_{max}$. The computations of the P values are as follows:

$$^1P_{\min} = A - 1 \tag{4.39}$$

and

$$\frac{^1P_{\max} = A \times (A-1)}{2} \tag{4.40}$$

$$^2P_{min} = A - 2 \tag{4.41}$$

and

$$^2P_{max} = \frac{(A-1) \times (A-2)}{2} \tag{4.42}$$

Here, $^1\kappa$ gives information about the number of cycles in or the complexity of a molecule. For a graph with no cycles, $^1\kappa = A$, and the presence of cycles in molecular graph tends to reduce the value of ${}^{1}\kappa$. For the second-order Kappa index, the ${}^{2}P_{max}$ value is computed from a star type of graph, where all but one vertex are adjacent to a central vertex. Here, ${}^{2}\kappa$ provides information regarding the spatial density of atoms in a molecule. A twin-star type of graph is contemplated for ${}^{3}P_{max}$. The parameter ${}^{3}\kappa$ gives information regarding the centrality of molecular branchedness. Kier [36] also proposed modified Kappa-shape parameters by incorporating information on shape and hybridization. These are known as *Kier alpha-modified shape indices* and are defined as follows:

$$\frac{{}^{1}\kappa_{\alpha m} = (A+\alpha)\times(A+\alpha-1)^2}{({}^{1}P+\alpha)^2} \tag{4.43}$$

$${}^{2}\kappa_{\alpha m} = \frac{(A+\alpha-1)\times(A+\alpha-2)^2}{({}^{2}P+\alpha)^2} \tag{4.44}$$

$$\begin{aligned} {}^{3}\kappa &= \frac{(A+\alpha-3)\times(A+\alpha-2)^2}{({}^{3}P+\alpha)^2} \quad \text{for even values of } A\ (A>3) \\ &= \frac{(A+\alpha-1)\times(A+\alpha-3)^2}{({}^{3}P+\alpha)^2} \quad \text{for odd values of } A\ (A>3) \end{aligned} \tag{4.45}$$

where α is defined as

$$\alpha = \sum_{i=1}^{A}\left(\frac{R_i}{R_{C_{sp3}}} - 1\right) \tag{4.46}$$

Here, the covalent radius of the ith atom and that of a sp^3-hybridized carbon atom are presented by R_i and $R_{C_{sp^3}}$, respectively. One can use tabulated values for the α ratio (Box 4.25).

4.4.5 Electrotopological state (E-state) indices

E-state indices encode information on electronic and topological features of atoms in a molecule. The E-state index S_i of atom i in a connected molecular graph can be defined as follows [37]:

$$S_i = I_i + \Delta I_i \tag{4.47}$$

where I_i represents the intrinsic factor of atom i and ΔI_i is a perturbation factor that may be defined as

$$\Delta I_i = \sum_{j=1}^{A}\frac{I_i - I_j}{(r_{ij}+1)^k} \tag{4.48}$$

BOX 4.25 Kappa Shape Indices Computation for Sample Molecules

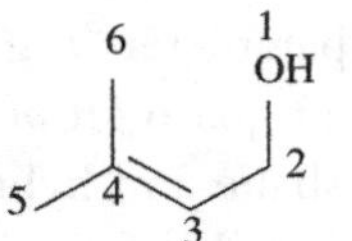

3-Methylbut-2-en-1-ol

Here,
$A = 6$
$^1P = 5$
$^2P = 5$
$^3P = 3$

Here, we would like to represent the common graphical connection to compute P_{max} and P_{min} applicable for $A = 6$.

The P_{min} connection graph for $A = 6$ would be like a normal six vertex chain giving $^1P_{min} = 5$, $^2P_{min} = 4$, $^3P_{min} = 3$

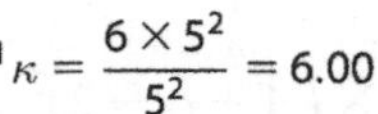

$$^1\kappa = \frac{6 \times 5^2}{5^2} = 6.00$$

$$^2\kappa = \frac{5 \times 4^2}{5^2} = 3.20$$

$$^3\kappa = \frac{3 \times 4^2}{3^2} = 5.333$$

The P_{max} connection graph for $A = 6$ would be as follows:

Order	P_{max}	P_{min}	Index value
1	=15	5	$^1\kappa = 2 \times \frac{15 \times 5}{5^2} = 6$
2	=10	4	$^2\kappa = 2 \times \frac{10 \times 4}{5^2} = 3.2$
3	=4	3	$^3\kappa = 4 \times \frac{4 \times 3}{3^2} = 5.333$

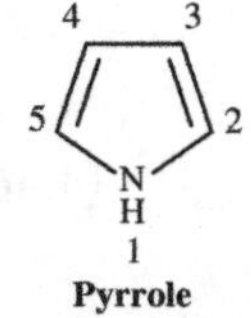

Pyrrole

Here,
$A = 5$
$^1P = 5$
$^2P = 5$
$^3P = 5$

The P_{min} connection graph for $A = 5$ would be like a normal five vertex chain giving $^1P_{min} = 5$, $^2P_{min} = 3$, $^3P_{min} = 2$.

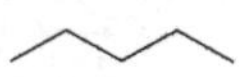

The P_{max} connection graph for $A = 5$ would be as follows:

$$^1\kappa = \frac{5 \times 4^2}{5^2} = 3.2$$

$$^2\kappa = \frac{4 \times 3^2}{5^2} = 1.44$$

$$^3\kappa = \frac{4 \times 2^2}{5^2} = 0.64$$

Order	P_{max}	P_{min}	Index value
1	=10	4	$^1\kappa = 2 \times \frac{10 \times 4}{5^2} = 3.2$
2	=6	3	$^2\kappa = 2 \times \frac{6 \times 3}{5^2} = 1.44$
3	=2	2	$^3\kappa = 4 \times \frac{2 \times 2}{5^2} = 0.64$

Here, the topological distance between the ith and jth atom is denoted using r_{ij}, and A represents the total number of atoms (i.e., vertices). The term k is used for modifying distance-based influences, and usually its value is considered to be 2. The intrinsic state of an atom can be defined as

$$I_i = \frac{(2/L_i)^2 \times \delta_i^v + 1}{\delta_i} \tag{4.49}$$

where L_i denotes the principal quantum number for atom i, while the number of sigma electrons (vertex degree) and valence shell electrons (vertex valence degree) are represented by δ_i and δ_i^v, respectively. It may be noted that ΔI_i can be computed by using a distance $+1$ matrix, where $+1$ has to be added to all the elements of the distance matrix.

The intrinsic state (I_i) denotes the partitioning of the nonsigma (σ) electronic influence. The valence electron becomes more available with less partitioning of the nonsigma (σ) electronic influence. The perturbation factor (ΔI_i), on the other hand, gives a measure of electronegative gradient, and its sign denotes the direction of influence surrounding I_i. In QSAR studies, E-state parameters play an important role by providing good and interpretable chemical features. Usually, E-state values of substructures with respect to atoms are used as descriptors or predictor variables. For example, E-state value of several terminal methyl groups in a molecule can be summed and used to denote the contribution of $-CH_3$ groups. Different chemometric software platforms encode many such atom-based E-state fragments from the analysis of a molecule. Different software tools represent E-state fragments according to their own notations. Figure 4.5 shows an overview of some E-state indices with a sample notation, where S refers to the summed E-state value for a given atom/fragment type, s denotes a single bond, d corresponds to a double bond, t refers to a triple bond, and a depicts an aromatic bond. In the examples, we have attempted to highlight some of the E-state fragments (Box 4.26).

4.4.6 Extended topochemical atom indices

After the development of Kier and Hall connectivity indices, a significant amount of research was performed on topological descriptors, and many of the researchers attempted to develop better alternatives with good diagnostic potential. In the late 1980s, a group led by A. U. De at Jadavpur University, India, devised a new set of parameters named topochemically arrived unique (TAU) indices [38,39] by exploring the chemistry of atomic core and valence electronic environment of atoms. In 2003, the present authors' group developed another novel group of topochemical parameters by refinement of the TAU indices. These indices are known as extended topochemical atom (ETA) indices [40–43]. Currently, two generations of ETA indices are available

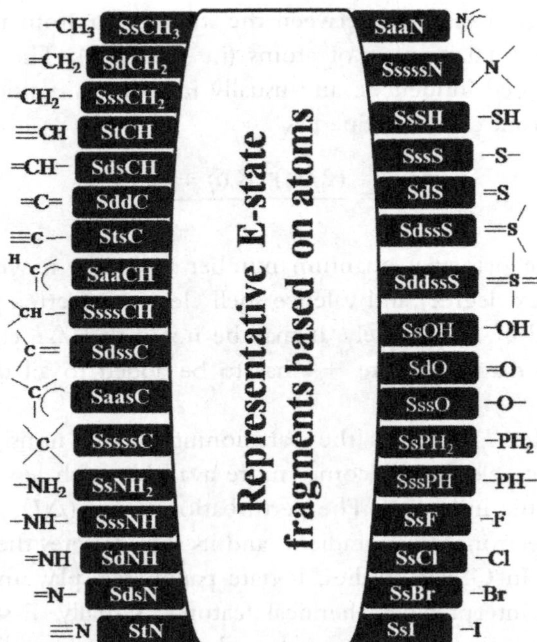

Figure 4.5 Representative electrotopological state (E-state) atom index fragments based on atoms.

for use. The ETA indices can be computed at the atomic level, as well as for the whole molecule. In keeping with the scope of this chapter, we have provided some details of the ETA indices in Table 4.4 so that readers can get an idea about these novel indices. For more elaborate explanation and examples, readers are advised to refer to articles on the ETA indices [40–43] (Box 4.27).

4.5 CONCLUSION AND POSSIBILITIES

Science has its own way of exploring core concepts to build a definite logic by bringing different disciplines under one umbrella. Chemistry is considered as one of the best-documented branches of science. Incorporation of mathematical functionalities has enabled the exploration of the quantitative chemical features of compounds. Topology and graph theoretical formalism present a unique opportunity of diagnosing the chemical structures using easily explainable algorithms. Since the development of Wiener and Platt indices, topological descriptors have been used extensively in modeling analyses by different research groups and have been modified by many of them. With the growing complexity of chemicals, the encoding of chemical information has become a difficult task. The task of a chemist lies in designing chemicals of interest with the desired features of the response parameter. The goal of predictive modeling analysis is to develop some

BOX 4.26 Electrotopological State Indices Computation for Sample Molecules

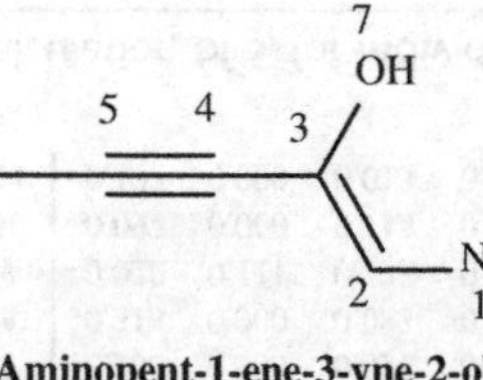

1-Aminopent-1-ene-3-yne-2-ol

Computation of I_i value:

i	L_i	Z	Z^v	δ_i^v	δ_i	I_i
1	2	7	5	3	1	4.0
2	2	6	4	3	2	2.0
3	2	6	4	4	3	1.667
4	2	6	4	4	2	2.5
5	2	6	4	4	2	2.5
6	2	6	4	1	1	2.0
7	2	8	6	5	1	6.0

Distance matrix elements:

	1	**2**	**3**	**4**	**5**	**6**	**7**
1	0	1	2	3	4	5	3
2	1	0	1	2	3	4	2
3	2	1	0	1	2	3	1
4	3	2	1	0	1	2	2
5	4	3	2	1	0	1	3
6	5	4	3	2	1	0	4
7	3	2	1	2	3	4	0

Computation of ΔI_i value (using values of I_i and distance matrix elements):

Atoms	1	2	3	4	5	6	7	Σ
1	0.000	0.500	0.259	0.094	0.060	0.056	−0.125	0.844
2	−0.500	0.000	0.083	−0.056	−0.031	0.000	−0.444	−0.948
3	−0.259	−0.083	0.000	−0.208	−0.093	−0.021	−1.083	−1.748
4	−0.094	0.056	0.208	0.000	0.000	0.056	−0.389	−0.163
5	−0.060	0.031	0.093	0.000	0.000	0.125	−0.219	−0.030
6	−0.056	0.000	0.021	−0.056	−0.125	0.000	−0.160	−0.375
7	0.125	0.444	1.083	0.389	0.219	0.160	0.000	2.420

Calculation of S_i for individual atom

i	I_i	ΔI_i	S_i
1	4.0	0.844	4.844
2	2.0	−0.948	1.052
3	1.667	−1.748	−0.081
4	2.5	−0.163	2.337
5	2.5	−0.030	2.470
6	2.0	−0.375	1.625
7	6.0	2.420	8.420

Selected E-state values:

$S(-NH_2)$ {$SsNH_2$} $= S_1 = 4.844$

$S(-CH_3)$ {$SsCH_3$} $= S_6 = 1.625$

$S(=CH-)${SdsCH} $= S_2 = 1.052$

$S(-OH)$ {SsOH} $= S_7 = 8.420$

$S(\equiv C-)$ {StsC} $= S_4 + S_5 = 4.807$

$S(=C<)$ = {SdssC} $= S_3 = -0.081$

(Continued)

BOX 4.26 Electrotopological State Indices Computation for Sample Molecules—cont'd

1 O 2 3 4 5 6 7 8 10 O 11 OH 9

4-Hydroxy-3-methoxybenzaldehyde

Computation of I_i value:

i	L_i	Z	Z^v	δ_i^v	δ_i	I_i
1	2	8	6	6	1	7.0
2	2	6	4	3	2	2.0
3	2	6	4	4	3	1.667
4	2	6	4	3	2	2.0
5	2	6	4	4	3	1.667
6	2	6	4	4	3	1.667
7	2	6	4	3	2	2.0
8	2	6	4	3	2	2.0
9	2	8	6	5	1	6.0
10	2	8	6	6	2	3.5
11	2	6	4	1	1	2.0

Distance matrix elements:

	1	**2**	**3**	**4**	**5**	**6**	**7**	**8**	**9**	**10**	**11**
1	0	1	2	3	4	5	4	3	6	5	6
2	1	0	1	2	3	4	3	2	5	4	5
3	2	1	0	1	2	3	2	1	4	3	4
4	3	2	1	0	1	2	3	2	3	2	3
5	4	3	2	1	0	1	2	3	2	1	2
6	5	4	3	2	1	0	1	2	1	2	3
7	4	3	2	3	2	1	0	1	2	3	4
8	3	2	1	2	3	2	1	0	3	4	5
9	6	5	4	3	2	1	2	3	0	3	4
10	5	4	3	2	1	2	3	4	3	0	1
11	6	5	4	3	2	3	4	5	4	1	0

Computation of ΔI_i value (using values of I_i and distance matrix elements):

i	**1**	**2**	**3**	**4**	**5**	**6**	**7**	**8**	**9**	**10**	**11**	Σ
1	0.000	1.250	0.593	0.313	0.213	0.148	0.200	0.313	0.020	0.097	0.102	3.249
2	−1.250	0.000	0.083	0.000	0.021	0.013	0.000	0.000	−0.111	−0.060	0.000	−1.304
3	−0.593	−0.083	0.000	−0.083	0.000	0.000	−0.037	−0.083	−0.173	−0.115	−0.013	−1.181
4	−0.313	0.000	0.083	0.000	0.083	0.037	0.000	0.000	−0.250	−0.167	0.000	−0.525
5	−0.213	−0.021	0.000	−0.083	0.000	0.000	−0.037	−0.021	−0.481	−0.458	−0.037	−1.352
6	−0.148	−0.013	0.000	−0.037	0.000	0.000	−0.083	−0.037	−1.083	−0.204	−0.021	−1.627
7	−0.200	0.000	0.037	0.000	0.037	0.083	0.000	0.000	−0.444	−0.094	0.000	−0.581
8	−0.313	0.000	0.083	0.000	0.021	0.037	0.000	0.000	−0.250	−0.060	0.000	−0.481
9	−0.020	0.111	0.173	0.250	0.481	1.083	0.444	0.250	0.000	0.156	0.160	3.090
10	−0.097	0.060	0.115	0.167	0.458	0.204	0.094	0.060	−0.156	0.000	0.375	1.279
11	−0.102	0.000	0.013	0.000	0.037	0.021	0.000	0.000	−0.160	−0.375	0.000	−0.566

Calculation of S_i for individual atom

Atoms	1	2	3	4	5	6	7	8	9	10	11
I_i	7.000	2.000	1.667	2.000	1.667	1.667	2.000	2.000	6.000	3.500	2.000
ΔI_i	3.249	−1.304	−1.181	−0.525	−1.352	−1.627	−0.581	−0.481	3.090	1.279	−0.566
S_i	10.249	0.696	0.486	1.475	0.314	0.040	1.419	1.519	9.090	4.779	1.434

Selected E-state values:

S(—CH₃) {SsCH₃} = S_{11} = 1.434

S( ) {SaasC} = $S_3 + S_5 + S_6$ = 0.840

S(=O) {SdO} = S_1 = 10.249

S(H)(SaaCH} = $S_4 + S_7 + S_8$ = 4.413

S(=CH—){SdsCH} = S_2 = 0.696

S(—O—) {SssO} = S_{10} = 4.779

S(—OH) {SsOH} = S_9 = 9.090

Table 4.4 Definition of the indices under the ETA formalism

First-generation indices			Second-generation indices	
Core count: $\alpha = \frac{Z - Z^v}{Z^v} \cdot \frac{1}{PN - 1}$ Defines molecular bulk. Z and Z^v are numbers of total and valence electrons, respectively. PN is periodic number.	Shape parameter: $(\Sigma\alpha)_p/\Sigma\alpha$ $(\Sigma\alpha)_Y/\Sigma\alpha$ $(\Sigma\alpha)_X/\Sigma\alpha$ Defines molecular shape and substitution pattern.	The VEM vertex count: $\gamma_i = \frac{\alpha_i}{\beta_i}$	Variants of core count α: $\Delta\alpha_A = \left\langle \frac{\Sigma\alpha - [\Sigma\alpha]_R}{N_v} \right\rangle$: Count of heteroatoms. N_v = number of vertices	$\Delta\alpha_B = \left\langle \frac{[\Sigma\alpha]_R - \Sigma\alpha}{N_v} \right\rangle$: Count of H-bond acceptor atoms and/or polar surface area.
Electronegativity count: $\varepsilon = -\alpha + 0.3 \times Z^V$ Gives information on electronegativity. Valence mobile electron (VEM) count (β): $\beta_s = \Sigma x\sigma$ and $\beta_{ns} = \Sigma y\pi + \delta$ $\beta = \Sigma x\sigma + \Sigma y\pi + \delta$ Provides information on sigma and pi bonded and lone pair electrons. σ, π, and δ presenting contribution of sigma, pi, and lone pair electrons respectively.		Composite index: $\eta = \sum_{i<j} \left[\frac{\gamma_i\gamma_j}{r_{ij}^2}\right]^{0.5}$ r_{ij} = topological distance between i and j. Composite index (reference alkane): $\eta_R = \left\{ \sum_{i<j} \left[\frac{\gamma_i\gamma_j}{r_{ij}^2}\right]^{0.5} \right\}_R$	Variants of electronegativity parameter ε: $\varepsilon_1 = \frac{\Sigma\varepsilon}{N}$ $\varepsilon_2 = \frac{\Sigma\varepsilon_{EH}}{N_v}$ $\varepsilon_3 = \frac{[\Sigma\varepsilon]_R}{N_R}$ $\varepsilon_4 = \frac{[\Sigma\varepsilon]_{SS}}{N_{SS}}$ $\varepsilon_5 = \frac{\Sigma\varepsilon_{EH} + \Sigma\varepsilon_{XH}}{N_v + N_{XH}}$ E_H = excluding H-atom E_{SS} = Saturated C-skeleton N_{XH} = H attached to heteroatom	$\Delta\varepsilon_A = \varepsilon_1 - \varepsilon_3$: Count of electronegative atom and unsaturation. $\Delta\varepsilon_B = \varepsilon_1 - \varepsilon_4$: Contribution of unsaturation. $\Delta\varepsilon_C = \varepsilon_3 - \varepsilon_4$: Measure of electronegativity. $\Delta\varepsilon_D = \varepsilon_2 - \varepsilon_5$: Measure of hydrogen bond donor atoms

(*Continued*)

Table 4.4 (Continued)

First-generation indices		Second-generation indices
Functionality index: $\eta_F = \eta_R - \eta$: Gives a measure of heteroatoms and multiple bonds. Local functionality contribution: $\eta_F^{\text{local}} = \eta_R^{\text{local}} - \eta^{\text{local}}$ Branching index: $\eta_B = \eta_N^{\text{local}} - \eta_R^{\text{local}} + 0.086 \times N_R$	Local composite index: $\eta^{\text{local}} = \sum_{i<j, r_{ij}=1} (\gamma_i \gamma_j)^{0.5}$ Only local contribution considered; that is, $r_{ij} = 1$.	Measure of H-bonding propensity: $\psi_1 = \dfrac{\Sigma\alpha}{[\Sigma\varepsilon]_{EH}} = \dfrac{\Sigma\alpha / N_v}{\varepsilon_2}$ $\Delta\psi_A = \langle 0.714 - \psi_1 \rangle$ and $\Delta\psi_B = \langle \psi_1 - 0.714 \rangle$ $\Delta\beta = \Sigma\beta_{ns} - \Sigma\beta_s$: Measure of relative unsaturation content

BOX 4.27 ETA Indices Computation for Sample Molecules

Benzaldehyde

Reference skeleton

Atom level indices

	1	2	3	4	5	6	7	8
α_i	0.333	0.500	0.500	0.500	0.500	0.500	0.500	0.500
ε_i	1.467	1.000	0.700	1.000	1.000	1.000	1.000	1.000
$[\beta_s]_i$	0.75	1.250	1.500	1.000	1.000	1.000	1.000	1.000
$[\beta_{ns}]_i$	1.500	1.500	2.000	2.000	2.000	2.000	2.000	2.000
β_i	2.25	2.75	3.500	3.000	3.000	3.000	3.000	3.000
γ_i	0.148	0.182	0.143	0.167	0.167	0.167	0.167	0.167
$[\eta]_i$	0.452	0.660	0.749	0.684	0.648	0.628	0.648	0.684
$[\eta_R]_i$	1.962	2.074	2.058	2.061	1.964	1.903	1.964	2.061

Whole molecular indices

$\Sigma\alpha/N_v$	0.479	$\Delta\alpha_B$	0.021	ε_1	0.583	$\Delta\varepsilon_A$	0.150	$\sum\beta'_{ns}$	0.938	$\Delta\psi_A$	0.112
$(\Sigma\alpha)_p/\Sigma\alpha$	0.087	η	2.576	ε_2	0.796	$\Delta\varepsilon_B$	0.085	$\sum\beta'$	1.469	$\Delta\psi_B$	0.000
$(\Sigma\alpha)_Y/\Sigma\alpha$	0.130	η_R	8.023	ε_3	0.433	$\Delta\varepsilon_C$	−0.065	$\Delta\beta'$	0.406	η'_B	0.009
$(\Sigma\alpha)_X/\Sigma\alpha$	0.000	η_F/N_v	0.681	ε_4	0.498	$\Delta\varepsilon_D$	0.000	$\sum\beta'_{ns(\delta)}$	0.000		
$\Delta\alpha_A$	0.000	η^{local}	1.303	ε_5	0.796	$\sum\beta'_s$	0.531	ψ_1	0.602		

definite chemical insight regarding the property/activity/toxicity of chemicals. It has been observed that sometimes an interpretation of topological descriptors becomes very difficult while dealing with complex chemicals. As a matter of fact, there is a longstanding argument regarding the use of topological variables in deriving a suitable mechanistic basis. The nonconsideration of 3D features that practically define any substance, like volume, surface area, and density, somehow creates loopholes in topological considerations of molecular structure representation. However, many authors have shown that topological properties are not entirely devoid of 3D features. The bonding schemes and connectivities identified by topological properties are related to the 3D bonding features and geometry commonly known as *topography* [26]. The chi (χ) indices have been shown to be a function of energy that depends upon the electron density of the molecules due to unsaturated π bonds [44]. There are also instances where the Randić connectivity index has been related to Hückel molecular orbital parameters to account for a measure of global π electron and the resonance energy [45]. Furthermore, both the Hückel molecular orbital theory and the valence bond theory use the concept of topological attributes [46]. Hence, it can be stated that 2D and 3D properties are internally linked.

Some researchers have found that combining 3D features with topological functionality can provide a suitable means of extracting chemical information, and this has led to the development of a series of related parameters: namely, quantum topological molecular similarity (QTMS), geometry, topology, and atom-weights assembly descriptors known as GEometric, Topological and Atomic Weighted AssemblY (GETAWAY). The Burden – CAS – University of Texas (BCUT) descriptors are derived by using a weighting scheme of 3D features on the molecular graph, thereby encoding information on topology and 3D geometry [47]. The symbiotic coherence of graph theory and topology had been found to be an interesting tool in chemistry more than 60 years ago. Molecular descriptors derived using graph theory and topology are designated by explicit algorithms, and they also consume less computational time. One of the interesting aspects of topological descriptors is their independence on receptor information, which allows them to be employed in ligand-based virtual screening (VS), a rational strategy for the selection of a desired chemical moiety by performing a systematic search operation on large databases of compounds. Topological indices can aid in the ligand-based similarity searching of chemicals in the VS paradigm for the identification of privileged structures containing the desired substructure or scaffold required for the chemical response. Various types of topological features like connectivity, atom path, branching, and common substructure can be employed as filtering tools or fingerprints in the virtual hunt for identical chemical moiety (i.e., similarity searching) from large databases of chemicals [48]. Figure 4.6 presents the fundamental advantages offered by topological indices in the realm of predictive modeling analysis. We strongly believe that there are still possibilities left unexplored in the realm of topological paradigm, and the discovery of novel parameters will continue.

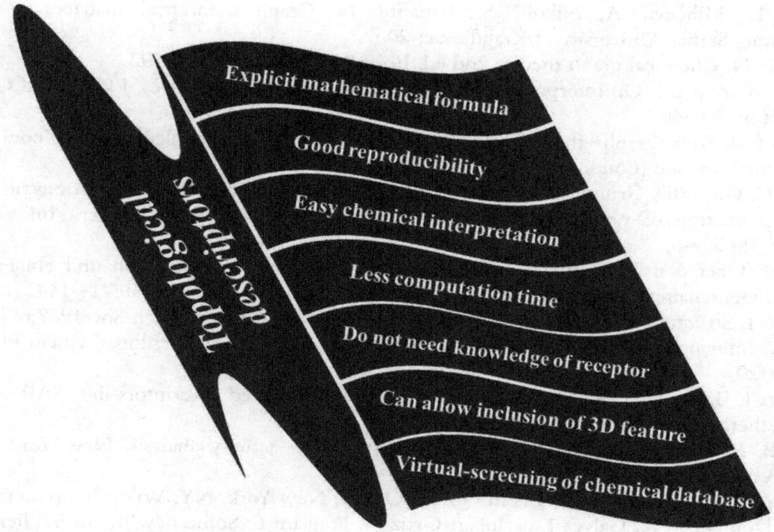

Figure 4.6 Advantages provided by the topological indices.

REFERENCES

[1] Testa B, Kier LB. The concept of molecular structure in structure–activity relationship studies and drug design. Med Res Rev 1991;11(1):35–48.

[2] Harary F. Graph theory. Reading, MA: Addision-Wesley; 1971.

[3] Euler L. Solutio problematis ad geometriam situs pertinentis. Comment Acad Scient Imper Petropolitane 1736;8:128–40.

[4] Kirchhoff GR. Über die Auflösung der Gleichungen, auf welche man bei der untersuchung der linearen verteilung galvanischer Ströme geführt wird. Ann Phys Chem 1847;72:497–508.

[5] Sylvester JJ. Chemistry and algebra. Nature 1877;17:284–309.

[6] Thackray A. Atoms and powers. Cambridge, MA: Harvard University Press; 1970.

[7] Higgins WA. Comparative view of the phlogistic and antiphlogistic theories. London: J. Murray; 1789.

[8] Dalton J. New system of chemical philosophy. London: S. Russell, for R. Bickerstaff, Cambridge Press; 1808.

[9] Wollaston WH. On super-acid and sub-acid salts. Phil Trans Roy Soc Lond 1808;98:96–102.

[10] Hein GE. Kekulé and the architecture of molecules. In: Kekulé Centennial. Advances in chemistry, Washington, DC 1966;61:1–12.

[11] van't Hoff JH. Sur les formules de structure dans l'espace. Arch Neerl Sci Exactes Nat 1874; 9:445–54.

[12] Le Bel JA. Sur les relations qui existent entre les formules atomiques des corps organiques et le pouvoir rotatoire de leurs dissolutions. Bull Soc Chim Fr 1874;22(2):337–47.

[13] Loschmidt J. Chemische Studien. Vienna: Gerold; 1861. (Reprinted as Ostwald's Klassiker No. 190, Engelmann Leipzig; 1913).

[14] Cayley A. On the mathematical theory of isomers. Phil Mag 1874;47(4):444–6.

[15] Henze HR, Blair CM. The number of structurally isomeric alcohols of the methanol series. J Am Chem Soc 1931;53(8):3042–6.

[16] Pólya G, Read RC. Combinatorial enumeration of groups, graphs and chemical compounds. New York, NY: Springer-Verlag; 1987.

[17] Janežič D, Miličević A, Nikolić S, Trinajstić N. Graph theoretical matrices in chemistry. Kragujevac, Serbia: University of Kragujevac; 2007.
[18] Trinajstić N. Chemical graph theory. 2nd ed. Boca Raton, FL: CRC; 1992.
[19] Randić M, Zupan J. On interpretation of well-known topological indices. J Chem Inf Comput Sci 2001;41(3):550–60.
[20] Mallion RB. Some graph–theoretical aspects of simple ring current calculations on conjugated systems. Proc Roy Soc (London) A 1975;341(1627):429–49.
[21] Basak SC, Gute BD, Grunwald GD. Use of topostructural, topochemical, and geometric parameters in the prediction of vapor pressure: a hierarchical QSAR approach. J Chem Inf Comput Sci 1997;37(4):651–5.
[22] Kopp H. Über den Zusammenhang zwischen der chemischen constitution und einigen physikalischen Eigenschaften bei ussigen Verbindungen. Ann Chem Pharm 1844;50:71–144.
[23] Wiener H. Structural determination of paraffin boiling points. J Am Chem Soc 1947;69(1):17–20.
[24] Platt JR. Influence of neighbor bonds on additive bond properties in paraffins. J Chem Phys 1947;15 (6):419–20.
[25] Devillers J, Balaban AT, editors. Topological Indices and related descriptors in QSAR and QSPR. The Netherlands: Gordon and Breach; 1999.
[26] Kier LB, Hall LH. Molecular connectivity in structure–activity analysis. New York, NY: John Wiley & Sons; 1986.
[27] Karelson M. Molecular descriptors in QSAR/QSPR. New York, NY: Wiley-Interscience; 2000.
[28] García-Domenech R, Gálvez J, de Julián-Ortiz JV, Pogliani L. Some new trends in chemical graph theory. Chem Rev 2008;108(3):1127–69.
[29] Roy K. Topological descriptors in drug design and modeling studies. Mol Diver 2004;8(4):321–3.
[30] Hosoya H. Topological index. A newly proposed quantity characterizing the topological nature of structural isomers of saturated hydrocarbons. Bull Chem Soc Jpn 1971;44(9):2332–9.
[31] Gutman I, Trinajstić N. Graph theory and molecular orbitals. Total π-electron energy of alternant hydrocarbons. Chem Phys Lett 1972;17(4):535–8.
[32] Balaban AT. Highly discriminating distance based topological index. Chem Phys Lett 1982;89(5): 399–404.
[33] Randić M. On characterization of molecular branching. J Am Chem Soc 1975;97(23):6609–15.
[34] Kier LB, Hall LH. The nature of structure–activity relationships and their relation to molecular connectivity. Eur J Med Chem 1977;12:307–12.
[35] Kier LB. A shape index from molecular graphs. Quant Struct-Act Relat 1985;4(3):109–16.
[36] Kier LB. Distinguishing atom differences in a molecular graph shape index. Quant Struct-Act Relat 1986;5(1):7–12.
[37] Kier LB, Hall LH. An electrotopological-state index for atoms in molecules. Pharm Res 1990;7(8): 801–7.
[38] Pal DK, Sengupta C, De AU. A new topochemical descriptor (TAU) in molecular connectivity concept: part I—aliphatic compounds. Indian J Chem 1988;27B:734–9.
[39] Pal DK, Sengupta M, Sengupta C, De AU. QSAR with TAU (τ) indices: part I—polymethylene primary diamines as amebicidal agents. Indian J Chem 1990;29B:451–4.
[40] Roy K, Ghosh G. QSTR with extended topochemical atom indices. 2. Fish toxicity of substituted benzenes. J Chem Inf Comput Sci 2004;44(2):559–67.
[41] Roy K, Ghosh G. Exploring QSARs with extended topochemical atom (ETA) indices for modeling chemical and drug toxicity. Curr Pharm Des 2010;16(24):2625–39.
[42] Roy K, Das RN. On some novel extended topochemical atom (ETA) parameters for effective encoding of chemical information and modeling of fundamental physicochemical properties. SAR QSAR Environ Res 2011;22(5–6):451–72.
[43] Roy K, Das RN. On extended topochemical atom (ETA) indices for QSPR studies. In: Castro EA, Hagi AK, editors. Advanced methods and applications in chemoinformatics: research progress and new applications. Hershey, PA: IGI Global; 2011. p. 380–411.
[44] Stankevich IV, Skovortsova MI, Zefirov NS. On a quantum chemical interpretation of molecular connectivity indices for conjugated hydrocarbons. J Mol Struct (Theochem) 1995;342:173–9.

[45] Gálvez J. On a topological interpretation of electronic and vibrational molecular energies. J Mol Struct (Theochem) 1998;429:255–64.
[46] Pilar FL. Elementary quantum chemistry. New York, NY: McGraw-Hill; 1968.
[47] Burden FR. A chemically intuitive molecular index based on the eigenvalues of a modified adjacency matrix. Quant Struct-Act Relat 1997;16(4):309–14.
[48] Bajorath J. Chemoinformatics: concepts, methods, and tools for drug discovery. Totowa, NJ: Humana Press Inc; 2004.

CHAPTER 5

Computational Chemistry

Contents

5.1 INTRODUCTION

Advancement in any scientific discipline proves fruitful when it is supplied with suitable media of operations that make the science unambiguous to all its users. The development of various computer applications has enriched the operations involved in different technical and scientific processes. As in other scientific disciplines, the deployment of computer

Understanding the Basics of QSAR for Applications in Pharmaceutical Sciences and Risk Assessment.
ISBN: 978-0-12-801505-6, DOI: http://dx.doi.org/10.1016/B978-0-12-801505-6.00005-3

workstations has instituted a revolution in the research and development of chemistry. Modern medicinal chemistry employs several computational applications in solving simple to complex problems with a high level of accuracy. Nowadays, computers have become an inevitable tool in drug discovery and drug development. The use of desktop computers has enabled the solving of complex chemical problems while requiring little specialist expertise at the laboratory-scale operations. The computer technology has enhanced the research in theoretical chemistry by allowing not only a platform for solving complex chemical equations and models, but also suitable graphical interfaces for a better understanding of the involved chemical phenomena. The quantitative structure–activity relationship (QSAR) methodology employs the quantification of molecular structures followed by the development of mathematical correlation with the aim of predicting the activity/property/toxicity of untested or new chemicals. The entire operation, starting from encoding of structural information to model development, and validation as well as prediction, employs a significant amount of data that can be reliably operated using suitable computer programs. At times, the predicted features have been found to be more accurate and reliable than experiments considering a higher degree of error involved in experimental studies. There are different technical aspects that must be considered while using computers as an essential component in the molecular modeling epitome, and it is thus obvious that the assistance of an expert in computational chemistry would be necessary while dealing with such *in silico* tools. However, it will be very helpful to have some basic insight regarding the fundamental theory involved in such operations based on how developers design their products. Hence, we shall highlight the basic theories involved in defining some of the chemical attributes, like molecular orbital (MO) theory, principles of molecular mechanics (MM), and quantum mechanics along with a focus on the avenues of their implementation in various types of algorithms.

5.2 COMPUTER USE IN CHEMISTRY

Discoveries and developments in chemistry have come a long way since the time of the Greek philosopher Thales (sixth century BC), who hypothesized that simple elements (earth, water, air, and fire) form chemical substances. With the passage of time, knowledge of the molecular composition, structural features, arrangement, and properties of chemicals have been developed, and computers have become an essential part of it by acting as a tool of documentation, analysis, and representation. It is not preposterous to state that the incorporation of computer technology has added significant momentum to the research of theoretical chemistry. However, it should be remembered that discovery and development of the theoretical bases are of primary importance, and computers act as an implementation tool. By the use of suitable software and hardware technologies, developers encode the theoretical information by applying definite algorithms, which makes the theory easily applicable to the users. Hence, any limitations or approximations of a software platform entirely depend upon the developer, not the theory itself. Now, with the incorporation of various applications of computers in solving chemical problems, several terms are used. *Theoretical chemistry* broadly corresponds to the mathematical depiction of chemical information, while *computational chemistry* is used to denote a collection of techniques employed to solve problems of chemistry using computers.

Now, it is evident that computers have played an essential part in almost all types of technical operations, including various chemical analysis systems like spectroscopy and chromatography, which provide analog support to the system. However, in this chapter, we shall focus on the use of computers in enhancing the theoretical aspect of chemistry. Another term, *molecular modeling*, is also used to define the same formalism encompassed by computational chemistry. Technically, the word *model* refers to an idealized depiction of a system, and if we consider mathematical formalism, a model is a way of providing the calculations and predictions of a system [1]. Hence, molecular modeling covers several aspects of theoretical chemical computation and the reasonable prediction thereof. The sphere of theoretical chemistry can be computational as well as noncomputational, depending upon the mathematical basis developed to encode a chemical problem. Hence, the noncomputational part concerns the formulation of analytical expressions for molecular properties, and when sufficient mathematical background is developed in addressing a chemical problem, the algorithm is executed using computational tools. Therefore, we can observe an interdisciplinary embellishment of chemical theory put into strong mathematical formalism, followed by computational encoding. The implementation of computational technology in theoretical chemistry can be broadly viewed in three aspects: namely, visualization, computation, and analysis. In the next sections, we shall present a brief overview of different molecular modeling operations performed with the assistance of computers.

5.2.1 Visualization

Computers strengthen general understanding of chemicals by providing a suitable graphical visualization interface. This encompasses the visualization of single chemical structures to the hypothetical interaction pattern between the receptor and ligand.

5.2.1.1 Structure drawing

Such tools allow the drawing of a chemical structure in a workspace within the desktop. By using the sketching tool, a user can draw structures employing various chemical bond tools, atoms, chains, ring-template, and other items. The structures are encoded in the form of coordinates that are graphically converted into images on the computer screen. The same structure can be displayed in different graphical forms, some of which include Corey–Pauling–Koltun (CPK), stick, ball-and-stick, space fill, mesh, and ribbon [2]. Of these, the ribbon type of representation is usually employed for large molecules like proteins and nucleic acids. Figure 5.1 shows several graphical depictions of the paracetamol (*p*-acetamidophenol) molecule. Most of the commercial structure-drawing packages assign a specific color coding to each type of atom, a system that is editable by the user. Examples of some chemical-drawing packages are ChemDraw (http://www.cambridgesoft.com/Ensemble_for_Chemistry/ChemDraw/), IsisDraw (a product of MDL Information Systems, Inc.), ChemSketch (http://www.acdlabs.com/products/draw_nom/draw/chemsketch/), and MarvinSketch (https://www.chemaxon.com). Many of these packages also allow the computation of various properties along with the drawing facility. Not only that, most of the software packages provide other tools that perform functions such as checking the structure (valence, bond order, etc.) and generating IUPAC names.

5.2.1.2 3D visualization

By using a suitable graphical conversion package, the user can obtain a three-dimensional (3D) visualization of the structure. Many of the molecular modeling packages allow the simple and direct conversion of a two-dimensional (2D) structural format into 3D when a 2D structure is opened or pasted into its drawing area. Examples of some software platforms that allow 3D viewing of molecular structures include Chem3D (http://www.cambridgesoft.com/Ensemble_for_Chemistry/ChemDraw/), Discovery Studio (http://accelrys.com/products/discovery-studio/), Sybyl (http://tripos.com/index.php), Hyperchem

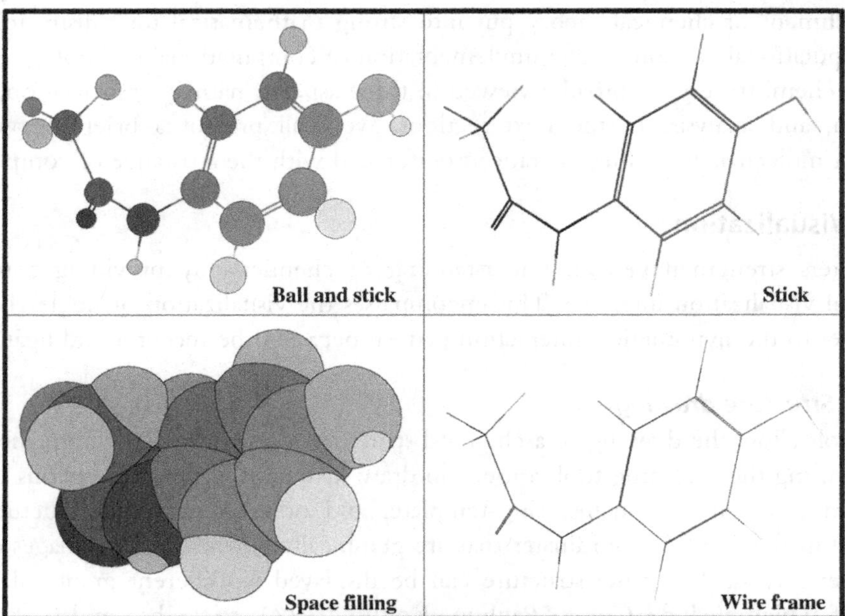

Figure 5.1 Different model representations of the paracetamol molecule.

(http://www.hyper.com/), and Maestro (http://www.schrodinger.com/Maestro/). However, it may be observed that the visualization plane of the computer is 2D, and hence a 3D molecular view is generated by making some modifications to the axes. This is achieved by making less dense coloring of the atoms/bonds away from the viewer or by reducing their visualization bond length.

5.2.1.3 Visualization of ligand–receptor interactions

Visualization of ligand–receptor interactions is a very useful functionality that provides a 3D graphical presentation of a hypothetical interaction between the ligand and the receptor molecule to the viewer. Since the biological system encountered by a query molecule is entirely 3D in nature, such visualization helps in predicting the nature of molecular interaction at the receptor binding site. Hence, by providing a suitable interface to the user, computers allow the storage of compound information in terms of their structure. Various formats are available to save the molecules, including .cdx, .mol, .skc, and .rxn. Drawing chemical structures is the beginning of any molecular modeling operation, since the drawings are used as input queries to carry out further analyses. It can be observed that the visualization of a chemical structure in a computer window is entirely a part of graphical conversion. The structures are represented by Cartesian/polar coordinates, which are being processed by software algorithms to be portrayed in different forms and shapes. Moreover, the user must understand that any kind of visualization under the molecular modeling paradigm is basically a form of representation for designing and communication purposes only, not a realistic depiction.

5.2.2 Calculation and simulation

Following the drawing/sketching of chemical structures, the next most important part of molecular modeling analysis involves the quantification of chemical information. These include a number of simple to complex theoretical analyses. Simply stated, with the aim of exploring the chemical attributes at the atomic and electronic levels, scientists have developed different theories on molecular environment by combining their knowledge of physics, chemistry, and mathematics. Such theories involve lengthy and intricate molecular mechanical and quantum chemical calculations to characterize the chemical nature at the electronic level. The use of computational programs has enabled such calculations to be done in less time with a good amount of reliability and accuracy. In other words, computational chemistry tools allow users to perform complex analysis just by providing some simple commands and other interfaces. Following the analysis, the derived features can be exploited in several aspects of analysis, like in a chemical characterization project, or as independent variables in QSAR analysis. With the progress of research in chemistry, various other theories of quantitative structural depiction have evolved. By the use of a suitable logical algorithm, computers can easily calculate many such molecular attributes—namely, molecular topology, geometric features, thermodynamic properties, and others. One more potential application of using computer technology to explore the chemical field is in drug–receptor studies. A number of techniques [namely, molecular docking studies, pharmacophore development, 3D-QSAR like comparative molecular field analysis (CoMFA) and comparative molecular similarity indices analysis (CoMSIA), etc.] attempt to find the essential structural requirements necessary for eliciting the biological activity of a ligand in a hypothetical 3D environment. Hence, the calculation of chemical features by employing computer applications can be viewed in the following four divisions:

1. Conformational analysis and energy minimization
2. MM- and quantum mechanics–based calculations
3. Miscellaneous molecular feature determination (charge, electrostatic potential, topological properties, thermodynamic properties, etc.)
4. Exploring drug–receptor interaction studies and structure–activity relationships (docking, pharmacophore development, CoMFA, etc.)

It can be observed that the abovementioned operations are linked to each other; for example, the computation of properties like charge, electrostatic potential, and molar refractivity is done after the energy minimization operation. In this chapter, we shall discuss the different aspects of conformational analysis and energy minimization using molecular and quantum mechanical calculations.

5.2.3 Analysis and storage of data

Computers are well known for their ability to process and analyze a large amount of data using a provided mathematical algorithm. Quantification of chemical information and the analysis thereof yield a significant amount of mathematical data, and these operations are properly done using various computational applications. Before the 1960s, the documentation and analyses of the QSAR technique was practiced without the use of computers. However, with the passage of time, the number of chemicals, end points, and descriptors has increased and needed a suitable platform for (i) storage, (ii) processing, and (iii) online availability of data. In order to pursue the analysis of chemical data, several mathematical techniques and suitable statistical measures are combined and used as *in silico* computational tools. Many of these tools allow the development of quantitative mathematical models employing techniques such as multiple linear regression (MLR), partial least squares (PLS), linear discriminant analysis (LDA), and genetic function approximation (GFA), followed by statistical validation; that is, computation of different validation metrics to judge the quality of the developed equation. Hence, the support provided by computers toward the analysis of chemical data can be categorized in the following ways:

1. Processing of data
2. Development of predictive models

3. Numerous statistical analyses
4. Storage of data

Many commercial software packages (e.g., Accelrys software) combine different features of molecular modeling like computation of chemical properties (descriptors), followed by an option for model development and validation, and finally storage of the analyzed data in a specified format. Currently, with the availability of suitable computers, it is possible to carry out virtual screening of library data that contains several thousands to millions of chemicals.

Finally, we would like to comment that by the use of suitable computer programs, it is possible to carry out various molecular modeling operations in a more rational and reliable way, eliminating possible sources of error. Using an efficient computer facility, a large amount of data can easily be processed in a short period of time. However, remember that computers do not and cannot replace any chemical experimentation or synthesis methodology; rather, it promotes molecular modeling analysis by providing a suitable platform to the experimental results toward the design and development of a desired, better chemical entity. Figure 5.2 depicts the privileges provided by various computational tools to facilitate computational chemistry analysis.

While performing complex chemical calculations, such as molecular mechanical, quantum chemical, and semiempirical, remember that the numerical solution provided by any platform cannot be assumed to be the exact or ultimate one, since each of these operations is being executed under several postulates or approximations. Hence, it is wise to decipher the results (i.e., extracted chemical information) with a

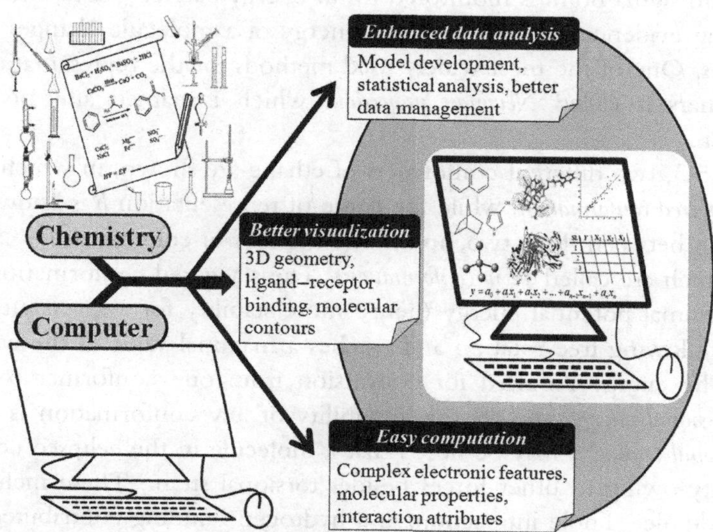

Figure 5.2 Computer technology enhancing the study of chemistry.

consideration of the assumptions involved during the calculations. If the chemist identifies any error in the calculation, that fact can be attributed to the algorithm employed or, more specifically, to the platform used but not to computers, which are blind boxes that process information based on the instruction fed to them.

5.3 CONFORMATIONAL ANALYSIS AND ENERGY MINIMIZATION

5.3.1 The concept

The term *conformation* refers to an arrangement of atoms in a molecule, which is interconvertible by rotation about single bonds. The nature of a covalent bond depends upon the state of orbital hybridization between the participating atoms. Since we know that different types of chemical bonds are characterized by specific energy values, free rotation about the sigma bond (σ), such as the carbon–carbon single bond, might induce changes in energy of the whole molecule, leaving it in a favorable or unfavorable energy condition. Now, if a molecule undergoes various molecular arrangements in space, questions might be asked regarding the actual structure, which basically contains all the possible conformers. Considering the ethane molecule, for example, the sigma bond (σ) between the two sp^3-hybridized carbon atoms is considered to be cylindrically symmetrical about a line joining both nuclei, and the bond strength is also expected to be same in all different arrangements.

The molecule can perform a free change of conformation from one to another only if the energy of different arrangements is the same or similar. However, considering certain physical properties, it has been observed that the rotation about the carbon–carbon sigma bond is monitored by an energy barrier (about 3 kcal/mole for ethane), giving evidence that the potential energy of a molecule changes in different conformations. One of the most widely used methods for the representation of structural conformers is called *Newman projection*, which is named after its developer, M.S. Newman.

In Figure 5.3, two different conformers of ethane are shown, in which the form *a* is termed *staggered conformation*, while the name of representation *b* is known as *eclipsed conformation*. In between these two, an infinite number of conformations can theoretically exist, which are called *skew conformations*. The staggered conformation is characterized by minimal potential energy (hence more stability for a given molecule); the energy rises following free rotation and reaches a maximal value at the eclipsed conformation. The energy required for conversion from one conformer to another is defined as *torsional energy*, and relative instability of any conformation is depicted in terms of *torsional strain*. It may be noted that a molecule in the eclipsed conformation faces instability owing to other forces besides torsional strain. These include van der Waals force, dipole–dipole interaction, and hydrogen bonding contributed by neighboring atoms or groups (this does not apply in the case of ethane). We would like to

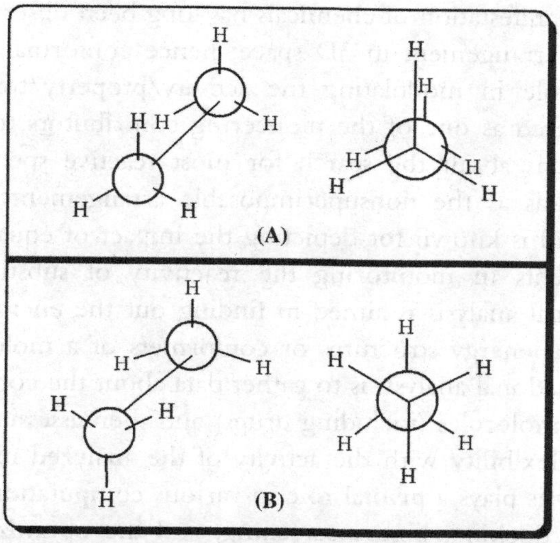

Figure 5.3 Staggered and eclipsed conformations of a ethane molecule. (A) Staggered conformations; (B) eclipsed conformations.

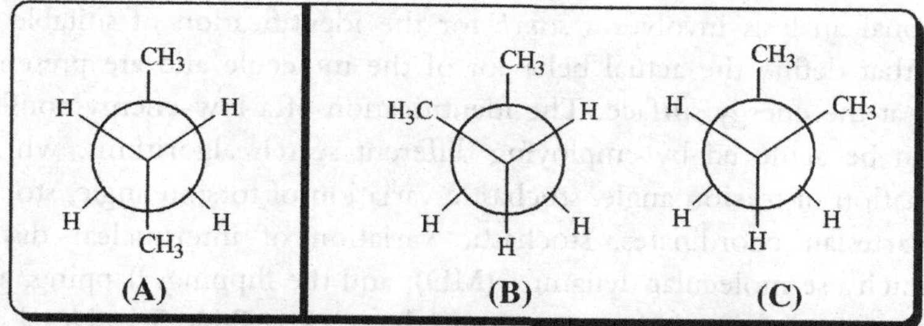

Figure 5.4 Staggered and eclipsed conformations of an *n*-butane molecule.

elaborate this point with one additional example, concerning *n*-butane. Unlike ethane, *n*-butane contains two terminal methyl groups attached to each of the carbon atoms number 2 and 3. As a result, *n*-butane is characterized by three staggered conformations (Figure 5.4). Here, the arrangement *i* is termed *anti*, as both the methyl substituents are placed farthest apart, while the rest two conformers are named *gauche*, where the substituent methyl groups are close to each other. The anti conformer has been observed to be more stable because of the absence of the steric van der Waals repulsion caused by the closely placed methyl groups of the gauche form [3]. Note that the energy required for interconversion of various conformers in case of ethane or butane is easily supplied from the collisions among the molecules at room temperature, and the individual conformers cannot be isolated.

The behavioral manifestation of chemicals has long been observed to depend upon a suitable molecular arrangement in 3D space; hence conformation is considered to play an important role in modulating the activity/property/toxicity of chemicals. Barton [4] is considered as one of the pioneering contributors to the exploration of conformational analysis about the search for most reactive species. Barton defined conformational analysis as the nonsuperimposable arrangements of the atoms of a molecule in space and is known for depicting the impact of equatorial and axial orientation of substituents in monitoring the reactivity of substituted cyclohexanes. Hence, conformational analysis is aimed in finding out the energetically stable form; that is, the minimum energy structures or conformers of a molecule. The principal objective of conformational analysis is to gather data about the conformational features of flexible bioactive molecules (including drugs) and then assessing the correlation of the conformational flexibility with the activity of the analyzed molecules. Therefore, conformational analysis plays a pivotal role in various computational chemistry operations like molecular docking, library screening, and the optimization and design of lead molecules.

5.3.2 Conformational search

Conformational analysis involves a *search* for the identification of suitable molecular conformers that define the actual behavior of the molecule and are present at minimum points at the energy surface. The identification of a low-energy conformer of a molecule can be achieved by employing different search algorithms, which involve systemic variation of torsion angle, stochastic variation of torsion angle, stochastic variation of Cartesian coordinates, stochastic variation of internuclear distances and methods, which use molecular dynamics (MD); and the flipping, flapping, and flexing of rings or mapping of the rings onto generic shapes. [5]. Table 5.1 gives a representative overview of various "search" methods [6] usually employed for the purpose of conformational analysis, while different experimental techniques (noncomputational) used to characterize conformational analysis [7] are briefly presented in Table 5.2.

5.3.3 Minimization of energy

Energy minimization is essential to determining the proper molecular arrangement in space since the drawn chemical structures are not energetically favorable. The potential energy of a molecule contains different energy components like stretching, bending, and torsion; hence, when an energy minimization program is run, it will immediately reach a minimum local energy value, and it might stop if the employed program is not exhaustive. In other words, an energy minimization might stop after it finds the first stable conformer that is structurally closest to the starting molecular arrangement. At this point, identified as the *local energy minimum*, structural variation

Table 5.1 An overview of different conformational search methods

Sl. No.	**Name of the search method**	**Brief description**
1	Systematic search	*Grid search*: Considering a dihedral angle to be the dominating parameter for differentiating conformers, conformers are generated by systematically varying the dihedral angle by some increment while keeping bond angle and length fixed, thereby obtaining all combinatorial possibilities of dihedral angles for the molecule. This type of systemic searching of conformers, termed as *grid search* or *grid scan*, generates an intractable number of conformers without identifying the unique low-energy local minima on the conformational hypersurface. *Custom search*: Here, specific values are assigned to the torsion angles. Such approach is advantageous if favorable states of torsion angles are known from a previous knowledge (study) so that one can limit the systemic search. Furthermore, this method can operate simultaneous changes in several torsion angles.
2	Model-building method	This method uses molecular fragments or larger building blocks, considering each fragment to be independent of the other. Hence, it is a substructure-based method and is applicable to molecules in which fragments are available.
3	Random approach	Following the generation of an initial structure, a random movement in Cartesian space occurs, leading to minimization. This minimized conformer is added to a list, the operation moves to the next starting structure, and the method stops after obtaining desired structures or completion of sampling of all conformers or the finish of a predefined number of steps.
4	Distance geometry	In this method, a matrix of all pairwise atomic distance values in a molecule is used to form a series of Cartesian coordinates. Standard geometries are used for some of the distances, while the others are gathered from experimental data and random number generation, as provided by the upper- and lower-bound range of the known distance. This method is suitable for the search of both small molecules and macromolecules.

(*Continued*)

Table 5.1 (Continued)

Sl. No.	Name of the search method	Brief description
5	Monte Carlo method	Here, simulation of the dynamic behavior of a molecule is done by randomly making changes to the system like rotation of dihedral angles or displacement of atoms. The newly generated atomic configuration is accepted if its energy is less than the previous one. However, in the case of a higher energy value of the conformer, acceptance is made using an algorithmic probability, such as the Metropolis algorithm. The probability is defined by the Boltzmann distribution as follows: $\exp\left(-\frac{\Delta E_i}{kT}\right)$, where k is the Boltzmann constant and T is the absolute temperature. If a randomly generated number is smaller than the Boltzmann factor, the configuration is accepted.

Table 5.2 Some representative experimental methods employed for characterizing conformational analysis

Sl. No.	Experimental techniques for conformational analysis	Brief notes
1	Gas-phase electron diffraction (GED)	A powerful old technique. Limitation includes interpretation of the experimental data. GED has been used by the researchers for the conformational analysis of ethane, cyclohexane, chlorocyclohexane, etc.
2	Electronic circular dichroism (ECD)	A chirooptical method. Useful in analyzing conformers that are different in the relative character of the chromophoric parts, giving different ECD spectra.
3	Vibrational circular dichroism (VCD)	Uses the infrared (IR) technique and is more advantageous than ECD since conformational changes are more sensibly reflected by IR bands and it does not necessitate chromophoric groups.
4	Raman optical activity (ROA)	Rarely used. Studies have been carried out on chiral deuterated [$^2H_1$, $^2H_2$, $^2H_3$]-neopentane.
5	Dynamic nuclear magnetic resonance (DNMR)	Allows wide signal dispersion and high sensitivity of chemical shifts toward conformational change. Can be operated at different NMR frequencies (e.g., ^1H, ^{19}F, ^{13}C, ^{29}Si, ^{31}P), as well as in a wide temperature range.
6	Nuclear overhauser effect (NOE)	Proton−proton intramolecular NOE determines the H-atoms in a molecule that are reciprocally close. It has been employed for determining stereochemical features of taxane derivatives.

yields a low change of energy; hence, minimization can stop. However, this may not be (and usually is not) the most stable conformer since the structural minimization stops before an energy barrier. This encumber of energy can be overcome by the use of suitable algorithms, which can increase the strain energy of the structure and finally lead to the most stable conformer, called *global energy minimum*. Hence, the identification of the energy minima (i.e., the potential energy hypersurface of a stable molecule) is crucial to determining its behavior. Molecular modeling operation (namely, MD) allows achieving the most stable conformational stage. Figure 5.5 shows different possible phases of an energy minimization operation. Now, since we are interested in finding the behavior of bioactive molecules, our intention will be finding the *bioactive conformer.* Although the most active conformer seems to be biologically potent, studies have shown that the bioactive conformer might differ from it. However, the bioactive conformer remains in a zone close to the most active conformer. Usually, if the cocrystal geometry of a molecule is present (i.e., geometry a ligand bound to a receptor pocket determined by experimental study like X-ray crystallographic analysis), that conformation of the ligand is considered as the bioactive molecular arrangement or conformation. In the absence of any cocrystal geometric structure, one can consider the most stable conformer as the bioactive conformer. It might be interesting to note that various studies have focused on the determination of the global energy minimum even if the cocrystal geometry of the molecule is present, thereby allowing a comparative assessment of molecular geometry.

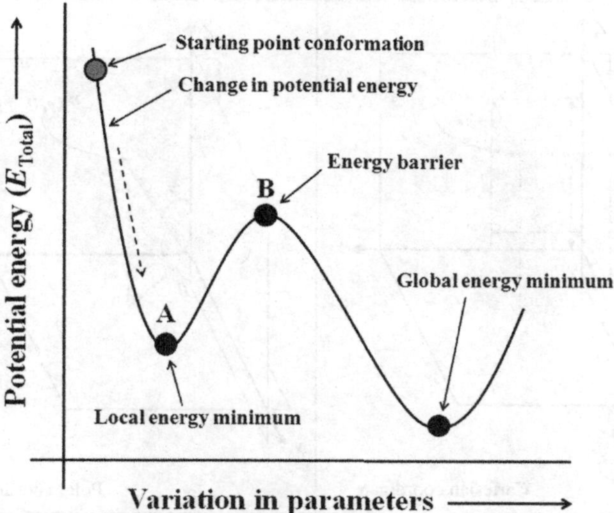

Figure 5.5 Different phases of a molecule during minimization of its energy.

The energy minimization methodology needs to involve identification of the point closest to the starting structure. It might involve a separate algorithmic support for the generation of initial starting structures toward ensuing minimization. It is necessary to understand the difference between conformation searches and other simulation operations like MD and Monte Carlo simulation. Conformational analysis aims to identify minimum energy structures, while simulation operations give an assembly of states that includes structures not at energy minima. However, both MD and Monte Carlo methods can be deployed as part of the conformational search mechanism. Therefore, minimization of energy of 3D structures is crucial to identifying the molecular behavior, but the level of analysis purely depends on the employed algorithm.

Two most important methods facilitating the computational aspects of theoretical chemistry are calculations involving MM and quantum mechanics. The approaches are directed toward the development of energy equations for the total structure of a molecule under investigation. One of the important aspects of these analyses is the position of the atoms in a molecular structure, which is defined by Cartesian or polar coordinates. The initial values of the coordinates can either be set by the modeler or can be obtained from preexisting structural fragments where computer programs set up the coordinates from the program database. Computer programs also can adjust the coordinates if additional fragments are added considering their relative positions. After running a job of MM or quantum mechanics (i.e., the establishment of an energy equation), a final set of coordinates for the minimized structure is calculated by computer. This final coordinate set is converted by using a suitable graphics package for the visualization of the energy-minimized structure. Figure 5.6 presents

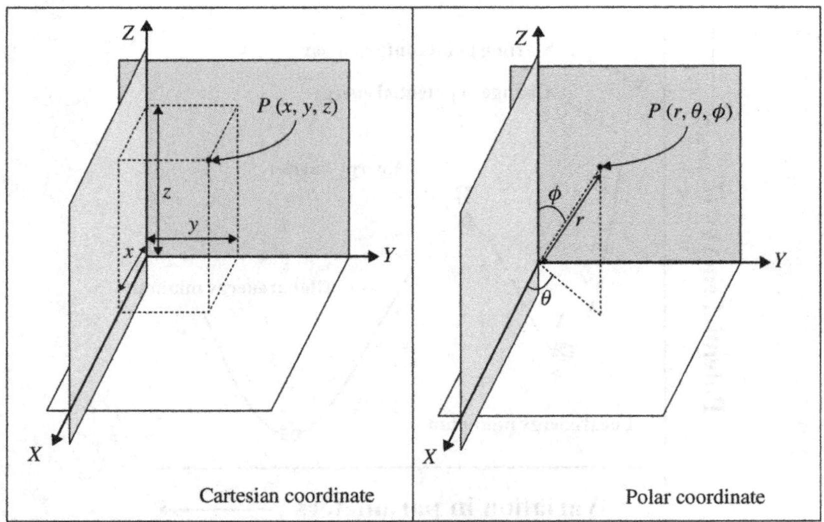

Figure 5.6 Representation of Cartesian and polar coordinates of an arbitrary point.

arbitrary Cartesian and polar coordinates in a 3D plane. Now, it should be noted that although calculations made using computer programs are likely to yield precise results, the conditions or constraints at which computations are made need to be considered. In many cases, the default calculations are based on a molecule defined at 0 K in vacuum instead of considering the actual influences of molecular vibration or the effects of the medium. Quantum mechanical calculations consume considerably more computation power than molecular mechanical calculations [8]. The choice of method depends upon the desire of the modeler and (more often) the available information.

5.4 MOLECULAR MECHANICS

MM assumes that the relative positions of the nuclei of the atoms forming a structure are a function of operating attractive and repulsive forces [9]. Different types of bond stretching, angle bending, torsional energy, and other nonbonded attributes are computed by employing equations of classical physics, giving various interactions and energies also known as *force fields.* Thus, the total potential energy of a molecule is expressed as the sum of all different types of attractive and repulsive forces between the atoms in the structure, considering the impact of nuclei and avoiding the impact of electrons. A hypothetical mechanical model is employed that considers spheres joined by mechanical springs, where the sphere and spring represent the atom and covalent bond, respectively, thereby allowing the application of laws of classical mechanics. A general form of the equation showing components of the total energy can be represented as follows:

$$E_{\text{Total}} = \sum E_{\text{Stretching}} + \sum E_{\text{Bend}} + \sum E_{\text{van der Waals}} + \sum E_{\text{Coulombic}} + \sum E_{\text{Torsion}} \tag{5.1}$$

It is beyond the scope of this chapter to provide detailed discussions on all different energy terminologies. A brief explanation on the force and energy terminologies presented in Eq. (5.1) has been provided in Table 5.3.

The steric energy of the molecules is first computed using force fields, followed by adjustment of the conformation for the minimization of steric energy. One of the methods of calculation in MM employs atom types for the determination of the functions and parameters that comprise the force field. A single element such as a carbon atom can be defined by different MM atom types, the selection of which depends upon various features such as hybridization and chemical environment. Examples of some MM force fields include MM2, MM3, MMFF, Amber, Dreiding, and UFF, all of which are implemented in different software packages [10–19]. Table 5.4 lists the basic features that are implemented in various force fields.

Table 5.3 Formal definition of different energy terms that define the total energy of a molecule

Phenomenon	Equation	Brief explanation
Torsion	$E_{Torsion} = \frac{1}{2} k_{\phi}[1 + \cos m(\phi + \phi_{offset})]$ where ϕ_{offset} is the ideal torsion angle relative to a staggered conformation of two atoms and k_{ϕ} represents the energy barrier for rotation about the torsion angle ϕ. The periodicity of rotation is denoted by *m*.	Torsional energy presents the energy required for the free rotation of a sigma bond. Torsion is about the atoms that are separated by three bonds from each other. The torsion angle represents the dihedral angle defining the relative orientation of the atoms. The following figure shows the torsion angle ϕ between two sample atoms in a staggered conformation.
Bond stretching	$E_{Stretching} = \frac{1}{2} k_{stretch} \times (r - r_0)^2$ where the ideal and stretched bond lengths are denoted by r_0 and *r*, respectively, and $k_{stretch}$ is a force constant giving a measure of the strength of the spring; that is, the bond. Hence, a double bond will have a larger value of $k_{stretch}$ than a single bond.	Considering a covalent bond made up of a spring, Hooke's law can be employed for the computation of bond stretching energy. However, the Morse function containing complex mathematical terms also allows computation of bond stretching.
Angle bending	$E_{Bend} = \frac{1}{2} k_{\theta} \times (\theta - \theta_0)^2$ where the ideal bond angle is denoted by θ_0 and θ is the bond angle in the bending position.	The ideal bond angle corresponds to the angle formed by three consecutive atoms at their minimum energy position. Bending angle θ can be represented as follows, where the arrows show movement of atoms:

van der Waals force	$E_{vdW} = \varepsilon \times \left[\left(\frac{r_{min}}{r}\right)^{12} - 2 \times \left(\frac{r_{min}}{r}\right)^{6}\right]$ Here, at minimum energy value ε, r_{min} presents the distance between atoms i and j while the actual distance between the atoms is r.	The van der Waals force of interaction can be represented by the Lennard–Jones potential equation, where the first term bearing power 6 $\{()^6\}$ represents forces of attraction, and the term with 12th power $\{()^{12}\}$ denotes the short-range repulsive forces involved.
Coulombic force	$E_{Coulombic} = \frac{q_i \times q_j}{D \times r_{ij}}$ where q_i and q_j represent the point charges on atoms i and j, respectively, with r_{ij} being the distance between them. D denotes the dielectric constant of the medium.	Measures the effect of a charge between two points. The attractive or repulsive interaction between two atoms i and j separated by distance r_{ij} can be represented as> 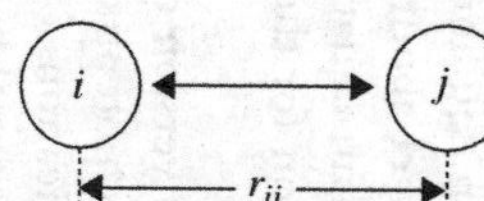

Table 5.4 Representative examples of various force fields that are employed in MM/dynamics studies

Sl. No.	Name	Characteristics
1	MM2	It is applicable for simple molecular structures containing common functional groups like ketones, ethers, and aromatic compounds. However, MM2 is more applicable to nonheteroatom-containing organic compounds. In order to characterize the real potential function of a chemical bond, MM2 adds terms to the bonded interaction considering anharmonic breakage of bonds. The MM2 force field considers the hybridization pattern and bonding partners in depicting the change in equilibrium bond lengths and angles. One more important fact about the MM2 force field is that it employs the Buckingham equation instead of the Lennard–Jones equation for the computation of van der Waals interactions.
2	MM3	It is a more sophisticated version of the MM2 force field incorporating complex potential functions. It considers several corrections and modifications over the MM2 algorithm, like correction of high rotational barriers in congested hydrocarbons, changes in the van der Waals parameter to circumvent strong H/H nonbonded repulsion when placed at a short distance, torsion–stretch interaction differentiating bond length between eclipsed and staggered conformations, and application of bond dipole moment correction to define crystal packing in benzene.
3	MM4	It performs improved calculation of vibrational frequencies, rotational barriers, etc. for compounds like alkanes and cycloalkanes, excluding small ring systems. It includes special interactions like torsion–bend and the bend–torsion–bend.
4	MMFF	Merck molecular force field (MMFF) is a force field comprising of high-quality data of wide range employed for MM/dynamics simulation operation. MMFF is supposed to present the structures of organic compounds in the Merck index or the Fine Chemicals Directory. This force field comprises several updated versions; however, the basic parameters include attributes of bond stretching, angle bending, stretch–bend interactions, out-of-plane bending at tri-coordinate centers, van der Waals force, torsion, and electrostatic interactions.
5	AMBER	Assisted model building with energy refinement (AMBER) algorithm uses an empirical energy approach, allowing the modeling of small molecules and polymers. AMBER comprises of various subunits, namely, PREP (residue preparation), LINK (residue joining), EDIT (structural modification, change in charges, etc.), PARM (adds parameter), MINM (energy partitioning minimization), ANAL (comparison of rms), etc. for the effective processing of the data.

(*Continued*)

Table 5.4 (Continued)

Sl. No.	Name	Characteristics
6	DREIDING	It aims at the use of general force constants and geometry parameters considering the state of hybridization instead of the information derived from combination of atoms. DREIDING uses atomic radii to compute all bond distances, as well as a single force constant, to denote each bond, angle and inversion accompanied by six values for the torsional strain. Atom types defined by a five-character mnemonic label are used as the components of the DREIDING force field, and the potential energy is considered to be summation of valence (E_{val}) and nonbonded (E_{nb}) interaction that depends on atomic distance. The bond stretch is defined either considering harmonic oscillator or using the Morse function.
7	UFF	Universal force field (UFF) focuses on the element, its state of hybridization, and the connectivity possessed by it. UFF allows large amplitude displacements for the functional forms that define angular distortion. Apart from being a molecular mechanical force field, UFF can be employed in an MD energy computation algorithm. Atomic bond radii dependent on the state of hybridization, hybridization angles, parameters defining van der Waals interaction, torsional and inversion barriers, and a set of effective nuclear charges are used as parameters in the UFF formalism.
8	CHARMM	Chemistry at HARvard Macromolecular Mechanics (CHARMM) presents a suitable simulation program allowing a versatile suit application for conformational and path sampling methods, free energy estimates, molecular minimization, MD, analysis techniques, as well as model-building capabilities involving many-particle systems. CHARMM can be employed for the study of biomolecules like peptides, proteins, prosthetic groups, small molecule ligands, nucleic acids, lipids, and carbohydrates. It can be used involving various energy functions and models.
9	OPLS	Optimized potentials for liquid simulations (OPLS) atomic nucleus are appended with interaction site with the exception of CH_n groups that are considered to be united atoms centered on the carbon. Special functions are used to denote H-bonding, and standard combination rules are employed for the Lennard–Jones interaction potential.
10	ECEPP	Empirical conformational energy program for peptides (ECEPP) defines the geometry of amino acid residues and the functions for interatomic interaction by employing a set of internally consistent and standardized parameters. ECEPP is characterized by experimental data and is updated following the development of new data.

The development of a molecular model by using MM force field can be achieved by two means: namely, (i) employment of a commercial force field program in a computer and (ii) use of a database of a molecular modeling program to assemble suitable structural fragments. In the first case, users can select the appropriate molecular mechanical force field from the available packages. In this case, the relevant values of the force field equation are provided as input. Computers calculate an initial value of E_{Total} for the model, which undergoes energy minimization, and then a final set of coordinates corresponding to the minimized structure is calculated. Coordinates of this final structure undergo suitable graphical conversion for the visualization of the energy minimized structure.

In the second method, the user collects fragments of desired configuration (hybridization, etc.) from the available database of a suitable molecular modeling program, which are assembled in a form that allows no steric hindrance. Now, the whole structure may not be at the minimized energy conformation that can be processed further to reach the state. It may be noted that during the process of minimization, any molecule is twisted, allowing steric hindrance, and the coordinates are changed accordingly. The graphical packages are designed such that they show the entire process of energy minimization (i.e., the twisting of the molecule in a computer screen), and some of these packages allow the user to record a video of the entire phenomenon.

5.5 MOLECULAR DYNAMICS

The foundation of life involves the dynamic evolution of a complex network of chemicals at the molecular level: namely, folding of proteins, nucleic acids, transport of ions through membrane, catalysis of biochemical reactions by enzymes, etc. In order to address the complexity and the dynamic nature of the biological systems, computational simulation methodologies have become increasingly important with the growth and development of powerful *in silico* workstations. The previous techniques discussed so far consider a static molecule during investigation; for example, MM calculations are performed at 0 K considering a frozen molecule. Hence, the natural motion of the atoms in a molecule is not considered when these studies are initiated. Hence, there is a need of a theoretical simulation system that can provide us with a hypothetical dynamic behavior of chemicals and biomolecules.

5.5.1 Definition

MD can be defined as a computer simulation technique that permits the prediction of time evolution of an interacting particular system involving the generation of atomic trajectories of a system using numerical integration of Newton's equation of motion for a specific interatomic potential defined by an initial condition and boundary condition. The dynamic simulation also provides information on molecular kinetics and thermodynamics. The determination of time-dependent motion of individual particles of a system allows quantification of the properties of the given system on a definite time scale that is otherwise unattainable.

5.5.2 Development and components

The base concept of MD emerged from the experiments carried out by theoretical physicists. Alder and Wainwright [20] are considered to be the first to study the dynamics of liquid using the "hard-sphere" model where atomic interaction took place through perfect collisions. This study was followed by Rahman's [21] simulation experiment impersonating the real atomic interactions by the use of smooth and continuous potential. One more important aspect about the development of MD simulation can be attributed to the revolutionary advancements of computational algorithm and technology, which actually allowed the application of MD in several areas of chemistry and physics. From 1970 onward, MD simulation has become a widely practiced simulation method for the study of structure and dynamics of macromolecules: namely, protein and nucleic acids among various research groups.

MD techniques are pursued in two major families to address a physical system considering the nature of the model and the mathematical formalism involved. The approaches include classical mechanics and quantum chemical formalisms, as described here:

1. *Classical mechanics approach:* In this treatment, molecules are considered as classical objects resembling that of the ball-and-stick model, where atoms denote soft balls and the bonds represent elastic sticks. The dynamics of a given system here is judged by the laws of classical mechanics.
2. *Quantum mechanics approach:* This is also termed the *first-principles* MD simulation and originated from the pioneering studies of Car and Parinello, who considered the quantum nature of the chemical bonds. The bonding in a system as defined by the electron density function of the valence electrons is determined employing quantum equations while the dynamics of ions (nuclei with their inner electrons) is subjected to classical treatment. Quantum MD simulations are the necessary enhancement of the classical formalism and they provide valuable information on several biological problems at the cost of consuming more computational resources.

The core requirement for MD simulation is actually simple; it involves a set of conditions defining the initial positions and velocities of all particles and the interaction potential that defines the forces among all the particles. Second, the determination of the evolution of the system in time is done by solving a set of equations of motion for all particles considered in the system. In the case of classical mechanics, Newton's law is applied to define the motion of classical particles. It may be noted that even a classical MD simulation for biomolecular systems consisting of thousands of atoms over a nanosecond time scale consumes a significant amount of computational resources [22].

The MD simulation formalism may be considered to be comprised of five conditions: namely, boundary condition, initial condition, force calculation, integrator/ensemble, and property calculation.

5.5.3 The algorithm

Considering a classical mechanics approach, the force F_i acting upon the ith particle possessing mass m_i at time t among a set of interacting particles will be given as follows:

$$F_i = m_i \frac{d^2 r_i(t)}{dt^2} \tag{5.2}$$

where $r_i(t)$ is the position vector of the ith particle and can be represented as $r_i(t) = \{x_i(t), y_i(t), z_i(t)\}$. Here, the term *particles* usually refer to atoms though distinct entity; for example, chemical groups can also be represented. Now, Eq. (5.2) is a differential equation of second order that can be integrated by providing specific values of the initial position of particles, their velocities, and the instantaneous force acting on them. The equation of motion is discretized followed by numerical solution because of the many-body system comprised of the particles. The trajectories in MD simulation are defined by position and velocity vector components, and the time evolution of the system is depicted in phase space. The position and velocities components are promulgated with a finite time interval by employing numerical integrators. The examples include the Verlet algorithm. The position of each particle in space is designated by $r_i(t)$, while the kinetic energy and temperature of the system is determined by velocity $v_i(t)$. The specialty of MD simulation is that it allows a direct tracing of the dynamic events that might be influential to the functional properties of the system.

The integration of Newton's force equation is performed to obtain an expression that gives the position $r_i(t + \Delta t)$ at time $t + \Delta t$ in terms of the already-known positions at time t. By employing the Taylor series, the mentioned position can be mathematically represented as follows [Eq. (5.3)]:

$$r_i(t + \Delta t) \cong 2r_i(t) - r_i(t - \Delta t) + \frac{F_i(t)}{m_i}\Delta t^2 \tag{5.3}$$

The calculation of velocity can be done using the positions or by the use of explicit methods as implemented in systems like alternative *leapfrog* and *velocity* Verlet scheme. It may be noted that an infinitesimally small integration step is obtained by the trajectories, although it is necessary to have larger time steps for sampling longer trajectories. In reality, determination of Δt involves the fastest motion. For example, the Δt value resides in a sub-femtosecond scale while simulating bonds bearing light atoms, ensuring the stability of the integration. However, coarse-grained simulations use atoms of larger mass, thereby leading to an increased integration time, as well as the trajectory length. One more important aspect of MD simulation is its behavioral nature with statistical mechanics, thereby allowing averaging of values obtained at a microscopic level. The Newtonian dynamics follows the conservation of energy, and MD trajectories give a set of microcanonical ensemble distribution of configurations. This permits the measurement of physical quantities by taking arithmetic average over instantaneous values from the trajectories in a MD simulation job. MD allows simulation of a wide range of experimental conditions; for example, simulation of protein in vacuum, explicit water environment, and crystal environment. Furthermore, the efficiency of MD simulation can be enhanced by the incorporation of improvements in algorithms. Examples of such improvements include RESPA, SHAKE, RATTLE, and LINCS. A larger time step (Δt) without any significant degradation in the trajectory can be obtained by the use of RESPA coupled with a fixed bond length involving H-atoms with SHAKE, RATTLE, or LINCS. Among other methods, adiabatic mapping is an example of studying motion in proteins.

5.6 QUANTUM MECHANICS

With the progress of scientific research, Erwin Schrödinger [23] developed the theory of quantum mechanics in 1926 while studying on the mathematical expression of the motion of electron in terms of its energy. Before going into the details of the quantum mechanical formalism, we would like to present a necessary look back at the electronic picture of atoms and molecules so that readers can have an overview of the essential theories and assumptions involved in formulating electronic models (Box 5.1).

The electron was assumed to depict the property of waves along with being particles and hence the mathematical equations developed by Schrödinger were termed as *wave equations*. A wave equation possesses a series of solutions termed as *wave functions*, each of which depicts a different energy level for the electron. A wave function is designated as a time-dependent state function since it defines the nature as well as the properties of the system. Even for a simple system, solving all of the wave equations is cumbersome. The basic principle of the Schrödinger wave equation can be mathematically depicted as given in Eq. (5.4):

$$H\psi = E\psi \tag{5.4}$$

BOX 5.1 A Necessary Look at the Assumptions and Theories That Define the Electronic Attributes of Atoms (and Molecules)

Theories and explanations on the fundamental basis of the chemical structures allow the building of a framework of ideas regarding the arrangement of atoms, their order, compatibility, electronic configuration, and possible interaction with neighboring moieties. Electrons are characterized by both the wave and particle nature. However, the wave equations are unable to show the exact position of an electron at a particular moment or the exact velocity at which it is moving; instead, they depict the probability of finding the electron at any particular space.

- *Different hypothesis/models/rules characterizing the nature of electrons*
  - *Thompson*: Proposed that electrons and protons are uniformly mixed throughout an atom and represent a "plum pudding" arrangement.
  - *Rutherford*: Proposed that the nucleus at the center of an atom carries a positive charge and contains the maximum mass, while electrons having minimum mass and negative charge orbit the nucleus at a certain distance. This is also termed the *planetary model.*
  - *Bohr*: Proposed that electrons are moving around the nucleus in specific circular quantized orbits having a definite angular momentum. The angular momentum of electrons is quantized (using Planck's theory), and the amount of energy depends upon the size of orbit. Electrons can absorb (gain) or release (lose) energy in the form of defined quanta while moving in between orbits.
  - *De Broglie*: Postulated a *wave-particle* duality of matter; that is, particles could have properties of a wave. The de Broglie wavelength was proposed to show that the wavelength is inversely proportional to the momentum of a particle using Planck's constant.
  - *Heisenberg uncertainty principle*: It is impossible to know the position and the momentum of an electron simultaneously at a given time.
  - *Aufbau principle*: Electrons occupy the lowest-energy orbital available.
  - *Hund's rule*: The spin of electrons filling orbitals of the same energy level remains parallel (aligned) until the formation of electron pairs. Aligned spins represent more stable forms considering quantum mechanical reasons.
  - *Pauli exclusion principle*: An orbital can only be filled with two electrons possessing opposite spin. Electrons of opposite spin are termed "paired" while those having "like" spin tend to get as far as possible and constitute the basis for shape and other molecular properties.
- *Wave nature of electrons*

  The wave property that describes an electron cloud is very similar to that of a standing or stationary wave. A sample stationary wave generated by the vibration of a string secured at both ends (for example) can be characterized by several segments when observed horizontally along its length as shown in Figure B5.1.

  The amplitude of the wave increases in one direction and passes through a maximum, followed by a gradual decrease into zero. Then it again increases in the reverse direction and follows a similar path. The places depicting zero amplitude are termed

(Continued)

BOX 5.1 A Necessary Look at the Assumptions and Theories That Define the Electronic Attributes of Atoms (and Molecules)—cont'd

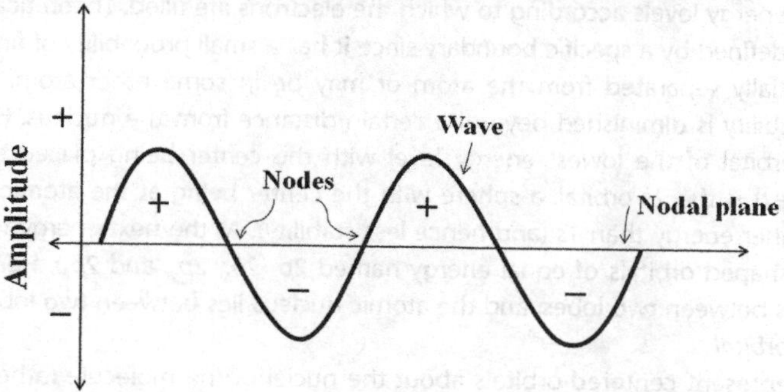

Figure B5.1 Example of a sample stationary wave generated by the vibration of a string that is secured at both ends.

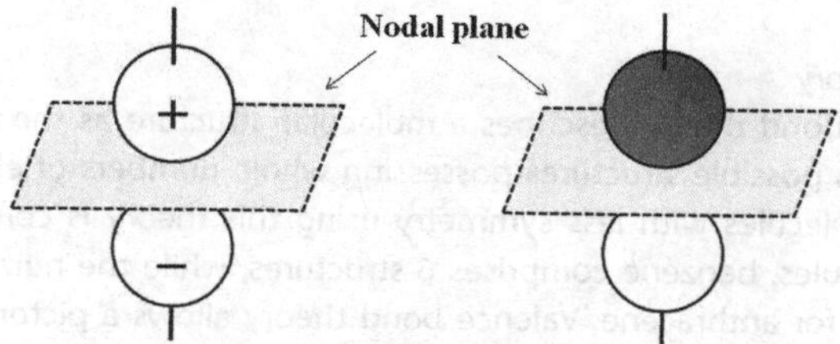

Figure B5.2 Representation of a *p*-orbital with the lobes being placed above and below the nodal plane.

nodes, and the corresponding plane is referred to as the *nodal plane*, while the upward and downward displacements denote opposite wave phases. A wave equation is a differential equation that can be solved in terms of the amplitude ψ as a function of the distance x along the wave; that is, $f(x)$. The amplitude (ψ) for the wave of an electron is represented by a function of three coordinates providing a 3D view of the motion. An electron wave is also characterized by nodes; that is, zero amplitude zone accompanied with upward and downward displacements. In the case of *p*-orbitals, these displacements are denoted by lobes (using + and − or shades) being above and below the nodal plane as given in Figure B5.2.

The wave function ψ represents an MO and is defined by the specific energy value required to move that electron from the molecule. The orbitals are polycentric in nature and considering a normalized solution of ψ, square of the amplitude (ψ^2) corresponds to the probability of finding an electron at any particular point in space. This allows a pictorial visualization of contours of constant probability of finding electron and regions with high and low probability.

- *Orbital*

Orbital represents the region in space where an electron is likely to be observed. Different kinds of orbitals (*s*, *p*, *d*, *f*) possess characteristic shapes and sizes and correspond

(*Continued*)

BOX 5.1 A Necessary Look at the Assumptions and Theories That Define the Electronic Attributes of Atoms (and Molecules)—cont'd

to specific energy levels according to which the electrons are filled. Theoretically, an orbital cannot be defined by a specific boundary since it has a small probability of finding an electron essentially separated from the atom or may be in some other atom. Nevertheless, such probability is diminished beyond a certain distance from the nucleus. Here, 1*s* is the spherical orbital of the lowest energy level with the center being placed at the atomic nucleus. Next is the 2*s* orbital, a sphere with the center being at the atomic nucleus possessing higher energy than 1*s* (and hence less stability). At the next energy level are three dumbbell-shaped orbitals of equal energy named 2*p* ($2p_x$, $2p_y$, and $2p_z$). Here, the atomic nucleus lies between two lobes, and the atomic nucleus lies between two lobes.

- *Molecular orbital*

  MOs represent centered orbitals about the nuclei of the molecule rather the individual nuclei. This theory is exhaustively mathematical and employs less pictorial depiction. In the case of MOs, each pair of electrons remains localized near the two nuclei and their shapes and disposition are related to those of the atomic orbitals of component atoms.

- *Valence bond theory*

  The valence bond theory describes a molecular structure as the weighted contribution of numerous possible structures possessing whole numbers of electrons. The depiction of larger molecules with less symmetry using this theory is complex. For instance, for simple molecules, benzene comprises 6 structures, while the number is 42 for naphthalene and 429 for anthracene. Valence bond theory allows a pictorial depiction of the most probable contributions.

- *LCAO approximation*

  The linear combination of atomic orbital (LCAO) method employs a linear mathematical relationship of combining atomic orbitals. For a molecule comprising atoms *A* and *B*, the MO ψ can be represented as the summed contribution of the atomic orbitals ψ_A and ψ_B, respectively, where c_a and c_b are the coefficients denoting the weights of the atomic orbitals *A* and *B*, respectively, as follows: $\psi = c_a\psi_a + c_b\psi_b$

  An MO ψ is considered to be more stable than the atomic orbitals ψ_A and ψ_B if the latter overlap to a considerable extent, possess comparable energy, and have symmetry about the bond axis.

- *Bonding and antibonding orbitals*

According to the rules of quantum mechanics, a linear combination of two functions yields two combinations instead of one. Hence, combination of two atomic orbitals will give two MO. Bonding orbitals are more stable than the component atomic orbitals, while antibonding orbital are less stable. In other words, a bonding orbital tends to stabilize a molecule, whereas an antibonding orbital tends to destabilize it. Mathematically, they can be represented as follows:

Bonding orbital: $\psi_+ = \psi_A + \psi_B$

Antibonding orbital: $\psi_- = \psi_A - \psi_B$

(Continued)

BOX 5.1 A Necessary Look at the Assumptions and Theories That Define the Electronic Attributes of Atoms (and Molecules)—cont'd

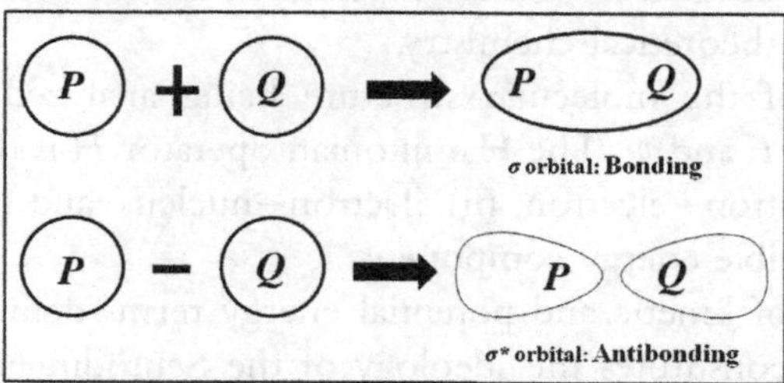

Figure B5.3 Two sample *s* orbitals *P* and *Q* forming bonding and antibonding orbitals.

An example of bonding and antibonding orbital formation by two *s* orbitals *P* and *Q* can be represented as shown in Figure B5.3.

where ψ denotes the time dependent wave function, H is the Hamiltonian operator, and $E\psi$ represents the total potential and kinetic energy of all the particles belonging to the molecular structure. Considering the movement in a 3D space bound by the x-, y-, and z-axes, the wave equation is represented by the following differential form:

$$\frac{\partial^2\psi}{\partial x^2}+\frac{\partial^2\psi}{\partial y^2}+\frac{\partial^2\psi}{\partial z^2}+\frac{8\pi^2 m}{h^2}(E-V)\psi=0 \tag{5.5}$$

where m is the mass, h denotes the Planck's constant term, and E and V represent the total and potential energy, respectively. Equation (5.5) can be represented in a shorter form by using a Laplacian operator ∇^2 for the partial differentials as follows:

$$\nabla^2\psi+\frac{8\pi^2 m}{h^2}(E-V)\psi=0 \tag{5.6}$$

However, we shall stick to Eq. (5.4) in order to maintain simplicity. The quantum mechanical calculations are performed employing theories of quantum physics, which account the interaction between nuclei and electrons. The approximations considered during quantum mechanical calculations are provided here:

1. Allowing the fast motion of electrons, nuclei are considered motionless, thereby differentiating nuclear energy from the energy of the electrons.
2. The movement of electrons is assumed to be independent, considering the influence of other electrons and nuclei as average.

The depiction of many-particle systems remains an essential and crucial task for scientists. The exact analytical solution to the Schrödinger equation can be formulated for only a very few simple systems comprising a small number of atoms. The deployment of the Hamiltonian model, however, provides an option of finding a solution to the equation. The Schrödinger equation actually defines a fundamental relationship of logical coherence to the experimental observations by providing a conceptual scaffold to theoretical chemistry.

The complexity of the molecular structure being analyzed defines the specific mathematical form of E and ψ. The Hamiltonian operator H is defined by interaction terms between (i) electron–electron, (ii) electron–nucleus, and (iii) nucleus–nucleus, accounting for all possible energy components.

Since summation of kinetic and potential energy terms defining the electron and nuclei in a structure constitutes the ideology of the Schrödinger equation, it can be represented as follows:

$$H\psi = (K + U) \times \psi \tag{5.7}$$

Here, E is defined as the summed contribution of kinetic energy term K and potential energy U. The H term for a simple molecule bearing two electron and two nuclei, such as hydrogen (H_2), will be represented by eight different terms, as depicted in Eq. (5.8):

$$H = -\frac{1}{2} \times \overline{V}_1^2 - \frac{1}{2} \times \overline{V}_2^2 + \frac{1}{R_1 R_2} - \frac{1}{R_1 r_1} - \frac{1}{R_1 r_2} - \frac{1}{R_2 r_1} - \frac{1}{R_2 r_2} + \frac{1}{r_1 r_2} \tag{5.8}$$

where $\frac{1}{2}\overline{V}_1^2$ and $\frac{1}{2}\overline{V}_2^2$ represent the kinetic energies of electrons 1 and 2, respectively. The positions of two electrons 1 and 2 are represented by r_1 and r_2, while R_1 and R_2 denote the positions of the nuclei 1 and 2, respectively. Computation of H becomes complex with the increased number of atoms in a molecule, and it becomes economically less viable for compounds possessing more than 50 atoms.

Different approaches for performing quantum mechanical calculations include the *ab initio* method, density function theory (DFT) technique, and semiempirical analysis. The quantum chemical *ab initio* (i.e., from the beginning) methods aim at providing the absolute solution by employing a convergent approach that gives high-quality, accurate results. However, considering the high operation cost and time consumption, such methods are limited to small molecules. Methods other than *ab initio* avoid many less important terms and attempts to hasten the computational procedure by applying several assumptions. The DFT approach provides a favorable performance, considering the cost, and gives reasonably accurate results for medium-sized molecules, while semiempirical computations are very efficient and applicable to large systems, although the accuracy is hindered owing to integral parameterizations. In the pursuit of finding a suitable solution of the Schrödinger wave equation, scientists have developed different approximations in order to reduce the computational burden. In the following sections, we shall highlight some of these approximations, as well as potential techniques that are widely used in quantum mechanical computations.

5.6.1 The Born–Oppenheimer approximation

In order to reduce the computation burden while dealing with various wave functions, the famous Born–Oppenheimer (BO) approximation (named after the contributors Max Born and J. Robert Oppenheimer) is employed to provide a solution to the time-dependent Schrödinger equation [24]. The BO approximation assumes the nucleus to be stationary with respect to the electrons and thereby leaves the kinetic energy of the nuclei out of the relationship, making it simpler. In other words, BO approximation separates the electronic motion and nuclear motion, considering the electronic wave functions to be dependent on the position of nucleus and not its velocity, and a tarnished potential of the speedy electrons is observed by the nuclear motion. Mathematically, the following equation can be written, where r_i denotes position of the electron and R_j represents nuclear position:

$$\psi_{\text{molecule}}(r_i, R_j) = \psi_{\text{electrons}}(r_i, R_j) \cdot \psi_{\text{nuclei}}(R_j) \quad (5.9)$$

In order to derive the energy and molecular wave functions employing the Schrödinger equation for the benzene molecule, which comprises 42 electrons and 12 nuclei, a partial differential eigenvalue equation of 162 variables has to be considered. The BO approximation can make the computation process less demanding, so it is important while dealing with quantum chemical problems.

5.6.2 The Hartree–Fock approximation

The Hartree–Fock (HF) approximation, also known as the *self-consistent field (SCF)* method, is attributed to the seminal work by Hartree [25] and Fock [26]. Considering an interacting particle system, a many-electron wave function can be defined as $\psi(r_1, r_2, \ldots, r_n)$, in which r_i represents the coordinates and spins of the particles. Hartree has provided a useful approximation of a many-electron wave function in terms of the product of single-particle functions, which can be represented as in Eq. (5.10):

$$\psi(r_1, r_2, \ldots, r_n) = \phi_1(r_1) \times \phi_2(r_2) \times \cdots \times \phi_n(r_n) \quad (5.10)$$

where each function $\phi_i(r_i)$ corresponds to a one-electron Schrödinger equation with a potential term belonging to the average field of the other electrons. The following equation for the one-particle function $\phi_i(r_i)$ was proposed by Hartree:

$$\left[-\frac{1}{2}\Delta + v(r) + \sum_{j=1,\, j\neq i}^{N} \int \frac{|\phi_j(r')|^2}{|r - r'|} dr'\right] \phi_i(r) = E_i \phi_i(r) \quad (5.11)$$

where N represents the total number of electrons. The term $v(r)$ is related to a nuclear charge parameter Z as follows: $v(r) = -Z/r$. Here, an electron is considered to be under the SCF at the *i*th state, which is determined by all electrons but the *i*th one. The two main deviations of the HF approximation from the Schrödinger equation include the presence of nonlinear and nonlocal parameters in the former. Because of the nonorthogonal nature of the functions $\phi_i(r)$, the HF equation suffers from the violation of exclusion principle, characterized by the nonorthogonal nature of the functions $\phi_i(r)$ since the self-consistent potential of the *i*th electron depends upon *i*. Various modifications and extensions have been made by researchers to eliminate the problems of the HF equation: namely, antisymmetrized modification, Fermi-statistics inclusion, configuration interaction (CI), etc. The HF equation is iteratively solved by employing a suitable computational platform. Investigation of dynamic properties of multielectron objects (such as atoms, molecules, clusters, and fullerene) by computing ground state energy and employing methods such as random phase approximation (RPA) and the random phase approximation with exchange (RPAE) uses HF as a basis [27].

5.6.3 Density functional theory

The ideological root of the DFT stems from the hypothesis of Thomas [28] and Fermi [29], who considered the employment of electron density to characterize the many-particle systems. It assumes the electronic motions to be uncorrelated, and the kinetic energy of the electrons is depictable by using a local approximation on the free electrons. The Thomas–Fermi equation presents a primitive approach to the density function-based theories and can be described by the following integral: $n(r) = N \int dr_2 \cdots \int dr_N \psi * (r, r_2, ..., r_N) \times \psi(r, r_2, ..., r_N)$, where $n(r)$ presents density of the electron. Following Thomas–Fermi, various developments in the DFT theory took place through the notable contributions of Dirac, Slater, and Gáspár. It is interesting to note that the explorations in the DFT formalism took place by filling the loopholes of the HF formalism. For example, Gáspár obtained better values of the HF eigenfunctions while studying the Cu^+ ion. Slater showed that the approximation of exchange potential in a system of variable density can be performed by incorporating a term possessing local dependence ($[n(r)]^{1/3}$) on the density. Such dependence on density relishes an idea of exchange known as *Fermi-hole* representing a region near an electron that is being avoided by the electron of the same spin and not on the exchange potential in a homogeneous system [30]. The simple local density (LD) approximation has been a very useful tool for the study of solids. Hohenberg and Kohn [31] provided the actual theorem for the DFT in 1964, which was later simplified and modified by Levy [32]. The Hamiltonian operator for *N* electrons moving in an external potential $V_{ext}(r)$ can be represented as follows:

$$H = T + V_{ee} + \sum_{i=1}^{N} V_{ext}(r_i) \tag{5.12}$$

where T and V_{ee} respectively denote the kinetic and electron–electron interaction operators. Considering ψ_{GS} as the wave-function and $n_{GS}(r)$ as the density, the ground-state energy E_{GS} can be represented as follows:

$$\begin{aligned} E_{GS} &= \int \mathrm{d}r V_{ext}(r) n_{GS}(r) + \langle \psi_{GS} | T + V_{ee} | \psi_{GS} \rangle \\ &= \int \mathrm{d}r V_{ext}(r) n_{GS}(r) + F[n_{GS}] \end{aligned} \tag{5.13}$$

where $V_{ext}(r)$ is the external potential and the term $F[n]$ represents a density that is functionally independent of any specific system or the external potential. It is interesting to observe that the Kohn–Sham theory presents another famous derivation in the realm of DFT for solving the Schrödinger equation for a fictitious system of noninteracting particles. Kohn and Sham depicted the application of an LD approximation to the limiting case of a slowly varying density using an exchange and correlation energy term (Eq. (5.14)):

$$E_{xc}^{LD} = \int \mathrm{d}r\ n(r) \varepsilon_{xc}[n(r)] \tag{5.14}$$

where $\varepsilon_{xc}[n]$ denotes the exchange and correlation energy per particle of a homogeneous electron gas characterized by density n. It was observed that use of the Kohn–Sham theory for the HF-like calculation of finite electron system leads to a ground energy value smaller than the actual HF method. The drawbacks of the HF theory are actually solved in the DFT formalism; for example, the nonlocality of single particle exchange potential in HF is overcome by LD approximation in the KS theory.

Many molecular attributes (namely, vibrational frequencies, atomization energies, ionization energies, electric and magnetic properties, reaction paths, etc.) are computable using the DFT.

5.6.4 Semiempirical analysis

5.6.4.1 Concept

Technically the term *semiempirical* refers to methods or techniques that employ assumptions, generalizations, or approximation in order to simplify complex calculations. Semiempirical analysis of the quantum chemical methods uses integral approximations and parameterizations to simplify large calculations of solving the Schrödinger wave equation. Because of the incorporation of several assumptions, the results obtained from semiempirical analysis can be characterized as less accurate, although it attempts to provide a realistic strategy for dealing with large molecules. The semiempirical methods begin with the *ab initio* formalism, followed by assumptive avoidance of several less important terms for the sake of speeding up the calculations. However, empirical parameters are utilized in the formalism with calibration against reliable theoretical or experimental data as a measure of compensation toward the errors of assumptions.

Some *ab initio* and DFT methods employ a number of empirical assumptions, and hence can be categorized into semiempirical analysis.

5.6.4.2 Developmental background

The parameterization of the MO-based valence electron methods are widely employed to address the semiempirical analysis with the aim of enhancing the accuracy of the *ab initio* HF results by the use of a minimal basis set. The primitive semiempirical approach to address electronic structure of chemical compounds includes the Hückel MO (HMO) method [33], which involves a π-electronic formalism for the generation of MO values of unsaturated molecules using a connectivity matrix. A citable enhancement of this method is Hoffman's [34] extended Hückel theory, which uses all valence electrons for computation. These methods make a significant contribution toward the development of qualitative MO theory, which accounts for orbital interactions. It should be noted here that Hückel methods are noniterative in nature, involving one-electron integrals. The Pariser—Parr—Pople [35] formalism describes the electronic spectra of unsaturated molecules that use antisymmetrized products of quantitative atomic orbital integrals possessing the core Hamiltonian and introduces an approximation of zero differential overlap, along with an optional, uniformly charged sphere depiction of atomic orbitals. This theory also allows the incorporation of σ-electron adjustment to the π-electronic distribution. Pople et al. [36] did bring in a hierarchy of integral approximations satisfying various consistency criteria, including the rotational invariance. They showed that the results obtained by neglecting a differential overlap in electron interaction integral without further adjustments are not constant to simple transformation of the atomic orbital basis set, such as the *s*, *p* orbital replacement by hybrids or the rotation of axes. This study led to the development of two schemes that are invariant to transformation among atomic orbitals: namely, the complete neglect of differential overlap (CNDO) and the neglect of diatomic differential overlap (NDDO). Modern semiempirical analyses largely employ the formalism of NDDO and INDO (intermediate neglect of differential overlap) in order to get successful computational results. Exploration of this differential overlap concept has led to the development of a number of schemes, the most frequently employed of which are discussed next, while Table 5.5 gives an overview of different such models.

5.6.4.3 Modified neglect of diatomic overlap

The modified neglect of diatomic overlay (MDNO) approach was proposed and developed by Dewar and Thiel [37] and is based on the NDDO algorithm for the parameterization of one-center, two-electron integrals from the spectroscopic data for isolated atoms. It is aimed at the estimation of other two-electron integrals using the formalism of multipole—multipole interactions from classical electrostatics. Classical MNDO models employ *s* and *p* orbitals as basis sets, while *d* orbitals are added in the

Table 5.5 A representative view of different schemes which have been implemented in semiempirical/self-consistent quantum chemical calculations

Sl. No.	Abbreviated name	Full form of the formalism	Notes
1	LCAOSCF	LCAO self-consistent function	It provides self-consistent function approximation using the LCAO method. Here energy minimization is facilitated by the coefficient of the orbitals. Application is limited due to computational difficulty.
2	CNDO	Complete neglect of differential overlap	CNDO and NDDO represent the simplification of LCAOSCF by employing the approximation of neglecting differential overlap. CNDO does not consider any differential overlap in all the basis sets. Here, a product of two different atomic orbitals corresponding to a specific electron is always "neglected" in electron interaction integrals.
3	NDDO	Neglect of diatomic differential overlap	This corresponds to the product of pairs of atomic orbitals of different atoms that have been neglected in certain electron repulsion integral. For a specific electron, the product of atomic orbitals will be neglected if they are on separate centers.
4	INDO	Intermediate neglect of differential overlap	This corresponds to the neglect of the differential overlap in the integral of all electron interaction except those using one center only; that is, the retention of a one-center product of different atomic orbitals in only one-center integral. It presents an intermediate complexity between the CNDO and NDDO methods.
5	MINDO	Modified intermediate neglect of differential overlap	This algorithm considers a common value in order to represent the two-center electron repulsion integral between the atomic orbitals of a chosen atomic pair.

(*Continued*)

Table 5.5 (Continued)

Sl. No.	Abbreviated name	Full form of the formalism	Notes
6	MNDO	Modified neglect of diatomic overlap	It gives better results in depicting the heat of formation of hydrocarbons, as well as radicals. Here, the approximation has been applied to the closed-shell molecules and their valence electrons, which are assumed to move in a constant core-field composed of the nuclei and inner shell electrons. It improves the computational results obtained from MINDO/3.

latest MNDO/d method for the depiction of hypervalent sulfur species and transition metals. The drawbacks of the MNDO formalism include its inability in describing H-bonding caused by strong intermolecular repulsion and poor consistency in predicting heats of formation. By applying the MNDO method, instability in prediction is shown for highly substituted stereoisomers with respect to the linear isomers, which can be attributed to the overestimation of repulsive forces in a sterically crowded system.

5.6.4.4 Austin model 1

Dewar et al. [38] developed the parametric Austin model 1 (AM1) as an approximation of the NDDO algorithm. Unlike MNDO, the two-electron integrals have been approximated here by using a modified version of the nuclear–nuclear core repulsion function (CRF) that mimics the van der Waals interactions as a nonphysical attraction force. This modification reparameterized the model by instituting changes in dipole moments, ionization potentials, and molecular geometries. The problem of reproducing hydrogen bonds in the MNDO scheme has been overcome in the AM1 method without any increase in computing time. Other advantages include the improvement of computation of some properties, such as the heats of formation with respect to the MNDO method. The disadvantages of the AM1 method include systemic overestimation of basicities and incorrect prediction of the lowest-energy geometry of water dimer.

5.6.4.5 Parametric method 3

The parametric method 3 (PM3) has been developed by Stewart [39] by using a similar Hamiltonian operator like that of AM1, but a separate parameterization strategy.

The PM3 formalism is parameterized in reproducing a large number of molecular properties,, unlike the AM1 strategy, which uses a relatively small number of atomic data. Hydrogen bonds are well assessed in PM3 method due to its specific parameterization protocol and nuclear repulsion treatment. However, the nonphysical hydrogen–hydrogen attraction forces are sometimes expressed, leading to trouble while computing intermolecular interactions. For example, methane is falsely predicted as a strongly bound dimer; and the determination of conformers of flexible molecules such as a hydroxyl group of 1-pentanol is strongly attracted to the methyl group. The PM3 method has a wider application for the computation of electronic attributes and yields more accurate thermochemical data than AM1, and the recent extended versions allow the inclusion of transition metals.

5.6.4.6 PDDG/PM3 and PDDG/MNDO

William Jorgensen and coworkers [40] developed two new formalisms in the realm of semiempirical quantum chemical calculations by using a pairwise distance directed Gaussian (PDDG) modification of the existing MNDO and PM3 methods. The PDDG/PM3 and PDDG/MNDO methods use reparameterized functional group-specific enhancement of the CRF and improve the accuracy of the previous NDDO methods (namely, PM5, PM3, AM1, and MNDO formalisms). Incorporation of the PDDG modification has led to improved computation of van der Waals attraction between atoms, accurate estimation of heat of formation values, and trustworthy calculation of intermolecular complexes, overcoming relative stability of hydrocarbon isomers, energetics of small rings and molecules containing multiple heteroatoms, and other issues. Improvement of the internal consistency of PDDG isomerization energy enjoys better results than the B3LYP/6-31G* method, a hybrid level (density functional) in which Gaussian computations are carried out depending upon the usage.

5.7 OVERVIEW AND CONCLUSION

The application of computer technology is a very significant and crucial element contributing to the exploration of theoretical chemistry. Computers have provided the necessary momentum to pursue studies in theoretical chemistry at a potentially higher level. Moving from visualization to computation is easily done using suitable *in silico* platforms. Moreover, the promising features of MD simulation were derivable only after the development of higher-capacity computer systems. Today, several commercial and open-access molecular modeling software/packages provide users with encouraging, user-friendly interfaces for carrying out modeling operations. Most of these packages offer tutorials describing the operational characteristics of the platform in order to run a specific molecular modeling job (computation or visualization), thereby making the operations easier. A user can perform various such analyses using the default specified values without using so-called expert knowledge. However, it is always helpful to gather some theoretical knowledge behind a major operation. It is also obvious that the basis of several computational chemistry operations stem from the depth of classical physics, mechanics, knowledge on mathematics, biology, and, of course, chemistry. Hence, instead of giving any cumbersome description of theory, we have attempted to provide some basic information defining various molecular modeling operations so that readers can get an overview of the process constraints. Figure 5.7 presents different facets of operations attained by molecular modeling algorithms involving MM, MD, and quantum mechanics.

Molecular mechanical methods are not concerned with the properties and distribution of electrons. Quantum mechanical methods should be used for computation of electron density at various atoms and energies of the highest occupied MO (HOMO) and lowest unoccupied MO (LUMO) and for understanding of the possible orientation of the transition state geometries during reaction. These calculations also provide information on possible reaction pathway and thermodynamic data like heat of formation. The choice of using a suitable molecular modeling technique depends upon the nature of the chemicals and also on the objective of the analysis. Although *ab initio* models provide a theoretical possibility of obtaining most accurate results, they are practiced far less owing to the unfeasible computation power required. In spite of the limitations and accuracy problems, semiempirical methods are quite often used to address the computation of quantum mechanical electronic attributes of chemicals

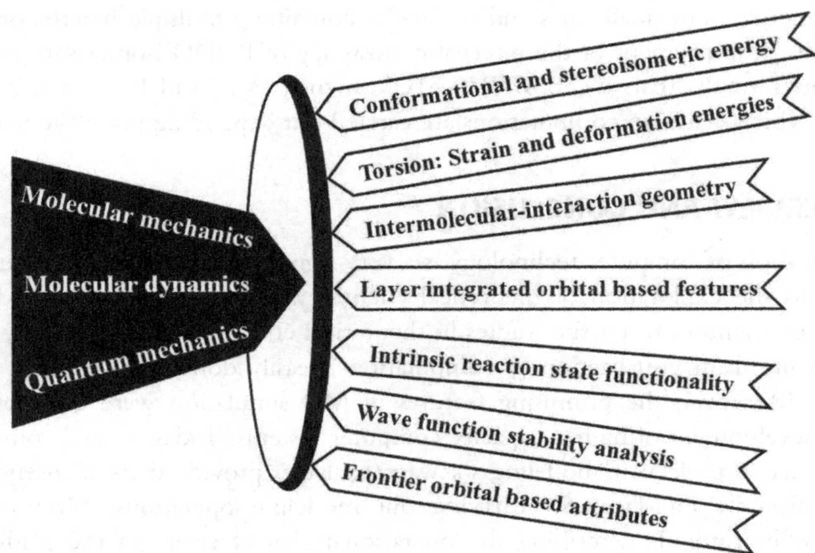

Figure 5.7 Different molecular attributes determined by MM, MD, and quantum chemical calculations.

possessing a relatively large structure, which are impractical to model using more accurate methods. Actually, large systems are either subjected to MM operation or semiempirical analysis for the structural optimization, as well as computation of conformational energy.

Molecular mechanical methods are comparatively faster and generate accurate (or nearly accurate) molecular geometries and conformational energies. Sometimes the prediction of thermochemical data of stable chemical species is obtained with appreciable reliability employing the MM3 or MM4 method. On the other hand, semiempirical analysis becomes valuable while addressing systems like reactive intermediates or transition states owing to the absence of any suitable force field program. Furthermore, a compromise is made between choosing semiempirical and *ab initio* methods while dealing with small molecules. We would like to add that the selection of a suitable technique also depends on the knowledge of the modeler regarding the nature of chemicals employed—for example, semiempirical methods elicit good results for chemical systems that are similar to those used in the parameterization set. Similarly, care should be taken where semiempirical analysis is prone to failure like the prediction of activation barriers. Finally, we would like to say that it is better to study a little regarding the pros and cons and applicability of a particular energy optimization scheme instead of placing blind faith in it; for example, the semiempirical method may not be applicable to a particular large chemical system, although they are known to produce good results in many such other systems. In this context, we would like to mention that among various molecular modeling platforms, Gaussian software (http://www.gaussian.com/) is one of the oldest, and it allows meticulous calculation involving *ab initio* formalism (HF, MP2, etc.), density functional theory (HFB, PW91, PBE, G96, LYP, VWN5, etc.), semiempirical techniques (AM1, MNDO, PM3, PM6, etc.), MM (Amber, Dreiding, UFF), and other hybrid methods (G1, G2, G2MP2, G3, G3B3, G4, G4MP2, MPW1PW91, B2PLYP, B3LYP, etc.). Gaussian software also allows the use of various set of functions in the form of basis sets (namely, STO-3G, 3-21G, 6-21G, 4-31G, 6-31G, etc.) to characterize the wave-function using the approximations obtained from different research outcomes. The development of this chemometric program is credited to John Pople and his research group, which released the first version, Gaussian70, in 1970. This software has undergone continual updates since then, and Gaussian 09 is the latest one [41].

One last issue to be discussed here is the fact that the study of molecules using suitable computer platforms and programs provides the user with only a hypothetical overview of the actual phenomenon involved. Hence, we prefer to use the term *simulation* since it is not a real-time situation and in fact may not represent the reality if all the constraints are not addressed properly. Instinctively, it may be observed that with the increased complexity of the system, less accurate approximations become foreseeable. Consideration of all real-time constraints, or even most of them, has yet not been feasible for large systems. However, computers facilitate considerably less drastic approximations, thereby allowing an association of experimental and theoretical insights that give a reasonable, realistic representation of problems.

REFERENCES

[1] Lewars EG. Computational chemistry: introduction to the theory and applications of molecular and quantum mechanics. Heidelberg, Germany: Springer; 2003.

[2] Corey RB, Pauling L. Molecular models of amino acids, peptides, and proteins. Rev Sci Instrum 1975;24:621–7.

[3] Morrison RT, Boyd RN. Organic chemistry. Upper Saddle River, NJ: Prentice-Hall Inc; 2002.

[4] Barton DHR. Principles of conformational analysis. Nobel lectures, chemistry 1963–1970. Amsterdam, the Netherlands: Elsevier Publishing Company; 1972.

[5] Kolossváry I, Guida WC. Low mode search. An Efficient, automated computational method for conformational analysis: application to cyclic and acyclic alkanes and cyclic peptides. J Am Chem Soc 1996;118:5011–19.

[6] Leech A. In: Lipkowitz KB, Boyd DB, editors. Reviews in computational chemistry, vol. 2. New York, NY: VCH; 1991.

[7] Mazzanti A, Casarini D. Recent trends in conformational analysis. WIREs Comput Mol Sci 2012;2:613–41.

[8] Golebiewski A, Parczewski A. Theoretical conformational analysis of organic molecules. Chem Rev 1974;74:519–30.

[9] Hendrickson JB. Molecular geometry. I. Machine computation of the common rings. J Am Chem Soc 1961;83:4537–47.

[10] Allinger NL. Conformational analysis. 130. MM2. A hydrocarbon force field utilizing V_1 and V_2 torsional terms. J Am Chem Soc 1977;99:8127–34.

[11] Allinger NL, Yuh YH, Lii J-H. Molecular mechanics. The MM3 force field for hydrocarbons. 1. J Am Chem Soc 1989;111:8551–66.

[12] Halgren TA. Merck molecular force field. I. Basis, form, scope, parameterization, and performance of MMFF94. J Comput Chem 1996;17:490–519.

[13] Allinger NL, Chen K, Lii J-H. An improved force field (MM4) for saturated hydrocarbons. J Comput Chem 1996;17:642–68.

[14] Mayo SL, Olafson BD, Goddard III WA. DREIDING: a generic force field for molecular simulations. J Phys Chem 1990;94:8897–909.

[15] Rappe AK, Casewit CJ, Colwell KS, Goddard III WA, Skiff WM. UFF, a full periodic table force field for molecular mechanics and molecular dynamics simulations. J Am Chem Soc 1992;114:10024–35.

[16] Weiner PK, Kollman PA. AMBER: assisted model building with energy refinement. A general program for modeling molecules and their interactions. J Comput Chem 1981;2:287–303.

[17] Jorgensen WL, Tirado-Rives J. The OPLS [optimized potentials for liquid simulations] potential functions for proteins, energy minimizations for crystals of cyclic peptides and crambin. J Am Chem Soc 1988;110:1657–66.

[18] Vanommeslaeghe K, Hatcher E, Acharya C, Kundu S, Zhong S, Shim J, et al. CHARMM general force field: a force field for drug-like molecules compatible with the CHARMM all-atom additive biological force fields. J Comput Chem 2010;31:671–90.

[19] Nemethy G, Gibson KD, Palmer KA, Yoon CN, Paterlini G, Zagari A, et al. Energy parameters in polypeptides. 10. Improved geometrical parameters and nonbonded interactions for use in the ECEPP/3 algorithm, with application to proline-containing peptides. J Phys Chem 1992;96:6472–84.

[20] Alder BJ, Wainwright TE. Phase transition for a hard sphere system. J Chem Phys 1957;27:1208–9.

[21] Rahman A. Correlations in the motion of atoms in liquid argon. Phys Rev 1964;136:A405–11.

[22] Petrenko R, Jaroszaw M. Molecular dynamics. Encyclopedia of life sciences (ELS). Chichester: John Wiley & Sons; 2010.
[23] Schrödinger E. Quantisierung als eigenwertproblem (erste Mitteilung). Ann Phys 1926;79:361–76.
[24] Born M, Oppenheimer R. Zur quantentheorie der molekeln. Ann Phys 1927;389:457–84.
[25] Hartree DR. The wave mechanics of an atom with a non-Coulomb central field. I. Theory and methods. Proc Cambridge Philos Soc 1928;24:89–110.
[26] Fock V. Näherungsmethode zur Lösung des Quantenmechanischen Mehrkörperproblems. Z Phys 1930; 61:126–48.
[27] Amusia MY. Atomic photoeffect. New York, NY: Plenum Press; 1990.
[28] Thomas LH. The calculation of atomic fields. Proc Cambridge Philos Soc 1927;23:542–8.
[29] Fermi E. Z Phys 1928;48:73–9.
[30] Jones RO, Gunnarsson O. The density functional formalism, its applications and prospects. Rev Mod Phys 1989;61:689–746.
[31] Hohenberg P, Kohn W. Inhomogeneous Electron Gas. Phys Rev 1964;136:B864.
[32] Levy M. Universal variational functionals of electron densities, first-order density matrices, and natural spin-orbitals and solution of the v-representability problem. Proc Natl Acad Sci (USA) 1979;76:6062–5.
[33] Hückel E. Quantum contributions to the benzene problem. Z Phys 1931;70:204–86.
[34] Hoffmann R. An extended Hückel theory. I. Hydrocarbons. J Chem Phys 1963;39:1397–412.
[35] Pariser R, Parr RG. A semi-empirical theory of the electronic spectra and electronic structure of complex unsaturated molecules. J Chem Phys 1953;21:466–71.
[36] Pople JA, Santry DP, Segal GA. Approximate self consistent molecular orbital theory. I. Invariant procedures. J Chem Phys 1965;43:S129–35.
[37] Dewar MJS, Thiel W. Ground states of molecules. 38. The MNDO method. Approximations and parameters. J Am Chem Soc 1977;99:4899–907.
[38] Dewar MJS, Zoebisch E, Healy EF, Stewart JJP. Development and use of quantum mechanical molecular models. 76. AM1: a new general purpose quantum mechanical molecular model. J Am Chem Soc 1985;107:3902–9.
[39] Stewart JJP. Optimization of parameters for semiempirical methods I. Method. J Comput Chem 1989;10:209–20.
[40] Repasky MP, Chandrasekhar J, Jorgensen WL. PDDG/PM3 and PDDG/MNDO: improved semi-empirical methods. J Comput Chem 2002;23:1601–22.
[41] Frisch MJ, Trucks GW, Schlegel HB, Scuseria GE, Robb MA, Cheeseman JR, et al. Gaussian 09, Revision D.01. Wallingford, CT: Gaussian, Inc.; 2009.

CHAPTER 6

Selected Statistical Methods in QSAR

Contents

6.1 INTRODUCTION

Quantitative structure–activity relationship (QSAR) models are developed using one or more statistical model building tools, which may be broadly categorized into regression- and classification-based approaches. Machine learning methods, which use artificial intelligence, may also be useful for predictive model development. Note that the latter may also be used for regression and classification problems. Apart from model development, statistical methods are needed for feature selection from a large pool of computed descriptors. As QSAR is a statistical approach, there should be a number of rigorous tests for checking the reliability of the developed models, which

Understanding the Basics of QSAR for Applications in Pharmaceutical Sciences and Risk Assessment.
ISBN: 978-0-12-801505-6, DOI: http://dx.doi.org/10.1016/B978-0-12-801505-6.00006-5

may otherwise be proved to be a statistical nuisance if proper care is not taken at every step of its development.

6.2 REGRESSION-BASED APPROACHES

Regression-based approaches are used when both the response variable and independent variables are quantitative. The generated regression model can compute quantitative response data from the model.

6.2.1 Multiple linear regression

Multiple linear regression (MLR) [1] is one of the most popular methods of QSAR due to its simplicity in operation, reproducibility, and ability to allow easy interpretation of the features used. This is a regression approach of the dependent variable (response property or activity) on more than one descriptor. The generalized expression of an MLR equation is as follows:

$$Y = a_0 + a_1 \times X_1 + a_2 \times X_2 + a_3 \times X_3 + \cdots + a_n \times X_n \quad (6.1)$$

In Eq. (6.1), Y is the response or dependent variable; $X_1, X_2, \ldots, X_n$ are descriptors (features or independent variables) present in the model with the corresponding regression coefficients $a_1, a_2, \ldots, a_n$, respectively; and a_0 is the constant term of the model.

6.2.1.1 Model development

Now consider the method for development of an MLR equation using the least squares method. Say that we have a set of m observations of n descriptors and the corresponding Y values (Table 6.1).

If we want to develop an MLR equation from this data set, then in the ideal case, the developed model should fit the data in a perfect way for all the observations. This

Table 6.1 A representative QSAR table

Compound No.	Response (Y)	Descriptor 1 (X_1)	Descriptor 2 (X_2)	Descriptor 3 (X_3)	...	Descriptor n (X_n)
1	$(Y)_1$	$(X_1)_1$	$(X_2)_1$	$(X_3)_1$	...	$(X_n)_1$
2	$(Y)_2$	$(X_1)_2$	$(X_2)_2$	$(X_3)_2$	...	$(X_n)_2$
3	$(Y)_3$	$(X_1)_3$	$(X_2)_3$	$(X_3)_3$	...	$(X_n)_3$
4	$(Y)_4$	$(X_1)_4$	$(X_2)_4$	$(X_3)_4$	...	$(X_n)_4$
...	...	...	...	...	...	...
m	$(Y)_m$	$(X_1)_m$	$(X_2)_m$	$(X_3)_m$	...	$(X_n)_m$

means that the calculated Y value (Y_{calc}) for a particular observation from the model should be exactly the same as the corresponding observed Y value (Y_{obs}).

Thus, in the ideal case, for compound 1,

$$[(Y)_1]_{obs} = [(Y)_1]_{calc} = a_0 + a_1 \times (X_1)_1 + a_2 \times (X_2)_1 + a_3 \times (X_3)_1 + \cdots + a_n \times (X_n)_1 \tag{6.2-1}$$

Similarly,

$$[(Y)_2]_{obs} = [(Y)_2]_{calc} = a_0 + a_1 \times (X_1)_2 + a_2 \times (X_2)_2 + a_3 \times (X_3)_2 + \cdots + a_n \times (X_n)_2 \tag{6.2-2}$$

$$\vdots$$

$$[(Y)_m]_{obs} = [(Y)_m]_{calc} = a_0 + a_1 \times (X_1)_m + a_2 \times (X_2)_m + a_3 \times (X_3)_m + \cdots + a_n \times (X_n)_m \tag{6.2-m}$$

In reality, however, there will be some difference between the observed and calculated response values for most (if not all) of the observations. The objective of the model development should be to minimize this difference (or the residual). However, some of the compounds (observations) will have positive residuals, and others will have negative residuals. Thus, squared residuals are considered while defining the objective function of the model development, which is actually the sum of the squared residuals $[\Sigma(Y_{obs} - Y_{calc})^2]$ for all the observations used in the model development; if the model is good, this should attain a low value. Hence, the method is also known as the *method of least squares*.

Now, while considering a problem such as MLR model development, the unknowns are a_0, a_1, a_2, a_3, ..., a_n, while X_1, X_2, X_3,...X_n, and Y are all known quantities. The constant a_0 can be easily found once the regression coefficients a_1, a_2, a_3..., a_n are known. Hence, here we have n unknowns. In case of solution of simultaneous equations, we would have needed only n equations (n observations). However, in our problem, a "perfect solution" is not desired as we must consider that errors are inherent in the biological measurements which will affect the "solutions." Hence, we adopt a statistical approach of regression, which uses the information from as many observations as possible to give an overall reflection of the contribution of each feature to the response. Equations (6.2-1)–(6.2-m) may be summed to give the following equations:

$$\sum Y = m \times a_0 + a_1 \times \sum X_1 + a_2 \times \sum X_2 + a_3 \times \sum X_3 + \cdots + a_n \times \sum X_n \tag{6.3}$$

Dividing both sides of Eq. (6.3) with the number of observations m, we get

$$\overline{Y} = a_0 + a_1 \times \overline{X_1} + a_2 \times \overline{X_2} + a_3 \times \overline{X_3} + \cdots + a_n \times \overline{X_n} \tag{6.4}$$

If we subtract Eq. (6.4) from each of Eqs. (6.2-1)−(6.2-m), we will get a series of equations with the centered values of the response and descriptors:

$$(y)_1 = a_1 \times (x_1)_1 + a_2 \times (x_2)_1 + a_3 \times (x_3)_1 + \cdots + a_n \times (x_n)_1 \quad (6.5\text{-}1)$$

$$(y)_2 = a_1 \times (x_1)_2 + a_2 \times (x_2)_2 + a_3 \times (x_3)_2 + \cdots + a_n \times (x_n)_2 \quad (6.5\text{-}2)$$

$$(y)_3 = a_1 \times (x_1)_3 + a_2 \times (x_2)_3 + a_3 \times (x_3)_3 + \cdots + a_n \times (x_n)_3 \quad (6.5\text{-}3)$$

$$\vdots$$

$$(y)_m = a_1 \times (x_1)_m + a_2 \times (x_2)_m + a_3 \times (x_3)_m + \cdots + a_n \times (x_n)_m \quad (6.5\text{-}m)$$

such that $y_i = Y_i - \overline{Y}$, $(x_1)_i = (X_1)_i - \overline{X_1}$, $(x_2)_i = (X_2)_i - \overline{X_2}$, $(x_3)_i = (X_3)_i - \overline{X_3}$, etc.

Now, multiplying each of Eqs. (6.5-1)−(6.5-m) by the x_1 term of the corresponding observation, we get

$$(y)_1 \times (x_1)_1 = a_1 \times [(x_1)_1]^2 + a_2 \times (x_2)_1 \times (x_1)_1 + a_3 \times (x_3)_1 \times (x_1)_1 + \cdots + a_n \times (x_n)_1 \times (x_1)_1 \quad (6.6\text{-}1)$$

$$(y)_2 \times (x_1)_2 = a_1 \times [(x_1)_2]^2 + a_2 \times (x_2)_2 \times (x_1)_2 + a_3 \times (x_3)_2 \times (x_1)_2 + \cdots + a_n \times (x_n)_2 \times (x_1)_2 \quad (6.6\text{-}2)$$

$$(y)_3 \times (x_1)_3 = a_1 \times [(x_1)_3]^2 + a_2 \times (x_2)_3 \times (x_1)_3 + a_3 \times (x_3)_3 \times (x_1)_3 + \cdots + a_n \times (x_n)_3 \times (x_1)_3 \quad (6.6\text{-}3)$$

$$\vdots$$

$$(y)_m \times (x_1)_m = a_1 \times [(x_1)_m]^2 + a_2 \times (x_2)_m \times (x_1)_m + a_3 \times (x_3)_m \times (x_1)_m + \cdots + a_n \times (x_n)_m \times (x_1)_m \quad (6.6\text{-}m)$$

Summing the respective terms in Eqs. (6.6-1)−(6.6-m),

$$\sum x_1 y = a_1 \times \sum x_1^2 + a_2 \times \sum x_1 x_2 + a_3 \times \sum x_1 x_3 + \cdots + a_n \times \sum x_1 x_n \quad (6.7\text{-}1)$$

Similarly, multiplying each of Eqs. (6.5-1)−(6.5-m) with the x_2 term of the corresponding observation and then summing the obtained equations, we have

$$\sum x_2 y = a_1 \times \sum x_1 x_2 + a_2 \times \sum x_2^2 + a_3 \times \sum x_2 x_3 + \cdots + a_n \times \sum x_2 x_n \quad (6.7\text{-}2)$$

In a similar manner, we can have

$$\sum x_3y = a_1 \times \sum x_1x_3 + a_2 \times \sum x_2x_3 + a_3 \times \sum x_3^2 + \cdots + a_n \times \sum x_3x_n \tag{6.7-3}$$

$$\vdots$$

$$\sum x_ny = a_1 \times \sum x_1x_n + a_2 \times \sum x_2x_n + a_3 \times \sum x_3x_n + \cdots + a_n \times \sum x_n^2 \tag{6.7-n}$$

Equations (6.7-1)–(6.7-*n*) are called *normal equations.* These equations are now used to *solve* the values for n unknowns, a_1 to a_n. Note that each of these normal equations contains information from all m observations, and hence this method of *solving* is not heavily affected by the possible error in the response value of a particular observation.

In a matrix notation, the problem may now be denoted as follows:

$$\begin{bmatrix} \sum x_1y \\ \sum x_2y \\ \sum x_3y \\ \vdots \\ \sum x_ny \end{bmatrix} = \begin{bmatrix} \sum (x_1)^2 & \sum x_1x_2 & \sum x_1x_3 & \cdots & \sum x_1x_n \\ \sum x_1x_2 & \sum (x_2)^2 & \sum x_2x_3 & \cdots & \sum x_2x_n \\ \sum x_1x_3 & \sum x_2x_3 & \sum (x_3)^2 & \cdots & \sum x_3x_n \\ \vdots & \vdots & \vdots & \ddots & \vdots \\ \sum x_1x_n & \sum x_2x_n & \sum x_3x_n & \cdots & \sum (x_n)^2 \end{bmatrix} \begin{bmatrix} a_1 \\ a_2 \\ a_3 \\ \vdots \\ a_n \end{bmatrix}$$

Let us call these three matrices **U**, **V**, and **W**, respectively. Note that the matrix **V** is a square and symmetric matrix of dimension n (which is equal to the number of unknowns), while the matrices **U** and **W** are columns of n rows, n being the number of unknowns. Thus, as the number of unknowns (regression coefficients of descriptors) increases, the complexity of calculation also increases.

The unknown matrix **W** can be computed by inverting the matrix **V** and then multiplying by **U**:

$$\mathbf{W} = \mathbf{V}^{-1}\mathbf{U} \tag{6.8}$$

A matrix can be inverted by the Gauss–Jordan method, where elementary operations are applied to both the matrix to be inverted and a unit matrix with the same dimensions such that the matrix to be inverted becomes a unit matrix. With the same sets of elementary operations, the original unit matrix becomes the inverted **V** matrix ($\mathbf{V}^{-1}$). The matrix $\mathbf{V}^{-1}$ is then multiplied by **U**. Note that the dimension of $\mathbf{V}^{-1}$ is $n \times n$, while that of **U** is $n \times 1$. Thus, on multiplication, we get a matrix of dimension $n \times 1$, which is actually the matrix **W** containing n unknowns (a_1, a_2, a_3, … , a_n). Once the values of the regression coefficients are known, one can use Eq. (6.4) to calculate the value of a_0.

With all the unknowns being known, one can compute the response values (Y_{calc}) for all the observations and can also check the residual values ($Y_{obs}-Y_{calc}$) in order to examine the quality of fits. The analysis of residuals can also identify the outliers, which are different from the rest of the data. A compound having a residual value that lies more than three standard deviations from the mean of the residuals may be considered an outlier. If a residual plot shows that all or most of the residuals are on one side of the 0 residual line, the residuals vary regularly with increasing measured values, or both, it indicates a systemic error. It is also possible to graphically plot the observed experimental values against the calculated values, and the degree of scatter (deviation from the 45° line) will be a measure of lack of fit (LOF). Now, the model having been developed, it is necessary to check the quality of the developed models using different criteria.

6.2.1.2 *Statistical metrics to examine the quality of the developed model*

6.2.1.2.1 Mean average error

Mean average error (MAE) can be easily determined from the following expression:

$$MAE = \frac{|Y_{obs} - Y_{calc}|}{n} \tag{6.9}$$

where n is the number of observations. Obviously, the value of MAE should be low for a good model. However, the MAE value will largely depend on the unit of the Y observations.

6.2.1.2.2 Determination coefficient (R^2)

In order to judge the fitting ability of a model, we can consider the average of the observed Y values ($\overline{Y}_{obs}$) as the reference, such that the model performance should be more than $\overline{Y}_{obs}$. For a good model, the residual values (or the sum of squared residuals) should be small, while the deviation of most of the individual observed Y values from $\overline{Y}_{obs}$ is expected to be high. Thus, the ration $\frac{\sum (Y_{obs}-Y_{calc})^2}{\sum (Y_{obs}-\overline{Y}_{obs})^2}$ should have a low value for a good model. We can define the determination coefficient (R^2) in the following manner:

$$R^2 = 1 - \frac{\sum (Y_{obs} - Y_{calc})^2}{\sum (Y_{obs} - \overline{Y}_{obs})^2} \tag{6.10}$$

For the ideal model, the sum of squared residuals being 0, the value of R^2 is 1. As the value of R^2 deviates from 1, the fitting quality of the model deteriorates. The square root of R^2 is the multiple correlation coefficient (R).

6.2.1.2.3 Adjusted R^2 (R_a^2)

If we examine the expression of the determination coefficient, we can see that it only compares the calculated Y values with the experimental ones, without considering the number of descriptors in the model. If one goes on increasing the number of descriptors in the model for a fixed number of observations, R^2 values will always increase, but this will lead to a decrease in the degree of freedom and low statistical reliability. Thus, a high value of R^2 is not necessarily an indication of a good statistical model that fits the available data. If, for example, one uses 100 descriptors in a model for 100 observations, the resultant model will show $R^2 = 1$, but it will not have any reliability, as this will be a perfectly fitted model (a *solved system*) rather than a statistical model. For a reliable model, the number of observations and number of descriptors should bear a ration of at least 5:1. Thus, to better reflect the explained variance (the fraction of the data variance explained by the model), a better measure is adjusted R^2, which is defined in the following manner:

$$R_a^2 = \frac{(N-1) \times R^2 - p}{N-1-p} \tag{6.11}$$

In Eq. (6.11), p is the number of predictor variables used in model development. For a model with a given number of observations (N), as the number of predictor variables increases, the value of R^2 increases, while the adjusted R^2 value is penalized due to an increase in the number of predictor variables.

6.2.1.2.4 Variance ratio (F)

In an MLR model, the deviations of Y from the population regression plane have mean 0 and variance σ^2, which can be shown by the following expression:

$$\sigma^2 = \frac{\sum (Y_{obs} - Y_{calc})^2}{N-p-1} \tag{6.12}$$

The sum of squares of deviations of the Y from their mean $[\sum (Y_{obs} - \overline{Y})^2]$ can be split into two parts: (i) the sum of squares of deviations of the fitted values from their mean $[\sum (Y_{calc} - \overline{Y})^2]$, with the corresponding degree of freedom being the number of predictor variables (source of variation being regression); and (ii) the sum of squares of deviations of the fitted values from the observed ones $[\sum (Y_{obs} - Y_{calc})^2]$ with the corresponding degree of freedom of $N-p-1$ (with the source of variations being deviations). To judge the overall significance of the regression coefficients, the variance ratio (the ratio of regression mean square to deviations mean square) can be defined as

$$F = \frac{\sum (Y_{calc} - \overline{Y})^2 / p}{\sum (Y_{obs} - Y_{calc})^2 / (N-p-1)} \tag{6.13}$$

The F value has two degrees of freedom: p and $N-p-1$. The computed F value of a model should be significant at $p<0.05$. For overall significance of the regression coefficients, the F value should be high.

The F value also indicates the significance of the multiple correlation coefficient R, and they are related by the following expression:

$$F = \frac{(N-p-1)\times R^2}{p\times(1-R^2)} \tag{6.14}$$

6.2.1.2.5 Standard error of estimate (s)

For a good model, the standard error of estimate of Y should be low, which is defined as

$$s = \sqrt{\frac{(Y_{\text{obs}}-Y_{\text{calc}})^2}{N-p-1}} \tag{6.15}$$

It has a degree of freedom of $N-p-1$.

6.2.1.2.6 Root mean square error of calibration

The root mean square error of calibration (RMSEC) can be computed from the following expression:

$$\text{RMSEC} = \sqrt{\frac{\sum(y_{\text{obs(training)}}-y_{\text{calc(training)}})^2}{n_{\text{training}}}} \tag{6.16}$$

The value of RMSEC should be low for a good model.

6.2.1.2.7 The "t" test for each regression coefficient

It is possible to examine the significance of each regression coefficient in an MLR model by computing the corresponding standard error. In the inverted **V** matrix ($\mathbf{V}^{-1}$), if the diagonal elements are $c11$, $c22$, $c33$, etc., then the standard error of the regression coefficients are given by

$$s_{X_1} = s\times\sqrt{c_{11}} \tag{6.17-1}$$

$$s_{X_2} = s\times\sqrt{c_{22}} \tag{6.17-2}$$

$$s_{X_3} = s\times\sqrt{c_{33}} \tag{6.17-3}$$

⋮

$$s_{X_n} = s\times\sqrt{c_{nn}} \tag{6.17-n}$$

The t value of the regression coefficient can be calculated from the regression coefficient value divided by the standard error of the regression coefficient.

Each regression coefficient (r.c. in the following equation) should be significant at $p < 0.05$. The 95% confidence intervals of regression coefficients can be computed as

$$\text{r.c.} \pm t_{0.05} \times s \tag{6.18}$$

6.2.1.2.8 Intercorrelation among descriptors

The descriptors present in an MLR model should not be intercorrelated very much. This can be determined by studying an intercorrelation table. The problem of multicollinearity may be checked from the variance inflation factor (VIF), which can be calculated as follows:

$$\text{VIF} = \frac{1}{1 - R_i^2} \tag{6.19}$$

where R_i^2 is the unadjusted R^2 when one regresses X_i against all the other explanatory variables in the model. It is a measure of how much the variance of an estimated regression coefficient enhances because of collinearity. If the VIF value is greater than 5, multicollinearity is very high.

These noted metrics are used to check the statistical quality of an MLR model, but they do not convey anything about the possible performance of the model on a new set of data. Thus, a few tests of validation are required to examine the predictive potential of the model. These tests are described in Chapter 7.

Note that the development of MLR models and computation of various statistical metrics can be done by using an open access tool called MLR plus Validation, available at http://dtclab.webs.com/software-tools and http://teqip.jdvu.ac.in/QSAR_Tools/, or the Apt Software website (http://aptsoftware.co.in/DTCMLRWeb/index.jsp).

6.2.1.3 Example of an MLR model development

Tables 6.2–6.6 give an example of MLR model development.

Normal equations:

$$1.089 = 3.779a_1 + 0.652a_2 - 0.035a_3$$

$$1.253 = 0.652a_1 + 1.999a_2 + 0.847a_3$$

$$-0.308 = -0.035a_1 + 0.847a_2 + 4.444a_3$$

Table 6.2 Example of a small QSAR table (the response variable and descriptors to be used in model development), along with the calculated response and residual values

Sl. No.	Response variable	Descriptors			Y_{calc}	Res $(=Y_{obs}-Y_{calc})$	Res^2
	pIC_{50} (Y_{obs})	MR (X_1)	σ (X_2)	Ind (X_3)			
1	−2.279	0.103	0	0	−2.174	−0.105	0.011
2	−2.447	0.103	0	1	−2.366	−0.081	0.007
3	−2.342	0.103	0	0	−2.174	−0.168	0.028
4	−2.204	0.787	−0.27	0	−2.232	0.028	0.001
5	−2.255	0.787	−0.27	1	−2.424	0.169	0.029
6	−2.322	0.787	−0.27	0	−2.232	−0.09	0.008
7	−1.785	0.786	0.35	0	−1.829	0.044	0.002
8	−1.763	0.603	0.23	0	−1.939	0.176	0.031
9	−1.929	0.092	0.06	0	−2.137	0.208	0.043
10	−1.892	1.382	0	0	−1.954	0.062	0.004
11	−1.491	1.349	0.72	0	−1.491	0	0
12	−2.255	1.03	−0.15	0	−2.112	−0.143	0.02
13	−2.204	1.382	0	1	−2.146	−0.058	0.003
14	−1.748	1.349	0.72	1	−1.683	−0.065	0.004
15	−1.663	0.736	0.78	1	−1.75	0.087	0.008
16	−2	0.603	0.23	1	−2.131	0.131	0.017
17	−2.301	0.092	0.06	1	−2.329	0.028	0.001
18	−2.146	0.502	0.54	1	−1.946	−0.2	0.04
	$\overline{Y}=-2.057$	$\overline{X_1}=0.699$	$\overline{X_2}=0.152$	$\overline{X_3}=0.444$			$\Sigma Res^2=0.256$

Table 6.3 Centered response and descriptor values

Sl. No.	$y_i = Y_i - \overline{Y}$	$x_{1\_i} = X_{1\_i} - \overline{X_1}$	$x_{2\_i} = X_{2\_i} - \overline{X_2}$	$x_{3\_i} = X_{3\_i} - \overline{X_3}$
1	−0.222	−0.596	−0.152	−0.444
2	−0.390	−0.596	−0.152	0.556
3	−0.285	−0.596	−0.152	−0.444
4	−0.147	0.088	−0.422	−0.444
5	−0.198	0.088	−0.422	0.556
6	−0.265	0.088	−0.422	−0.444
7	0.272	0.087	0.198	−0.444
8	0.294	−0.096	0.078	−0.444
9	0.128	−0.607	−0.092	−0.444
10	0.165	0.683	−0.152	−0.444
11	0.566	0.650	0.568	−0.444
12	−0.198	0.331	−0.302	−0.444
13	−0.147	0.683	−0.152	0.556
14	0.309	0.650	0.568	0.556
15	0.394	0.037	0.628	0.556
16	0.057	−0.096	0.078	0.556
17	−0.244	−0.607	−0.092	0.556
18	−0.089	−0.197	0.388	0.556

Table 6.4 Preparing normal equations (part 1)

Sl. No.	$y_i \times x_{1\_i}$	$x_{1\_i} \times x_{1\_i}$	$x_{2\_i} \times x_{1\_i}$	$x_{3\_i} \times x_{1\_i}$
1	0.132	0.355	0.09	0.265
2	0.232	0.355	0.09	−0.331
3	0.17	0.355	0.09	0.265
4	−0.013	0.008	−0.037	−0.039
5	−0.017	0.008	−0.037	0.049
6	−0.023	0.008	−0.037	−0.039
7	0.024	0.008	0.017	−0.039
8	−0.028	0.009	−0.007	0.043
9	−0.078	0.368	0.056	0.27
10	0.113	0.467	−0.104	−0.304
11	0.368	0.423	0.37	−0.289
12	−0.066	0.11	−0.1	−0.147
13	−0.1	0.467	−0.104	0.38
14	0.201	0.423	0.37	0.361
15	0.015	0.001	0.023	0.021
16	−0.005	0.009	−0.007	−0.053
17	0.148	0.368	0.056	−0.337
18	0.018	0.039	−0.076	−0.109
$\sum =$	1.089	3.779	0.652	−0.035

Table 6.5 Preparing normal equations (part 2)

Sl. No.	$y_i \times x_{2\_i}$	$x_{1\_i} \times x_{2\_i}$	$x_{2\_i} \times x_{2\_i}$	$x_{3\_i} \times x_{2\_i}$
1	0.034	0.09	0.023	0.067
2	0.059	0.09	0.023	−0.084
3	0.043	0.09	0.023	0.067
4	0.062	−0.037	0.178	0.187
5	0.083	−0.037	0.178	−0.234
6	0.112	−0.037	0.178	0.187
7	0.054	0.017	0.039	−0.088
8	0.023	−0.007	0.006	−0.035
9	−0.012	0.056	0.008	0.041
10	−0.025	−0.104	0.023	0.067
11	0.322	0.37	0.323	−0.253
12	0.06	−0.1	0.091	0.134
13	0.022	−0.104	0.023	−0.084
14	0.176	0.37	0.323	0.316
15	0.248	0.023	0.395	0.349
16	0.004	−0.007	0.006	0.044
17	0.022	0.056	0.008	−0.051
18	−0.035	−0.076	0.151	0.216
$\sum =$	1.253	0.652	1.999	0.847

Table 6.6 Preparing normal equations (part 3)

Sl. No.	$y_i \times x_{3\_i}$	$x_{1\_i} \times x_{3\_i}$	$x_{2\_i} \times x_{3\_i}$	$x_{3\_i} \times x_{3\_i}$
1	0.099	0.265	0.067	0.198
2	−0.217	−0.331	−0.084	0.309
3	0.127	0.265	0.067	0.198
4	0.065	−0.039	0.187	0.198
5	−0.11	0.049	−0.234	0.309
6	0.118	−0.039	0.187	0.198
7	−0.121	−0.039	−0.088	0.198
8	−0.131	0.043	−0.035	0.198
9	−0.057	0.27	0.041	0.198
10	−0.073	−0.304	0.067	0.198
11	−0.252	−0.289	−0.253	0.198
12	0.088	−0.147	0.134	0.198
13	−0.082	0.38	−0.084	0.309
14	0.172	0.361	0.316	0.309
15	0.219	0.021	0.349	0.309
16	0.032	−0.053	0.044	0.309
17	−0.136	−0.337	−0.051	0.309
18	−0.049	−0.109	0.216	0.309
$\sum =$	−0.308	−0.035	0.847	4.444

Matrix notation:

$$\begin{bmatrix} 1.089 \\ 1.253 \\ -0.308 \end{bmatrix} = \begin{bmatrix} 3.779 & 0.652 & -0.035 \\ 0.652 & 1.999 & 0.847 \\ -0.035 & 0.847 & 4.444 \end{bmatrix} \begin{bmatrix} a_1 \\ a_2 \\ a_3 \end{bmatrix}$$

Thus,

$$\begin{bmatrix} a_1 \\ a_2 \\ a_3 \end{bmatrix} = \begin{bmatrix} 3.779 & 0.652 & -0.035 \\ 0.652 & 1.999 & 0.847 \\ -0.035 & 0.847 & 4.444 \end{bmatrix}^{-1} \begin{bmatrix} 1.089 \\ 1.253 \\ -0.308 \end{bmatrix}$$

$$= \mathbf{V}^{-1}\mathbf{W}$$

Inversion of the matrix **V** *using the Gauss–Jordan method*:

$$\begin{bmatrix} 3.779 & 0.652 & -0.035 \\ 0.652 & 1.999 & 0.847 \\ -0.035 & 0.847 & 4.444 \end{bmatrix} : \begin{bmatrix} 1 & 0 & 0 \\ 0 & 1 & 0 \\ 0 & 0 & 1 \end{bmatrix}$$

Dividing $R1$ by 3.779, we get

$$\begin{bmatrix} 1 & 0.172 & -0.009 \\ 0.652 & 1.999 & 0.847 \\ -0.035 & 0.847 & 4.444 \end{bmatrix} : \begin{bmatrix} 0.265 & 0 & 0 \\ 0 & 1 & 0 \\ 0 & 0 & 1 \end{bmatrix}$$

Operating $R2 - 0.652R1$ and $R3 + 0.035R1$, we get:

$$\begin{bmatrix} 1 & 0.172 & -0.009 \\ 0 & 1.887 & 0.853 \\ 0 & 0.853 & 4.444 \end{bmatrix} : \begin{bmatrix} 0.265 & 0 & 0 \\ -0.172 & 1 & 0 \\ 0.009 & 0 & 1 \end{bmatrix}$$

Dividing $R2$ by 1.887, we get:

$$\begin{bmatrix} 1 & 0.172 & -0.009 \\ 0 & 1 & 0.452 \\ 0 & 0.853 & 4.444 \end{bmatrix} : \begin{bmatrix} 0.265 & 0 & 0 \\ -0.091 & 0.53 & 0 \\ 0.009 & 0 & 1 \end{bmatrix}$$

Operating $R1 - 0.172R2$ and $R3 - 0.853R2$, we get:

$$\begin{bmatrix} 1 & 0 & -0.087 \\ 0 & 1 & 0.452 \\ 0 & 0 & 4.059 \end{bmatrix} : \begin{bmatrix} 0.280 & -0.091 & 0 \\ -0.091 & 0.53 & 0 \\ 0.087 & -0.452 & 1 \end{bmatrix}$$

Dividing $R3$ by 4.059, we get:

$$\begin{bmatrix} 1 & 0 & -0.087 \\ 0 & 1 & 0.452 \\ 0 & 0 & 1 \end{bmatrix} : \begin{bmatrix} 0.280 & -0.091 & 0 \\ -0.091 & 0.53 & 0 \\ 0.022 & -0.111 & 0.246 \end{bmatrix}$$

Operating $R1 + 0.087R3$ and $R2 - 0.452R3$, we get:

$$\begin{bmatrix} 1 & 0 & 0 \\ 0 & 1 & 0 \\ 0 & 0 & 1 \end{bmatrix} : \begin{bmatrix} 0.282 & -0.101 & 0.022 \\ -0.101 & 0.580 & -0.111 \\ 0.022 & -0.111 & 0.246 \end{bmatrix}$$

Therefore,

$$\mathbf{V}^{-1} = \begin{bmatrix} 0.282 & -0.101 & 0.022 \\ -0.101 & 0.580 & -0.111 \\ 0.022 & -0.111 & 0.246 \end{bmatrix}$$

$$\begin{bmatrix} a_1 \\ a_2 \\ a_3 \end{bmatrix} = \begin{bmatrix} 0.282 & -0.101 & 0.022 \\ -0.101 & 0.580 & -0.111 \\ 0.022 & -0.111 & 0.246 \end{bmatrix} \begin{bmatrix} 1.089 \\ 1.253 \\ -0.308 \end{bmatrix}$$

$$= \begin{bmatrix} 0.282 \times 1.089 - 0.101 \times 1.253 + 0.022 \times (-0.308) \\ -0.101 \times 1.089 + 0.580 \times 1.253 - 0.111 \times (-0.308) \\ 0.022 \times 1.089 - 0.111 \times 1.253 + 0.246 \times (-0.308) \end{bmatrix}$$

$$= \begin{bmatrix} 0.174 \\ 0.651 \\ -0.192 \end{bmatrix}$$

$$a_1 = 0.174, a_2 = 0.651, a_3 = -0.192$$

$$a_0 = \overline{Y} - a_1\overline{X}_1 - a_2\overline{X}_2 - a_3\overline{X}_3 = -2.192$$

The MLR equation for the data set is

$$\text{pIC}_{50} = -2.192 + 0.174\text{MR} + 0.651\sigma - 0.192\text{Ind}$$

A scatter plot of the observed and calculated pIC_{50} values based on the abovementioned MLR equation is shown in Figure 6.1, while a residual plot is shown in Figure 6.2.

The quality metrics for the equation are computed here:

MAE $= \sum[|Y_{obs} - Y_{calc}|]/n = 0.102$

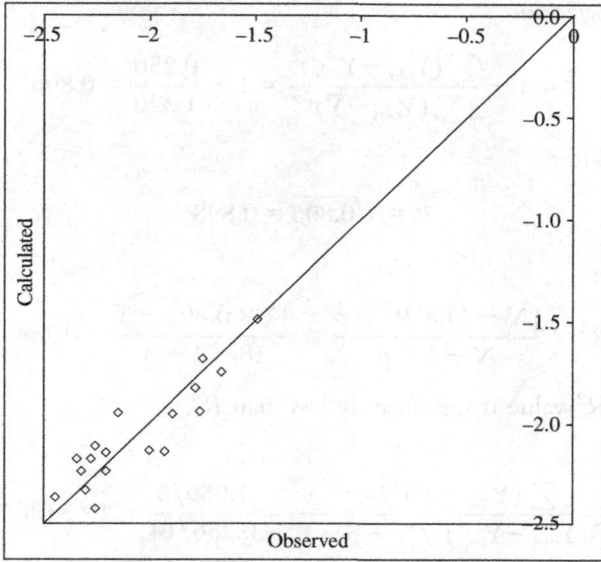

Figure 6.1 A scatter plot of the observed and calculated activity (pIC_{50}) for the MLR equation described in Section 6.2.1.3.

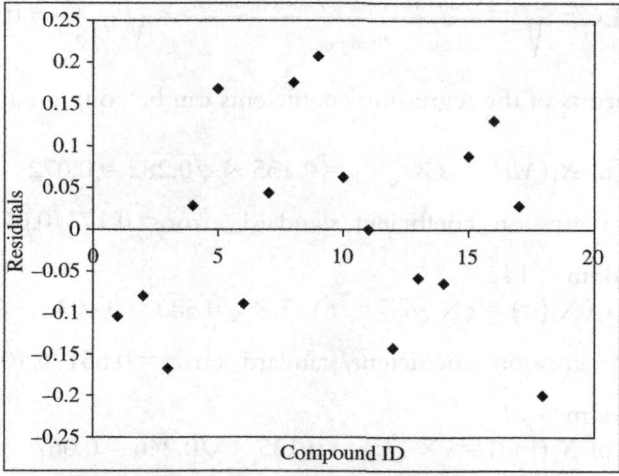

Figure 6.2 A residual plot for the MLR equation described in Section 6.2.1.3.

Determination coefficient:

$$R^2 = 1 - \frac{\sum (Y_{obs} - Y_{calc})^2}{\sum (Y_{obs} - \overline{Y})^2} = 1 - \frac{0.256}{1.320} = 0.806$$

Correlation coefficient:

$$R = \sqrt{0.806} = 0.898$$

Adjusted R^2:

$$R_a^2 = \frac{(N-1) \times R^2 - p}{N-1-p} = \frac{17 \times 0.806 - 3}{18-1-3} = 0.764$$

Note that the R_a^2 value is significantly less than R^2.
Variance ratio:

$$F = \frac{\sum (Y_{calc} - \overline{Y})^2 / p}{\sum (Y_{obs} - Y_{calc})^2 / N - p - 1} = \frac{1.059/3}{0.256/14} = 19.3 \text{ (df } 3, 14)$$

Standard error of estimate:

$$s = \sqrt{\frac{\sum (Y_{obs} - Y_{calc})^2}{N-p-1}} = \sqrt{0.256/14} = 0.135$$

RMSEC:

$$\text{RMSEC} = \sqrt{\frac{\sum (y_{obs(training)} - y_{calc(training)})^2}{n_{training}}} = \sqrt{\frac{0.256}{18}} = 0.119$$

The standard errors of the regression coefficients can be computed in the following manner:
Standard error of $X_1(MR) = s \times \sqrt{c_{11}} = 0.135 \times \sqrt{0.282} = 0.072$

$$t_{X_1} = \text{regression\_coefficient/standard\_error} = 0.174/0.072 = 2.417$$

Degree of freedom = 14
Standard error of $X_2(\sigma) = s \times \sqrt{c_{22}} = 0.135 \times \sqrt{0.580} = 0.103$

$$t_{X_2} = \text{regression\_coefficient/standard\_error} = 0.651/0.103 = 6.320$$

Degree of freedom = 14
Standard error of $X_3(\text{Ind}) = s \times \sqrt{c_{33}} = 0.135 \times \sqrt{0.246} = 0.067$

$$t_{X_1} = \text{regression\_coefficient/standard\_error} = 0.192/0.067 = 2.866$$

Degree of freedom = 14

From the t table, the theoretical t value at $p = 0.05$ and at df $14 = 2.145$, suggesting that all of the regression coefficients are significant at $p < 0.05$:

$$pIC_{50} = -2.192 + 0.174(\pm 0.072)MR + 0.651(\pm 0.103)\sigma - 0.192(\pm 0.067)Ind$$

Another possible representation is to use 95% confidence intervals of the regression coefficients, which can be obtained by multiplying $t_{0.05}(=2.145$ here) with corresponding standard error:

$$pIC_{50} = -2.192 + 0.174(\pm 0.154)MR + 0.651(\pm 0.221)\sigma - 0.192(\pm 0.144)Ind$$

When the 95% confidence interval value is higher than the value of the corresponding regression coefficient, then obviously the coefficient is not significant at $p = 0.05$.

6.2.1.4 Data pretreatment and variable selection

Before a QSAR analysis can be undertaken, it is imperative to perform data set curation and some pretreatment process to obviate errors and redundancy. This is followed by the appropriate selection of descriptors for model development.

6.2.1.4.1 Data set curation

There is the possibility that either or both of the biological activity and descriptor values may be inaccurate in a QSAR table. The success of any QSAR modeling depends on the correctness of the input data. While preparing the QSAR table, care should be taken to ensure that the biological activity (or other response) data have been taken from an authentic source and the standard error of the observed data for each data point should be known to verify the precision of such data. If the experimental standard error value of any data point is high, that particular observation should be omitted. The compounds in the data set should follow a normal distribution pattern with respect to the response values. The researcher should also be careful about the use of data collected from different sources, because if the experimental protocols and conditions are not the same for the different sources, such data sets should not be clubbed into a single QSAR table. While clubbing two or more data sets, care should also be taken that a same compound may be present in two different names in two different data sets. If the molecular structures are imported from any database, this should be manually checked for correctness, as all the computed descriptors will be wrong in case of an inaccurate structural representation. The analyst should also pay attention to the correct tautomeric form of the structure of the compounds as the computed descriptors values will depend on the tautomeric structure. The descriptor values should be calculated using authentic and validated software tools. If three-dimensional (3D) descriptors are being used, this should be computed after necessary structure optimization has been carried out. The analyst should also be aware whether the software tool being used for descriptor calculation is capable of handling all kind of structural features present in the data set.

6.2.1.4.2 Data pretreatment

If a large number of descriptors have been calculated, a descriptor-thinning process may be applied. The descriptors with a constant value for all observations and the descriptors showing a very low variance should be omitted. Among the descriptors showing high mutual intercorrelation, only one should be retained discarding the others unless some specific interpretation or functional relationship (like parabolic relationship) is desired. Sometimes descriptors showing a very low correlation with the response are also omitted to thin the descriptor matrix. In some cases, it may be desirable to scale the descriptor values. One method of scaling may be the following:

$$x_{i\_\text{scaled}} = \frac{x_i - \overline{x}}{\text{sd}} \tag{6.20}$$

where $\overline{x}$ is the mean value of the x column and sd is the standard deviation.

6.2.1.4.3 Variable selection (feature selection)

The selection of the appropriate descriptors for model development from the pool of a large number of descriptors is an important step in QSAR modeling. Such selection may be done in a variety of ways, among which some common and popular methods are mentioned below.

6.2.1.4.3.1 Stepwise selection This is one of the popular methods of variable selection. When applied to MLR, this is carried out in the following steps [2]:

a. The descriptor from the pool, which shows the maximum correlation with the response is initially selected.

b. This descriptor is retained and an additional descriptor is selected such that its contribution is the maximum. The objective function (stepping criterion) of the selection may be "*F*-for-inclusion," which is actually the square of the *t* value of the incoming descriptor.

c. The process continues; that is, a third descriptor is incorporated retaining the first two descriptors in steps 1 and 2. A statistical check based on the *t* test is also performed whether any of the previously selected descriptors has become insignificant and in such case that descriptor may be omitted from the model based on the *F*-for-exclusion criterion.

d. The addition of descriptors continues unless no suitable descriptor is found with the stated stepping criteria or when a desired number of descriptors are already present in the model.

The stepwise process of variable selection may not be able to give the best combination of descriptors for a given data set, but it can be used for quick development of models. Readers may use the stepwise regression tool called Stepwise MLR, available at http://dtclab.webs.com/software-tools and http://teqip.jdvu.ac.in/QSAR_Tools/.

6.2.1.4.3.2 All possible subset selection This method can be used when the number of descriptors present in the pool is not very high. It is more time-consuming than the stepwise method. Additional filters like intercorrelation cutoff or minimum value of determination coefficient or cross-validated variance may be used to save the computational time. Readers may use the all possible subset regression tool called MLR Best Subset Selection, available at http://dtclab.webs.com/software-tools and http://teqip.jdvu.ac.in/QSAR_Tools/.

6.2.1.4.3.3 Genetic method Rogers and Hopfinger [3,4] first used the genetic algorithm (GA) technique in the QSAR study and proved it as a very efficient tool with many merits compared to other variable selection techniques. It investigates many possible solutions simultaneously, each of which explores different regions in the vector space defined by calculated descriptors. The first step in a typical GA procedure is to create a population of N descriptors. The fitness of each descriptor combination in this generation is determined. In the second step, a fraction of children of the next generation is produced by crossover (i.e., crossover children) and the rest by mutation (i.e., mutation children) from the parents on the basis of their scaled fitness scores. The new offspring contains characteristics from two or one of its parents. The genetic content of this individual simply moves to the next generation intact. These selection, crossover, and mutation processes are repeated until all of the N parents in the population are replaced by their children. The fitness score of each member of this new generation is again evaluated, and the reproductive cycle is continued until 80% of the generations show the same target fitness score. A combination of GA with multivariate adaptive regression splines (MARS) algorithm is used in genetic function approximation (GFA), which can handle data sets with a nonlinear relationship between the response and descriptors. GFA provides an error measure, called the *LOF score*, that automatically penalizes models with too many features [5,6]:

$$\mathrm{LOF} = \frac{\mathrm{LSE}}{[1-(c+dp)/M]^2} \tag{6.21}$$

where c is the number of basis functions (other than the constant term); d is the smoothing parameter (adjustable by the user); M is the number of samples in the training set; LSE is least squares error; p is the total number of features contained in all basis functions.

A distinctive feature of GFA is that it produces a population of models (e.g., 100), instead of generating a single model, as do most other statistical methods. The range of variations in this population gives added information on the quality of fit and importance of the descriptors. The model with proper balance of all statistical terms can be used to explain variance in the response. For examples of the use of GFA in QSAR model development, see Refs. [5,6].

6.2.1.4.3.4 Factor analysis Factor analysis (FA) is basically a data reduction tool, but it can also be used for variable selection when it is applied to the descriptor matrix along with the response values [7,8]. In a typical FA procedure, the data matrix is first standardized, and the correlation matrix and subsequently reduced correlation matrix are constructed. An eigenvalue problem is then solved, and the factor pattern can be obtained from the corresponding eigenvectors. The principal objectives of FA are to display multidimensional data in a space of lower dimensionality with minimum loss of information (explaining >95% of the variance of the data matrix) and to extract the basic features behind the data with ultimate goal of interpretation, prediction, or both. For variable selection in MLR, FA is performed on the data set containing the response and all descriptor variables, which are to be considered. The factors are extracted by the principal component (PC) method and then rotated by VARIMAX rotation, a kind of rotation that is used in principal component analysis (PCA) so that the axes are rotated to a position in which the sum of the variances of the loadings is the maximum possible to obtain Thurston's simple structure. The simple structure is characterized by the property that as many variables as possible fall on the coordinate axes when presented in common factor space, so that largest possible number of factor loadings becomes zero. This is done to obtain a numerically comprehensive picture of the relatedness of the variables. Only variables with nonzero loadings in such factors where biological activity also has nonzero loading are considered important in explaining variance of the response. Further, variables with nonzero loadings in different factors are combined in a multivariate equation [9]. For examples of the use of FA in QSAR model development, see Refs. [6,9].

6.2.1.4.3.5 Other methods There are several other methods for variable selection in QSAR model development [10], some of which are mentioned in the next sections.
Particle swarm optimization Particle swarm optimization (PSO) is a population-based optimization algorithm that initializes with a population of random solutions and searches for optima by updating generations [11]. In PSO, each single solution is a particle in the search space. The potential solutions, called *particles*, are "flown" through the problem space by following the current optimum particles. This method simulates the behaviors of bird flocking involving the scenario of a group of birds randomly looking for food in an area. Not all of the birds know where the food is located, only the individual that is closest to the food location. Therefore, the effective strategy for the birds to find food is to follow the bird that is closest to the food. The algorithm models the exploration of a problem space by a population of individuals or particles. All of the particles have fitness values that are evaluated by a fitness function to be optimized. Similar to the other evolutionary computation, the population of individuals is updated by applying some kind of operators according to the fitness information so that the individuals of the population can be expected to move toward better solution areas.

Ant colony optimization The ant colony optimization (ACO) algorithms are stochastic search techniques inspired by the behavior of real ants [12]. In nature, it is observed that real ants are capable of finding the shortest path between a food source and their nest without visual information. The deposition of pheromone is the key feature in enabling real ants to find the shortest paths over a period of time. Each ant probabilistically prefers to follow a direction rich in this chemical. The pheromone decays over time, resulting in much less pheromone on less popular paths. On the basis of this idea, artificial ants can be deployed to solve complex optimization problems via the use of artificial pheromone deposition. ACO is particularly attractive for descriptor selection. Descriptors are recognized with space dimensions defining the available paths followed by ants, with permitted coordinates of 1 or 0 (selected and unselected descriptors respectively, as in GA). In this way, a given path is connected to a number of selected descriptors, which in turn corresponds to a given prediction error. In each generation, ants deposit a certain amount of pheromone, which increases with decreasing values of the objective function defined by each path.

k-*Nearest neighborhood method* The *k*-nearest neighborhood (kNN) as a tool for variable selection in QSAR studies was first used by Zheng and Tropsha [13]. A subset of variables is selected randomly as a hypothetical descriptor pharmacophore (HDP). One compound is eliminated and its *k*-nearest neighbors in the HDP are identified. The activity of the eliminated compound is predicted by weighted kNN. This is repeated over all molecules of interest and the leave-one-out (LOO) Q^2 is found out. The number of variables selected is set to different values to obtain the best LOO Q^2 possible. A method of simulated annealing with the Metropolis-like acceptance criteria is used to optimize the variable selection. The kNN method optimizes the number of descriptors to achieve a QSAR regression equation with the highest LOO Q^2 as a fitness function.

6.2.2 Partial least squares

Partial least squares (PLS) is a generalization of MLR [14]. It can analyze data with strongly collinear, correlated, noisy, and numerous *X*-variables, and it can also simultaneously model several response variables *Y*. If the number of descriptors gets too large (e.g., close to the number of observations) in MLR, it is likely to get a model that fits the sampled data perfectly in a phenomenon called *overfitting*. The general idea of PLS is to try to extract the latent variables (LVs) accounting for as much of the manifest factor variation as possible while modeling the responses well. This is achieved indirectly by extracting the latent variables **T** and **U**, from sampled factors (descriptors) and responses, respectively. The extracted factors **T** (also referred to as X-*scores) are used to predict the* Y-*scores* **U**, *and then the predicted* Y-*scores are used to construct predictions for the responses.*

6.2.2.1 The method

Before analysis, the *X*- and *Y*-variables are often transformed to make their distributions fairly symmetrical. The response variables are usually logarithmically transformed or fourth root transformed. The *X*-variables should be scaled appropriately [see Eq. (6.20)]. Let us consider a training set of *N* observations with *K X*-variables denoted by $\mathbf{x}_k$ ($k = 1, \ldots, K$), and *M Y*-variables $\mathbf{y}_m$ ($m = 1,2, \ldots, M$). These training data form the two matrices **X** and **Y** of dimensions (N^*K) and (N^*M), respectively. Figure 6.3 shows schematically some basic features of PLS model development.

The linear PLS finds a few new variables (latent variables), denoted by t_a ($a = 1, 2, \ldots, A$), which are linear combinations of the original variables x_k with the coefficients w^*_{ka} ($a = 1, 2, \ldots, A$):

$$t_{ia} = \sum_k w^*_{ka} X_{ik} \tag{6.22}$$

The *X*-scores are few ($A < K$) and orthogonal.

Again, it can be written that

$$X_{ik} = \sum_a t_{ia} p_{ak} + e_{ik} \tag{6.23}$$

where p_{ak} represents the loadings and e_{ik} the *X* residuals.

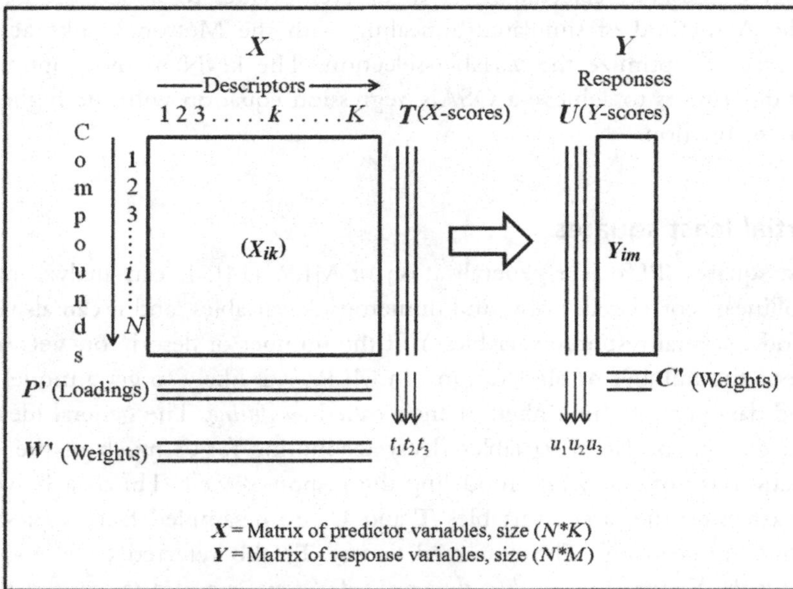

Figure 6.3 Schematic representation of some basic features of PLS model development.

Similarly, the Y responses may be expressed as Y-scores (u_a) such that

$$y_{im} = \sum_a u_{ia} c_{am} + g_{im} \tag{6.24}$$

where c_{am} is the weight and g_{im} the Y-residual (the deviation between the observed and modeled responses).

The X-scores are good predictors of Y. Thus, it can be written that

$$y_{im} = \sum_a c_{ma} \sum_k w^*_{ka} x_{ik} + f_{im} = \sum_k b_{mk} x_{ik} + f_{im} \tag{6.25}$$

where the PLS-regression coefficient b_{mk} can be written as

$$b_{mk} = \sum_a c_{ma} w^*_{ka} \tag{6.26}$$

Note that when $A = K$, the PLS model becomes the same as the MLR model. A strict test of the predictive significance of each PLS component is necessary, and then the addition of further components must stop when they start to be insignificant. Cross-validation is a practical and reliable way (see Chapter 7) to test this predictive significance. The weights w_a are essential for the understanding of which X-variables are important (numerically large w_a values), and which X-variables provide the same information (i.e., similar profiles of w_a values). Large Y-residuals indicate that the model is poor, and X-residuals are useful for identifying outliers in the X-space; that is, molecules with structures that do not fit the model. In PLS modeling, important variables for the modeling of $\mathbf{Y}$ may be identified by large PLS-regression coefficients, b_{mk}. However, a variable may also be important for the modeling of $\mathbf{X}$, which is identified by large loadings, p. A summary of the importance of an X-variable for *both* $\mathbf{Y}$ and $\mathbf{X}$ is given by the variable importance in projection (VIP), which is a weighted sum of squares of the PLS weights, w^*_{ak}, with the weights calculated from the amount of Y variance of each PLS component, a. A PLS score plot (t_1 versus t_2) may show the object similarity or dissimilarity while a PLS loading (weight) plot (component 1 versus component 2) may identify which PLS component is dominated by which features. For determination of the applicability domain of PLS models, usually distance to the model (DModX) approach is used.

6.2.2.2 An example

In this section, we present an example of PLS modeling using the data given in Table 6.2. Taking the number of latent variables as 1, the derived PLS equation gives $R^2 = 0.740$ and LOO $Q^2 = 0.611$ (see Chapter 7 for a definition of LOO Q^2), while taking the number of latent variables as 2, the derived PLS equation gives $R^2 = 0.803$, $Q^2 = 0.691$. The 5%-rule states that an addition of a latent variable is permitted only when it results in an increase in the value of Q^2 by 5% or more [15]. Thus, in this case, the number of latent variables should be set at 2. Note that here, we cannot use LV = 3, as the total number of descriptors present in the QSAR table is 3 and the resulting PLS equation will be the same as the MLR model already derived. Setting LV = 2, the following model is obtained:

$$pIC_{50} = -2.205 + 0.203MR + 0.621\sigma - 0.199Ind$$

$$n = 18,\ R^2 = 0.691,\ F = 30.5\ (df\ 2, 15),\ Q^2 = 0.691,\ PRESS = 0.408$$

This PLS model can be interpreted in a similar manner to an MLR model

6.2.3 Principal component regression analysis

To avoid the multicollinearity problem (existence of near-linear relationships among the independent variables) in MLR, principal component regression analysis (PCRA) may be used [16]. In PCRA, instead of regressing the dependent variable on the explanatory variables [X] directly, the PCs of the explanatory variables are used as regressors. PCA is a data reduction tool that allows the identification of the principal directions in which the data varies. In computational terms, the PCs are found by calculating the eigenvectors and eigenvalues of the data covariance matrix. Let us now explain the terms *eigenvalue* and *eigenvector.*

Let **A** be an $n \times n$ matrix. The eigenvalues of **A** are defined as the roots of the determinant $|\mathbf{A} - \lambda\mathbf{I}| = 0$, where **I** is the $n \times n$ identity matrix. This equation (characteristic polynomial) has n roots. Let λ be an eigenvalue of **A**. Then there exists a vector x such that $\mathbf{A}x = \lambda x$. The vector x is called an eigenvector of **A** associated with the eigenvalue λ.

The first step in PCRA is to standardize the variables (both dependent and independent) by subtracting their means and dividing by their standard deviations. The observed data matrix for the explanatory variables is subjected to PCA to obtain the PCs, and then a subset of PCs is selected, based on appropriate criterion (i.e., explained variance), for further use.

To perform PCA, one needs to transform the independent variables (X) to their PCs (**Z**). Mathematically, one can write

$$\mathbf{X'X} = \mathbf{PDP'} = \mathbf{Z'Z} \tag{6.27}$$

where **D** is a diagonal matrix of the eigenvalues of **X′X** (the correlation matrix **R** of the independent variables), **P** is the eigenvector matrix of **X′X**, and **Z** is a data matrix (similar in structure to **X**) made up of the PCs. **P** is orthogonal so that $\mathbf{P'P} = \mathbf{I}$. The new variables **Z** are weighted averages of the original variables **X**. Since these new variables are PCs, their correlations with each other are all zero. If one begins with variables X_1, X_2, and X_3, three PCs (Z_1, Z_2, and Z_3) will be generated. Eigenvalues near zero indicate a multicollinearity problem in the data. One should omit the components (the Zs) associated with small eigenvalues (<1) for the regression.

When one regresses the response **Y** on the selected PCs (after omitting PCs with low eigenvalues), multicollinearity is no longer a problem. The results can then be transformed back to the **X** scale to obtain estimates of the original regression coefficients. These estimates will be biased, but the size of this bias is more than compensated for by the decrease in variance.

6.2.4 Ridge regression

Ridge regression is another method for analyzing multiple regression data that suffer from multicollinearity [17]. In ridge regression, the first step is to standardize the variables (both dependent and independent) by subtracting their means and dividing by their standard deviations.

Now, following the usual notation, let us represent the regression equation in the matrix form as

$$\mathbf{Y} = \mathbf{XB} + \mathbf{e} \tag{6.28}$$

where **Y** is the matrix of the dependent variable, **X** represents the matrix of the independent variables, **B** is the matrix of the regression coefficients to be estimated, and **e** represents the errors that are residuals.

In ordinary least squares, the regression coefficients are estimated using the formula

$$\mathbf{B} = (\mathbf{X'X})^{-1}\mathbf{X'Y} \tag{6.29}$$

Note that since the variables are standardized, $\mathbf{X'X} = \mathbf{R}$, where **R** is the correlation matrix of independent variables. Now, ridge regression proceeds by adding a small value, k, to the diagonal elements of the correlation matrix:

$$\mathbf{B}^{\text{ridge}} = (\mathbf{R} + k\mathbf{I})^{-1}\mathbf{X'Y} \tag{6.30}$$

where k is a positive quantity less than 1 (usually <0.3) and **I** is the identity matrix.

One of the main obstacles in using ridge regression is in choosing an appropriate value of k. This can be done from a plot (ridge trace) of the ridge regression coefficients as a function of k. One should choose the smallest possible value of k after which the regression coefficients seem to remain constant.

6.3 CLASSIFICATION-BASED QSAR

It is possible to use graded response data (like active–inactive and positive–negative) for classification-based QSAR models when the descriptor values are quantitative.

6.3.1 Linear discriminant analysis

Linear discriminant analysis (LDA) [18] separates two or more classes of objects and can thus be used for classification problems and for dimensionality reduction. LDA undertakes the same task as MLR by predicting an outcome when the response property has categorical values and molecular descriptors are continuous variables. LDA explicitly attempts to model the difference between the classes of data. The form of LDA equation is as follows:

$$\mathrm{DF} = c_1 \times X_1 + c_2 \times X_2 + \cdots + c_m \times X_m + a \tag{6.31}$$

where DF is the discriminate function, which is a linear combination (sum) of the discriminating variables; c is the discriminant coefficient or weight for that variable; X is the respondent's score for that variable; a is a constant; m is the number of predictor variables.

The c's are unstandardized discriminant coefficients analogous to the beta coefficients in the regression equation. These c's maximize the distance between the means of the criterion (dependent) variable. Standardized discriminant coefficients can also be used as beta weight in regression. Good predictors tend to have a large weight. After using an existing set of data to calculate the discriminant function and classify cases, any new cases (test samples) can then be classified. The number of discriminant functions is 1 minus the number of groups. There is only one function for the basic two-group discriminant analysis.

In a two-group situation (Figure 6.4), the predicted membership is calculated by first producing a score for DF for each case using the discriminate function. Then, cases with DF values smaller than the cutoff value are classified as belonging to one group while those with larger values are classified into the other group. The group centroid is the mean value of the discriminant score for a given category of the dependent variable. There are as many centroids as there are groups or categories. The cutoff is the mean of the two centroids. If the discriminant score of the function is less than or equal to the cutoff the case is classed as 0, whereas if it is greater, it is classed as 1.

In stepwise discriminant function analysis, a model of discrimination is built step by step. Specifically, at each step, all the variables are reviewed and evaluated to determine which one will contribute most to the discrimination between groups. That variable will be included in the model, and the process starts again. The stepwise procedure is guided by the respective F to enter and F to remove values. The F value for a variable indicates its statistical significance in the discrimination between groups; that is, it is a measure of the extent to which a variable makes a unique contribution to the prediction of group membership.

6.3.2 Logistic regression

Logistic regression [19] is a statistical classification model that measures the relationship between a categorical-dependent variable (having only two categories) and one or

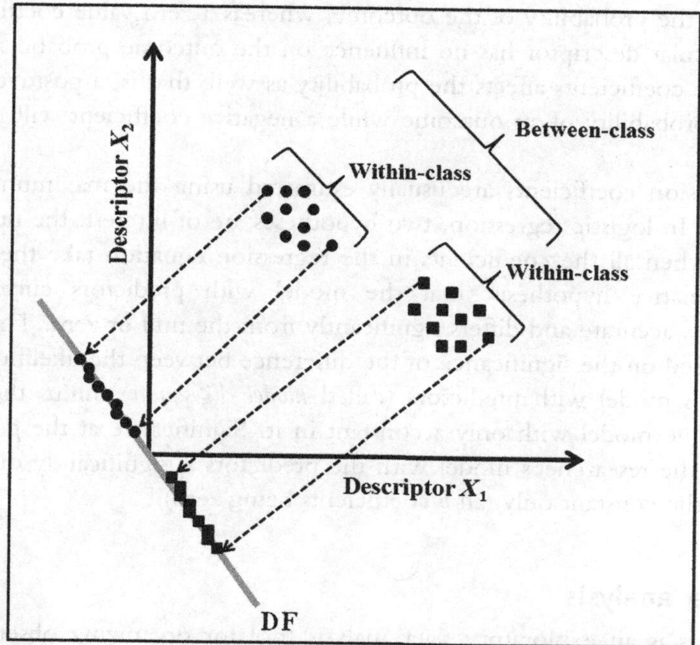

Figure 6.4 Distribution of compounds in two groups using a discrimination function DF.

more independent variables, which are usually (but not necessarily) continuous, by using probability scores as the predicted values of the dependent variable. Logistic regression does not assume a linear relationship between the dependent and independent variables. The independent variables need neither be normally distributed, nor linearly related, nor of equal variance within each group.

The form of the logistic regression equation is

$$\text{logit}\left[p(x)\right] = \log\left[\frac{p(x)}{1 - p(x)}\right] = a + b_1x_1 + b_2x_2 + b_3x_3 + \cdots \tag{6.32}$$

where logit$[p(x)]$ is the log (to base e) of the likelihood ratio that the dependent variable is 1, and p can only range from 0 to 1. In Eq. (6.32), a is the model's intercept, and $X_1, \ldots, X_k$ are molecular descriptors with their corresponding regression coefficients $b_1, \ldots, b_k$ (for molecular descriptors 1 through k). For an unknown compound, LR calculates the probability that the compound belongs to a certain target property (say, active or inactive). LR estimates the probability of the compound being an active substance. If the calculated logit$[p(x)]$ is greater than 0.5, then it is more probable that the compound is active. Similar to MLR, the regression coefficients in LR can describe the influence of a molecular descriptor on the outcome of the prediction. When the coefficient has a large value, it shows that the molecular descriptor strongly affect the probability of the outcome, whereas a zero value coefficient shows that the molecular descriptor has no influence on the outcome probability. Likewise, the sign of the coefficients affects the probability as well; that is, a positive coefficient increases the probability of an outcome while a negative coefficient will result in the opposite.

The regression coefficients are usually estimated using the maximum likelihood (ML) method. In logistic regression, two hypotheses are of interest: the null hypothesis, which is when all the coefficients in the regression equation take the value zero; and the alternative hypothesis, that the model with predictors currently under consideration is accurate and differs significantly from the null or zero. The likelihood ratio test is based on the significance of the difference between the likelihood ratio for the researcher's model with predictors (called *model chi square*) minus the likelihood ratio for baseline model with only a constant in it. Significance at the $p = 0.05$ level or less means the researcher's model with the predictors is significantly different from the one with the constant only (all b coefficients being zero).

6.3.3 Cluster analysis

Cluster analysis is an exploratory data analysis tool for organizing observed data or cases into two or more groups [20]. Unlike LDA, cluster analysis requires no prior knowledge of which elements belong to which clusters. The clusters are defined through an analysis of the data. Cluster analysis maximizes the similarity of cases within each cluster while maximizing the dissimilarity between groups that are initially unknown (Figure 6.5).

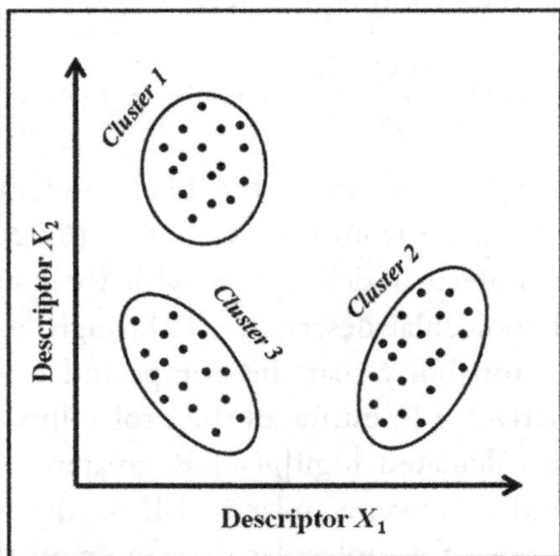

Figure 6.5 Example of clustering of compounds based on two descriptors, X_1 and X_2.

6.3.3.1 *Hierarchical cluster analysis*

Hierarchical cluster analysis is a statistical method for finding relatively homogeneous clusters of cases based on dissimilarities or distances between objects. It starts with each case as a separate cluster (i.e., there are as many clusters as cases), and then combines the clusters sequentially, reducing the number of clusters at each step until only one cluster is left. A hierarchical tree diagram or dendrogram (Figure 6.6) can be generated to show the linkage points: the clusters are linked at increasing levels of dissimilarity.

The most straightforward and generally accepted way of computing distances between objects in a multidimensional space is to compute Euclidean distances or the squared Euclidean distance (in order to place progressively greater weight on objects that are farther apart). Euclidean (and squared Euclidean) distances are usually computed from raw data, not from standardized data. In the case of p variables $X_1, X_2, \ldots,$ X_p measured on a sample of n subjects, the observed data for subject i can be denoted by $X_{i1}, X_{i2}, \ldots, X_{ip}$, and the observed data for subject j by $X_{j1}, X_{j2}, \ldots, X_{jp}$, while the Euclidean distance between these two subjects is given by

$$d_{ij} = \sqrt{(x_{i1}-x_{j1})^2 + (x_{i2}-x_{j2})^2 + \cdots + (x_{ip}-x_{jp})^2} \tag{6.33}$$

6.3.3.2 *k-Means clustering*

This section discusses *k*-means clustering, a non-hierarchical method of clustering that can be used when the number of clusters present in the objects or cases is known. It is an unsupervised method of centroid-based clustering. In general, the *k*-means method will produce exactly *k* different clusters. The main idea is to define *k* centroids, one for each cluster. These centroids should be placed as far away from each other as possible. The next step is to take each point belonging to a given data set and associate it with the nearest centroid. When no point is pending, the positions of the *k* centroids are recalculated. This procedure is repeated until the centroids no longer move (Figure 6.7).

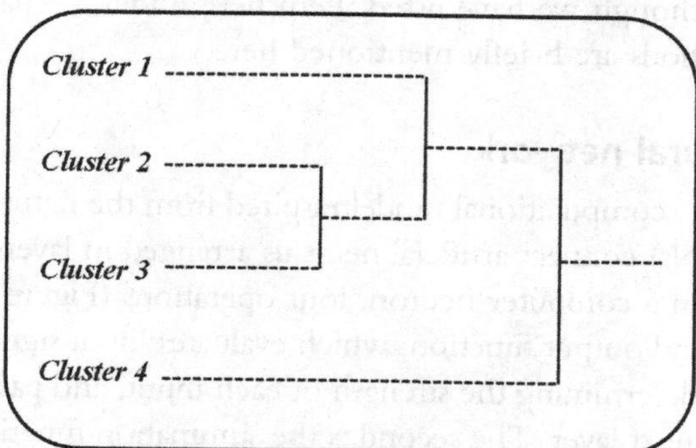

Figure 6.6 Example of a dendogram.

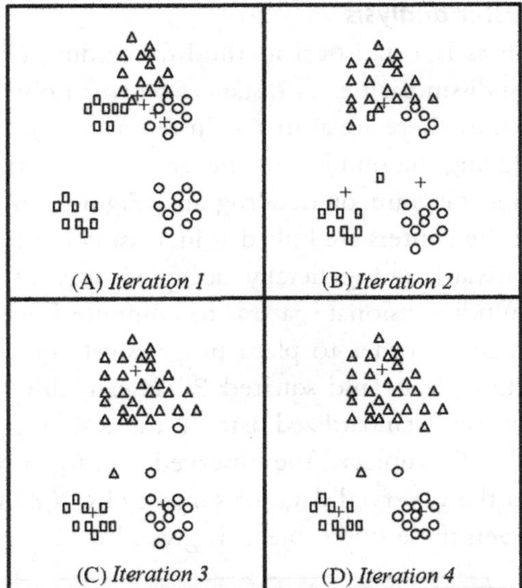

Figure 6.7 Separation of data points into three clusters using *k*-means clustering: (A) Iteration 1, (B) Iteration 2, (C) Iteration 3, (D) Iteration 4.

6.4 MACHINE LEARNING TECHNIQUES

Machine learning, using the knowledge of computer science and statistics, deals with the construction and study of systems that can learn from data, rather than following only explicitly programmed instructions. It is also related to artificial intelligence and optimization techniques. A supervised learning algorithm analyzes the training data and produces an inferred function, which can be used for mapping new examples. In unsupervised learning, no labels are given to the learning algorithm, leaving it on its own to group similar inputs (clustering) and project high-dimensional data that can be visualized effectively. Machine learning methods can be used for classification and regression problems, though we have listed them here under a separate heading. Some of the important methods are briefly mentioned here.

6.4.1 Artificial neural network

An artificial neuron is a computational model inspired from the natural neurons. Artificial neural networks (ANNs) connect artificial neurons arranged in layers in order to process information [21,22]. In a computer neuron, four operations (Figure 6.8) are performed. The first is the input and output function, which evaluates input signals from the neurons of the previous layer, determining the strength of each input, and passes the output signal to the neurons of the next layer. The second is the summation function, which calculates a total for the combined input signals according to the equation

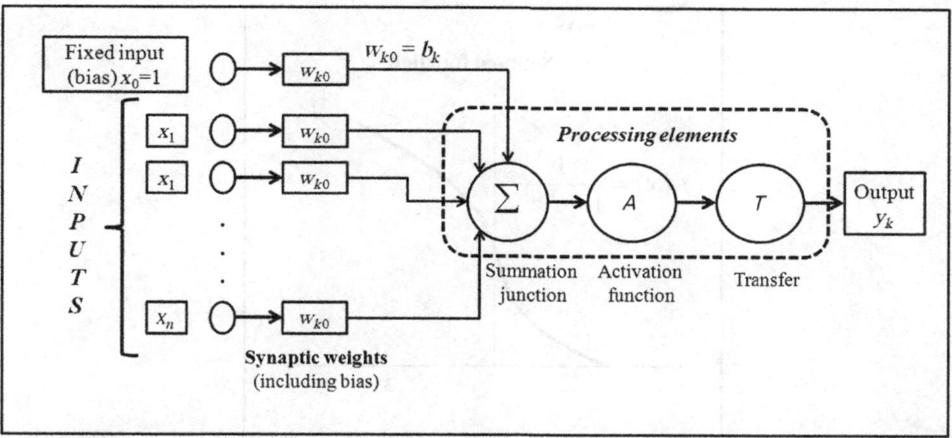

Figure 6.8 Schematic representation of a computer neuron.

$$i_j = \sum w_{ji} o_i \tag{6.34}$$

where i_j is the net input in node j (of, say, layer λ), while o_i is the output of node i in the previous layer ($\lambda - 1$); and w_{ji} is the weight associated with the nodes i and j. Third is the activation function, which allows the outputs to vary with respect to time. The result of summation is passed to this function before it is input to the transfer function. The final element is the transfer function, which maps the summed input to an output value. The most commonly used transfer function is the logistic function (sigmoidal), which incorporates the nonlinearity feature (Figure 6.9) in the mapping process:

$$o_j = f(i_j) = \frac{1}{1 + e^{-i_j}} \tag{6.35}$$

By adjusting the weights of an artificial neuron, one can modify the output for specific inputs. This process of adjusting the weights is called *learning* or *training*.

Neural networks are typically organized in layers. Layers are made of a number of interconnected nodes that contain an activation function. Patterns are presented to the network via the input layer, which communicates to one or more hidden layers where the actual processing is done via a system of weighted connections. The hidden layers then link to an output layer, where the answer is the output.

Figure 6.10 represents architecture of a simple neural network. It is made up from an input, an output, and one hidden layer. Each input layer node corresponds to a single independent variable, with the exception of the bias node. Similarly, each output layer node corresponds to a different dependent variable. Each node from the input layer is connected to a node from the hidden layer and every node from the hidden layer is connected to a node in the output layer. There is usually some weight associated with every connection.

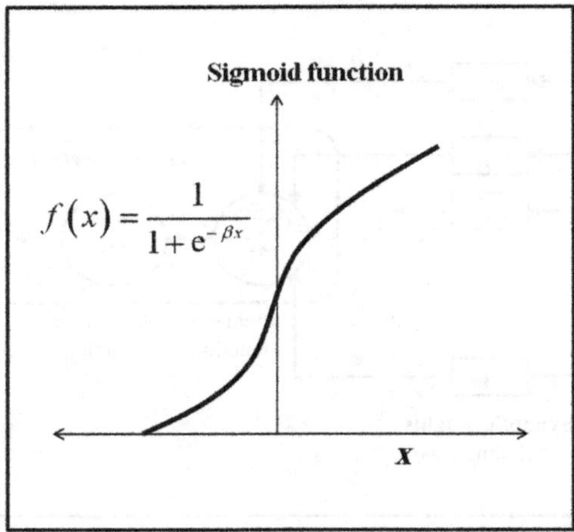

Figure 6.9 Sigmoidal function.

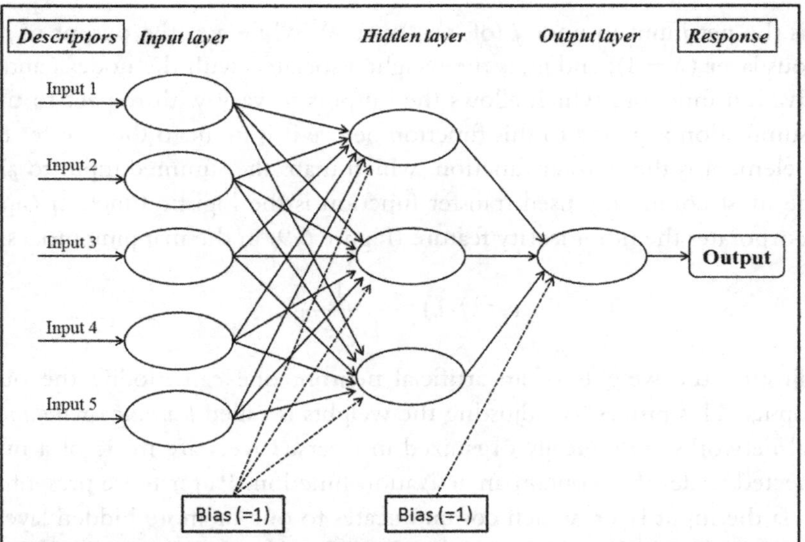

Figure 6.10 Architecture of a three-layer ANN.

Associated with each node is an internal state designated by s_i, s_h, and s_o for the input, hidden, and output layers, respectively. Each of the input and hidden layers has an additional unit, termed a *bias unit*, whose internal state is assigned a value of 1. The input layer's s_i values are related to the corresponding independent variables by the scaling equation

$$s_i = 0.8\frac{X_i - X_{i,\min}}{X_{\max} - X_{\min}} + 0.1 \tag{6.36}$$

where X_i is the value of the ith independent variable, and $X_{i,\min}$ and $X_{i,\max}$ are its minimum and maximum values, respectively. The state S_h of each hidden unit is calculated by the sigmoidal function

$$s_h = \frac{1}{1 + e^{-i_h}} \tag{6.37}$$

where

$$i_h = \sum w_{hi} s_i + \theta_h \tag{6.38}$$

Note that w_{hi} is the weight of the bond that connects the hidden unit h with input unit i and θ_h is the weight of the bond connecting hidden unit h to the input layer bias unit. The state s_o of the output unit o is calculated by

$$s_o = \frac{1}{1 + e^{-i_o}} \tag{6.39}$$

where

$$i_o = \sum w_{oh} s_h + \theta_o \tag{6.40}$$

Note that w_{oh} is the weight of the bond that connects output unit o to the hidden unit h and θ_o is the weight of the bond that connects output unit o to the hidden-layer bias unit. The network-calculated s_o have values in the range [0, 1].

Training of the neural network of Figure 6.10 is achieved by minimizing an error function E with respect to the bond weights (w_{hi}, w_{oh}):

$$E = \sum E_p = 0.5 \sum (t_p - s_{o_p})^2 \tag{6.41}$$

where E_p is the error of the pth training pattern, defined as the set of independent and dependent variables corresponding to the pth data point, or chemical compound; and t_p corresponds to the experimentally measured value (i.e., the *target value*) of the pth pattern, scaled by

$$t_p = 0.8\frac{Y_p - Y_{p,\min}}{Y_{p,\max} - Y_{p,\min}} + 0.1 \tag{6.42}$$

To summarize the learning process, an input is fed into the network to calculate the error with respect to the desired target. This error is then used to compute the weight corrections layer by layer, backward through the net. The supervised training process is repeated until the errors for the entire training set are minimized. Typically, this involves thousands of iterations. After the training process is over, the network is fully operational.

Backpropagation is a widely used supervised learning method for multiple-layer nets, which seems to be the best for solving pattern recognition problems. This technique is the most widely used generalization of the δ rule, and the procedure involves two phases. The forward phase occurs when the input is presented and propagated forward through the network to compute an output value for each processing element based on its current set of weights.

The backward phase is a recurring difference computation performed in a backward direction. The error, δ, for neurons in the output layer is given by

$$\delta_o = (t_o - s_o)f'(i_o) \tag{6.43}$$

where $f'(i_o)$ is the first derivative of the transfer function and t_o is the target output. For the units in the hidden layer, a specific target value is unknown; it is computed in terms of the errors in the units in the next layer:

$$\delta_h = \sum(\delta_o w_{oh})f'(i_h) \tag{6.44}$$

The weight between the hidden unit h and the output unit o is then modified according to the equation

$$\Delta w_{oh} = \eta\delta_o s_h + \alpha(\Delta w_{oh})_{previous} \tag{6.45}$$

where η is an empirical parameter known as the *learning rate.* Theoretically, η needs to be infinitesimally small for true gradient descent of error, but in practice, it typically takes values from 0.1 to 1.0 and is gradually reduced during the training process. A problem often occurs in the training process: namely, the system gets stuck in a local minimum and fails to reach the global minimum state. To rectify this, researchers often add a momentum term α, which considers past weight changes in the calculation of weight adjustments.

To summarize the learning process, an input is fed into the network to calculate the error with respect to the desired target. This error is then used to compute the weight corrections layer by layer, backward through the net. The supervised training process is repeated until the errors for the entire training set are minimized. Typically, this involves thousands of iterations.

The number of input and output nodes depends on the training set. There are two advantages of adopting networks with a small number of hidden units. First, the efficiency of each node increases, and consequently, the time of the computer simulation is significantly reduced. Second, and more important, the network can generalize the input patterns better, and this results in superior predictive power. However, a network with insufficient hidden units will not be able to extract all the relevant correlation between physicochemical parameters and biological activity.

While the numbers of nodes in the input and output layers are likely to be predetermined by the nature of experimental data, the freedom of the analyzer lies in fixing the number of hidden units. It has been suggested that a ratio, ρ, plays a crucial role in determining the number of hidden units being employed. The definition of ρ is

$$\rho = \frac{\text{number\_of\_data\_points\_in\_the\_training\_set}}{\text{number\_of\_variables\_controlled\_by\_the\_network}} \tag{6.46}$$

The number of variables is simply the sum of the number of connections in the network and the number of biases. The suggested range of $1.8 < \rho < 2.2$ is perhaps empirical, and it is also likely to be implementation-dependent. The method to control neural networks is by setting and adjusting weights between nodes. Initial weights are usually set at some random numbers and then they are adjusted during neural-network training. The neural-network fitting may suffer from overfitting, thus requiring strict tests of validation before they can be applied for prediction purposes.

6.4.2 Bayesian neural network

A Bayesian neural network is a probabilistic graphical model [23]. Bayesian methods are complementary to neural networks, as they overcome the tendency of an over-flexible network to discover nonexistent or overly complex data models. Unlike a standard backpropagation neural network training method, where a single set of parameters (weights, biases, etc.) is used, the Bayesian approach to neural-network modeling considers all possible values of network parameters weighted by the probability of each set of weights. The nodes in a Bayesian network represent a set of random variables, $X = X_1, X_2, \ldots, X_n$, from the domain. A set of directed arcs (or links) connects pairs of nodes, $X_i \to X_j$, representing the direct dependencies between variables. Assuming discrete variables, the strength of the relationship between variables is quantified by conditional probability distributions associated with each node. The only constraint on the arcs allowed in a Bayesian network is that there must not be any directed cycles: one cannot return to a node simply by following directed arcs. In a Bayesian model, all model parameters are explicitly expressed as probability distributions. The posterior distributions of the model parameters are estimated from their prior probability distribution given the training data set. Training the network amounts to estimating the posterior distributions of the network parameters. These are then used to estimate the distribution of the model output $p(t)$ when given new data x. Using the Bayesian framework, all the data can be utilized to estimate and tune the model parameters; hence, there is no requirement for splitting the data set. This is important when the data set is small or difficult to obtain.

6.4.3 Decision tree and random forest

A *decision tree* [24] is a graphical decision support tool that searches for rules that are able to classify objects on the basis of descriptors. Each event is assigned a subjective probability; the sum of probabilities for the events in a set must equal 1. A major goal of the analysis is to determine the best decisions. The rules are inferred from objects in the training set. After the training process is over, the trees can be applied to new objects for their classification. A decision tree is a structure with a hierarchical arrangement of nodes and branches.

Decision trees have three kinds of nodes (Figure 6.11): a root node, internal nodes, and terminal nodes. The tree starts from a root node, which does not have any incoming branches, while an internal node has one incoming branch and two or more outgoing branches. Finally, the terminal nodes have one incoming branch and no outgoing branches. Each terminal node is assigned a target property, while a non-terminal node (root or internal node) is assigned a molecular descriptor that becomes a test condition that branches out into groups of differing properties. The root node in a tree corresponds to the best predictor. Decision trees create an iterative branching topology in which the branch taken at each intersection is determined by a rule related to a descriptor of the molecule.

Finally, each terminating leaf of the tree is assigned to a class. A binary decision tree consists of three steps that are carried out iteratively. First, for each descriptor, a numerical value is determined that represents a threshold dividing the compounds into two groups. This threshold is chosen in a way so that the number of compounds assigned to an incorrect group is minimal. In the second step, the descriptor showing the lowest possible false classification is chosen as the branching point (node). In cases

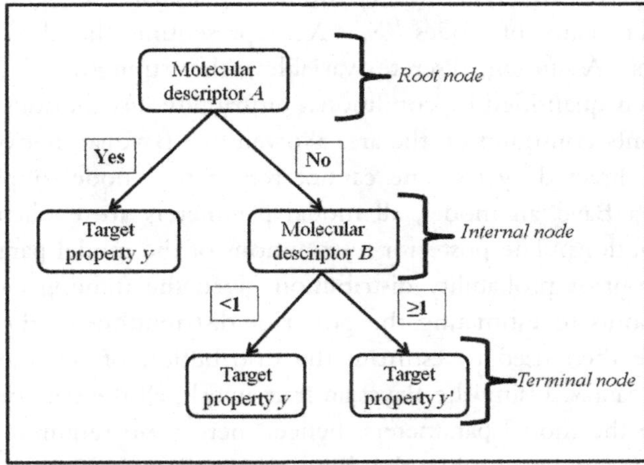

Figure 6.11 Example of a decision tree.

where two or more descriptors yield identical errors, the descriptor showing the lowest variance among its numerical range is chosen, which leads to better results. The third step is comprised of the partitioning of the compound data set into two parts according to the determined threshold at this node. For these two partial sets of the original set, the algorithm is applied recursively, while excluding descriptors that have already been used in the path up to the preceding node to avoid redundancies. However, the multiple use of one descriptor at different nodes in the tree is allowed. The algorithm is terminated if either all remaining compounds are sorted correctly or if no descriptor is available that would lead to an improved partitioning. To avoid excessive partitioning, branching is also terminated if the maximum branching depth as specified by the user is reached. The analysis of the branching topology is performed with an independent data set, whereby the descriptors and margins obtained with the training set are kept unchanged. A decision tree can easily be transformed to a set of rules by mapping from the root node to the leaf (terminal) nodes one by one.

Random forest (RF), an ensemble learning method, uses consensus classification to reduce the problem of overfitting while improving accuracy [25,26]. The algorithm works by growing multiple decision trees (collectively known as a *forest*) that make a final prediction based on the majority prediction from each of the trees. To construct each tree, a training sample of a reduced size is selected at random with replacement from original data. Using the new training sample, a tree is grown with randomly selected descriptors, and it is not pruned. The remaining training data are used to estimate error and variable importance. RF is easy to use, as the user needs to fix only two parameters: the number of trees in the forest and the number of descriptors in each tree. A large number of trees should be grown, and the number of descriptors to be taken is the square root of the total number of descriptors. RF can handle a large number of training data and descriptors. Besides classifying an unknown compound, it can be extended for unsupervised clustering and outlier detection. RF can also be used to infer the influence of the descriptors in a classification task and to estimate missing data. The performance of RF can be influenced by an imbalanced data set or small sample size, as well as by the number of trees and features selected. Therefore, the parameters for RF should be carefully selected through the use of cross-validation.

6.4.4 Support vector machine

Support vector machines (SVMs) are supervised learning models that analyze data and recognize patterns, used for classification and regression analysis [27]. SVM works by constructing hyperplanes in a multidimensional space that separates cases of different class labels. SVM supports both regression and classification tasks and can handle multiple continuous and categorical variables.

SVMs are effective in high-dimensional spaces, even when the number of dimensions is greater than the number of samples. They are memory-efficient and versatile. However, if the number of features is much greater than the number of samples, the method is likely to result in poor performance. Although SVMs were originally developed for classification problems; they can also be extended to solve nonlinear regression problems by the introduction of ε-insensitive loss function. In support vector regression, the input x is first mapped into a higher-dimensional feature space by the use of a kernel function, and then a linear model is constructed in this feature space. The kernel functions often used in SVM include linear, polynomial, radial basis function, and sigmoid function. The linear model $f(x,\omega)$ in the feature space is given by

$$f(x, \omega) = \sum_{j=1}^{m} \omega_j g_j(x) + b \tag{6.47}$$

where $g_j(x)$ represents a set of nonlinear transformations and b is the bias term.

The quality of estimation is measured by a loss function known as *ε-insensitive loss function*. The advantages of SVM and support vector regression include that they can be used to avoid the difficulties of using linear functions in the high-dimensional feature space, and the optimization problem is transformed into dual convex quadratic programs. In the case of regression, the loss function is used to penalize errors that are greater than the threshold ε. Such loss functions usually lead to the sparse representation of the decision rule, giving significant algorithmic and representational advantages. The disadvantage of SVM is that SVMs do not directly provide probability estimates; rather, these are calculated using an expensive, fivefold cross-validation.

6.5 CONCLUSION

QSAR models are developed using statistical approaches; thus, a sound knowledge of chemometrics is essential for good QSAR practices. The statistical techniques employed in QSAR may be regression-based or use linear or nonlinear techniques for classification. The proper choice of a technique for modeling purposes depends on the particular problem to analyze, the nature of the training set data, objective of the analysis, and type and number of the descriptors involved.

REFERENCES

[1] Snedecor GW, Cochran WG. Statistical methods. New Delhi: Oxford and IBH; 1967.
[2] Darlington RB. Regression and linear models. New York, NY: McGraw-Hill; 1990.
[3] Rogers D, Hopfinger AJ. Application of genetic function approximation to quantitative structure–activity relationships and quantitative structure–property relationships. J Chem Inf Comput Sci 1994;34 (4):854–66.

[4] Fan Y, Shi LM, Kohn KW, Pommier Y, Weinstein JN. Quantitative structure–antitumor activity relationships of camptothecin analogues: cluster analysis and genetic algorithm-based studies. J Med Chem 2001;44(20):3254–63.

[5] Bhattacharya P, Leonard JT, Roy K. Exploring QSAR of thiazole and thiadiazole derivatives as potent and selective human adenosine A3 receptor antagonists using FA and GFA techniques. Bioorg Med Chem 2005;13(4):1159–65.

[6] Roy K, Leonard JT. QSAR by LFER model of cytotoxicity data of anti-HIV 5-phenyl-1-phenylamino-1*H*-imidazole derivatives using principal component factor analysis and genetic function approximation. Bioorg Med Chem 2005;13:2967–73.

[7] Franke R. Theoretical drug design methods. Amsterdam, the Netherlands: Elsevier; 1984.

[8] Franke R, Gruska A. In: van de Waterbeemd H, editor. Chemometric methods in molecular design. Weinheim, Germany: VCH; 1995. pp. 113.

[9] Leonard JT, Roy K. QSAR by LFER model of HIV protease inhibitor mannitol derivatives using FA-MLR, PCRA, and PLS techniques. Bioorg Med Chem 2006;14(4):1039–46.

[10] Shahlaei M. Descriptor selection methods in quantitative structure–activity relationship studies: a review study. Chem Rev 2013;113(10):8093–103.

[11] Kennedy J., Eberhart R. Particle swarm optimization. In: Proc. IEEE international conference on neural network; New Jersey, 1995. P. 1942.

[12] Dorigo M, Stützle T. Ant colony optimization. Cambridge, MA: The MIT Press; 2004.

[13] Zheng W, Tropsha A. A novel variable selection quantitative structure–property relationship approach based on the *k*-nearest-neighbor principle. J Chem Inf Comput Sci 2000;40:185–94.

[14] Wold S, Sjöström M, Eriksson L. PLS-regression: a basic tool of chemometrics. Chemom Intell Lab Syst 2001;58:109–30.

[15] Wold S, Johansson E, Cocchi M. PLS: partial least squares projections to latent structures. In: Kubinyi H, editor. 3D QSAR in drug design: theory methods and applications. Leiden, the Netherlands: ESCOM; 1993. p. 523–50.

[16] Frank LE, Friedman JHA. Statistical view of some chemometrics regression tools. Technometrics 1993;35(2):109–35.

[17] Hoerl AE. Application of ridge analysis to regression problems. Chem Eng Prog 1958;54–9.

[18] Agresti A. An introduction to categorical data analysis. New Jersey: John Wiley & Sons; 1996.

[19] Harrell FE. Regression modeling strategies. Springer-Verlag; 2001.

[20] Everitt BS, Landau S, Leese M. Cluster analysis. 4th ed. Arnold; 2001.

[21] So S, Richards WG. Application of neural networks: quantitative structure–activity relationships of the derivatives of 2,4-diamino-5-(substituted-benzyl)pyrimidines as DHFR inhibitors. J Med Chem 1992;35:3201–7.

[22] Andrea TA, Kalayeh H. Applications of neural networks in quantitative structure–activity relationships of dihydrofolate reductase inhibitors. J Med Chem 1991;34(9):2824–36.

[23] Ben-Gal I. Bayesian networks. In: Ruggeri F, Faltin F, Kenett R, editors. Encyclopedia of statistics in quality & reliability. New York: John Wiley & Sons; 2007.

[24] Andres C, Hutter MC. CNS permeability of drugs predicted by a decision tree. QSAR Comb Sci 2006;25(4):305–9.

[25] Amit Y, Geman D. Shape quantization and recognition with randomized trees. Neural Comput 1997; 9:1545–88.

[26] Yee LC, Wei YC. Current modeling methods used in QSAR/QSPR. In: Dehmer M, Varmuza K, Bonchev D, editors. Statistical modelling of molecular descriptors in QSAR/QSPR. Weinheim: Wiley VCH; 2012. pp. 1–31.

[27] Vapnik VN. Statistical learning theory. New York, NY: John Wiley & Sons; 1998.

CHAPTER 7

Validation of QSAR Models

Contents

7.1 INTRODUCTION

A large amount of *in silico* research worldwide has been oriented toward the rational drug discovery, property prediction, toxicity, and risk assessment of new drug molecules, as well as chemicals [1]. Quantitative structure–activity relationship (QSAR) analysis has gained great popularity recently in order to fulfill the following objectives [2]: (a) prediction of new analogs with better activity; (b) improved understanding and investigation of the mode of action of chemicals and pharmaceuticals; (c) optimization of the lead compound to congeners with decreased toxicity; (d) rationalization of wet laboratory experimentation (QSAR offers an economical and time-effective alternative to the medium-throughput in vitro and low-throughput in vivo assays); (e) reduction of cost, time, and manpower requirements by developing more effective compounds using a scientifically less exhaustive approach; and finally, (f) to develop alternative methods to animal experimentation in conformity to the Registration, Evaluation, and Authorization of Chemicals (REACH) guidelines [3] and the 3R concept [4], which signifies "reduction, replacement, and refinement" of animal

Understanding the Basics of QSAR for Applications in Pharmaceutical Sciences and Risk Assessment.
ISBN: 978-0-12-801505-6, DOI: http://dx.doi.org/10.1016/B978-0-12-801505-6.00007-7

experiments. As a consequence, the QSAR technique emerges as an alternative tool to use for the design, development, and screening of new drug molecules and chemical substances.

The QSAR models are principally applied to predict the activity/property/toxicity of new classes of compounds falling within the domain of applicability of the developed models. Again, to check the acceptability and reliability of the QSAR models' predictions, validation of the QSAR model has been recognized as one of the key elements [5]. It is now accepted that validation is a more holistic process for assessing the quality of data, applicability, and mechanistic interpretability of the developed model [6]. Various methodological aspects of validation of QSARs have been the subject of much debate within the academic and regulatory communities. The following questions are often raised before successful validation and succeeding appliance of a QSAR model:

1. Which of the validation approaches should be performed to evaluate the quality and the predictive power of the QSAR model?
2. What is the foremost criterion for establishing the scientific validity of a QSAR model?
3. How should one use QSAR models for regulatory purposes?
4. Is it possible to use any QSAR model for any given set of new untested chemicals?

The Organisation for Economic Cooperation and Development (OECD) [7] has agreed to five principles that should be followed to set up the scientific validity of a QSAR model, thereby facilitating its recognition for regulatory purposes. OECD principle 4 refers to the need to establish "appropriate measures of goodness-of-fit, robustness, and predictivity" for any QSAR model. It identifies the need to validate a model internally (as represented by goodness-of-fit and robustness) as well as externally (predictivity). Validation strategies largely depend on various metrics. The statistical quality of regression- and classification-based QSAR models can be examined by different statistical metrics developed over the years [8].

Another important aspect of the validation of the QSAR model is the need to define an applicability domain (AD)—that is, OECD principle 3—of the developed QSAR model. The AD expresses the fact that QSARs are inescapably associated with restrictions in the categories of chemical structures, physicochemical properties, and mechanisms of action for which the models can generate reliable predictions [9]. The AD of a QSAR model has been defined as the response and chemical structure space, characterized by the properties of the molecules in the training set. The developed model can predict a new molecule confidently only if the new compound lies in the AD of the QSAR model. It is extremely helpful for the QSAR model user to have information about the AD of the developed model to identify interpolation (true prediction) or extrapolation (less reliable prediction) [10].

Bearing in mind the magnitude of QSAR validation approaches and different validation parameters in the development of successful and acceptable QSAR models, this chapter will focus on classical as well as relatively new validation metrics used to judge the quality of the QSAR models. Along with the validation metrics, the important concepts of the AD approach to build reliable and acceptable QSAR models are discussed thoroughly.

7.2 DIFFERENT VALIDATION METHODS

With the introduction of fast computational approaches, it is now feasible to calculate a large number of descriptors using various software tools. However, one cannot ignore the risk of chance correlations with the increased number of variables included in the final model as compared to the number of compounds for which the model is constructed [11]. Again, employing diverse optimization procedures, it is possible to obtain models that can fit the experimental data well, but there is always a chance of overfitting. Fitting of data does not confirm the predictability of a model, as it does for the quality of the model. This is the main basis behind the necessity of validation of the developed models in terms of robustness and predictivity. A QSAR model is fundamentally judged in terms of its predictivity; that is, representing how well it is able to forecast end-point values of molecules that are not employed to develop the correlation.

Apart from the use of fitness parameters to judge the statistical quality of the model, validation of QSAR models is carried out using two major strategies [12]: (i) internal validation using the training set molecules, and (ii) external validation based on the test set compounds by splitting the whole data set into training and test sets. However, there is another technique called *true external validation*, which uses the developed QSAR model to predict an external data set. It is important to mention that many times, an external data set is absent for the same end point. In such a case, the data set is divided into a training and a test set for external validation. Here, for better understanding of the validation methods, we are including true external validation in the discussion of the basic external validation approach. Both the internal and external validation methods have been considered by different groups of researchers for evaluating the predictability of the models. Besides these techniques, randomization or *Y*-scrambling (again, which can be regarded as a type of internal validation) executed on the data matrix provides a valuable technique for evaluating the existence of any chance correlation in the QSAR model. Along with these validation techniques, determination of the AD of the model and selection of outliers are other vital aspects in the course of developing a reliable QSAR model with the spirit of OECD principles. The steps for development of reliable and acceptable QSAR model along with the currently employed validation methods are demonstrated in Figure 7.1.

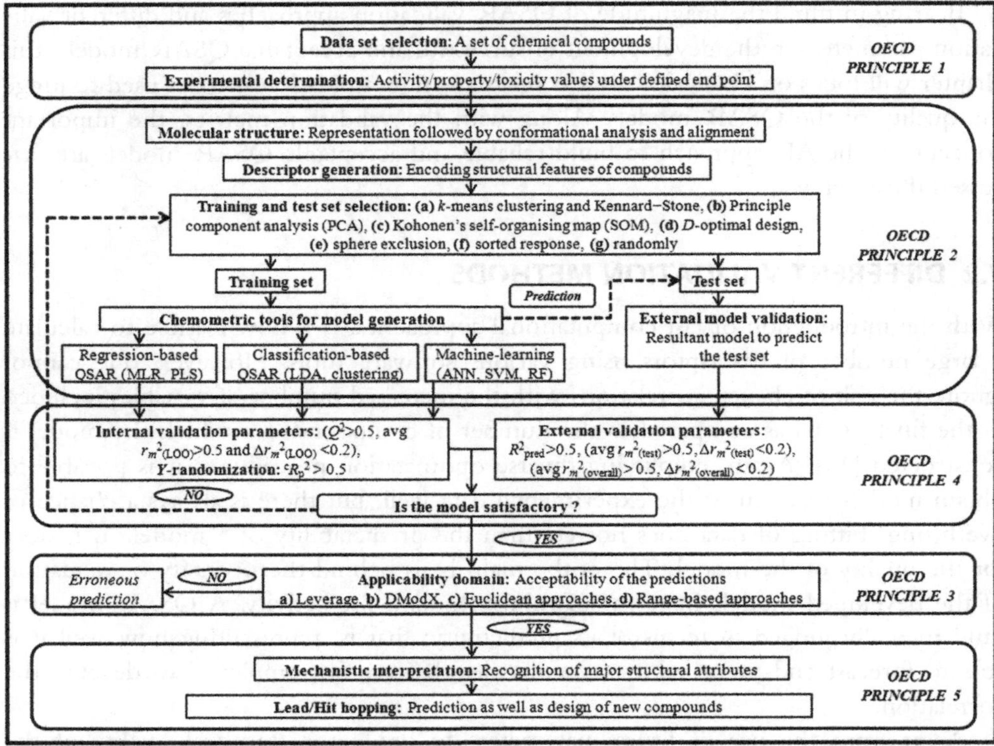

Figure 7.1 Steps for the construction of a QSAR model, along with employed validation methods in spirit of OECD guidelines.

7.2.1 The OECD principles

A meeting of QSAR experts was held in Setúbal, Portugal, in March 2002 to formulate guidelines for the validation of QSAR models, particularly for regulatory purposes [13]. These principles were approved by the OECD member countries, QSAR, and regulatory communities at the 37th Joint Meeting of the Chemicals Committee and Working Party on Chemicals, Pesticides, and Biotechnology in November 2004. These principles are meant to be the best feasible outline of the most imperative points that must be addressed to find consistent, dependable, and reproducible QSAR models [14]. The five guidelines adopted by the OECD, denoting validity of the QSAR model, are as follows:

i. *Principle 1—A defined end point*: The intent of a defined end point is to certify that clarity in the end point can be predicted by a given model, since a given end point could be determined by different experimental protocols and under different experimental conditions. It is therefore important to identify the experimental protocol used for the end point that is being modeled by the QSAR. Laboratory-to-laboratory variance in the experimental method may lead to erroneous model development.

ii. *Principle 2—An unambiguous algorithm*: The intent of having an unambiguous algorithm is to guarantee transparency in the model algorithm that generates predictions of an end point from information on chemical structure, physicochemical properties, or both. It is identified that the information regarding commercially developed models is not always publicly available. Therefore, reproducibility is a major issue for regulatory acceptance. The algorithms used in developing QSAR modeling should be mentioned properly so that individual developers can reproduce the model. Compound structure pretreatment (energy minimization, partial charge calculation, addition or suppression of hydrogen, conformer generation, etc.), calculation of the descriptors, the software employed, and the variable selection procedure for QSAR model development should be considered as imperative parts of the overall definition of an unambiguous algorithm.

iii. *Principle 3—A defined domain of applicability*: The need to define an AD reflects the fact that QSARs are unavoidably associated with limitations in terms of the types of chemical structures, physicochemical properties, and mechanisms of action for which the models can generate reliable predictions. The AD of a QSAR model has been defined as the response and chemical structure space that is defined by the nature of the chemicals in the training set. If a new compound exists in the AD of the developed model, only then can the developed model predict the compound precisely. It is extremely useful for QSAR developers to have information about the AD of the developed model to identify interpolation (true predictions) or extrapolation (less reliable predictions).

iv. *Principle 4—Appropriate measures of goodness-of-fit, robustness, and predictivity*: The appropriate measures of goodness-of-fit, robustness, and predictivity identify the need to validate a model internally (as represented by goodness-of-fit and robustness) as well as externally (predictivity).

v. *Principle 5—A mechanistic interpretation, if possible*: Providing a mechanistic interpretation of a given QSAR model is not always possible from a scientific viewpoint. The absence of a mechanistic interpretation for a model does not mean that a model is not potentially useful in the regulatory context. The intent of principle 5 is not to reject models that have no apparent mechanistic basis, but to ensure that some consideration is given to the possibility of a mechanistic association between the descriptors used in a model and the end point being predicted, and that this association is documented.

The OECD has also presented a checklist to offer direction on the interpretation of these principles. Thus, the existing challenge in the process of development of a QSAR model is no longer developing a model that is able to predict the activity within the training set in a statistically sound fashion, but developing a model with the capacity to precisely predict the activity of untested chemicals [15].

7.2.2 Internal validation

Internal validation of a QSAR model is done based on the molecules involved in QSAR model development [16,17]. It involves activity prediction of the studied molecules, followed by the estimation of parameters for detecting the precision of predictions. The cross-validation technique mainly involves internal validation, where a sample of n observations is partitioned into calibration (i.e., training) and validation (i.e., test) subsets. The calibration subset is used to construct a model, while the validation subset is used to test how well the model predicts the new data—that is, the data points not used in the calibration procedure. To judge the quality and goodness-of-fit of the model, internal validation is ideal. But the major drawback of this approach is the lack of predictability of the model when it is applied to a completely new data set.

7.2.3 External validation

Internal validation considers only chemicals belonging to the same set of compounds. As a consequence, one cannot judge the predictive capability of the developed model when it has been employed to predict a completely new set of compounds. In many cases, where truly external data points are unavailable for prediction purposes, the original data set compounds are divided into training and test sets [18], thus enabling external validation. This subdivision of the data set can be accomplished in many ways. The details about the division of the data set into training and test sets are illustrated in Section 7.2.3.1. In the case of external validation, the data set is initially divided into training and test sets, and subsequently, a model is developed with the training set and the constructed model is employed to check the external validation by utilizing the test set molecules that are not used in the model development process. The external validation ensures the predictability and applicability of the developed QSAR model for the prediction of untested molecules. A series of both classical and newly introduced validation metrics and model stability parameters are discussed in Section 7.2.4.

7.2.3.1 Division of the data set into training and test sets

The selection of training and test sets should be based on the immediacy of the test set members to representative points of the training set in the multidimensional descriptor space [19,20]. Ideally, this division must be performed such that points representing both training and test sets are distributed within the whole descriptor space occupied by the whole data set and each point of the test set is near at least one compound of the training set. This approach ensures that the similarity principle can be employed for the activity prediction of the test set [19]. There are several possible approaches available for the selection of the training and test sets. The following approaches are largely employed by the QSAR practitioners:

i. *Random selection*: In this method, the data set is divided into training and test sets by a mere random selection.

ii. *Based on Y-response*: One more frequently used approach is based on the activity (Y-response) sampling. The whole range of activities is divided into bins, and compounds belonging to each bin are randomly (or in some regular way) assigned to the training or test sets [21].

iii. *Based on X-response*: Another approach is selection of the training and test sets on the basis of compound similarity. In this method, physicochemical properties and structural similarity of the compounds are considered for the grouping of similar or homologous compounds. Thereafter, a predecided portion of compounds is manually or in some regular way assigned to the training or test set.

The test set thus selected may vary in size depending upon the number of compounds in the data set. The selection of molecules in the training and test sets, as well as their size, are the prime criteria for development of a statistically significant QSAR model [22]. From this perspective, the most generally employed tools for rational division of the data set into training and test sets are discussed in the following list:

a. k-*Means clustering*: The k-means clustering is one of the best known nonhierarchical clustering techniques [23]. This approach is based on clustering a series of compounds into several statistically representative classes of chemicals. At the end of the analysis, the data are split into k clusters. As the result of k-means clustering analysis, one can examine the means for each cluster on each dimension to assess how distinct the k clusters are. This procedure ensures that any chemical class is represented in both series of compounds (i.e., training and test sets) [23].

b. *Kohonen's self-organizing map selection*: Kohonen's self-organizing map (SOM) considers the closeness between data points. One has to remember that these points, which are close to each other in the multidimensional descriptor space, are also close to each other on the generated map by the SOM. Representative points falling into the identical areas of the SOM are arbitrarily chosen for the training and test sets. The shortcoming of this method is that the quantitative methods of prediction use accurate values of distances between representative points: as SOM is a nonlinear projection method, the distances between points in the map are distorted [24].

c. *Statistical molecular design*: Statistical molecular design may be employed for the training set selection [25]. It uses a large number of molecular structures for which the response variable (Y) is not required. Molecular descriptors are computed for all compounds, and principal component analysis (PCA) is performed. The principal components (PCs) that are combinations of the molecular properties signify the principal properties of the data set explaining the variation among the molecules in an optimal way. The design is then executed with respect to the principal properties by picking a subset of compounds that are most competent in spanning the substance space and, thus, are the best selection of training set for a QSAR model. The selection can be done manually from the score plots if the number of PCs is less than 3 or 4 [26].

d. *Kennard–Stone selection*: To pick a representative subset from a data set, hierarchical clustering and maximum dissimilarity approach also can be employed. The Kennard–Stone method selects a subset of samples from N that offers unvarying coverage over the data set and includes samples on the boundary of the data set. The method begins by finding the two samples that are farthest apart in terms of geometric distance. To add another sample to the selection set, the algorithm selects from the remaining samples the one that has the greatest separation distance from the selected samples. The separation distance of a candidate sample from the selected set is the distance from the candidate to its closest selected sample. This most-separated sample is then added to the selection set, and the process is repeated until the required number of samples, x, has been added to the selection set. The drawbacks of clustering methods are that different clusters contain different numbers of points and have different densities of representative points. Therefore, the closeness of each point of the test set to at least one point of the training set is not guaranteed. Maximum dissimilarity and Kennard–Stone methods guarantee that the points of the training set are distributed more or less evenly within the whole area occupied by representative points, and the condition of closeness of the test set points to the training set points is satisfied [27].

e. *Sphere exclusion*: In the sphere exclusion method, a compound with the highest activity is selected and included in the training set. A sphere with the center in the representative point of this compound with radius $r = d(V/N)^{1/P}$ is built, where P is the number of variables that represents the dimensionality of descriptor space, d is the dissimilarity level, N is the total number of compounds in the data set, and V is the total volume occupied by the representative points of compounds. The dissimilarity level is varied to create different training and test sets. The molecules corresponding to representative points within this sphere (except for the center) are incorporated in the test set. All points within this sphere are excluded from the initial set of compounds. Let n be the number of remaining compounds. If $n = 0$, splitting is stopped [28]. If $n > 0$, the next compound is randomly selected. Otherwise, distances of the representative points of the remaining compounds to the sphere centers are calculated, and a compound with the smallest or greatest distance is selected.

f. *Extrapolation-oriented test set selection*: Extrapolation-oriented test set selection is an external validation method that performs better than those constructed by random selection and uniformly distributed selection. This algorithm selects pairs of molecules from those available that have the highest Euclidean distance in the descriptor space and then moves them to the external validation set, one after the other, until the set is complete [29].

The OECD members did not prepare any general rules regarding the impact of training and test set size on the quality of prediction, but it is important to point out that the training set size should be set at an optimal level so that the model is developed with a reliable and acceptable number of training set compounds and it is able to satisfactorily predict the activity values of the test set compounds. Note that the division of a data set using some common algorithms can be easily done by the use of an open-access tool called Dataset Division GUI 1.0, available at http://dtclab.webs.com/software-tools and http://teqip.jdvu.ac.in/QSAR_Tools/.

7.2.3.2 Applicability domain

7.2.3.2.1 Concept of the AD

The AD [30] is a theoretical region in the chemical space surrounding both the model descriptors and modeled response. In the construction of a QSAR model, the AD of molecules plays a deciding role in estimating the uncertainty in the prediction of a particular compound based on how similar it is to the compounds used to build the model. Therefore, the prediction of a modeled response using QSAR is applicable only if the compound being predicted falls within the AD of the model, as it is impractical to predict an entire universe of chemicals using a single QSAR model. Again, AD can be described as the physicochemical, structural, or biological space information based on which the training set of the model is developed, and the model is applicable to make predictions for new compounds within the specific domain [31].

One has to remember that the selection process of the training and test sets has a very important effect on the AD of the constructed QSAR model. Thus, while splitting a data set for external validation, the training set molecules should be selected in such a way that they span the entire chemical space for all the data set molecules. In order to obtain successful predictions, a QSAR model should always be used for compounds within its AD.

7.2.3.2.2 History behind the introduction of the AD

A QSAR model is essentially valued in terms of its predictability, indicating how well it is able to predict the end-point values of the compounds that are not used to develop the correlation. Models that have been validated internally and externally can be considered reliable for both scientific and regulatory purposes [32]. As decided by the OECD, QSAR models should be validated according to the OECD principles for reliable predictions (elaborated previously in this chapter in Section 7.2.1). Thus, the present challenge in the procedure of developing a QSAR model is no longer ensuring that the model is statistically able to predict the activity within the training set, but developing a model that can predict accurately the activity of untested chemicals.

In this context, QSAR model predictions are most consistent if they are derived from the model's AD, which is broadly defined under OECD principle 3. The OECD includes AD assessment as one of the QSAR acceptance criteria for regulatory purposes [14]. The Setubal Workshop report [13] presented the following regulation for AD assessment: "The applicability domain of a (Q)SAR is the physicochemical, structural, or biological space, knowledge, or information on which the training set of the model has been developed, and for which it is applicable to make predictions for new compounds. The applicability domain of a (Q)SAR should be described in terms of the most relevant parameters, i.e. usually those that are descriptors of the model. Ideally the (Q)SAR should only be used to make predictions within that domain by interpolation not extrapolation." This depiction is useful for explaining the instinctive meaning of the "applicability domain" approach.

7.2.3.2.3 Types of AD approaches

The most common approaches for estimating interpolation regions in a multivariate space include the following [10]:

- Ranges in the descriptor space
- Geometrical methods
- Distance-based methods
- Probability density distribution
- Range of the response variable

The first four approaches are based on the methodology used for interpolation space characterization in the model descriptor space. The last one, however, depends solely on the response space of the training set molecules. A compound can be identified as being out of the domain of applicability in a simple way; namely, (a) at least one descriptor is out of the span of the ranges approach and (b) the distance between the chemical and the center of the training data set exceeds the threshold for distance approaches. The threshold for all kinds of distance methods is the largest distance between the training set data points and the center of the training data set. Classification of the AD approaches is graphically presented in Figure 7.2. In order to better explain the theory, criteria, and drawbacks of each type of AD approaches [9,10,30,33–48], we have depicted all the methods in Table 7.1.

The domain of applicability for the bounding box method is the smallest axis-aligned rectangular box containing all the data points, as presented in Figure 7.3A. The AD space for the PCA bounding box approach is presented in Figure 7.3B. In explanation of Figure 7.3B, the QSAR model training set is represented by the biggest circle and the predictions of the query molecules within the training space are

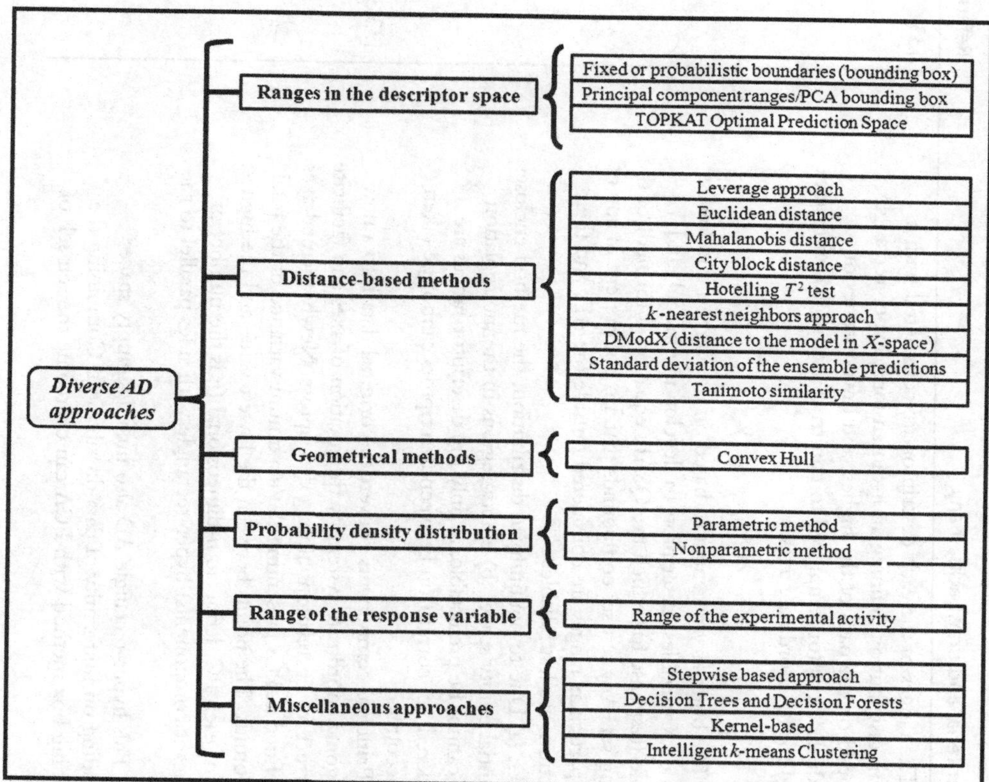

Figure 7.2 Classification of the AD approaches.

considered reliable. Again, query compounds that are located outside the training model space would be expected to be less reliably predicted. Both these approaches are the part of the "ranges in the descriptor space" approach. The AD of the "convex hull" method (geometrical approach) is the smallest axis-aligned convex region containing all the data points presented in Figure 7.3C. In Figure 7.4A, a graphical illustration of the basic "distance-to-centroid" approach is illustrated. Under this method, a $k-$nearest neighbors plot is presented in Figure 7.4B, where the distance of a point to the domain is taken as the average distance to the k-nearest data points; and a graphical illustration of the standard deviation (STD) approach has been given in Figure 7.4C. Here, reliable prediction has a low prediction spread of the drawn curve, and unreliable prediction has a higher prediction of the drawn curve. The most commonly used methods, like the leverage approach (Williams plot) and Euclidean distance approach, are plotted and explained employing a real data set in Section 7.3 of this chapter.

Table 7.1 Hypotheses of diverse AD methods

Types	Subtypes	Theory, criteria, and drawbacks, if any	Reference
Ranges in the descriptor space approach	Fixed or probabilistic boundaries/ bounding box	*Theory*: The ranges of the each descriptor are considered with a uniform distribution defining an *n*-dimensional hyper-rectangle developed on the basis of the highest and lowest values of individual descriptors employed to construct the model with sides parallel to the coordinate axes. $$d(x, y) = x - y$$ *Criteria*: The boundary is generated based on the highest and lowest values of *X* variables (descriptors to develop the model) and *Y* variable (response for which the QSAR equation is formed) of the training set. Any test set compounds that are not present in any of these particular ranges are considered outside the AD, and their predictions are less reliable. *Drawbacks*: (a) Due to nonuniform distribution, the method encloses substantial empty space; (b) empty regions in the interpolation space cannot be predictable, as only the descriptor ranges are considered; (c) correlation between descriptors cannot be taken into account.	[33]
	PC ranges/PCA bounding box	*Theory*: Principal components convert the original data into a new orthogonal coordinate system by the rotation of axes and facilitate to correct for correlations among descriptors. Newly formed axes are defined as PCs presenting the maximum variance of the total compounds. The points between the lowest value and the highest value of each PC define an *n*-dimensional (*n* is the number of significant components) hyper-rectangle with sides parallel to the PCs. *Criteria*: This hyper-rectangle AD also includes empty spaces depending on uniformity of data distribution. Combining the bounding box method with PCA can overcome the setback of	[33,34]

		correlation between descriptors, but the issue of empty regions within the interpolation space remains. It is interesting to point out that the empty space is smaller than the hyper-rectangle in the original descriptor ranges.	
	TOPKAT optimal prediction space	*Theory*: A variation of PCA is implemented by the optimum prediction space (OPS) from TOPKAT OPS 2000. In the PCA approach, instead of the standardized mean value, the data is centered around the mean of individual parameter range ($[x_{max}-x_{min}]/2$). Thus, it establishes a new orthogonal coordinate system which is known as OPS coordinate system. Here, the basic process is the same, extracting eigenvalues and eigenvectors from the covariance matrix of the transformed data. The OPS boundary is defined by the minimum and maximum values of the generated data points on each axis of the OPS coordinate system. *Criteria*: The property sensitive object similarity (PSS) is implemented in the TOPKAT as a heuristic solution to replicate the the data set's dense and spare regions, and it includes the response variable (y). Accuracy of prediction between the training set and queried points is assessed by the PSS. Similarity, a search method is used to evaluate the performance of TOPKAT in predicting the effects of a chemical that is structurally similar to the training structure.	[35]
Geometrical methods	Convex hull	*Theory*: This estimates the direct coverage of an n-dimensional set employing convex hull calculation, which is performed based on complex but efficient algorithms. The approach recognizes the boundary of the data set considering the degree of data distribution. *Criterion*: Interpolation space is defined by the smallest convex area containing the entire training set. *Drawbacks*: (a) Implementing a convex hull can be challenging, as an increase in dimensions contributes to the order of complexity.	[33,36]

(*Continued*)

Table 7.1 (Continued)

Types	Subtypes	Theory, criteria, and drawbacks, if any	Reference
		Convex hull calculation is efficient for two and three dimensions. The complexity swiftly amplifies in higher dimensions. For n points and d dimensions, the complexity is of order O, which can be defined as $O = [n^{[d/2]+1}]$. (b) The approach only analyzes the set boundaries without considering the actual data distribution. (c) It cannot identify the potential internal empty regions within the interpolation space.	
Distance-based methods (based on the distance-to-centroid principle)	Leverage approach	*Theory*: The leverage (h) of a compound in the original variable space is calculated based on the HAT matrix as $$H = (X^T(X^TX)^{-1}X)$$ where H is an $[n \times n]$ matrix that orthogonally projects vectors into the space spanned by the columns of X. The AD of the model is defined as a squared area within the ± 3 band for standardized cross-validated residuals (σ), and the leverage threshold is defined as $h^* = 3(p+1)/n$, where p is the number of variables and n is the number of compounds. The leverage values (h) are calculated (in the X-axis) for each compound and plotted versus cross-validated standardized residuals (σ) (in the Y-axis), referred to as the *Williams plot*. The leverage approach assumes normal data distribution. It is interesting to point out that when high leverage points fit the model well (having small residuals), they are called *good high leverage points* or *good influence points*. Those points stabilize the model and make it more accurate. On the contrary, high leverage points, which do not fit the model (having large residuals), are called *bad high leverage points* or *bad influence points*. *Criteria*: The Williams plot confirms the presence of response outliers (when the compound bears a standardized cross-validated residual	[30,37]

		value greater than $\pm 3\sigma$ units, but it lies within the critical HAT [h^*]) and training set chemicals that are structurally very influential (higher leverage value than h^*, but lie within the fixed $\pm 3\sigma$ limit of the ordinate) in determining model parameters. It is interesting to point out that although the chemical is influential one for the model, it is not a response outlier (not a *Y*outlier). The data predicted for high leverage chemicals in the prediction set are extrapolated and could be less reliable.	
	Euclidean distance	*Theory*: This approach calculates the distance from every other point to a particular point in the data set. A distance score, d_{ij}, for two different compounds X_i and X_j can be measured by the Euclidean distance norm. The Euclidean distance can be expressed by the following equation: $$d_{ij} = \sqrt{\sum_{k=1}^{m} (x_{ik} - x_{jk})^2}$$ The mean distances of one sample to the residual ones are calculated as follows: $$\overline{d}_i = \sum_{j=1}^{n} d_{ij}/n - 1,$$ where $i = 1,2,\ldots,n$. The mean distances are then normalized within the interval of zero to 1. It is applicable only for statistically independent descriptors. *Criteria*: Compounds with distance values adequately higher than those of the most active probes are considered to be outside the domain of applicability. The mean normalized distances are measured for both training and test set compounds. The boundary region created by normalized mean distance scores of the training set are considered as the AD zone for test set compounds. If the	[38]

(*Continued*)

Table 7.1 (Continued)

Types	Subtypes	Theory, criteria, and drawbacks, if any	Reference
		test set compounds are inside the domain, then these compounds are inside the AD; otherwise, they are not.	
	Mahalanobis distance	*Theory*: The approach considers the distance of an observation from the mean values of the independent variables, but not the impact on the predicted value. It offers one of the distinctive and simple approaches for identification of outliers. The approach is unique because it automatically takes into account the correlation between descriptor axes. *Criterion*: Observations with values much greater than those of the remaining ones may be considered to be outside the domain.	[39]
	City block distance	City block distance is the summed difference across dimensions and is computed employing the following equation: $$d(x, y) = \sum_{i=1}^{n} \lvert x_i - y_i \rvert$$ It examines the complete differences between coordinates of a pair of objects (x_i and y_i) and it assumes a triangular distribution. The method is predominantly useful for the distinct type of descriptors. It is used only for training sets that are uniformly distributed with respect to count-based descriptors.	[38]
	Hotelling T^2 test	*Theory*: The Hotelling T^2 method is a multivariate student's t test and proportional to leverage and Mahalanobis distance approach. It presumes a normal data distribution like the leverage approach. The method is used to evaluate the statistical impact of the difference on the means of two or more variables between two groups. Hotelling T^2 corrects for collinear descriptors through the use of the covariance matrix. Hotelling T^2 measures the distance of an observation from the center of a set of X observations. A tolerance volume is derived for Hotelling T^2.	[39]

		Criterion: Based on the *t* value, the significant compounds within the domain are determined.	
	k-nearest neighbors approach	*Theory*: The approach is based on a similarity search for a new chemical entity with respect to the space shaped by the training set compounds. The similarity is identified by finding the distance of a query chemical from the nearest training compound or its distances from *k*-nearest neighbors in the training set. Thus, similarity to the training set molecules is significant for this approach in order to associate a query chemical with reliable prediction. *Criterion*: If the calculated distance values of test set compounds are within the user-defined threshold set by the training set molecules, then the prediction of these compounds are considered to be reliable.	[40]
	DModX (distance to the model in X-space)	*Theory*: This approach is usually applied for the partial least squares (PLS) models. The basic theory lies in the residuals of *Y* and *X*, which are of diagnostic value for the quality of the model. As there are a number of *X*-residuals, one needs a summary for each observation. This is accomplished by the residual standard deviation (SD) of the *X*-residuals of the corresponding row of the residual matrix *E*. As this SD is proportional to the distance between the data point and the model plane in *X*-space, it is usually called DModX (distance to the model in *X*-space). Here, *X* is the matrix of predictor variables, of size (N^*K); *Y* is the matrix of response variables, of size (N^*M); *E* is the (N^*K) matrix of *X*-residuals; *N* is number of objects (cases, observations); *k* is the index of *X*-variables ($k = 1, 2, \ldots, K$); and *m* is the index of *Y*-variables ($m = 1, 2, \ldots, M$). *Criteria*: A DModX value larger than around 2.5 times the overall SD of the *X* residuals (corresponding to an *F*-value of 6.25) signifies	[9,41]

(*Continued*)

Table 7.1 (Continued)

Types	Subtypes	Theory, criteria, and drawbacks, if any	Reference
		that the observation is outside the AD of the model. In the DModX plot, the threshold line is attributed as a D-critical line, and this plot can be drawn in SIMCA-P software.	
	Tanimoto similarity	The Tanimoto index measures similarity between two compounds based on the number of common molecular fragments. In order to calculate the Tanimoto similarity, all single fragments of a particular length in two compounds are computed. The Tanimoto similarity between the compounds J and I is defined as $$\text{TANIMOTO}\ (J,K) = \frac{\sum_{i=1}^{N}(x_{J,i}\cdot x_{K,i})}{\sum_{i=1}^{N}(x_{J,i}\cdot x_{J,i}) + \sum_{i=1}^{N}(x_{K,i}.x_{K,i}) - \sum_{i=1}^{N}(x_{J,i}.x_{K,i})}$$ where N is the number of unique fragments in both the compounds, $x_{J,i}$ and $x_{K,i}$ are the counts of the ith fragment in the compounds J and K. Based on this equation, the distance between two compounds J and K is $1-$ TANIMOTO(J, K), and the distance of a compound to the model is the least distance between the query compound and compounds from the training set.	[42]
	Standard deviation of the ensemble predictions (STD)	The method depicts that if dissimilar models give appreciably different predictions for a particular molecule, then the prediction is more likely to be erratic. The sample standard deviation is preferably employed as an estimator of model uncertainty. The method has been confirmed to offer stupendous results for discrimination of highly accurate predictions for regression models. For example, consider that $Y(J) = \{y_i(J),\ i = 1, \ldots, N\}$ is a set of predictions for a compound J given by a set of N trained models,	[42,43]

		the corresponding distance to model STD can be defined by the following equation: $$d_{STD}(J) = \mathrm{stdev}(Y(J)) = \sqrt{\frac{\sum (y_i(J) - \bar{y})^2}{N-1}}$$ The STD approach can be classified into numerous subtypes considering the type of an ensemble used to evaluate the standard deviation. (a) Consensus STD (CONS-STD) for models developed based on different machine-learning techniques. (b) Associative neural networks (ASNN-STD) for an ensemble of neural network models. (c) BAGGING-STD for an ensemble of models formed utilizing the bagging technique.	
Probability density distribution	Parametric and nonparametric methods	*Theory*: Probability density distribution is one of the most advanced approaches for defining the AD, based on estimating the probability density function of the given data. The approach is categorized into two classes. The first is a parametric method that assumes a standard distribution, such as Gaussian and Poisson distributions; and the second is a nonparametric method that does not rely on such assumptions considering the data distribution. These methods are carried out by estimating the probability density of the compounds, followed by identifying the highest-density region that consists of a known fraction from the total probability mass. A potential is formed for each compound in the training set such that it is uppermost for that molecule and decreases with increasing distance. Once the potential is evaluated for all the compounds, global potential is obtained by summing up the individual potentials, thus indicating the probability density. The method has the capability to identify the internal empty space.	[10,33,44]

(*Continued*)

Table 7.1 (Continued)

Types	Subtypes	Theory, criteria, and drawbacks, if any	Reference
		The actual data distribution can be revealed by generating concave regions around the interpolation space borders. *Criteria*: Here, a Gaussian function is verified. Given two compounds x_i and x_j, it can be determined as follows: $$\varphi = \frac{1}{\sqrt{(2\pi)}s}.\exp\left[\frac{-1}{(2s^2)(x_i - x_j)^2}\right]$$ where Φ (x_i and x_j) is the potential induced on x_j by x_i and the width of the curve is defined by smoothing parameter s. The cutoff value associated with Gaussian potential functions; namely, f_p can be calculated by methods based on a sample percentile: $$f_p = f_i + (q - j)(f_{j+1} - f_j)$$ with $q = p \times n/100$, where p is the percentile value of probability density, n is the number of compounds in the training set, and j is the nearest integer value of q. Test compounds with potential function values below the set threshold are considered outside the AD.	
Range of the response variable	N/A	Creating the distribution plot or scrutinizing the range of the response variable, query molecule can be identified as outside the AD generated by the training set of compounds. In a data set, if the response value of a particular test compound is significantly diverse from the mean response value of the training set compounds, then the compound can be considered as outside the AD.	–
Miscellaneous approaches	Stepwise-based approach	*Theory*: This method reflects mechanistic rationality and transparency of the QSAR model. This approach is practiced in four stages in a sequential manner. The first step, *general requirements domain*,	[45]

		consists of examining the variation of the physicochemical properties of the query compounds in the training set. The second stage, *structural domain*, signifies the structural similarity which is found within the chemicals that are appropriately predicted by the model. The third stage, *mechanistic domain*, takes into account of the mechanistic interpretation of the modeled phenomenon to define the domain of applicability. In the fourth and final stage, *domain of metabolic stimulator*, if stimulated metabolism of chemicals is a part of the developed QSAR model, then the dependability of simulated metabolism is considered in assessing the dependability of the predictions. *Criterion*: An external compound is obligatory to gratify all the conditions specified within the stated four steps to be considered within the AD. The approach is a painstaking one, as a chemical is examined for similarity and a metabolic and mechanistic check is performed to address the reliability of predictions and allow a superior assessment of the model's AD.	
	Decision trees and decision forests	This approach identifies the AD in terms of prediction confidence and domain extrapolation based on the consensus prediction of decision trees (DTs) and decision forests (DFs). The basic principle is to diminish overfitting, which can be achieved by merging the DTs and keeping the differences within various DTs to the maximum. Predictions from all the combined DTs are averaged in order to find the prediction confidence for a particular molecule, while domain extrapolation provides the prediction precision for that compound outside the training space.	[10,46]
	Kernel-based AD	Most machine learning approaches for QSAR greatly depend on a vectorial illustration of the molecules. Thus, the AD is expressed as a subspace of the vector space with one dimension for	[47]

(*Continued*)

Table 7.1 (Continued)

Types	Subtypes	Theory, criteria, and drawbacks, if any	Reference
		individual descriptor used. However, this vectorial concept cannot be straightforwardly applied to kernel-based techniques like support vector machines. Thus, these methods have to rely on an inherent feature space that is only defined by the applied kernel similarity and with unknown dimensions. Therefore, the domain of applicability of a kernel-based model has to be defined by means of the kernel. This also permits the use of structured similarity measures like the optimal assignment kernel and its extension, instead of a numerical encoding.	
	Intelligent *k*-means clustering	An intelligent version of the *k*-means clustering algorithm-based measure of distance-to-domain for QSAR models has been designed to avert the difficulties of existing methods (like convex hull, and bounding box) in terms of primitiveness and computational complexity. This measure combines the modeling of the training set as a collection of the intelligent *k*-means clusters algorithm in the descriptor space with a new interpretation of a conventional optimization criterion in fuzzy clustering which leads to a modified harmonic mean measure. A test compound is assigned fuzzy membership of each individual cluster, from which an overall distance may be calculated.	[48]

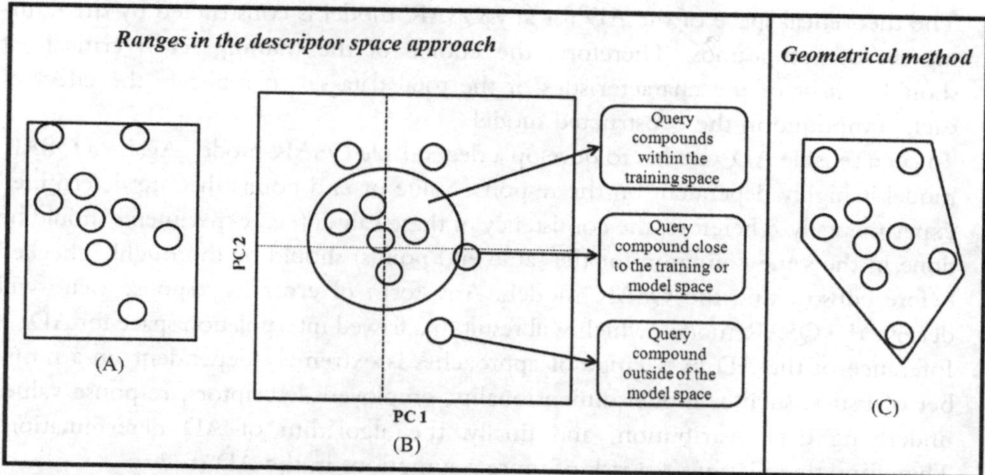

Figure 7.3 (A) Bounding box plot, (B) PCA bounding box plot, and (C) convex hull plot.

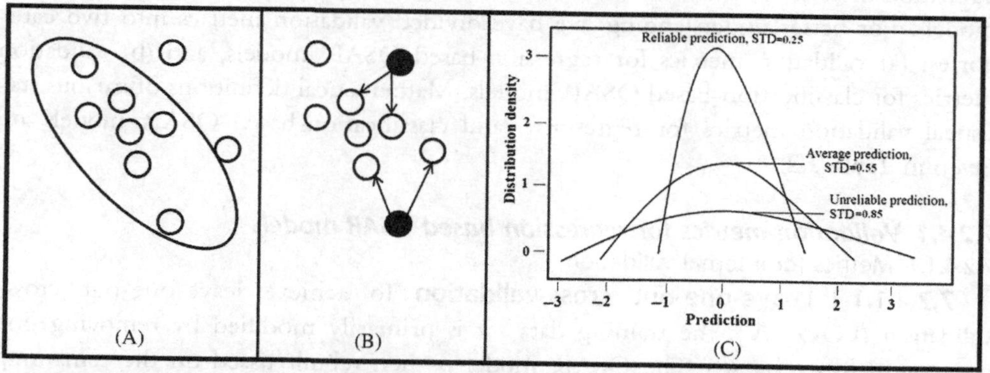

Figure 7.4 (A) Distance-to-centroid approach, (B) *k*—nearest neighbor plot, and (C) STD plot.

7.2.3.2.4 Checklist and importance of the AD study in validation

To make the QSAR model predictive and reproducible, these points should be followed:

a. The ultimate criterion of any QSAR model is its predictability for new sets of compounds. From this perspective, the QSAR fraternity has accepted the AD study as one of the compulsory validation criteria considering the reliability of the predictive capability of the QSAR model.

b. One has to solely depend on the AD of the QSAR model before estimating the activity/property/toxicity of any chemical or pharmaceutical employing the developed model.

c. The theoretical space of the AD for any QSAR model is constructed by the training set of compounds. Therefore, the choice of the training set is critical—it should consist of the characteristics of the total data set to replicate the effect of each compound in the constructed model.

d. To get a reliable AD, one has to develop a dependable QSAR model. Again, a QSAR model is highly dependent on the response value or end points that are determined experimentally. Therefore, the consistency of these values (i.e., experiments should be done in the same condition for the same end points) should be thoroughly checked before constructing the QSAR models. Any form of error in response value will deceive the QSAR model, which will result in a flawed interpolation space for AD.

e. Inference of the AD by a range of approaches is extremely dependent on a number of issues, such as model dimensionality, employed descriptors, response value, underlying data distribution, and finally, the algorithm of AD determination. Therefore, there is always a risk of more assumptions in the AD study.

7.2.4 Validation metrics

Validation metrics are the ultimate criteria to judge the quality of the validated QSAR models. For better understanding, we have divided validation metrics into two categories: (a) validation metrics for regression-based QSAR models, and (b) validation metrics for classification-based QSAR models. Mathematical definitions of various statistical validation metrics for regression- and classification-based QSAR models are given in Table 7.2.

7.2.4.1 Validation metrics for regression-based QSAR models

7.2.4.1.1 Metrics for internal validation

7.2.4.1.1.1 Leave-one-out cross-validation To achieve leave-one-out cross-validation (LOO-CV), the training data set is primarily modified by removing one compound from the set. The QSAR model is then rebuilt based on the remaining molecules of the training set using the descriptor combination originally selected, and the activity of the deleted compound is measured based on the resulting QSAR equation. This cycle is repeated until all the molecules of the training set have been deleted once, and the predicted activity data obtained for all the training set compounds are used for the calculation of various internal validation parameters. Finally, model predictivity is judged using the predicted residual sum of squares (*PRESS*) and cross-validated R^2 (Q^2) [49] for the model. *PRESS* is the sum of squared differences between experimental and LOO predicted data, and the value of standard deviation of error of prediction (*SDEP*) [50] is calculated from *PRESS*. Equations (7.1)–(7.3) give the expressions for *PRESS*, *SDEP*, and Q^2, respectively:

$$\text{PRESS} = \sum (Y_{\text{obs}} - Y_{\text{pred}})^2 \tag{7.1}$$

Table 7.2 Mathematical definition of various statistical validation metrics for the regression- and classification-based QSAR models

Type of metric	Metrics defining statistical quality of the regression-based models	Type of metric	Metrics defining statistical quality of the classification-based QSAR models
Goodness-of-fit and quality measures	$s=\sqrt{\frac{(Y_{obs}-Y_{calc})^2}{N-p-1}}$	*Goodness-of-fit and quality measures*	$\lambda=\det\left(\frac{W_g}{B_g+W_g}\right)$
	$R^2=1-\frac{\sum(Y_{obs}-Y_{calc})^2}{\sum(Y_{obs}-\overline{Y}_{training})^2}$		$R_c=\sqrt{\frac{\lambda_i}{1+\lambda_i}}$
	$R_a^2=\frac{\{(n-1)\times R^2\}-p}{n-p-1}$		$\chi^2=\sum_{i=1}^{t}\frac{(f_i-F_i)^2}{F_i}$
	$\text{RMSE}_c=\sqrt{\frac{\sum(Y_{obs(training)}-Y_{calc(training)})^2}{n_{training}}}$		$F=\frac{s_1^2/\sigma_1^2}{s_2^2/\sigma_2^2}$
	$\text{RMSE}_p=\sqrt{\frac{\sum(Y_{obs(test)}-Y_{pred(test)})^2}{n_{test}}}$		$d_{Mahalanobis}(x_i,x_j)=\sqrt{(x_i-x_j)^T\Sigma^{-1}(x_i-x_j)}$
	$\rho=\frac{n_{training}}{p}$		$\rho=\frac{n_{training}}{p}$
Internal parameters for robustness checking	$Q^2(Q^2_{Loo})=1-\frac{\sum(Y_{obs(training)}-Y_{pred(training)})^2}{\sum(Y_{obs(training)}-\overline{Y}_{training})^2}$	*Internal and external validation metrics*	$\text{Sensitivity}=\frac{TP}{TP+FN}$
	${}^cR_p^{22}=R_{nonrandom}\times\sqrt{(R^2_{nonrandom}-R^2_{random})}$		$\text{Specificity}=\frac{TN}{TN+FP}$
External predictivity parameters	$Q^2_{(F1)}=1-\frac{\sum(Y_{obs(test)}-Y_{pred(test)})^2}{\sum(Y_{obs(test)}-\overline{Y}_{training})^2}$		$\text{Accuracy}=\frac{TP+TN}{TP+FN+TN+FP}$
	$Q^2_{F2}=1-\frac{\sum(Y_{obs(test)}-Y_{pred(test)})^2}{\sum(Y_{obs(test)}-\overline{Y}_{test})^2}$		$\text{Precision}=\frac{TP}{TP+FP}$
	$Q^2_{(F3)}=1-\frac{\left[\sum(Y_{obs(test)}-Y_{pred(test)})^2\right]/n_{test}}{\left[\sum(Y_{obs(train)}-\overline{Y}_{train})^2\right]/n_{train}}$		$F-\text{measure}=\frac{2}{1/\text{Precision}+1/\text{Sensitivity}}$
	$\text{CCC}=\overline{\rho}_c=\frac{2\sum_{i=1}^{n}(x_i-\overline{x})(y_i-\overline{y})}{\sum_{i=1}^{n}(x_i-\overline{x})^2+\sum_{i=1}^{n}(y_i-\overline{y})^2+n(\overline{x}-\overline{y})}$		$\text{MCC}=\frac{(TP\times TN)-(FP\times FN)}{\sqrt{(TP+FP)\times(TP+FN)\times(TN+FP)\times(TN+FN)}}$

(Continued)

Table 7.2 (Continued)

Type of metric	Metrics defining statistical quality of the regression-based models	Type of metric	Metrics defining statistical quality of the classification-based QSAR models
	Golbraikh and Tropsha criteria: i. $Q^2_{training} > 0.5$. ii. $R^2_{test} > 0.6$. iii. $\frac{r^2 - r_0^2}{r^2} < 0.1$ and $0.85 \le k \le 1.15$ **or** $\frac{r^2 - r_0'2}{r^2} < 0.1$ and $0.85 \le k' \le 1.15$. iv. $\lvert r_0^2 - r_0'2 \rvert < 0.3$.		$\text{Cohen's } \kappa = \frac{P_r(a) - P_r(e)}{1 - P_r(e)}$ $P_r(a) = \frac{(\text{TP} + \text{TN})}{(\text{TP} + \text{FP} + \text{FN} + \text{TN})}$ $P_r(e) = \frac{\{(\text{TP} + \text{FP}) \times (\text{TP} + \text{FN})\} + \{(\text{TN} + \text{FP}) \times (\text{TN} + \text{FN})\}}{(\text{TP}+\text{FN}+\text{FP}+\text{TN})^2}$
r_m^2 *Rank metrics*	$r^2_{m(rank)} = r^2_{(rank)} \times \left(1 - \sqrt{r^2_{(rank)} - r^2_{0(rank)}}\right)$		$G - \text{means} = \sqrt{\text{Sensitivity} \times \text{Specificity}}$
Scaled r_m^2 *metrics for internal, external and overall predictivity*	r_m^2 *metric* $\overline{r}^2_m = (r^2_m + r'_m2)/2$ and $\Delta r^2_m = \lvert r^2_m - r'_m2 \rvert$, where $r^2_m = r^2 \times (1 - \sqrt{r^2 - r_0^2})$ $r'_m2 = r^2 \times (1 - \sqrt{(r^2 - r'_02)})$ The parameters r^2 and r_0^2 are defined as $r_0^2 = 1 - \frac{\sum (Y_{obs} - k \times Y_{pred})^2}{\sum (Y_{obs} - \overline{Y}_{obs})^2}$ and $r'_02 = 1 - \frac{\sum (Y_{pred} - k \times Y_{obs})^2}{\sum (Y_{pred} - \overline{Y}_{pred})^2}$	*Parameters for ROC analysis*	$\text{tp rate} \approx \frac{\text{Positives (active molecules) correctly classified}}{\text{Total postives}}$ $= \text{Sensitivity}$ $\text{fp rate} = \frac{\text{Negatives (inactive compounds) incorrectly classified}}{\text{Total negatives}}$ $= 1 - \text{specificity}$ $d_i = \sqrt{(1 - Se_r)^2 + (1 - Sp_r)^2}$ $\text{ROCED} = (\lvert d_{training} - d_{test} \rvert + 1) \times (d_{training} + d_{test}) \times (d_{test} + 1)$ $\text{FIT}(\lambda) = \frac{(1 - \lambda) \times (n - p - 1)}{(n + p^2) \times \lambda}$ $\text{ROCFIT} = \frac{\text{ROCED}}{\text{FIT}(\lambda)}$ $\text{AUC} - \text{ROC} = 1 - \frac{\sum_{i=1}^{n} r_i}{n \times (N - n)} + \frac{n + 1}{2 \times (N - n)}$

The terms k and k' are defined as $k = \frac{\sum (Y_{obs} \times Y_{pred})}{\sum (Y_{pred})^2}$ and $k' = \frac{\sum (Y_{obs} \times Y_{pred})}{\sum (Y_{obs})^2}$ The Y_{obs} and Y_{pred} values are scaled at the beginning using the following formula: $Y_{i(scaled)} = \frac{Y_i - Y_{min(obs)}}{Y_{max(obs)} - Y_{min(obs)}}$	*Metrics for PDD analysis*	$E_{active} = \frac{\% \text{ of actives}}{\% \text{ of inactives} + 100}$ $E_{inactive} = \frac{\% \text{ of inactives}}{\% \text{ of actives} + 100}$

Each notation is mentioned in the text.

$$\mathrm{SDEP} = \sqrt{\frac{\mathrm{PRESS}}{n}} \tag{7.2}$$

$$Q^2 = 1 - \frac{\sum (Y_{\mathrm{obs(train)}} - Y_{pred(train)})^2}{\sum (Y_{\mathrm{obs(train)}} - \overline{Y}_{\mathrm{training}})^2} = 1 - \frac{\mathrm{PRESS}}{\sum (Y_{\mathrm{obs(train)}} - \overline{Y}_{\mathrm{training}})^2} \tag{7.3}$$

In Eq. (7.1), Y_{obs} and Y_{pred} correspond to the observed and LOO predicted activity values, while in Eq. (7.2), n refers to the number of observations. In Eq. (7.3), $Y_{\mathrm{obs(train)}}$ is the observed activity, $Y_{\mathrm{pred(train)}}$ is the predicted activity of the training set molecules based on the LOO technique. A model is considered acceptable if the value of Q^2 exceeds the predetermined value of 0.5.

In spite of its wide acceptance, a high value of Q^2 alone is not enough of a criterion to evaluate the predictive potential of a QSAR model. Structural redundancy of the training set may be a reason for overestimation of the value of Q^2 [51]. The models developed using LOO-CV may undergo the problem of overfitting. Therefore, despite bearing a noteworthy correlation between the descriptors and response parameter, the developed model may fail to predict correctly the activity of new compounds. LOO-Q^2 can serve only as a basic (but not sufficient) criterion to judge the predictive ability of a model; external validation plays a prime role in detecting the ability of the model to predict the activity of a new set of molecules.

7.2.4.1.1.2 Leave-many-out cross-validation The basic principle of the leave-many-out (LMO) technique or leave-some-out (LSO) technique is that a definite portion of the training set is held out and eliminated in each cycle [52]. For each cycle, the model is constructed based on the remaining molecules (and using the originally selected descriptors), and then the activity of the deleted compounds is predicted using the developed model. Thus, after all the cycles have been completed, the predicted activity values of the compounds are used to calculate LMO-Q^2. Based on the predicted activity values of the deleted compounds in each of the cycles, the values of predictive R^2 (R^2_{pred}) may be calculated for each cycle. Thus, in light of internal validation, the LMO technique partially reflects a form of external validation. The fundamental steps for LOO and LMO cross-validation are presented in Figure 7.5.

7.2.4.1.1.3 True Q^2 The procedure of choice of the training- and test-set compounds from the total data set may be performed in a biased manner, although external validation is largely accepted as the ultimate validation tool by various research groups. Moreover, the splitting of a data set in this manner may result in loss of

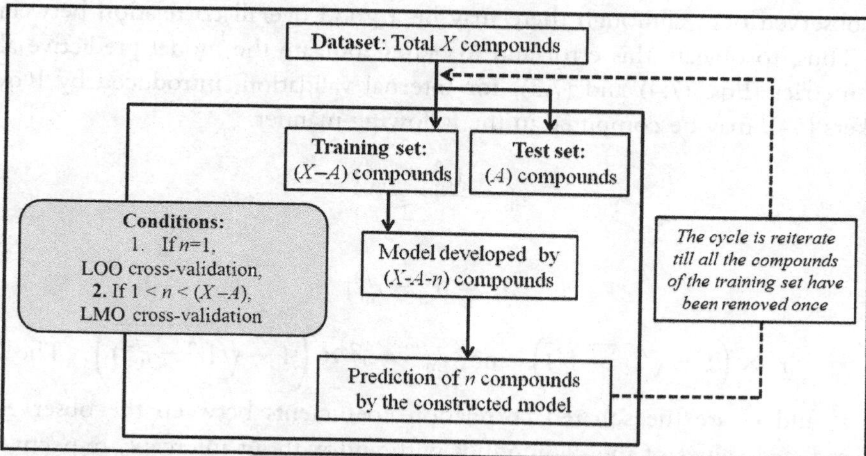

Figure 7.5 Key steps for the calculation of LOO and LMO cross-validation metrics.

valuable chemical information that otherwise could have been utilized for creating the QSAR model. According to Hawkins et al. [53], holding out a fraction of the data set is unnecessary in the case of a small data set. For external validation, the data set is to be divided into training and test sets, and such reduction of the training-set size may result in loss of information because of the small size of the data set. Again, in the case of cross-validation, the model is built using the entire data set and the division is done internally. If cross-validation is to attain the desired goal of providing a check of model fit, it is critical that each compound should be eliminated for prediction so that it is not used in any way in the model fitting applied to the remaining retained $n-1$ compounds. The activity of the deleted compound is then predicted using the equation developed for the remaining retained $n-1$ compounds. Therefore, Hawkins et al. [53] proposed the concept of "true Q^2" parameter, calculated based on the application of the variable selection strategy at each validation cycle. They showed that cross-validation employing all available compounds properly may be a better tool for assessing model predictivity, chiefly in the case of small data sets, compared to the traditional approach of the splitting of the data set into training and test sets [53].

7.2.4.1.1.4 The r_m^2 metric for internal validation The mean response value of the training set molecules and the distance of the mean from the response values of the individual molecules play a crucial role in determining the value of Q^2. As the value of the denominator $(\Sigma(Y_{obs(train)} - \overline{Y_{training}})^2)$ on the right side of Eq. (7.3) increases, the value of Q^2 also increases. Thus, even for large differences in the predicted and observed response values, acceptable Q^2 values may be obtained if the molecules exhibit a significantly wide range of response data. Hence, a large value of Q^2 does not necessarily indicate that the predicted activity data lie in close proximity to the observed ones, although there may be a good overall correlation between the values. Thus, to obviate this error and to better indicate the model predictive ability, the r_m^2 metrics (Eqs. (7.4) and (7.5)) for internal validation, introduced by Roy and coworkers [54], may be computed in the following manner:

$$\overline{r_m^2} = \frac{(r_m^2 + r_m'^2)}{2} \quad (7.4)$$

$$\Delta r_m^2 = |r_m^2 - r_m'^2| \quad (7.5)$$

where $r_m^2 = r^2 \times \left(1 - \sqrt{(r^2 - r_0^2)}\right)$ and $r_m'^2 = r^2 \times \left(1 - \sqrt{(r^2 - r_0'^2)}\right)$. The parameters r^2 and r_0^2 are the squared correlation coefficients between the observed and LOO predicted values of the compounds with and without intercept, respectively. In the initial studies, the observed values were considered in the *y*-axis, whereas predicted values were considered in the *x*-axis; and $r_0'^2$ bears the same meaning but uses the reversed axes. It is interesting to note that during the change of axes, the value of r^2 remains the same, while it changes in the case of r_0^2. When the observed values of the training set compounds (*y*-axis) are plotted against the estimated values of the compounds (*x*-axis), setting the intercept to zero, the slope of the fitted line gives the value of *k*. Interchange of the axes gives the value of *k′*. The following equations are employed for the calculation of r^2, r_0^2, *k*, and *k′*:

$$r_0^2 = 1 - \frac{\sum (Y_{obs} - k \times Y_{pred})^2}{\sum (Y_{obs} - \overline{Y_{obs}})^2} \quad (7.6)$$

$$r_0'^2 = 1 - \frac{\sum (Y_{pred} - k' \times Y_{obs})^2}{\sum (Y_{pred} - \overline{Y_{pred}})^2} \quad (7.7)$$

$$k = \frac{\sum (Y_{obs} \times Y_{pred})}{\sum (Y_{pred})^2} \quad (7.8)$$

$$k' = \frac{\sum (Y_{obs} \times Y_{pred})}{\sum (Y_{obs})^2} \quad (7.9)$$

Here, $\overline{r_m^2}$ is the average value of r_m^2 and $r_m'^2$, and Δr_m^2 is the absolute difference between r_m^2 and $r_m'^2$. In general, the difference between r_m^2 and $r_m'^2$ values of the training set should be low for good models. The $\overline{r_{m(LOO)}^2}$ and $\Delta r_{m(LOO)}^2$ parameters can be used for the internal validation of the training set, and it has been shown that the value of $\Delta r_{m(LOO)}^2$ should be less than 0.2, provided that the value of $\overline{r_{m(LOO)}^2}$ is more than 0.5.

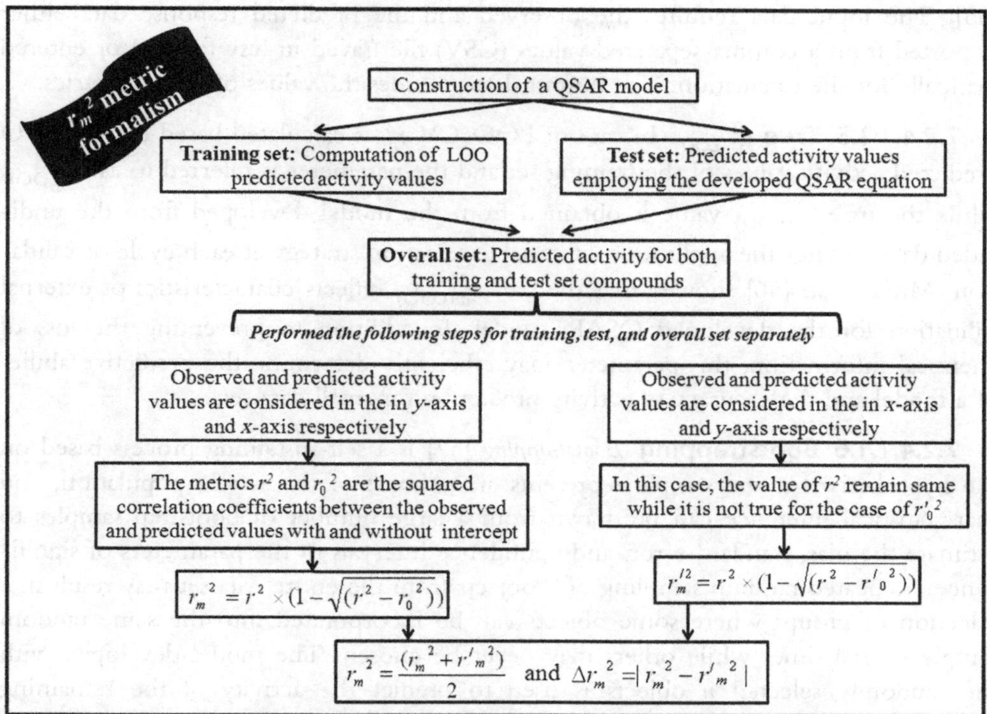

Figure 7.6 Fundamental steps for the calculation of r_{m}^2 metrics.

In Figure 7.6, we have tried to demonstrate the major steps for the calculation of r_{m}^2 metrics.

Roy et al. [55] proposed that the calculation of the r_{m}^2 metrics should be based on the scaled values of the observed and the predicted response data to obviate any form of discrepancy based on the unit of measurement of the same response data. Scaling is done based on the maximum and the minimum experimental (observed) values of the response parameter as follows:

$$\text{Scaled } Y_i = \frac{Y_i - Y_{\mathrm{min(obs)}}}{Y_{\mathrm{max(obs)}} - Y_{\mathrm{min(obs)}}} \tag{7.10}$$

where Y_i refers to the observed/predicted response for the ith (1, 2, 3, ..., n) compound in the training/test set. In addition, $Y_{\mathrm{max(obs)}}$ and $Y_{\mathrm{min(obs)}}$ indicate the maximum and minimum values, respectively, for the observed response in the training set compounds.

A web application known as the r_{m}^2 *calculator* (http://aptsoftware.co.in/rmsquare) has been developed for easy calculation of all variants of the r_{m}^2 metrics by Roy et al.

[55]. The input data requires the observed and the predicted response data either imported from a comma-separated values (CSV) file (saved in .csv format) or entered manually for the calculation. The output data provides the values of the r^2_m metrics.

7.2.4.1.1.5 True $r^2_{m(LOO)}$ In case of LOO-CV, r^2_m is calculated based on the LOO predicted activity values of the training set and the parameter is referred to as $r^2_{m(LOO)}$, while the true $r^2_{m(LOO)}$ value is obtained from the model developed from the undivided data set after the application of variable selection strategy at each cycle of validation. Mitra et al. [56] showed that the true $r^2_{m(LOO)}$ reflects characteristics of external validation for the developed QSAR model. In addition to preventing the loss of chemical information, this parameter may efficiently determine the predictive ability of a model and the accuracy of activity prediction for small data sets.

7.2.4.1.1.6 Bootstrapping *Bootstrapping* [57] is a self-sustaining process based on the hypothesis that the sample represents an estimate of the whole population, and that statistical inference can be drawn from a large number of bootstrap samples to estimate the bias, standard error, and confidence intervals of the parameters of significance. Repeated random sampling of n objects from the entire data set may result in a selection of groups where some objects can be incorporated into the same random sample several times while others may never be chosen. The model developed with the randomly selected n objects is used to predict the activity of the remaining excluded compounds and the average Q^2 value is calculated. A high value of bootstrapped Q^2 reflects statistical significance of the developed QSAR model [58]. A basic difference between cross-validation and bootstrapping is that in the case of bootstrapping, random resampling of the available data is done with replacement, whereas in the case of cross-validation, sampling is done without replacement.

7.2.4.1.1.7 Metrics for chance correlation: *Y*-randomization *Y*-randomization is performed in order to ensure the robustness of the developed QSAR model. In *Y*-randomization, validation is performed by permuting the response values (Y) with respect to the X matrix, which has been kept unaltered. This method is generally performed in two different ways: (a) process randomization and (b) model randomization performed at varying confidence levels. In process randomization, the values of the dependent variable are randomly scrambled, and the choice of descriptors is done again from the total pool of the descriptor matrix. In contrast, for model randomization, the Y column data points are scrambled and new QSAR models are developed employing the already selected set of variables present in the nonrandom model.

The degree of variation in the values of the squared mean correlation coefficient of the randomized model (R^2_r) and squared correlation coefficient of the nonrandom model (R^2) is reflected in the value of the ${}^cR_p{}^2$[59] parameter. This metric penalizes the model R^2 for a small difference between the values of the squared correlation coefficients of the nonrandom (R^2) and the randomized (R_r^2) models, as per Eq. (7.11):

$$^cR_p^2 = R \times \sqrt{R^2 - R_r^2} \tag{7.11}$$

The threshold value of $^cR_p^2$ is 0.5, and the fact that a QSAR model has the corresponding value above the stated limit might be considered to indicate that the model is not obtained by chance.

7.2.4.1.2 Metrics for external validation

7.2.4.1.2.1 Predictive R^2 (R^2_{pred}) External validation of a QSAR model begins by splitting the data set into training and test sets. Then the QSAR models are constructed using the training set molecules and the activity of the test set molecules is predicted based on the developed model. Thus, the value of R^2_{pred} [32] reflects the degree of correlation between the observed and predicted activity data:

$$R^2_{pred} = 1 - \frac{\sum (Y_{obs(test)} - Y_{pred(test)})^2}{\sum (Y_{obs(test)} - \overline{Y}_{training})^2} \tag{7.12}$$

In Eq. (7.12), $Y_{obs(test)}$ and $Y_{pred(test)}$ are the observed and predicted activity data for the test set compounds, while $\overline{Y}_{training}$ indicates the mean observed activity of the training set molecules. Thus, models with values of R^2_{pred} above the stipulated value of 0.5 are considered to be well predictive.

7.2.4.1.2.2 Validation based on Golbraikh and Tropsha's criteria Golbraikh and Tropsha [32] proposed several parameters for determining the external predictability of the QSAR model. An acceptable QSAR model should be close to ideal in order to exert high predictive ability. For an ideal model, the value of correlation coefficient (R) between the observed (y) and predicted (y') activities should be close to 1. According to Golbraikh and Tropsha [32], regressions of y against y' or y' against y through the origin should be characterized by either k or k' (slopes of the corresponding regression lines) being close to 1. Subsequently, the regression lines through the origin are defined by $y^{r_0} = ky'$ and $y'^{r_0} = k'y$, while the slopes k and k' are given by Eqs. (7.13) and (7.14), respectively:

$$k = \frac{\sum y_i y_i'}{\sum y_i'^2} \tag{7.13}$$

$$k' = \frac{\sum y_i y_i'}{\sum y_i^2} \tag{7.14}$$

A more strict condition for the QSAR model to have high predictive ability was further proposed by Golbraikh and Tropsha [32]. They showed that either of the squared correlation coefficients of these two regression lines (y against $y^{/}$ or $y^{/}$ against y through the origin) r_0^2 or $r_0^{/2}$ (given by Eqs. (7.15) and (7.16), respectively) should be close to the value of r^2 for the developed model. The values of r^2 and r_0^2 indicate the squared correlation coefficients between the observed and the predicted activity values with and without intercept, respectively, while $r_0^{/2}$ represents the same information as r_0^2 does, but with inverted axes:

$$r_0^2 = 1 - \frac{\sum (y_i^{/} - y_i^{r_0})^2}{\sum (y_i^{/} - \overline{y^{/}})^2} \qquad (7.15)$$

$$r_0^{/2} = 1 - \frac{\sum (y_i - y_i^{/r_0})^2}{\sum (y_i - \overline{y})^2} \qquad (7.16)$$

where $\overline{y}^{/}$ and $\overline{y}$ refer to the mean values of the predicted and observed activity data, respectively. Thus, according to Golbraikh and Tropsha [32], models are considered satisfactory if all of the following conditions are satisfied:

i. $Q^2_{\text{training}} > 0.5$
ii. $R^2_{\text{test}} > 0.6$
iii. $r^2 - r_0^2/r^2 < 0.1$ and $0.85 \le k \le 1.15$ or $r^2 - r_0'2/r^2 < 0.1$ and $0.85 \le k' \le 1.15$
iv. $|r_0^2 - r_0'2| < 0.3$.

7.2.4.1.2.3 The $r^2_{m(test)}$ metric for external validation Like Q^2, the value of R^2_{pred} relies on the mean activity value of the training set compounds. Hence, a high R^2_{pred} value may be obtained when the test set compounds possess a wide range of activity data; but this may not indicate that the predicted activity values are very close to the corresponding observed values. In order to verify the propinquity between the observed and predicted data, the parameter $r^2_{m(test)}$ [54], similar to $r^2_{m(LOO)}$ used in internal validation, was developed by Roy et al. [54]. The value of $r^2_{m(test)}$ is calculated using the squared correlation coefficients between the observed and predicted activity of the test set compounds. For an acceptable prediction, the value of $\Delta r^2_{m(test)}$ should be less than 0.2, provided that the value of $\overline{r^2_{m(test)}}$ is more than 0.5.

It is even more interesting to note that Roy and coworkers [54] established that this tool can be extended to the entire data set employing the LOO predicted activity for the training set and predicted activity for the test set compounds. These parameters have been referred to as $\overline{r^2_{m(overall)}}$ and $\Delta r^2_{m(overall)}$, which reflect the predictive ability of the model for the entire data set. The advantages of such a consideration include

i. Unlike external validation parameters, the $r^2_{m(overall)}$ metric involves both training- and test-set compounds, and thus the statistic is based on the predictions of a comparably hefty number of compounds, which provides greater reliability to the model.

ii. In many cases, comparable models are obtained, where some models may show greater reliability in terms of the internal validation parameters while others may exhibit superior values of external validation parameters. In such cases, selection of the best model becomes a difficult task.

Since $r^2_{\mathrm{m(overall)}}$ and $\Delta r^2_{\mathrm{m(overall)}}$ are based on the entire data set, the values of these parameters facilitate the selection of the best model based on an overall contribution of both internal and external validation measures.

7.2.4.1.2.4 RMSEP The external predictive ability of a QSAR model may further be determined by a comparison of the observed activity values and the model predictions of the test set molecules through calculation of a parameter referred to as *root mean square error of prediction (RMSEP)* [60] given by Eq. (7.17):

$$\mathrm{RMSEP} = \sqrt{\frac{\sum (y_{\mathrm{obs(test)}} - y_{\mathrm{pred(test)}})^2}{n_{\mathrm{ext}}}} \quad (7.17)$$

where n_{ext} refers to the number of test set compounds. The parameter depends solely on the deviations between the predicted and observed activity values and can also be calculated when there is only one test compound.

7.2.4.1.2.5 $Q^2_{(F2)}$ Another expression for the calculation of external Q^2 (i.e., $Q^2_{(F2)}$) is based on the prediction of test-set compounds ($Q^2_{(F2)}$) proposed by Schuurmann et al. [61], as given by Eq. (7.18):

$$Q^2_{(F2)} = 1 - \frac{\sum (Y_{\mathrm{obs(test)}} - Y_{\mathrm{pred(test)}})^2}{\sum (Y_{\mathrm{obs(test)}} - \overline{Y}_{\mathrm{test}})^2} \quad (7.18)$$

where $\overline{Y}_{\mathrm{test}}$ refers to the mean observed data of the test set compounds and $Q^2_{(F2)}$ differs from $Q^2_{(F1)}$ in the mean value used in the denominator for calculation. When the two values approach each other, it can be inferred that the training set mean lies in close proximity to that of the test set, indicating that the test set used for prediction spans the whole response domain of the model. A threshold value 0.5 is defined for this parameter.

7.2.4.1.2.6 $Q^2_{(F3)}$ One more parameter, $Q^2_{(F3)}$ with a threshold value of 0.5, used for validation of a QSAR model, has been proposed by Consonni et al. [60]. This parameter is defined as follows:

$$Q^2_{(F3)} = 1 - \frac{\left[\sum (Y_{\mathrm{obs(test)}} - Y_{\mathrm{pred(test)}})^2\right] / n_{\mathrm{ext}}}{\left[\sum (Y_{\mathrm{obs(train)}} - \overline{Y}_{\mathrm{train}})^2\right] / n_{\mathrm{tr}}} \quad (7.19)$$

where n_{tr} refers to the number of compounds in the training set. Here, the summation in the numerator deals with the external test set, while that in the denominator runs over the training set compounds. Considering that the number of test and training objects are usually different, divisions by n_{ext} and n_{tr} make the two values comparable. However, although the value of $Q^2_{(F3)}$ measures the model predictability, it is sensitive to training-set data selection and tends to penalize models fitted to a very homogeneous data set, even if predictions are close to the truth. Since this function includes information about the training set, it cannot be properly regarded as an external validation measure even if predictions are really obtained for the external test set [60,61].

7.2.4.1.2.7 Concordance correlation coefficient The concordance correlation coefficient (CCC) parameter [62] can also be calculated to check the model reliability by using the following equation:

$$\overline{\rho}_c = \frac{2\sum_{i=1}^{n}(x_{obs(test)} - \overline{x_{obs(test)}})(y_{pred(test)} - \overline{y_{pred(test)}})}{\sum_{i=1}^{n}(x_{obs(test)} - \overline{x_{obs(test)}})^2 + \sum_{i=1}^{n}(y_{pred(test)} - \overline{y_{pred(test)}})^2 + n(\overline{x_{obs(test)}} - \overline{y_{pred(test)}})} \tag{7.20}$$

Here, $x_{obs(test)}$ and $y_{pred(test)}$ correspond to the observed and predicted values of the test compounds, n is the number of chemicals, and $\overline{x_{obs(test)}}$ and $\overline{y_{pred(test)}}$ correspond to the averages of the observed and predicted values of the test compounds, respectively. The CCC measures both precision and accuracy, detecting the distance of the observations from the fitting line and the degree of deviation of the regression line from that passing through the origin, respectively. Any deviation of the regression line from the concordance line (line passing through the origin) gives a value of CCC smaller than 1.

7.2.4.1.2.8 The $r^2_{m(rank)}$ metric In order to measure the closeness between the order of the predicted activity data and corresponding observed activity data, the $r^2_{m(rank)}$ parameter was developed [63]. The $r^2_{m(rank)}$ metric is calculated based on the correlation of the ranks obtained for the observed and predicted response data. In this case, the observed and predicted response data of the compounds are ranked, and the Pearson's correlation coefficients of the corresponding ranks are determined with intercept ($r^2_{(rank)}$) and without intercept ($r^2_{0(rank)}$). The values of $r^2_{(rank)}$ and $r^2_{0(rank)}$, thus calculated based on the rank order, are used to determine the value of the $r^2_{m(rank)}$ metric. The values of $r^2_{(rank)}$ and $r^2_{0(rank)}$ differ from each other based on the difference in ranking of the two variables. An ideal ranking, where the observed and the predicted response data perfectly match each other, yields zero difference between the two values for each molecule, and the $r^2_{m(rank)}$ metric attains a value of unity. An increase in difference between the two rank orders for different molecules is marked by a decrease in the value of this metric, with the proposed threshold value for acceptance being 0.5. The calculation of the new $r^2_{m(rank)}$ metric serves the prediction of rank orders of the molecules and determination of correlation for the ranks obtained for the test-set predicted activity data:

$$r^2_{m(rank)} = r^2_{(rank)} \times \left(1 - \sqrt{r^2_{(rank)} - r^2_{0(rank)}}\right) \tag{7.21}$$

There are various other metrics available for checking statistical quality and internal and external validation tests of QSAR models. The information on metrics for model instability analysis, metrics for descriptive power of a model, metrics for predictive power of a model, and metrics for global modeling power of a model are available elsewhere [64,65].

7.2.4.2 Validation metrics for classification-based QSAR models

Validation metrics can assess the performance of the classification-based models in terms of accurate qualitative prediction of the dependent variable [66]. The validation for classification model is usually executed for two-class problems, where the compounds are categorized either as actives (positives) or as inactives (negatives). Majorly applied metrics for classification-based QSAR models are demonstrated in the next sections.

7.2.4.2.1 Goodness-of-fit and quality measures

7.2.4.2.1.1 Wilks lambda (λ) statistics The Wilks lambda (λ) is a metric for testing the significance of discriminant model functioning. It is a distance-based parameter calculated from the scalar transformations of the covariance matrices of between- and within-group variances. In a classification analysis, the Wilks λ is determined as the ratio of the within-group sum of squares and total sum of squares; that is, within-category to total dispersion [67]:

$$\text{Wilks } \lambda = \frac{\text{Within group sum of squares}}{\text{Total sum of squares}} \tag{7.22}$$

Let us consider a scenario where B_g and W_g are the random $p \times p$ independent variable matrix with the distribution $W_p(q, \Sigma)$ and $W_p(n, \Sigma)$, respectively, assuming that $n > p$. Then the Wilks λ will be given by Eq. (7.23):

$$\lambda = \det\left(\frac{B_g}{B_g + W_g}\right) \tag{7.23}$$

where det signifies the determinant of the generated matrix that employs descriptors. The Wilks λ focuses on the best discriminating property of the analyzed independent variables, and it spans from 0 to 1, where 0 corresponds to different values of group means signifying a good level of discrimination achieved by the variables and 1 refers to similar group mean values meaning that no discrimination achieved by the variables. Hence, the value of Wilks λ for a good discriminant model should preferably be less.

7.2.4.2.1.2 Canonical index (R_c) The quantification of the strength of the relationship between the two variates (dependent and independent variables) is articulated as a canonical correlation coefficient [68]:

$$R_c = \sqrt{\frac{\lambda_i}{1 + \lambda_i}} \tag{7.24}$$

Here, λ_i is referred to as the *eigenvalue* of the matrix.

7.2.4.2.1.3 Chi-square (χ^2) The quality of classification-based QSAR models has also been judged using the chi-square (χ^2) statistics that perceives the independence between two groups or classes signifying that higher values of this metric will indicate superior separability between groups; that is, good classification analysis [69]:

$$\chi^2 = \sum_{i=1}^{t} \frac{(f_i - F_i)^2}{F_i} \tag{7.25}$$

where f_i is observed response, F_i is predicted response, and t is the number of observations.

7.2.4.2.1.4 Squared Mahalanobis distance The squared Mahalanobis distance is calculated during linear discriminant analysis (LDA) for the determination of probability of a compound to be classified in a definite group in the discriminant space. In a referred discrimination space, Euclidean distances among data points become equal to Mahalanobis distances. In a multivariate normal distribution with covariance matrix Σ, the Mahalanobis distance between any two data points x_i and x_j can be defined as [67]

$$d_{\text{Mahalanobis}}(x_i, x_j) = \sqrt{(x_i - x_j)^{\text{T}} \sum^{-1} (x_i - x_j)} \tag{7.26}$$

where x_i and x_j are two random data points, T is the transpose of a matrix, and Σ^{-1} is the inverse of the covariance matrix.

7.2.4.2.2 Metrics for model performance parameters

7.2.4.2.2.1 Sensitivity, specificity, and accuracy The compounds classified employing the classification-based QSAR model can be divided into four categories based on a comparison between the predicted and observed activity values: (i) true positives (TPs), the active (positive) compounds that have been correctly predicted as actives based on the developed QSAR models; (ii) false positives (FPs), which include the inactive compounds that have been erroneously classified as actives; (iii) false negatives (FNs), which comprise the active compounds wrongly classified as negatives (i.e.,inactives); and (iv) true negatives (TNs), which account for the inactive compounds that have been accurately predicted as inactives by the QSAR models under validation [70]. Based on this classification and the number of test-set molecules, a two-by-two confusion matrix [71], also referred to as the *contingency table (confusion matrix)*, may be constructed that corresponds to the dispositions of the molecules under consideration. This is a matrix with two rows and two columns that reports the number of compounds belonging to each of the four classes. To evaluate the classifier model performance and classification capability, a number of statistical tests have been employed by several researchers:

$$\text{Sensitivity} = \text{Recall} = \frac{\text{TP}}{\text{TP} + \text{FN}} \tag{7.27}$$

$$\text{Specificity} = \frac{\text{TN}}{\text{TN} + \text{FP}} \tag{7.28}$$

$$\text{Accuracy} = \frac{\text{TP} + \text{TN}}{\text{TP} + \text{FP} + \text{TN} + \text{FN}} \tag{7.29}$$

7.2.4.2.2.2 *F*-measure and precision The *F*-measure (Eq. (7.30)) may also be computed, which refers to the harmonic mean of recall (Eq. (7.27)) and precision (Eq. (7.31)), where *recall* refers to the accuracy of real prediction and *precision* defines the accuracy of a predicted class. Higher values of recall and precision are associated with higher *F*-measure values, which in turn find a better classification capability of the model.

$$F\text{-measure} = \frac{2(\text{Recall})(\text{Precision})}{\text{Recall} + \text{Precision}} \tag{7.30}$$

$$\text{Precision} = \frac{\text{TP}}{\text{TP} + \text{FP}} = \text{fp rate} \tag{7.31}$$

7.2.4.2.2.3 G-means Merging sensitivity and specificity into a single parameter via the geometric mean (G-means) allows a straightforward way to assess the model's ability to perfectly classify active and inactive samples using the following formula [72]:

$$\text{G-means} = \sqrt{\text{Sensitivity} \times \text{Specificity}} \tag{7.32}$$

G-means measures the balanced performance of a learning algorithm between these two classes.

7.2.4.2.2.4 Cohen's κ Cohen's kappa (κ) can be utilized to determine the agreement between classification (predicted) models and known classifications [73]. It is defined as

$$\text{Cohen's } \kappa = \frac{P_r(a) - P_r(e)}{1 - P_r(e)} \quad (7.33)$$

$$P_r(a) = \frac{(\text{TP} + \text{TN})}{(\text{TP} + \text{FP} + \text{FN} + \text{TN})} \quad (7.34)$$

$$P_r(e) = \frac{\{(\text{TP} + \text{FP}) \times (\text{TP} + \text{FN})\} + \{(\text{TN} + \text{FP}) \times (\text{TN} + \text{FN})\}}{(\text{TP}+\text{FN}+\text{FP}+\text{TN})^2} \quad (7.35)$$

Here, $P_r(a)$ is the relative observed agreement between the predicted classification of the model and the known classification, and $P_r(e)$ is the hypothetical probability of chance agreement. The $P_r(a)$ and $P_r(e)$ values are calculated from the confusion matrix. Cohen's κ analysis returns values between −1 (no agreement) and 1 (complete agreement). The resultant Cohen's κ values between −1.0 and 0.4 indicate that the model is poor; values between 0.4 and 0.6 signify that the model is average; values between 0.6 and 0.8 imply that the model is acceptable; and values between 0.8 and 1.0 indicate that the model is highly predictive.

7.2.4.2.2.5 Matthews correlation coefficient The Matthews correlation coefficient (MCC) [74] is utilized as a measure of the quality of binary classifications. It considers true and false positives and negatives and is generally regarded as a balanced measure that can be used even if the classes have different sizes. The MCC is simply a correlation coefficient between the observed and predicted binary classifications, and it returns a value between −1 and 1. A coefficient of 1 indicates a perfect prediction, 0 an average random prediction, and −1 an inverse prediction.

The MCC can be calculated directly from the confusion matrix using the following formula:

$$\text{MCC} = \frac{\text{TP} \times \text{TN} - \text{FP} \times \text{FN}}{\sqrt{(\text{TP} + \text{FP})(\text{TP} + \text{FN})(\text{TN} + \text{FP})(\text{TN} + \text{FN})}} \quad (7.36)$$

In Eq. (7.36), TP is the number of true positives, TN the number of true negatives, FP the number of false positives, and FN the number of false negatives. If any of the four sums in the denominator is zero, the denominator can be arbitrarily set to 1; this results in a Matthews correlation coefficient of zero, which can be shown to be the correct limiting value. This metric in particular addresses the issue of improper explanation of a confusion matrix and the cases where the data set sizes are higher.

7.2.4.2.3 Parameters for receiver operating characteristics analysis

7.2.4.2.3.1 ROC curve The receiver operating characteristics (ROC) curve is a visual illustration of the success and error observed in a classification model. The curve is plotted taking the true positive rate (tp rate) on the *Y*-axis and false positive rate (fp rate) on the *X*-axis, and the characteristics of the curve provide easier recognition of the precision of prediction. Apart from classification problems, ROC curves have been a constructive measure in signal detection theory for determining the trade-off between hit rates and false alarm rates of classifiers [71]:

$$\text{tp rate} \approx \frac{\text{Positives (active molecules) correctly classified}}{\text{Total postives}} = \text{Sensitivity} \qquad (7.37)$$

$$\text{fp rate} = \frac{\text{Negatives (inactive compounds) incorrectly classified}}{\text{Total negatives}} = 1 - \text{specificity} \qquad (7.38)$$

The ROC curve is drawn by plotting the false positive rate and the true positive rate along the *X*- and *Y*-axes, respectively. It signifies the number of objects that the classifier identifies correctly, as well as the number wrongly identified. A sample picture of the ROC curve is presented in Figure 7.7. Most classifiers vary from

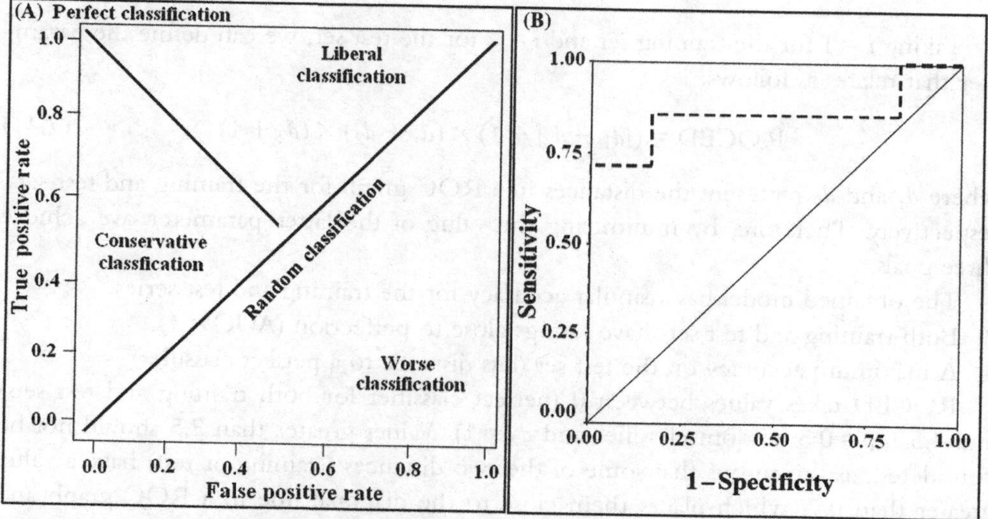

Figure 7.7 The ROC space (A) and a sample ROC curve (B).

"conservative" to "liberal." A perfect classification correctly classifies all positive cases and has no false positives. A conservative classification (lower-left region of the ROC space) requires strong evidence to classify a point as positive, while a liberal classification (upper-right region of the ROC space) does not require much evidence to classify an event as positive.

7.2.4.2.3.2 ROCED and ROCFIT Two metrics based on distances in a ROC curve for the selection of classification models with an correct balance in both training and test sets; namely, the ROC graph Euclidean distance (ROCED) and the ROC graph Euclidean distance corrected with fitness function (FIT(λ)) or Wilks λ (ROCFIT) are also used [75].

If the best model is one whose representation is positioned as close as possible to the upper-left corner in the ROC chart, a good indicator would be a measure of this distance. The Euclidean distance between the perfect and a real classifier (d_i), expressed as a function of their respective values of sensitivity and specificity, is

$$d_i = \sqrt{(Se_p - Se_r)^2 + (Sp_p - Sp_r)^2} \tag{7.39}$$

where Se_p and Se_r are the sensitivity values of the perfect and the real classifier, respectively; and Sp_p and Sp_r represent the specificity values of the perfect and real classifier, respectively. Since the sensitivity and specificity for a perfect classifier take values of 1, the Euclidean distance can be expressed as

$$d_i = \sqrt{(1 - Se_r)^2 + (1 - Sp_r)^2} \tag{7.40}$$

Taking $i = 1$ for the training set and $i = 2$ for the test set, we can define the parameter that relates as follows:

$$\text{ROCED} = (|d_1 - d_2| + 1) \times (d_1 + d_2) \times (d_2 + 1) \tag{7.41}$$

where d_1 and d_2 represent the distances in a ROC graph for the training and test sets, respectively. Therefore, by minimizing the value of the latter parameter, we achieve three goals:

1. The obtained model has a similar accuracy for the training and test series.
2. Both training and test sets have ratings close to perfection (AUC = 1).
3. A maximum accuracy on the test set (less distance to a perfect classifier).

ROCED takes values between 0 (perfect classifier for both training and test sets) and 4.5 ($d_1 = 0.5$ random classifier and $d_2 = 1$). Values greater than 2.5 should not be considered, as this means that some of the two distances (training or test) have a value greater than 0.7, which places them close to the diagonal line in a ROC graph and indicates that these models have random responses.

ROCFIT is defined as follows:

$$\text{ROCFIT} = \frac{\text{ROCED}}{\text{Wilks}(\lambda)} \tag{7.42}$$

7.2.4.2.3.3 AUC-ROC Area under curve-receiver operating characteristics (AUC-ROC) is equivalent to a simple average of the ranks of the actives; the good performance of *early recognitions* is offset quickly by *late recognitions* [76]. Let n be the number of actives and N be the total number of compounds; in that case, AUC-ROC is approximately normally distributed, with mean $\mu = 1/2 + 1/2(N - n)$ and variance $\sigma^2 = N + 1/12n(N - n)$. AUC-ROC, as defined in Eq. (7.43), is linearly related to the rank sum of actives, which is also called the *Mann–Whitney U test*.

$$\text{AUC-ROC} = 1 - \frac{\sum_{i=1}^{n} r_i}{n \times (N - n)} + \frac{n + 1}{2 \times (N - n)} \tag{7.43}$$

In this expression, r_i is the rank of the ith active.

7.2.4.2.4 Metrics for Pharmacological distribution diagram

Pharmacological distribution diagram (PDD) is a frequency distribution plot of a dependent variable where expectancy values of the variable is plotted in the Y-axis against numeric intervals of the variable in the X-axis. In a classification issue, *expectancy* refers to the probability of categorization of a compound in a specific group for a specific value of the discriminant function (DF). During the LDA, a DF is developed, which is a mathematical equation used to calculate discriminant scores of every individual compounds. Then the DF values of all compounds are taken in the abscissa in the form of range, and the expectancy values (probability of activity) are plotted in the ordinate against those ranges. Hence, this graph visually signifies the overlapping regions of the categories (e.g., positives and negatives), as well as the regions of DF values that possess maximal probability of finding actives and inactives [77]. For a classification case comprising of two classes like actives and inactives (or positives and negatives), two terms named *activity expectancy* and *inactivity expectancy* may be defined as shown here, where the denominator has a numerical value of 100 added to it to avoid division by zero [77]:

$$\text{Activity expectancy} = E_a = \frac{\text{Percentage of actives}}{(\text{Percentage of inactives} + 100)} \tag{7.44}$$

$$\text{Inactivity expectancy} = E_i = \frac{\text{Percentage of inactives}}{(\text{Percentage of actives} + 100)} \tag{7.45}$$

where the subscript a and i are the number of occurrences of active and inactive compounds at a specific range. It is obvious that for a perfect classification, the active

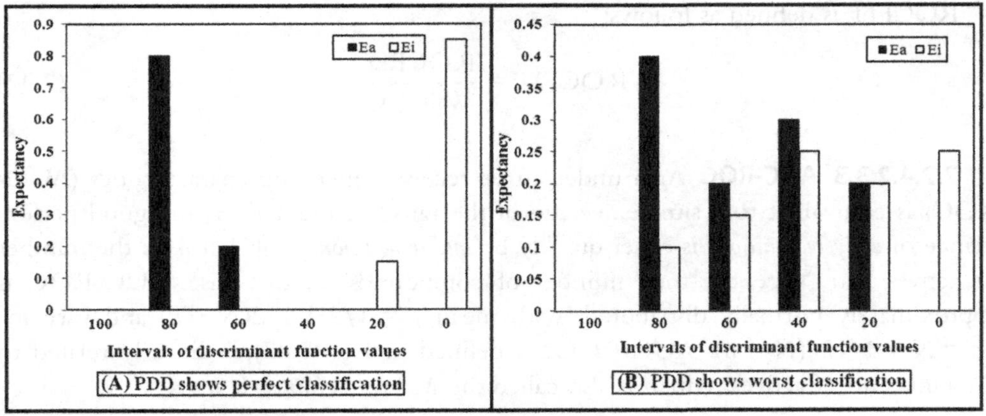

Figure 7.8 Sample PDDs showing perfect and worst classifications.

(positive) and inactive (negative) compounds will always be characterized by diverse ranges of DF values; hence, in an perfect discriminant study, the actives will always be alienated from the inactives, whereas overlapping them will correspond to errors in prediction (i.e., false positives and false negatives). A hypothetical picture of PDDs showing good and bad classifications is represented in Figure 7.8.

7.3 A PRACTICAL EXAMPLE OF THE CALCULATION OF COMMON VALIDATION METRICS AND THE AD

Chapter 6 described the 18 antimalarial cyclic peroxy ketals studied by Posner et al. [78] to develop a multiple linear regression (MLR) equation consisting of three descriptors. These descriptor values were taken from Roy et al. [79]. Here, the developed MLR equation was considered as the model equation for the further calculation of regression-based internal validation metrics. The test set was developed hypothetically to calculate different external validation metrics. In Table 7.3, we have demonstrated how one can easily calculate different metrics from an MLR-based QSAR model. Employing the same training and test sets, we have developed a classification-based QSAR model employing LDA. In Table 7.4, the methods of computation of different validation metrics for the classification-based QSAR model are demonstrated. A plot showing the method of calculation of the r^2, r_0^2, and $r_0^{\prime 2}$ for the mentioned test set is given in Figure 7.9.

In order to demonstrate how to determine the AD for the developed MLR-based QSAR model, we have illustrated simple AD approaches like leverage, Euclidean distance, fixed or probabilistic boundaries (bounding box), and range of the response variable approaches. All these methods can be used by any QSAR researchers without the use of any software.

Table 7.3 An example of computation of different internal and external validation metrics

General structure of cyclic peroxy ketals

					General structure of cyclic peroxy ketals					
Model equation (MLR)					$pIC_{50} = -2.192 + 0.174 \times MR + 0.651 \times \sigma - 0.192 \times Ind$					
Sl. No.	Substitution		Experimental value	Descriptors			Calculated/LOO predicted	$\sum(Y_{obs(train)} - Y_{calc(train)})2$	$\sum(Y_{obs(train)} - \overline{Y}_{training})^2$	$\sum(Y_{obs(train)} - Y_{LOO-pred(train)})2$
	R	*n*	pIC_{50} ($Y_{observed}$)	MR (*X1*)	σ (*X2*)	Ind (*X3*)	(Y_{calc}/Y_{LOO})			
Training set										
1	H	2	−2.279	0.103	0	0	−2.174/ − 2.409	0.011	0.049	0.017
2	H	3	−2.447	0.103	0	1	−2.366/ − 2.552	0.007	0.152	0.011
3	H	4	−2.342	0.103	0	0	−2.174/ − 2.551	0.028	0.081	0.044
4	CH_3O	1	−2.204	0.787	−0.27	0	−2.231/ − 2.172	0.001	0.022	0.001
5	CH_3O	3	−2.255	0.787	−0.27	1	−2.423/ − 2.016	0.028	0.039	0.057
6	CH_3O	4	−2.322	0.787	−0.27	0	−2.231/ − 2.432	0.008	0.070	0.012
7	CF_3O	4	−1.785	0.786	0.35	0	−1.827/ − 1.736	0.002	0.074	0.002
8	Cl	4	−1.763	0.603	0.23	0	−1.937/ − 1.565	0.030	0.086	0.039
9	F	4	−1.929	0.092	0.06	0	−2.137/ − 1.668	0.043	0.016	0.068
10	CH_3S	4	−1.892	1.382	0	0	−1.952/ − 1.813	0.004	0.027	0.006
11	CH_3SO_2	4	−1.491	1.349	0.72	0	−1.489/ − 1.495	0.000	0.320	0.000
12	CH_3CH_2	4	−2.255	1.03	−0.15	0	−2.110/ − 2.430	0.021	0.039	0.030
13	CH_3S	3	−2.204	1.382	0	1	−2.144/ − 2.295	0.004	0.022	0.008
14	CH_3SO_2	3	−1.748	1.349	0.72	1	−1.681/ − 1.846	0.005	0.095	0.010
15	NO_2	3	−1.663	0.736	0.78	1	−1.748/ − 1.545	0.007	0.155	0.014
16	Cl	3	−2	0.603	0.23	1	−2.129/ − 1.852	0.017	0.003	0.022
17	F	3	−2.301	0.092	0.06	1	−2.329/ − 2.265	0.001	0.060	0.001
18	CF_3	3	−2.146	0.502	0.54	1	−1.945/ − 2.395	0.040	0.008	0.062
			$\overline{Y}_{Training} = -2.057$	$\overline{X}_1 = 0.699$	$\overline{X}_2 = 0.152$	$\overline{X}_3 = 0.444$		$\Sigma = 0.256$	$\Sigma = 1.320$	$\Sigma = 0.406$

Sl. No.	R	n	pIC_{50} ($Y_{observed}$)	MR ($X1$)	σ ($X2$)	Ind ($X3$)	Predicted value (Y_{pred})	$\sum(Y_{obs(test)} - Y_{pred(test)})2$	$\sum(Y_{obs(test)} - \overline{Y}_{training})^2$	$\sum(Y_{obs(test)} - \overline{Y}_{test})^2$
Test set										
T1	Br	3	−2.053	0.888	0.23	1	−2.080	0.001	0.000	0.099
T2	OC_3H_7	3	−2.123	1.706	−0.25	1	−2.250	0.016	0.004	0.060
T3	NH_2	3	−2.934	0.542	−0.66	1	−2.719	0.046	0.769	0.321
T4	SO_2NH_2	3	−1.991	1.228	0.57	1	−1.799	0.037	0.004	0.141
T5	CH_3	3	−2.789	0.565	−0.17	1	−2.396	0.154	0.536	0.178
T6	CH_2Cl	3	−1.987	1.049	0.12	1	−2.123	0.019	0.005	0.144
T7	OH	3	−2.279	0.285	−0.37	1	−2.575	0.088	0.049	0.008
T8	$CONH_2$	3	−2.003	0.981	0.36	1	−1.979	0.001	0.003	0.132
T9	$NHCH_3$	3	−3.001	1.033	−0.84	1	−2.751	0.062	0.891	0.402
T10	C_2H_5	3	−2.505	1.03	−0.15	1	−2.302	0.041	0.201	0.019
			$\overline{Y}_{Test} = -2.367$					$\Sigma = 0.464$	$\Sigma = 2.463$	$\Sigma = 1.505$

Calculation of metrics

Standard error of estimate (S)

$$s = \sqrt{\frac{\sum(Y_{obs} - Y_{calc(train)})^2}{n-p-1}} = \sqrt{\frac{0.256}{18-3-1}} = 0.135$$

Determination coefficient (R^2)

$$R^2 = 1 - \frac{\sum(Y_{obs(train)} - Y_{calc(train)})^2}{\sum(Y_{obs(train)} - \overline{Y}_{training})^2} = 1 - \frac{0.256}{1.320} = 0.806$$

Adjusted R^2 (R_a^2)

$$R_a^2 = \frac{(n-1)R^2 - p}{n-p-1} = \frac{(18-1)\times 0.806 - 3}{18-3-1} = 0.764$$

$RMSE_c$

$$RMSE_c = \sqrt{\frac{\sum(Y_{obs(training)} - Y_{calc(training)})^2}{n_{training}}} = \sqrt{\frac{0.256}{18}} = 0.119$$

$RMSE_p$

$$RMSE_p = \sqrt{\frac{\sum(Y_{obs(test)} - Y_{pred(test)})^2}{n_{test}}} = \sqrt{\frac{0.464}{10}} = 0.215$$

Q^2

$$Q^2 = 1 - \frac{\sum(Y_{obs(train)} - Y_{LOO-pred(train)})^2}{\sum(Y_{obs(train)} - \overline{Y}_{training})^2} = 1 - \frac{0.406}{1.320} = 0.693$$

R^2_{pred}

$$R^2_{pred} = 1 - \frac{\sum(Y_{obs(test)} - Y_{pred(test)})^2}{\sum(Y_{obs(test)} - \overline{Y}_{training})^2} = 1 - \frac{0.464}{2.463} = 0.811$$

Calculation of metrics	
$Q^2_{(F2)}$	$Q^2_{(F2)} = 1 - \frac{\sum(Y_{obs(test)} - Y_{pred(test)})^2}{\sum(Y_{obs(test)} - \overline{Y}_{test})^2} = 1 - \frac{0.464}{1.505} = 0.692$
$Q^2_{(F3)}$	$Q^2_{(F3)} = 1 - \frac{\left[\sum(Y_{obs(test)} - Y_{pred(test)})^2\right]/n_{ext}}{\left[\sum(Y_{obs(train)} - \overline{Y}_{train})^2\right]/n_{tr}} = 1 - \frac{0.464/10}{1.320/18} = 0.630$
Scaled $\overline{r^2_{m(LOO)}}$ and $\Delta r^2_{m(LOO)}$	$r^2_m = r^2 \times \left(1 - \sqrt{(r^2 - r^2_0)}\right) = 0.806$
	$r'^2_m = r^2 \times \left(1 - \sqrt{(r^2 - r'^2_0)}\right) = 0.663$
	$\overline{r^2_{m(LOO)}} = \frac{(r^2_m + r'^2_m)}{2} = \frac{(0.806 + 0.663)}{2} = 0.734$
	$\Delta r^2_{m(LOO)} = \lvert r^2_m - r'^2_m \rvert = \lvert 0.806 - 0.663 \rvert = 0.143$
Scaled $\overline{r^2_{m(test)}}$ and $\Delta r^2_{m(test)}$	$r^2_m = r^2 \times \left(1 - \sqrt{(r^2 - r^2_0)}\right) = 0.625$
	$r'^2_m = r^2 \times \left(1 - \sqrt{(r^2 - r'^2_0)}\right) = 0.369$
	$\overline{r^2_{m(test)}} = \frac{(r^2_m + r'^2_m)}{2} = \frac{(0.625 + 0.369)}{2} = 0.497$
	$\Delta r^2_{m(test)} = \lvert r^2_m - r'^2_m \rvert = \lvert 0.625 - 0.369 \rvert = 0.255$
Scaled $\overline{r^2_{m(overall)}}$ and $\Delta r^2_{m(overall)}$	$r^2_m = r^2 \times \left(1 - \sqrt{(r^2 - r^2_0)}\right) = 0.690$
	$r'^2_m = r^2 \times \left(1 - \sqrt{(r^2 - r'^2_0)}\right) = 0.684$
	$\overline{r^2_{m(overall)}} = \frac{(r^2_m + r'^2_m)}{2} = \frac{(0.690 + 0.684)}{2} = 0.687$
	$\Delta r^2_{m(overall)} = \lvert r^2_m - r'^2_m \rvert = \lvert 0.690 - 0.684 \rvert = 0.006$

The developed MLR equation (see Chapter 6) for 18 antimalarial cyclic peroxy ketals is considered for the calculation of various regression-based internal validation metrics. A hypothetically developed test set is employed to calculate different external validation metrics.

[a]The r^2_m metrics can be easily calculated with the help of open-source software available from http://aptsoftware.co.in/rmsquare/. Here, in the case of $\overline{r^2_{m(test)}}$ and $\Delta r^2_{m(test)}$ calculation, $Y_{observed}$ and $Y_{predicted}$ values of the test set are considered; in the case of $\overline{r^2_{m(LOO)}}$ and $\Delta r^2_{m(LOO)}$ calculation, $Y_{observed}$ and Y_{LOO} predicted values of the training set are considered; and finally, for the calculation of $\overline{r^2_{m(overall)}}$ and $\Delta r^2_{m(overall)}$, $Y_{observed}$ for the training and test sets, and Y_{LOO} predicted and $Y_{predicted}$ for the training and test sets, respectively, are considered. It is important to mention that one can easily calculate the metrics manually even without using software. For complete mathematical expressions, see Table 7.2.

Table 7.4 Calculation of classification-based QSAR metrics employing confusion matrix generated from the training and test sets described in Table 7.3

Compound ID	Observed activity (pIC_{50})	Observed classification	Posterior probabilities (PP)	Predicted classification
		Threshold based on pIC_{50}: ($L < -2.05 < H$)		Threshold based on PP: ($L < 0.50 < H$)
Training set compounds				
1	−2.279	L	0.744	L
2	−2.447	L	0.969	L
3	−2.342	L	0.744	L
4	−2.204	L	0.906	L
5	−2.255	L	0.990	L
6	−2.322	L	0.906	L
7	−1.785	H	0.078	H
8	−1.763	H	0.211	H
9	−1.929	H	0.651	L
10	−1.892	H	0.367	H
11	−1.491	H	0.002	H
12	−2.255	L	0.739	L
13	−2.204	L	0.862	L
14	−1.748	H	0.026	H
15	−1.663	H	0.036	H
16	−2	H	0.743	L
17	−2.301	L	0.953	L
18	−2.146	L	0.236	H
Test set compounds				
T1	−2.053	L	0.669	L
T2	−2.123	L	0.965	L
T3	−2.934	L	1.000	L
T4	−1.991	H	0.090	H
T5	−2.789	L	0.985	L
T6	−1.987	H	0.792	L

T7	−2.279	L	0.998	L
T8	−2.003	H	0.400	H
T9	−3.001	L	1.000	L
T10	−2.505	L	0.968	L
Classification metrics	Training set		Test set	
	Confusion matrix: P row: P = 6, N = 2; N row: P = 1, N = 9		Confusion matrix: P row: P = 2, N = 1; N row: P = 0, N = 7	
TP	6		2	
FN	2		1	
FP	1		0	
TN	9		7	
Sensitivity (%) Sensitivity = $\frac{TP}{TP+FN}$	$\left(\frac{6}{6+2}\right) * 100 = 75$		$\left(\frac{2}{2+1}\right) * 100 = 66.67$	
Specificity (%) Specificity = $\frac{TN}{TN+FP}$	$\left(\frac{9}{9+1}\right) * 100 = 90$		$\left(\frac{7}{7+0}\right) * 100 = 100$	
Precision (%) Precision = $\frac{TP}{TP+FP}$	$\left(\frac{6}{6+1}\right) * 100 = 85.71$		$\left(\frac{2}{2+0}\right) * 100 = 100$	
Accuracy (%) Accuracy = $\frac{TP+TN}{TP+FN+TN+FP}$	$\left(\frac{6+9}{6+2+9+1}\right) * 100 = 83.33$		$\left(\frac{2+7}{2+1+7+0}\right) * 100 = 90$	
F-measure (%) $F-\text{measure} = \frac{2}{1/\text{Precision}+1/\text{Sensitivity}}$	$\left(\frac{2}{1/0.857+1/0.75}\right) * 100 = 80$		$\left(\frac{2}{1/1+1/0.667}\right) * 100 = 80$	
G-means $G-\text{means} = \sqrt{\text{Sensitivity} \times \text{Specificity}}$	$\sqrt{(0.75 \times 0.90)} = 0.822$		$\sqrt{(0.667 \times 1)} = 0.816$	

(*Continued*)

Table 7.4 (Continued)

Compound ID	Observed activity (pIC_{50})	Observed classification Threshold based on pIC_{50}: (L < −2.05 < H)	Posterior probabilities (PP)	Predicted classification Threshold based on PP: (L < 0.50 < H)
Cohen's κ $P_r(a) = \frac{(TP + TN)}{(TP + FP + FN + TN)}$ $P_r(e) = \frac{\{(TP + FP) \times (TP + FN)\} + \{(TN + FP) \times (TN \times FN)\}}{(TP+FN+FP+TN)^2}$ $\text{Cohen's } \kappa = \frac{P_r(a) - P_r(e)}{1 - P_r(e)}$ *MCC* $MCC = \frac{(TP \times TN) - (FP \times FN)}{\sqrt{(TP + FP) \times (TP + FN) \times (TN + FP) \times (TN + FN)}}$	$P_r(a) = \left(\frac{6+9}{6+1+2+9}\right) = 0.83$ $P_r(e) = \frac{\langle(6+1) \times (6+2)\rangle + \langle(9+1) \times (9+2)\rangle}{(6+2+1+9)^2}$ $= 0.512$ $\text{Cohen's } \kappa = \frac{0.83 - 0.512}{1 - 0.512} = 0.652$ $\left(\frac{(6 \times 9) - (1 \times 2)}{\sqrt{(6+1) \times (6+2) \times (9+1) \times (9+2)}}\right) = 0.663$		$P_r(a) = \left(\frac{2+7}{2+0+1+7}\right) = 0.90$ $P_r(e) = \frac{\langle(2+0) \times (2+1)\rangle + \langle(7+0) \times (7+1)\rangle}{(2+1+0+7)^2}$ $= 0.62$ $\text{Cohen's } \kappa = \frac{0.90 - 0.62}{1 - 0.62} = 0.737$ $\left(\frac{(2 \times 7) - (0 \times 1)}{\sqrt{(2+0) \times (2+1) \times (7+0) \times (7+1)}}\right) = 0.734$	

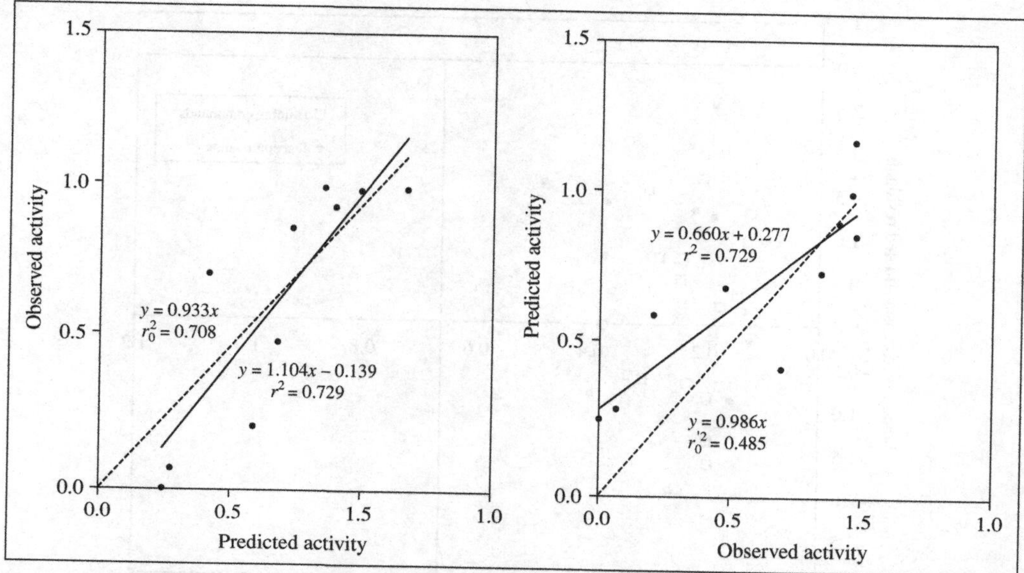

Figure 7.9 Regression plots obtained for the scaled data points with and without intercept: (A) predicted data is plotted along the *X*-axis, while the observed data is plotted along the *Y*-axis; (B) the axes are interchanged.

A. *Fixed or probabilistic boundaries (bounding box) and range of the response variable*: Both approaches strictly depend on the boundary created by independent and response variables of the training set compounds. As previously mentioned, the model consists of three descriptors (see Table 7.3). Scrutinizing the descriptor values for the training and test sets, one can easily identify that a test compound (T2) falls outside the AD boundary created by the independent variable MR. On the other hand, four compounds (T3, T5, T9, and T10) can be considered outside the AD boundary when one considers the response variable range. Therefore, one can conclude that considering both methods, five compounds reside outside the AD (see Table 7.3).

B. *Leverage approach*: Based on the calculated leverage (h) and standardized residual values, we have constructed a Williams plot (Figure 7.10). Here, the standardized cross-validated residual (SR) value is calculated based on the following equation:

$$\mathrm{SR} = \frac{\text{Residual value} - \text{Average Residual value}_{(\text{Training})}}{\text{Standard deviation of Residual value}_{(\text{Training})}} \qquad (7.46)$$

Then the Williams plot is constructed taking the SR values in the Y-axis and leverage values in X-axis (Table 7.5). As the number of descriptors is 3 and number of compounds in the training set is 18, the critical leverage (h^*) value is $[3^*(3+1)]/18 = 0.67$. Taking into consideration the criteria described in

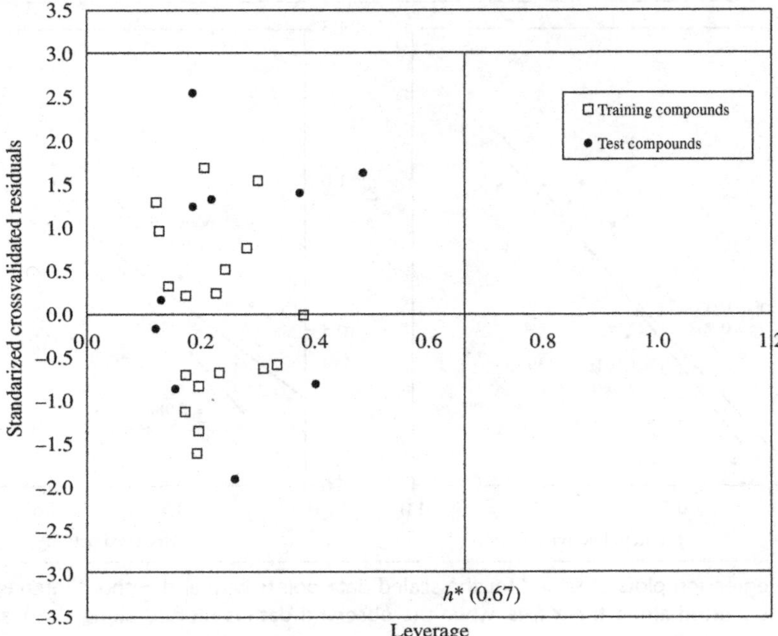

Figure 7.10 Williams plot for the developed QSAR model.

Table 7.1, one can firmly conclude that based on the leverage approach for the studied QSAR model, all the query compounds are within the AD.

C. *Euclidean distance-based approach*: First, the Euclidean distance scores and mean distance scores are calculated (see the equations mentioned in Table 7.1; and for computed values, see Table 7.5) for the training and test sets. The mean distances of the training set are then normalized within the interval of zero to 1. From the normalized mean distances of the test set, it is clear that three test compounds (T2, T3, and T9) reside outside the AD. Next, the Euclidean plot (Figure 7.11) is developed by taking the mean normalized distance in the *Y*-axis and compound numbers in the *X*-axis.

Merging the results of all methods, one can conclude that the prediction of the 5 test compounds are not reliable (out of a total of 10 test set compounds), as they fall outside the AD zone created by the descriptors and the response values. It is important to note that the results of one particular method may not be equivalent with those from another approach, as each method is based on dissimilar statistical algorithms for the determination of AD. Thus, multiple methods should be applied before coming to a final conclusion regarding AD of a QSAR model.

Table 7.5 Determination of the AD for the developed MLR-based QSAR model using leverage and Euclidean distance-based approaches

Compound ID	Y* (observed)	Y (LOO predicted)	h^a	Residual	Standardized, cross-validated residual	Distance score[b]	Mean distance[c]	Normalized mean distance
Training set								
1	−2.279	−2.409	0.20	−0.13	−0.838	16.889	0.938	0.347
2	−2.447	−2.552	0.23	−0.105	−0.676	18.375	1.021	0.557
3	−2.342	−2.551	0.20	−0.209	−1.349	16.889	0.938	0.347
4	−2.204	−2.172	0.17	0.032	0.211	15.57	0.865	0.16
5	−2.255	−2.016	0.30	0.239	1.552	17.539	0.974	0.439
6	−2.322	−2.432	0.17	−0.11	−0.708	15.57	0.865	0.16
7	−1.785	−1.736	0.14	0.049	0.321	14.947	0.83	0.072
8	−1.763	−1.565	0.12	0.198	1.286	14.44	0.802	0
9	−1.929	−1.668	0.20	0.261	1.694	16.966	0.943	0.357
10	−1.892	−1.813	0.24	0.079	0.515	18.596	1.033	0.588
11	−1.491	−1.495	0.38	−0.004	−0.022	20.863	1.159	0.909
12	−2.255	−2.430	0.17	−0.175	−1.129	15.921	0.885	0.21
13	−2.204	−2.295	0.33	−0.091	−0.585	19.879	1.104	0.77
14	−1.748	−1.846	0.31	−0.098	−0.631	21.506	1.195	1
15	−1.663	−1.545	0.28	0.118	0.768	18.912	1.051	0.633
16	−2	−1.852	0.13	0.148	0.962	15.707	0.873	0.179
17	−2.301	−2.265	0.23	0.036	0.237	18.348	1.019	0.553
18	−2.146	−2.395	0.19	−0.249	−1.608	17.142	0.952	0.382
Compound ID	**Y* (Observed)**	**Y (Predicted)**	**h^a**	**Residual**	**Standardized cross-validated residual**	**Distance score[b]**	**Mean distance[c]**	**Normalized mean distance**
Test set								
T1	−2.053	−2.080	0.12	−0.027	−0.171	16.304	0.906	0.264
T2	−2.123	−2.250	0.40	−0.127	−0.818	24.917	1.384	1.483
T3	−2.934	−2.719	0.37	0.215	1.396	21.736	1.208	1.032
T4	−1.991	−1.799	0.19	0.192	1.247	19.555	1.086	0.724
T5	−2.789	−2.396	0.18	0.393	2.549	16.963	0.942	0.357
T6	−1.987	−2.123	0.15	−0.136	−0.877	17.106	0.95	0.377
T7	−2.279	−2.575	0.26	−0.296	−1.913	19.599	1.089	0.73
T8	−2.003	−1.979	0.13	0.024	0.159	17.002	0.945	0.363
T9	−3.001	−2.751	0.48	0.25	1.623	24.705	1.373	1.453
T10	−2.505	−2.302	0.22	0.203	1.318	17.829	0.991	0.48

*Y is the response variable; *h* is defined as the leverage value.

a. Calculated by employing the equation $h = (X^T(X^TX)^{-1}X)$; $h^* = 0.67$.

b. Calculated by employing the equation $d_{ij} = \sqrt{\sum_{k=1}^{m}(x_{ik} - x_{jk})^2}$.

c. Calculated employing the equation $\overline{d}_i = \sum_{j=1}^{n} d_{ij}/n - 1$. For more detail, see Table 7.1.

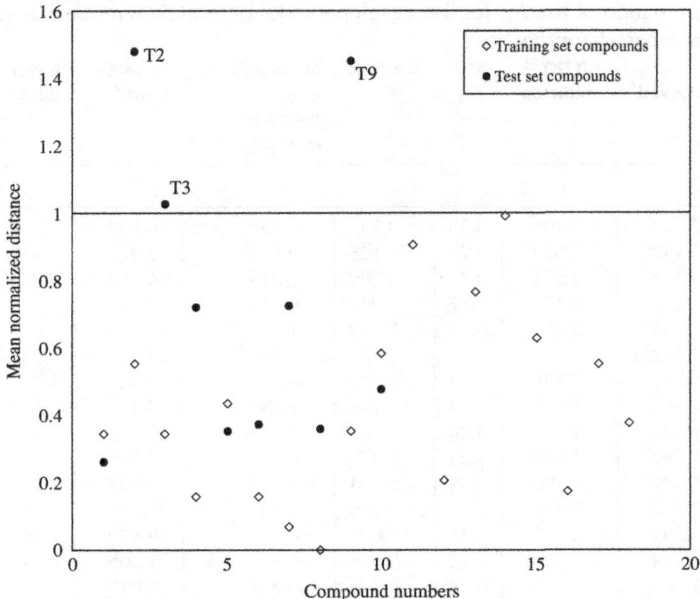

Figure 7.11 Euclidean distance plot for the developed QSAR model.

7.4 QSAR MODEL REPORTING FORMAT

7.4.1 Concept of the QMRF

The QSAR model reporting format (QMRF) is a harmonized template for summarizing and reporting the key information on ecotoxicological QSAR models, including the results of any validation studies. The information is structured according to the OECD QSAR validation principles (http://ihcp.jrc.ec.europa.eu/our_databases/jrc-qsar-inventory).

7.4.2 Why QMRF?

QMRF can be used as follows:

- Developers and users of QSAR models can submit information on QSAR models to the joint research center (JRC) using the QMRF.
- The JRC performs a quality control (i.e., adequacy and completeness of the documentation) of the QMRFs submitted.
- Properly documented summaries of QSARs are included in the JRC's QSAR Model Database.
- The QSAR Model Database helps to identify valid QSARs—for example, for the purposes of REACH.

- The QMRF is expected to be a communication tool between industry and the authorities under REACH.
- Responsibility for use of the models lies totally with the users.

7.4.3 How to construct QMRF

The QSAR Model Database is intended to provide information on QSAR models. These developed QSAR models can be submitted to JRC for peer review at http://qsardb.jrc.it/qmrf/search_catalogs.jsp.

7.4.4 Utility of the QMRF

The QMRF should be regarded as a communication tool. It describes some of the information provided by applying the OECD principles for QSAR validation, but it is not intended to be a complete characterization of the model in itself. The QMRF provides the user with details on the following:

a. The source of the model, including the developer
b. Model type
c. Model definition
d. The process of developing the model
e. The validation of the model
f. Possible applications of the model

It is important to point out that the QMRF should not be confused with the reporting formats used to provide QSAR estimates for chemicals that are registered within a given regulatory program, even though such formats are likely to contain similar information fields.

7.5 OVERVIEW AND CONCLUSION

QSAR-oriented research has advanced significantly in recent years with the growing number of chemical and pharmaceutical databases. A good number of successful applications of QSAR approaches in the process of drug design have communicated the effectiveness of this computational method. QSAR has been highly regarded as a scientifically trustworthy tool for predicting and classifying the biological activities/properties/toxicities of untested pharmaceuticals/chemicals for a long time. In order to make the models transferable and acceptable to the scientific community, validation aspects and the mechanistic interpretation are of paramount importance for any QSAR model. A wide range of validation techniques have been illustrated for detecting the capability of the QSAR model to predict the activity of new series of compounds. Here, we have discussed the most commonly used validation metrics for developing robust and externally predictive QSAR models. If sufficient consideration is given to the critical issues of QSAR model validation, the models could indeed be employed in large numbers successfully for virtual screening and to generate reliable computational hits.

The AD of a QSAR model is anticipated by determining interpolation regions as defined by the training set in a model descriptor space, but the region fluctuates depending on the adopted approach. Each implemented AD approach has its own prospective and flaws. Few approaches have multifaceted algorithms behind the detection of interpolation regions; on the other hand, some have strong and simple statistical background behind the AD estimation. Therefore, the model developer must decide how the specific approach is selected based on the requirement to define the AD for the model more accurately and in a robust way. It is imperative to note that if the researcher uses diverse AD approaches for the developed QSAR model from a single data set, the result may vary, and none of these recognized methods can be considered universal. Therefore, it is always recommended to assess the results from different available strategies before assessing a new compound set so that one can have confidence in the prediction result.

The discussed validation metrics and the concept about the AD should be helpful for both computational and synthetic chemists, as well as biologists doing biological screening of chemical libraries using QSAR models. We firmly believe that the provided examples for calculation of individual metrics and AD approaches from the practical data set also will be very helpful for the QSAR learner.

REFERENCES

[1] Helguera AM, Combes RD, Gonzalez MP, Cordeiro MN. Applications of 2D descriptors in drug design: a DRAGON tale. Curr Top Med Chem 2008;8(18):1628–55.

[2] Cronin MTD, Jaworska JS, Walker JD, Comber MHI, Watts CD, Worth AP. Use of QSARs in international decision-making frameworks to predict health effects of chemical substances. Environ Health Perspect 2003;111(10):1391–401.

[3] Worth AP, Bassan A, De Bruijn J, Saliner AG, Netzeva T, Patlewicz G, et al. The role of the European Chemicals Bureau in promoting the regulatory use of (Q)SAR methods. SAR QSAR Environ Res 2007;18(1–2):111–25.

[4] Russell WMS, Burch RL. The principles of humane experimental technique. London: Methuen; 1959.

[5] Balls M, Blaauboer BJ, Fentem JH, Bruner L, Combes RD, Ekwall B, et al. Practical aspects of the validation of toxicity test procedures—the report and recommendations of ECVAM workshop 5. Altern Lab Anim 1995;23:129–47.

[6] Aptula AO, Jeliazkova NG, Schultz TW, Cronin MTD. The better predictive model: high q^2 for the training set or low root mean square error of prediction for the test set? QSAR Comb Sci 2005;24 (3):385–96.

[7] Snedecor GW, Cochran WG. Statistical Methods. New Delhi, India: Oxford & IBH; 1967.

[8] OECD Document. Guidance Document on the Validation of (Quantitative) 1226 Structure Activity Relationships (Q)SARs Models, ENV/JM/MONO(2007)2; 2007.

[9] Wold S, Sjostrom M, Eriksson L. PLS-regression: a basic tool of chemometrics. Chemom Intell Lab Syst 2001;58:109–30.

[10] Netzeva TI, Worth AP, Aldenberg T, Benigni R, Cronin MTD, Gramatica P, et al. Current status of methods for defining the applicability domain of (quantitative) structure–activity relationships. Altern Lab Anim 2005;33(2):155–73.
[11] Topliss JG, Costello RJ. Chance correlation in structure-activity studies using multiple regression analysis. J Med Chem 1972;15(10):1066–8.
[12] Wold S, Eriksson L. In: van de Waterbeemd HE, editor. Chemometric methods in molecular design. Weinheim, Germany: VCH; 1995. p. 195–218.
[13] Jaworska JS, Comber M, Auer C, Van Leeuwen CJ. Summary of a workshop on regulatory acceptance of (Q)SARs for human health and environmental endpoints. Environ Health Perspect 2003; 111(10):1358–60.
[14] OECD, principles for the validation of (Q)SARs. Retrieved 31 August, 2014 from <http://www.oecd.org/dataoecd/33/37/37849783.pdf>; 2004.
[15] Tropsha A, Gramatica P, Gombar VK. The importance of being earnest: validation is the absolute essential for successful application and interpretation of QSPR models. QSAR Comb Sci 2003;22(1):69–77.
[16] Wold S. Cross-validation estimation of the number of components in factor and principal components models. Technometrics 1978;20:397–405.
[17] Wold S. Validation of QSAR's. Quant Struct-Act Relat 1991;10:191–3.
[18] Roy K. On some aspects of validation of predictive QSAR models. Expert Opin Drug Discov 2007; 2(12):1567–77.
[19] Golbraikh A, Tropsha A. Predictive QSAR modeling based on diversity sampling of experimental datasets for the training and test set selection. J Comput Aided Mol Des 2002;16:357–69.
[20] Guha R, Jurs PC. Determining the validity of a QSAR model—a classification approach. J Chem Inf Model 2005;45(1):65–73.
[21] Carlson R. Design and optimization in organic synthesis. Amsterdam: Elsevier; 1992.
[22] Roy PP, Leonard JT, Roy K. Exploring the impact of the size of training sets for the development of predictive QSAR models. Chemom Intell Lab Syst 2008;90(1):31–42.
[23] Everitt BS, Landau S, Leese M. Cluster Analysis. London: Edward Arnold; 2001.
[24] Gasteiger J, Zupan J. Neural networks in chemistry. Angew Chem 1993;32(4):503–27.
[25] Huuskonen J. QSAR modeling with the electrotopological state: TIBO derivatives. J Chem Inf Comput Sci 2001;41(2):425–9.
[26] Tetko IV, Kovalishyn VV, Livingstone DJ. Volume learning algorithm artificial neural networks for 3D QSAR studies. J Med Chem 2001;44(15):2411–20.
[27] Snarey M, Terrett NK, Willett P, Wilton DJ. Comparison of algorithms for dissimilarity-based compound selection. J Mol Graph Model 1997;15(6):372–85.
[28] Golbraikh A. Molecular dataset diversity indices and their applications to comparison of chemical databases and QSAR analysis. J Chem Inf Comput Sci 2000;40(2):414–25.
[29] Szàntai-Kis C, Kövesdi I, Kèri G, Orfi L. Validation subset selections for extrapolation oriented QSPAR models. Mol Divers 2003;7(1):37–43.
[30] Gramatica P. Principles of QSAR models validation: internal and external. QSAR Comb Sci 2007; 26(6):694–701.
[31] Weaver S, Paul Gleeson M. The importance of the domain of applicability in QSAR modeling. J Mol Graph Model 2008;26(8):1315–26.
[32] Golbraikh A, Tropsha A. Beware of q^2!. J Mol Graph Model 2002;20(4):269–76.
[33] Jaworska J, Nikolova-Jeliazkova N, Aldenberg T. QSAR applicability domain estimation by projection of the training set descriptor space: a review. Altern Lab Anim 2005;33(5):445–59.
[34] Nikolova-Jeliazkova N, Jaworska J. An approach to determining applicability domain for QSAR group contribution models: an analysis of SRC KOWWIN. Altern Lab Anim 2005;33(5):461–70.
[35] TOPKAT OPS. U.S. Patent 6, 036, 349; March 14, 2000.
[36] Preparata FP, Shamos MI. In: Preparata FP, Shamos MI, editors. Computational geometry: an introduction. New York, NY: Springer-Verlag; 1991.
[37] Eriksson L, Jaworska J, Worth AP, Cronin MT, McDowell RM, Gramatica P. Methods for reliability and uncertainty assessment and for applicability evaluations of classification- and regression-based QSARs. Environ Health Perspect 2003;111(10):1361–75.

[38] Jaworska JS, Nikolova-Jeliazkova N, Aldenberg T. Review of methods for applicability domain estimation. Ispra (Italy): Report, The European Commission-Joint Research Centre; 2004.
[39] Hair Jr JF, Anderson RE, Tatham RL, Black WC. Multivariate data analysis. Singapore: Pearson Education; 2005.
[40] Sheridan R, Feuston RP, Maiorov VN, Kearsley S. Similarity to molecules in the training set is a good discriminator for prediction accuracy in QSAR. J Chem Inf Comput Sci 2004;44(6): 1912–28.
[41] SIMCA-P 10.0. info@umetrics.com, UMETRICS, Umea, Sweden, <www.umetrics.com>; 2002.
[42] Tetko IV, Sushko I, Pandey AK, Zhu H, Tropsha A, Papa E, et al. Critical assessment of QSAR models of environmental toxicity against *Tetrahymena pyriformis*: focusing on applicability domain and overfitting by variable selection. J Chem Inf Model 2008;48(9):1733–46.
[43] Manallack DT, Tehan BG, Gancia E, Hudson BD, Ford MG, Livingstone DJ, et al. A consensus neural network-based technique for discriminating soluble and poorly soluble compounds. J Chem Inf Comput Sci 2003;43(2):674–9.
[44] Jouan-Rimbaud D, Bouveresse E, Massart DL, de Noord OE. Detection of prediction outliers and inliers in multivariate calibration. Anal Chim Acta 1999;388(3):283–301.
[45] Dimitrov S, Dimitrova G, Pavlov T, Dimitrova N, Patlewicz G, Niemela J, et al. Stepwise approach for defining the applicability domain of SAR and QSAR models. J Chem Inf Model 2005;45(4): 839–49.
[46] Tong W, Hong H, Xie Q, Xie L, Fang H, Perkins R. Assessing QSAR limitations—a regulatory perspective. Curr Comput Aided Drug Des 2004;1(2):195–205.
[47] Fechner N, Jahn A, Hinselmann G, Zell A. Atomic local neighborhood flexibility incorporation into a structured similarity measure for QSAR. J Chem Inf Model 2009;49(3):549–60.
[48] Stanforth RW, Kolossov E, Mirkin B. A measure of domain of applicability for QSAR modeling based on intelligent *K*-means clustering. QSAR Comb Sci 2007;26(7):837–44.
[49] Debnath AK. In: Ghose AK, Viswanadhan VN, editors. Combinatorial library design and evaluation. New York, NY: Marcel Dekker; 2001.
[50] Tichý M, Rucki M. Validation of QSAR models for legislative purposes. Interdisc Toxicol 2009;2 (3):184–6.
[51] Clark RD, Sprous DG, Leonard JM. In: Höltje HD, Sippl W, editors. Rational approaches to drug design, proceedings of the thirteenth European symposium on quantitative structure–activity relationships. Dusseldorf, Germany: Prous Science; 2001. p. 475–85.
[52] Geisser S. The predictive sample reuse method with application. J Amer Stat Ass 1975;70:320–8.
[53] Hawkins DM, Basak SC, Mills D. Assessing model fit, by cross-validation. J Chem Inf Comput Sci 2003;43(2):579–86.
[54] Roy K, Mitra I, Kar S, Ojha PK, Das RN, Kabir H. Comparative studies on some metrics for external validation of QSPR models. J Chem Inf Model 2012;52(2):396–408.
[55] Roy K, Chakraborty P, Mitra I, Ojha PK, Kar S, Das RN. Some case studies on application of "r_m^2" metrics for judging quality of QSAR predictions: emphasis on scaling of response data. J Comput Chem 2013;34(12):1071–82.
[56] Mitra I, Roy PP, Kar S, Ojha P, Roy K. On further application of r_m^2 as a metric for validation of QSAR models. J Chemom 2010;24(1):22–33.
[57] Wehrens R, Putter H, Buydens LMC. The bootstrap: a tutorial. Chemom Intell Lab Syst 2000;54(1): 35–52.
[58] Cramer III RD, Bunce JD, Patterson DE, Frank IE. Crossvalidation, bootstrapping, and partial least squares compared with multiple regression in conventional QSAR studies. Quant Struct-Act Relat 1988;7:18–25.
[59] Mitra I, Saha A, Roy K. Exploring quantitative structure–activity relationship (QSAR) studies of antioxidant phenolic compounds obtained from traditional Chinese medicinal plants. Mol Simul 2010;36(13):1067–79.
[60] Consonni V, Ballabio D, Todeschini R. Evaluation of model predictive ability by external validation techniques. J Chemom 2010;24(3–4):194–201.

[61] Schuurmann G, Ebert RU, Chen J, Wang B, Kuhne R. External validation and prediction employing the predictive squared correlation coefficient-test-set activity mean vs training set activity mean. J Chem Inf Model 2008;48(11):2140–5.
[62] Chirico N, Gramatica P. Real external predictivity of QSAR models: how to evaluate it? Comparison of different validation criteria and proposal of using the concordance correlation coefficient. J Chem Inf Model 2011;51:2320–35.
[63] Roy K, Mitra I, Ojha PK, Kar S, Das RN, Kabir H. Introduction of $r_m{}^2{}_{(rank)}$ metric incorporating rank-order predictions as an additional tool for validation of QSAR/QSPR models. Chemom Intell Lab Syst 2012;118(15):200–10.
[64] Roy K, Kar S. How to judge predictive quality of classification and regression based QSAR models? In: Haq Z, Madura JD, editors. Frontiers in computational chemistry. Bentham Science Publishers; 2014, [In press].
[65] Roy K, Mitra I. On various metrics used for validation of predictive QSAR models with applications in virtual screening and focused library design. Comb Chem High Throughput Screen 2011; 14:450–74.
[66] Walkera JD, Carlsenb L, Jaworskac J. Improving opportunities for regulatory acceptance of QSARs: the importance of model domain, uncertainty, validity and predictability. QSAR Comb Sci 2003;22:346–50.
[67] Gálvez-Llompart M, Recio MC, García-Domenech R. Topological virtual screening: a way to find new compounds active in ulcerative colitis by inhibiting NF-kB. Mol Divers 2011;15(4):917–26.
[68] Prado-Prado FJ, Uriarte E, Borges F, González-Díaz H. Multi-target spectral moments for QSAR and complex networks study of antibacterial drugs. Eur J Med Chem 2009;44(11):4516–21.
[69] Speck-Planche A, Kleandrova VV, Luan F, Cordeiro MNDS. Fragment-based QSAR model toward the selection of versatile anti-sarcoma leads. Eur J Med Chem 2011;46(12):5910–16.
[70] Afantitis A, Melagraki G, Sarimveis H, Koutentis PA, Igglessi-Markopoulou O, Kollias G. A combined LS-SVM & MLR QSAR workflow for predicting the inhibition of CXCR3 receptor by quinazolinone analogs. Mol Divers 2010;14(2):225–35.
[71] Fawcett T. An introduction to ROC analysis. Pattern Recognit Lett 2006;27:861–74.
[72] Kubat M, Holte R, Matwin S. Machine learning for the detection of oil spills in satellite radar images. Mach Learn 1998;30:195–215.
[73] Cohen JA. Coefficient of agreement for nominal scales. Educ Psychol Meas 1960;20:37–46.
[74] Matthews BW. Comparison of the predicted and observed secondary structure of T4 phage lysozyme. Biochim Biophys Acta 1975;405(2):442–51.
[75] Perez-Garrido A, Helguera AM, Borges F, Cordeiro MNDS, Rivero V, Escudero AG. Two new parameters based on distances in a receiver operating characteristic chart for the selection of classification models. J Chem Inf Model 2011;51:2746–59.
[76] Truchon JF, Bayly CI. Evaluating virtual screening methods: good and bad metrics for the "early recognition" problem. J Chem Inf Model 2007;47(2):488–508.
[77] Galvez J, Garcia-Domenech R, de Gregorio Alapont C, De Julian-Ortiz V, Popa L. Pharmacological distribution diagrams: a tool for *de novo* drug design. J Mol Graph 1996;14(5): 272–6.
[78] Posner GH, O'Dowd H, Ploypradith P, Cumming JN, Xie S, Shapiro TA. Antimalarial cyclic peroxy ketals. J Med Chem 1998;41:2164–7.
[79] Roy K, Pal DK, Sengupta C. Hansch analysis of antimalarial cyclic peroxy ketals with physicochemical and electrotopological parameters. Drug Des Discov 2000;17:183–90.

CHAPTER 8

Introduction to 3D-QSAR

Contents

Understanding the Basics of QSAR for Applications in Pharmaceutical Sciences and Risk Assessment.
ISBN: 978-0-12-801505-6, DOI: http://dx.doi.org/10.1016/B978-0-12-801505-6.00008-9

8.1 INTRODUCTION

The basic principle of a quantitative structure–activity relationship (QSAR) study is that the deviations in biological response among a series of compounds are accountable for the differences in the structural properties. In the classical QSAR studies, biological responses have been correlated with atomic, group, or molecular properties such as lipophilicity, polarizability, electronic, and steric properties (Hansch analysis) or with certain structural features (Free–Wilson analysis). However, in these techniques, one cannot ignore their limited utility for designing diverse functional new molecules due to the lack of consideration of the three-dimensional (3D) structures of the molecules. As a consequence, 3D-QSAR has emerged as a natural extension to the classical Hansch and Free–Wilson approaches that exploits the 3D properties of the ligands to predict their biological response by employing robust chemometric tools. The 3D-QSAR is a broad term encompassing all those QSAR methods that correlate macroscopic target properties with computed atom-based descriptors derived from the spatial representation of the molecular structures. These approaches have served as a valuable predictive tool in the design of pharmaceuticals and agrochemicals [1–3].

The prime goal of any 3D-QSAR method is to establish the relationship between biological activity and spatial properties of chemicals like steric, electrostatic, and lipophilic ones. The 3D-QSAR methodology is computationally more exhaustive and complex than 2D-QSAR approaches. Normally, it consists of several steps to acquire numerical descriptors from the compound structures:

1. The optimum (near bioactive) conformation of the compound has to be determined, either from experimental data (X-ray crystal structure or NMR) or a theoretical tool like molecular mechanics, and then optimization of the energy has to be performed.
2. An alignment of the conformers in the data set has to be generated in 3D-space.
3. The space with an immersed conformer is probed computationally for generating various descriptors.
4. Finally, the computed descriptors should be correlated with the experimental biological response of the studied compounds.

It is interesting to point out that some methods, independent of the alignment strategy, have also been developed with the progress of 3D-QSAR approaches [4].

One has to understand that the QSAR model is not a substitute for the experimental assays, although experimental techniques are also not free of inaccuracies. However, QSAR researchers are trying to develop a model that is as close as possible to the real one, and for this purpose, the 3D-QSAR techniques have to rely on some basic assumptions, which are illustrated here:

- Binding of a drug molecule or ligand with the receptor is considered directly related to the biological response. Effects on second messengers or other signaling effects between receptor binding and experimentally observed response are not normally considered.
- Molecular properties (physical, chemical, and biological) are encoded with a set of numbers or descriptors.
- It is believed in general that compounds with common structures have comparable properties, and thus they have similar binding modes and accordingly equivalent biological activities and vice versa.
- Structural properties leading to a biological response are usually determined by nonbonding forces, mainly steric and electrostatic ones.
- Another important assumption is that the biological response is shown by the ligand itself, not by its metabolite product.
- The lowest-energy conformation of the ligand is its bioactive conformation, which exerts binding effects.
- The geometry of the receptor binding site is considered rigid, though there are a few exceptions.
- The loss of translational and rotational degrees of freedom (entropy) upon binding is believed to follow a similar pattern for all these compounds.
- The protein binding site is assumed to be the same for all of the studied ligands.
- The major factors that contribute to the overall free energy of binding, like desolvation energy, temperature, diffusion, transport, pH, salt concentration, and plasma protein binding, are difficult to identify and thus are generally ignored.

The 3D-QSAR methods can be classified based on a variety of criteria, as given in Table 8.1. Most commonly and successfully employed 3D-QSAR methods are discussed in the following sections of this chapter.

8.2 COMPARATIVE MOLECULAR FIELD ANALYSIS

8.2.1 Concept of CoMFA

Comparative molecular field analysis (CoMFA) is a molecular field–based, alignment-dependent, ligand-based method developed by Cramer et al. [5], which helps in building the quantitative relationship of molecular structures and its response property. The method mostly focuses on ligand properties like steric and electrostatic ones, and the resulting favorable and unfavorable receptor–ligand interactions. As CoMFA is an

Table 8.1 Categorization of 3D-QSAR techniques

Basis of classification	Type	Examples of techniques
Based on employed chemometric techniques	Linear	CoMFA, CoMSIA, AFMoC, GERM, CoMMA, SoMFA
	Nonlinear	Compass
Based on the alignment criterion	Alignment-dependent	CoMFA, CoMSIA, MSA, RSA, GERM, AFMoC, HIFA, VFA, MQSM
	Alignment-independent	Compass, CoMMA, HQSAR, WHIM, GRIND, VolSurf, CoSA
Based on intermolecular modeling or the information employed to develop QSAR	Ligand-based	CoMFA, CoMSIA, MSA, RSA, Compass, GERM, CoMMA, SoMFA
	Receptor-based	AFMoC, HIFA

alignment-dependent, descriptor-based method, all aligned ligands are placed in an energy grid, and by placing an appropriate probe at each lattice point, energy is calculated. The resultant energy calculated at each unit fraction corresponds to electrostatic (Coulombic) and steric (van der Waals) properties. These computed values serve as descriptors for model development. These descriptor values are then correlated with biological responses employing a robust linear regression method like partial least squares (PLS). The PLS results serve as an important signal to identify the favorable and unfavorable electrostatic and steric potential and also correlate it with biological responses.

8.2.2 Methodology of CoMFA

The formalism of the CoMFA methodology is described next:

a. Structures of all molecules are drawn using any structure-drawing software.

b. The bioactive conformation of each molecule is generated and energy minimization is carried out.

c. All the molecules are superimposed or aligned using either manual or automated methods employed in the working software, in a manner defined by the supposed mode of interaction with the receptor.

d. Thereafter, the overlaid compounds are positioned in the center of a lattice grid with a spacing of 2 Å.

e. In the 3D space, the steric and electrostatic fields are calculated around the molecules with different probe groups positioned at all intersections of the lattice. Computation of the steric field uses the Lennard–Jones equation as follows:

$$V_{LJ} = 4\varepsilon\left[\left(\frac{\sigma}{r}\right)^{12} - \left(\frac{\sigma}{r}\right)^{6}\right] = \varepsilon\left[\left(\frac{r_m}{r}\right)^{12} - 2\left(\frac{r_m}{r}\right)^{6}\right] \tag{8.1}$$

In Eq. (8.1), ε is the depth of the potential well, σ is the finite distance at which the interparticle potential is zero, r is the distance between the particles, and r_m is the distance at which the potential reaches its minimum. At r_m, the potential function has the value $-\varepsilon$. The distances are given as $r_m = 2^{1/6}\sigma$.

Again, computation of electrostatic field follows the Coulombic interaction equation as follows:

$$E = \left[\frac{q_1 q_2}{4\pi\varepsilon r}\right] \tag{8.2}$$

where q_1 and q_2 denote point charges, r is the distance between charges, and ε is the dielectric constant of the medium.

f. The interaction energy or field values forming a pool of the descriptor/variable matrix are correlated with the biological response data employing the PLS technique, which identifies and extracts the quantitative influence of specific features of molecules on their activity.

g. The results may be expressed as correlation equations with the number of latent variable terms, each of which is a linear combination of original independent lattice descriptors.

h. For visual interpretation, the PLS output is illustrated in the form of interactive graphics consisting of colored contour plots of coefficients of the corresponding field variables at each lattice intersection, and showing the imperative favorable and unfavorable regions in the 3D space, which are closely associated with the biological activity.

The CoMFA formalism is schematically illustrated in Figure 8.1.

8.2.3 Factors responsible for the performance of CoMFA

There are diverse factors that can control the complete performance of the constructed CoMFA model. These are described in the next sections.

8.2.3.1 Biological data

Like any 2D-QSAR method, one has to use precise activity data in order to create a good 3D-QSAR model. The following conditions should be fulfilled for maintaining the accuracy and appropriateness of the biological response data [3,6]:

- All molecules should belong to a congeneric series.
- Compounds should possess the same mechanism of action and the same (or at least an equivalent) binding mode.
- The biological responses of molecules should correlate to their binding affinity, and their specified biological responses should be assessable.

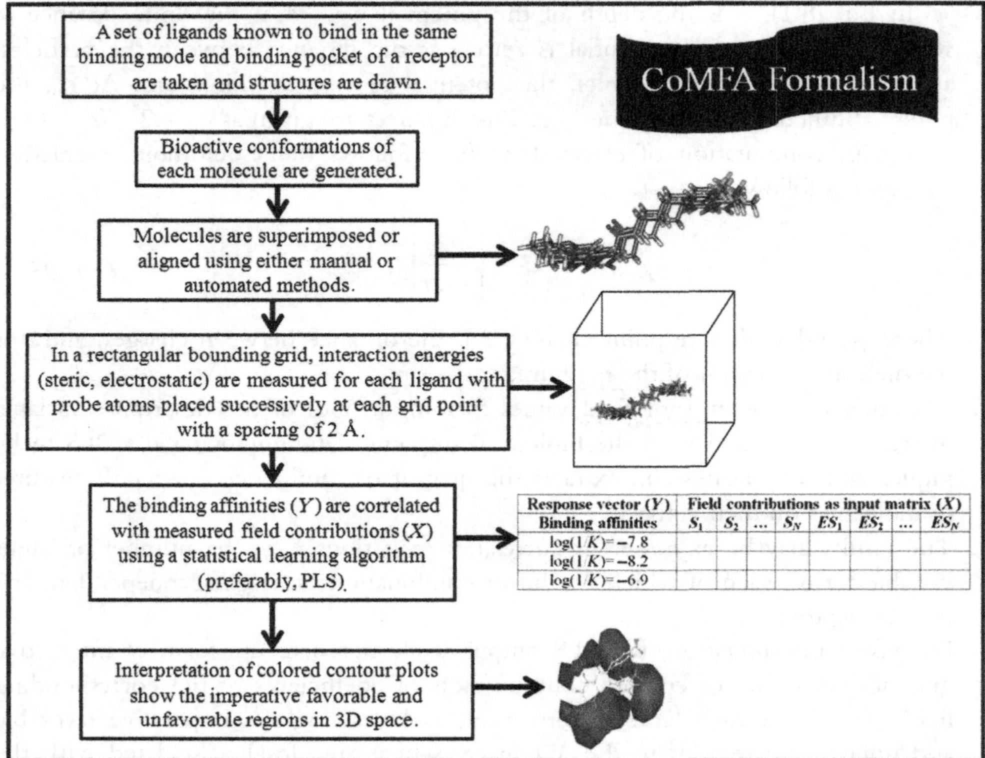

Figure 8.1 Fundamental steps of the CoMFA methodology.

- Experimental responses should be measured employing standardized and uniform protocols and preferably from a single source (organism/tissue/cell/protein) and a single laboratory.
- The activity values of all compounds should be in the same units of measure (binding/functional/IC_{50}/K_i). The K_i value is preferred over the IC_{50} data, as it is independent of the substrate concentration.
- The ranges of biological responses should be as large as possible, keeping the mode of action identical.
- Preferably, the biological response should be symmetrically distributed around the mean, and its accuracy should be evenly distributed over its range of variation.

8.2.3.2 Optimization of 3D structure of the compounds

Representing the initial molecular structure is an important issue in 3D-QSAR analysis. This can be done by both experimental and computational approaches. A huge number of experimentally determined crystal structures are accessible in databases like the Cambridge Structural Database [7] and the Protein Data Bank [8]. The obtainable crystal structures present the benefit that some conformational information about the flexible molecule is included. Computationally, the 3D structures can be generated by three methods:

- Manually, by drawing the structures in a 3D computer graphics interface or from an existing 3D structure included in the fragment libraries
- Numerically, by utilizing mathematical techniques like distance geometry and quantum or molecular mechanics
- Automatic methods that are often employed for creating 3D structure databases

Once the starting 3D molecular structures are generated, their geometries are refined by minimizing their conformational energies using following structure optimization techniques, including:

- *Molecular mechanics*: It does not explicitly consider the electronic motion, so they are fast, accurate, and can be employed for large molecules like enzymes.
- *Quantum mechanics* or *ab initio*: It takes into account the 3D distribution of electrons around the nuclei, and thus it is extremely precise. The identified major drawbacks of this methods are that they are time-consuming and computationally intensive, and they cannot handle large molecules.
- *Semiempirical*: Semiempirical quantum chemical methods attempt to address two restrictions—namely, slow speed and low accuracy of quantum mechanical (e.g., Hartree–Fock) calculations by omitting certain integrals based on experimental data, such as ionization energies of atoms or dipole moments of molecules. Thus, semiempirical methods are very fast, applicable to large molecules, and may give precise results when applied to molecules that are similar to the molecules used for parameterization. Molecules to be used for semiempirical calculations may contain hundreds of atoms. Modern semiempirical models are based on the neglect of diatomic differential overlap (NDDO) methods like MNDO, AM1, PM3, and PDDG/PM3.

8.2.3.3 Conformational analysis of compounds

The following conformational search methods can be implemented:

- *Systematic search (or grid search)*: It generates all probable conformations by systematically varying each of the torsion angles of a molecule by some increment, keeping the bond lengths and bond angles fixed.
- *Monte Carlo*: It simulates dynamic behavior of a compound and generates the conformations by making random changes in its structure, calculating and comparing its energy with that of the previous conformation, and accepting the result if it is unique.
- *Random search*: It generates a set of conformations by repetitively and arbitrarily changing either the Cartesian (*x*, *y*, *z*) or the internal (bond lengths, bond angles,

and torsion/dihedral angles) coordinates of a starting geometry of the molecule under consideration.

- *Molecular dynamics*: It employs Newton's second law of motion (force = mass × acceleration) to simulate the time-dependent movements and conformational changes in a molecular system, and results in a so-called trajectory showing how the positions and velocities of atoms in the molecular system vary with time.
- *Simulated annealing*: It theoretically heats up the molecular system under consideration to high temperatures to overcome huge energy barriers, and after equilibrating there for some time using molecular dynamics, cools down the system slowly and gradually to obtain low-energy conformations according to the Boltzmann distribution.
- *Distance geometry algorithm*: It generates a random set of coordinates by selecting random distances within each pair of upper and lower bounds to form constraints in a distance matrix, which are employed to create energetically feasible conformations of a set of molecules.
- *Genetic and evolutionary algorithms*: It is based on the concept of biological evolution and initially creates a population of promising solutions to the problem. The solutions with the best fitness scores undergo crossovers and mutations over a time, and proliferate their good distinctiveness down the generations resulting in better solutions in the form of new conformers.

8.2.3.4 Determination of bioactive conformations

The bioactive conformation defines a particular conformation of the molecule in which it is bound to the receptor. The intrinsic forces between the atoms in the molecule, as well as extrinsic forces between the molecule and its surrounding environment, considerably influence the bioactive conformation of the molecule [6]. Bioactive conformations of the compounds can be attained both by experimental and theoretical techniques. Experimental methods for creating bioactive conformations comprise the techniques described.

8.2.3.4.1 X-ray crystallography

The precise 3D structure of the macromolecules can be obtained by this method. Drug–receptor complexes generated by X-ray crystallography logically offer the exact information, but this method has several disadvantages:

- The protein needs to be crystallized, and the formation of crystallizing media is not typically like the physiological conditions.
- There is a chance of structural distortion due to crystal packing.
- Due to crystal instability and active-site occlusion, it is often not promising to disperse substrates or other biologically applicable molecules into the existing crystals.
- The positions of hydrogen atoms are tricky to be determined.
- There is a possibility of errors in determining the structure of the ligand.

8.2.3.4.2 NMR spectroscopy

The 3D structural data is obtained in the solution and is a method of selection when the molecule cannot be crystallized through experimental ways, as in the case of the membrane-bound receptors or receptors, which have not yet been isolated due to stability, resolution, or other issues. The imperative features of this method are:

- As no protein crystallization is required, the conformation of the protein is not influenced by packing forces of the crystal environment.
- The solution conditions (pH, ionic strength, substrate, temperature, etc.) can be accustomed to match the physiological conditions.
- Significant information regarding dynamic aspects of molecular motion can be obtained.
- It requires much less time but applicable to small molecules only.
- The positions of hydrogen atoms can be resolved.
- Apolar solvents may lead to an overprediction of hydrogen-bonding phenomena.
- Structures generated from NMR may not be comparable to the ones obtained from the experiment and frequently it may not signify the receptor-bound conformation.

8.2.3.5 Alignment of molecules

Various approaches have been used to superimpose the molecules as precisely as possible, some of the most commonly used methods are as follows:

- *Atom overlapping—based superimposition*: The basic principle involves atom-to-atom pairing between the molecules. It is known as the *pharmacophore approach* and is the most popular method, as it provides the best matching of the preselected atom positions. It is useful in identifying dissimilarity between similar molecules but cannot be applied to heterogeneous molecules.
- *Binding sites—based superimposition*: Molecular alignment is obtained by superimposing the receptor active sites or the receptor residues that interact with the ligands. This approach is believed to be more reliable, despite problems in conformational analysis due to enhanced degrees of freedom.
- *Fields/pseudofields-based superimposition*: This method performs superimposition by comparing the similarities in the computed interaction energy fields between the molecules. Electrostatic similarity and molecular surface similarity indices have also been used for molecular alignment.
- *Pharmacophore-based superimposition*: This method utilizes a hypothetical pharmacophore as a useful common target template. Each molecule is conformationally directed to assume the shape obligatory for its submolecular features to match with either a known pharmacophore or the one that is generated during the conformational analysis.
- *Multiple conformer-based superimposition*: It is helpful in cases where the ligands may bind to a receptor in multiple ways or when the correct binding mode is unidentified and the ligands have a fair degree of conformational flexibility.

8.2.3.6 Calculation of molecular interaction energy fields

Following superimposition, the overlaid set of compounds is placed in the center of a lattice or grid box to compute interaction energies between the ligands and different probe atoms placed at each intersection of the lattice [9]. The following aspects are required to be considered while computing the interaction energies in the CoMFA methodology:

- The usual size of the grid spacing is 2 Å. The grid spacing is inversely proportional to the meticulousness of calculations. As the grid spacing decreases to 1 Å or less, the calculations become more exhaustive.
- The distinctive size of the grid box is 3–4 Å larger than the union surface of the overlaid compounds. As the electrostatic/Coulombic interactions are long range in nature, a larger grid box may be required. It is true for steric/van der Waals interactions also.
- The position of the grid box significantly manipulates the statistics particularly the number of components in the final CoMFA model. Generally, the initial models are constructed at diverse locations to spot the best grid position.
- In CoMFA, the interaction energies are computed using probes. The probe may be a small molecule like water, or a chemical fragment such as a methyl group. The electrostatic energies are calculated with H^+ probe, whereas a sp^3 hybridized carbon atom with an effective radius of 1.53 Å and a 1.0 charge is used as probe for including the steric energies.
- A force field is a combination of bond lengths, bond angles, dihedral angles, inter-atomic distances, along with coordinates and other parameters that empirically fit the potential energy surface. Major forces encountered in the drug–receptor intermolecular interactions include electrostatic/Coulombic, hydrogen bonding, steric/van der Waals, and hydrophobic. The electrostatic and hydrogen bonding interactions are accountable for ligand–receptor specificity, whereas hydrophobic interactions usually provide the strength for binding. The steric and electrostatic interactions are mainly enthalpic in nature.
- In CoMFA, the standard Lennard–Jones function is utilized to model the van der Waals interactions, whereas electrostatic interactions are determined by Coulomb's law. The Lennard–Jones and Coulombic potentials depict singularities at the atomic positions. To avoid it, the cutoff values ($\pm$ 30 kcal/mol) for steric and electrostatic energy are defined.

8.2.3.7 Model generation

The computed interaction energies that are considered as variables are correlated to the biological responses of the compounds [10]. To extract a stable and robust QSAR model from a range of possible solutions, generally the PLS technique is employed. Other linear methods like principal component analysis (PCA) and principal component regression (PCR) can also be used. However, many times, the relationship between the dependent (y) and independent (x) variables is not linear or it cannot be predicted; in such cases, nonlinear chemometric methods like neural networks are employed.

8.2.4 Display and interpretation of results

For uncomplicated and easy visual interpretation, the results are displayed as coefficient contour (or scalar product of coefficients and standard deviation) plots, portraying vital regions in 3D-space around the compounds where specific structural modifications appreciably varies with the response. In CoMFA, two types of contours are shown for each interaction energy field: (i) positive and (ii) negative contours. Generally, the contours for steric fields are depicted in green (positive contours, with more bulk favored) and yellow (negative contours, with less bulk favored), while the electrostatic field contours are shown in red (positive contours, with electronegative substituents favored) and blue (negative contours, with electropositive substituents favored) colors. It is interesting to point out that researchers can change the color depiction considering the applicable requirements.

Along with the contour plots, CoMFA also offers two types of plots from PLS models: (i) score plots and (ii) loading/weight plots. The score plots between biological response (*Y*-scores) and latent variables (*X*-scores) show the relationship between the activity and the structures, whereas plots of latent variables (*X*-scores) display the similarity/dissimilarity between the molecules and their clustering predispositions.

8.2.5 Advantages and drawbacks of CoMFA

The CoMFA technique has been very successful in medicinal chemistry and allied fields due to the high interpretability of the models and ability to design new ligands in the structure–activity correlation problems. The major advantages of CoMFA are illustrated as follows:

- The CoMFA considers important physicochemical features like steric and electrostatic forces involved in ligand–receptor interactions.
- The technique appears extremely general, being directly applicable to any series of molecules for which alignable models can be constructed and whose desired property is believed to result from an alignment-dependent, noncovalent molecular interactions.
- Each CoMFA parameter represents the interaction energy of an entire ligand, not just the interaction of a more or less randomly selected substructure of the ligand.
- The only inputs needed are models of all the molecules, their lattice description, and usually, an explicit alignment rule. The most important outputs are the coefficient contour map displays and model predictions.

Although CoMFA offers many advantages over classical QSAR, it also has several limitations and defects [3,6]:

- Too many variables like overall orientation, lattice placement, step size, and probe atom type are considered.
- It is appropriate only with in vitro data.
- There is a low signal-to-noise ratio due to many ineffectual field variables.
- There is improbability in the choice of molecules and variables.
- There are fragmented contour maps with variable selection procedures.
- Some potential energy functions are flawed.
- Hydrophobicity is not well quantified.
- Cutoff limits are utilized.

In general, CoMFA results are highly dependent on the accuracy of the conformational analysis, determination of bioactive conformation, and method of alignment.

8.3 COMPARATIVE MOLECULAR SIMILARITY INDICES ANALYSIS

8.3.1 Concept of comparative molecular similarity indices analysis

Comparative molecular similarity indices analysis (CoMSIA) is a ligand-based, alignment-dependent, and linear 3D-QSAR method that is a modified version of CoMFA [11]. The approaches of CoMFA and CoMSIA are almost similar except for molecular similarity, which is also computed in the case of CoMSIA. CoMFA mostly focuses on the alignment of molecules and may lead to errors in alignment sensitivity and interpretation of electrostatic and steric potential. To address this, Gaussian potentials are employed in CoMSIA fields which are much softer than the CoMFA functions. The usual energy grid box is created, and similar probes are positioned throughout the grid lattice. In addition, the solvent reliant molecular entropic (hydrophobicity) term is also included in the CoMSIA. To analyze the property of a data set molecule, a common probe is placed and similarity at each grid point is calculated. The computation is mostly done on steric, electrostatic, hydrophobic, and hydrogen-bonding properties. The mentioned properties are computed at regularly spaced grid points corresponding to a particular descriptor, and these are significant in correlation with the biological response.

8.3.2 Methodology of CoMSIA

In CoMSIA, five different similarity fields are calculated at regularly spaced grid points for the aligned molecules: namely, steric, electrostatic, hydrophobic, hydrogen bond donor, and hydrogen bond acceptor. The interactions of the molecules with the probe atom under the influence of different similarity fields are correlated with the biological responses of the molecules using appropriate chemometric tool. The general formalism of the CoMSIA technique is illustrated as follows:

a. Initially, conformer generation is performed for the studied molecules employing one of the approaches mentioned in Section 8.2.3.3.

b. Energy minimization of the molecules is performed by any of the techniques mentioned in Section 8.2.3.2 (the choice of technique depends on the employed software, as well as the researchers' requirements), and then partial atomic charges of the molecules are calculated (using methods like the Gasteiger–Huckle method, Mulliken analysis, Coulson's charges, dipole charges, Voronoi deformation density, and density -derived electrostatic and chemical methods).

c. The training set molecules are aligned based on the points of alignment of the most active compound, which is used as the template molecule.

d. Thereafter, molecular interaction based on the five physicochemical properties should be calculated using a common probe atom with 1 Å radius, charge of 1, hydrophobicity of 1, and hydrogen bond donor and acceptor properties of 1. The grid can be extended beyond the molecular dimensions by 2.0 Å in all directions.

e. Subsequently, the PLS approach is employed to derive the 3D-QSAR models using the similarity (CoMSIA) factors as the independent variables and biological response as the dependent variable.

f. The results are represented in the form of contour maps that characterize the favorable and unfavorable regions for the five different interaction fields. Based on favorable interaction regions obtained from the contour map, the molecular fragments essential for the respective activity should be characterized. Figure 8.2 illustrates the steps involved in the CoMSIA formalism.

8.3.3 Advantages of CoMSIA

The CoMSIA technique shares a few drawbacks of CoMFA, but it also offers several distinguishing advantages:

- The utilization of the "Gaussian distribution of similarity indices" evades the unexpected changes in grid-based probe–atom interactions.
- The choice of similarity probe is not only limited to either steric or electrostatic potential fields, but also hydrogen bonding (hydrogen bond acceptors and donors) and hydrophobic fields.
- The effect of the solvent entropic provisions can also be incorporated by employing a hydrophobic probe.
- With CoMFA, a contour map highlights those regions in space where the aligned molecules would favorably or unfavorably interact with a probable receptor environment. On the other hand, the CoMSIA contours indicate those areas within the region occupied by the ligands that "favor" or "dislike" the occurrence of a group

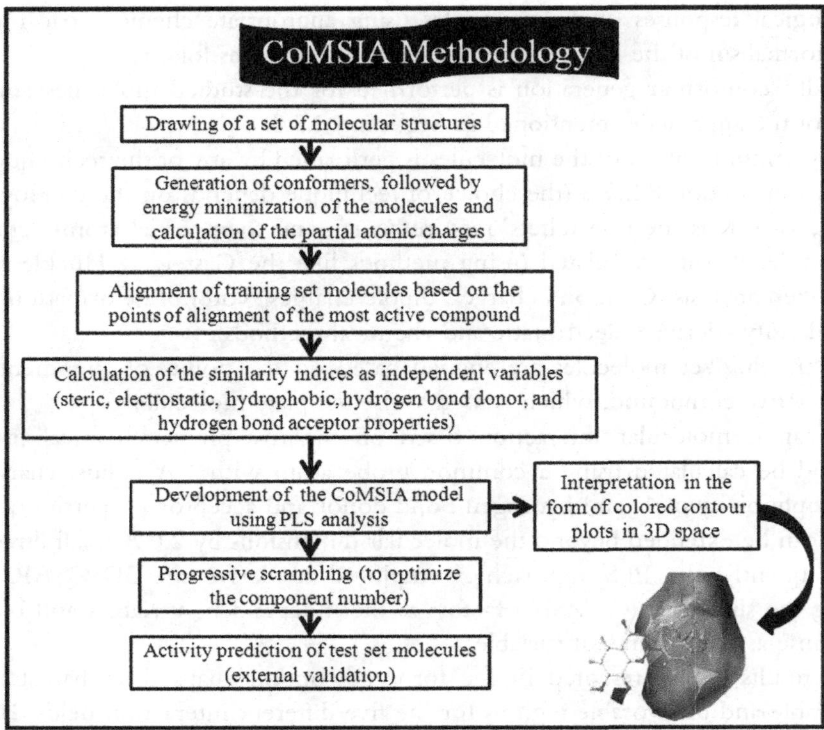

Figure 8.2 The complete methodology of the CoMSIA technique.

with a particular physicochemical property. This relationship between the requisite properties and a possible ligand shape is a more direct guide to authenticate whether all features crucial for response are present in the structures being considered.

8.4 MOLECULAR SHAPE ANALYSIS

8.4.1 Concept of molecular shape analysis

Molecular shape analysis (MSA) is a ligand-based 3D-QSAR approach that attempts to combine conformational analysis with the classical Hansch approach. It deals with the quantitative characterization, representation, and exploitation of molecular shape in the construction of a QSAR model. The overall aim of the MSA [2] is to identify the biologically relevant conformation without having to know the receptor geometry. The MSA, an alignment-dependent approach, incorporates conformational flexibility and shape data into the 3D-QSAR. Multiple conformations of each molecule can be generated using the conformational search method. A conformer of the most active compound is selected as a shape reference compound with which all the structures in the study compounds can be aligned through pairwise superpositioning. This alignment procedure looks at molecules as points and lines, and it uses the techniques of graph theory to identify patterns. It finds the largest subset of atoms in the shape reference compound that is shared by all the structures in the study table and uses this subset for alignment. A rigid fit of atom pairings is performed to superimpose each structure so that it overlays the shape reference compound. The MSA can be performed using Cerius2 software [12] from Accelrys Inc.

8.4.2 Methodology of the MSA

The MSA is an iterative process in which steps are repeated until the molecular shape similarities and other descriptors are checked and adjusted in order to generate a QSAR equation with optimal statistical significance. The goal of MSA is to generate a QSAR equation that incorporates spatial molecular similarity data. The process consists of seven major steps:

1. *Generating conformers and energy minimization*: The purpose of this step is to generate and analyze conformers for each structure to be investigated, and then to reduce the number of conformers to those that are likely to be relevant to biological activity.
2. *Hypothesizing an active conformer (global minimum of the most active compound)*: This step generates a structure that corresponds to the structure present in the rate-limiting step for the biological action. This step typically involves ligand–receptor binding, but it may also involve metabolic activation or deactivation, membrane transport, or formation of a transition state.
3. *Selecting a candidate shape reference compound*: The shape reference compound is the molecule that is used when shape descriptors are calculated for the study matrix. To select the reference compound, each compound in the data set is tested in one or more possible active conformations.
4. *Performing pairwise molecular superimposition*: In this step, pairwise molecular superpositions are performed to find out what and how atoms of data set compounds are equivalent to atoms in the shape reference compound.
5. *Measuring molecular shape commonality*: It involves the calculation of the MSA descriptors to compare the properties that two molecules have in common and to measure molecular shape commonality.
6. *Determining other molecular features*: One can add other molecular properties to the QSAR table by calculating spatial, electronic, and thermodynamic descriptors that comprise possible additional features that govern biological activity.
7. *Generating trial QSAR*: Mathematical equations are generated by the application of genetic function approximation (GFA) or genetic partial least squares (G/PLS) methods.

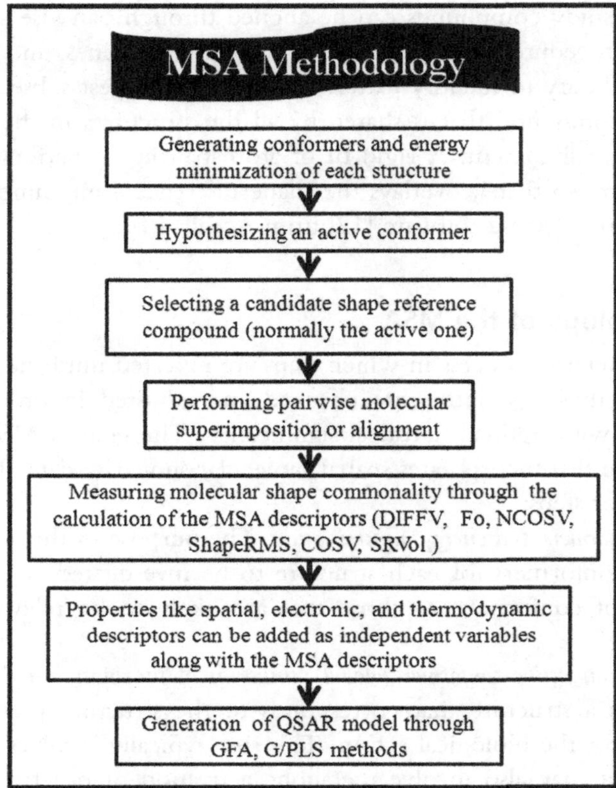

Figure 8.3 The principal steps of the MSA formalism.

A simple graphical illustration of the basic steps of the MSA approach is presented in Figure 8.3.

8.4.3 MSA descriptors

MSA descriptors are used to determine the molecular shape commonality. The most commonly used ones are described here:

- *Difference volume (DIFFV)*: This is the difference between the volume of the individual molecule and the volume of the shape reference compound.
- *Common overlap volume ratio (Fo)*: This is the common overlap steric volume descriptor divided by the volume of the individual molecule.
- *Noncommon overlap steric volume (NCOSV)*: This is the volume of the individual molecule and the common overlap steric volume.
- *RMS to shape reference (ShapeRMS)*: This is the root mean square (RMS) deviation between the individual molecule and the shape reference compound.

- *Common overlap steric volume (COSV)*: This is the common volume between each individual molecule and the molecule selected as the reference compound. This is a measure of how similar in steric shape the analogs are to the shape reference.
- *Volume of shape reference compound (SRVol)*: This is the volume of the shape reference compound.

8.5 RECEPTOR SURFACE ANALYSIS

8.5.1 Concept of receptor surface analysis

Receptor surface analysis (RSA) [13] is a useful tool in situations when the 3D structure of the receptor is unknown, since one can build a hypothetical model of the receptor site. RSA differs from pharmacophore models in that the former tries to capture essential information about the receptor, while the latter captures information about the commonality of compounds that bind to a receptor. A receptor surface model embodies essential information about the hypothetical receptor site as a 3D surface with associated properties, such as hydrophobicity, partial charge, electrostatic potential, van der Waals potential, and hydrogen-bonding propensity. Receptor surface models provide compact, quantitative descriptors that capture 3D information of interaction energies in terms of steric and electrostatic fields at each surface point.

8.5.2 Methodology of the RSA

The major steps of RSA are as follows:

1. The conformers of molecular structures are generated and optimized.
2. Molecules are superimposed in their bioactive conformation.
3. A receptor-complementary surface is generated using shape fields (defined by some distance-dependent function) that enclose a volume common to all the aligned molecules and that represent their aggregate molecular shape.
4. The putative chemical properties of the receptor at every surface point are computed.
5. Mathematical equations are developed by GFA or G/PLS, which correlate surface properties with molecular biological activities.

The principal steps of the RSA formalism are shown in Figure 8.4.

8.5.3 RSA descriptors

The RSA descriptors define the energy of interactions (known as *surface point energies*) between each point on the receptor surface and each model. Depending on the size of the drug molecules, the number of surface points varies. The technique resembles CoMFA, but instead of a rectangular grid, the points considered are taken from the hypothetical receptor surface. Therefore, they are probably more chemically relevant

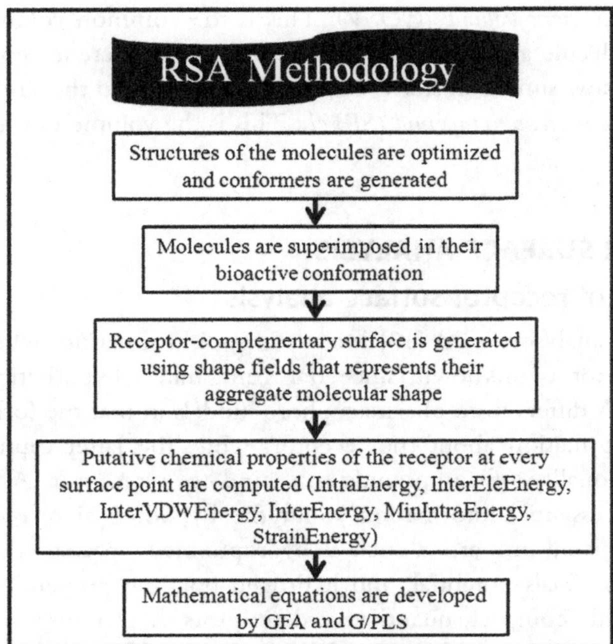

Figure 8.4 The principal steps of the RSA formalism.

than a rectangular grid, because they exist on a surface that is shaped like a molecule—and even better, a surface constructed from a subset of active molecules.

The most commonly used RSA descriptors are the following:

- *IntraEnergy*: Molecular internal energy inside the receptor
- *InterEleEnergy*: Nonbond electrostatic energy between a molecule and the receptor
- *InterVDWEnergy*: Nonbond van der Waals energy between a molecule and the receptor
- *InterEnergy*: Total nonbond energy between a molecule and the receptor
- *MinIntraEnergy*: Molecular internal energy minimized without the receptor
- *StrainEnergy*: Molecular strain energy within the receptor—that is, the difference in internal energy between the molecule minimized within the receptor model (*IntraEnergy*) and the molecule minimized without the receptor model (*MinIntraEnergy*)

8.6 OTHER APPROACHES

8.6.1 Alignment-based 3D-QSAR models

8.6.1.1 Self-organizing molecular field analysis

The self-organizing molecular field analysis (SOMFA) [14] technique has similarities to MSA and CoMFA, as well as to the hypothetical active-site lattice (HASL) method proposed by Doweyko [15]. The mean centered activity is crucial in SOMFA. The fundamental steps of SOMFA are as follows:

a. The mean activity of the training set is subtracted from the activity of each molecule to obtain their mean centered activity values.
b. A 3D grid around the molecules, with values at the grid points signifying the shape or electrostatic potential, is generated.
c. The shape or electrostatic potential value at every grid point for each molecule is multiplied by its mean centered activity.
d. The grid values for each molecule are summed to give the master grids for each property.
e. The so-called $SOMFA_{property,i}$ descriptors from the master grid values are calculated and correlated with the log-transformed molecular activities.

8.6.1.2 Voronoi field analysis

In the Voronoi field analysis (VFA) [16] technique, Voronoi field variables are assigned to each of the Voronoi polyhedra produced by dividing the superimposed molecular space, but not to each of the lattice points as CoMFA does. The methodology to construct VFA-based 3D-QSAR model consists of the following steps:

a. Conformational analysis, energy minimization, and superimposition of all the molecules are executed.
b. The volume occupied by a superimposed set of compounds is divided into subspaces referred to as *Voronoi polyhedrals*, each including a reference point (an atom) with certain coordinates explored in the next steps.
c. A template (the simplest) molecule is selected, and all the atoms of the template molecule are allocated as initial reference points.
d. The largest molecule in the data set is superimposed on the template in terms of the number of atoms, and new reference points are designated if this point is farther than 1 Å away from the reference points identified in step c.
e. Steps c and d are repeated with superimposition of other molecules in decreasing order of their size, each time defining isolated atoms as new reference points by the abovementioned criteria, until all compounds are superimposed.
f. A cuboid with six tangential planes divided into a 3D lattice with a spacing of 0.3 Å, surrounding the union volume of the superposed set of molecules is constructed. This creates the Voronoi polyhedral.
g. The potential and electrostatic energy indices at each lattice point are computed according to the hard-sphere potential model and Coulomb's law, respectively.
h. The PLS algorithm is then applied to correlate independent steric and electrostatic latent variables with the activity index.

8.6.1.3 Molecular quantum similarity measures

The molecular quantum similarity measure (MQSM) is defined by the vectors of the electronic density function as descriptors, which represent the similarity using MQSM [17]. MQSM is optimized by translating and rotating molecular pairs so as to maximize the overlap of their molecular electronic density. In this approach, since the independent variables are a square symmetric matrix consisting of MQSM between molecular pairs, PCA can be performed in order to reduce the number of variables. The methodology is based on the quantification of the similarity between two molecules using the first order density functions of both studied systems. Once the density functions have been calculated, MQSM between two molecules A and B can be computed by direct quantitative comparison, generally defined by the following integral:

$$Z_{AB}(\Omega) = \iint \rho_A(r_1)\Omega(r_1, r_2)\rho_B(r_2)dr_1 r_2 \qquad (8.3)$$

where $\{\rho_A(r_1),\ \rho_B(r_2)\}$ are the respective molecular first-order density functions and $\Omega(r_1,r_2)$ is a positive definite operator used as a weight.

8.6.1.4 Adaptation of the fields for molecular comparison

Adaptation of the fields for molecular comparison (AFMoC) is a 3D-QSAR method involving fields derived from the protein environments. It is also called a "reverse" CoMFA (=AFMoC) approach or "inverted CoMFA" derived from the potential scoring function (drug score) [18]. The methodology of AFMoC is comparable to that of CoMFA and CoMSIA, but the added benefit is the contribution of protein environment in the method. The protein-specific potential fields are created in binding sites, which are employed for the prediction of binding affinity. The basic methodology of AFMoC includes four steps:

1. *Potential field calculation and ligand alignment*: Drug score is a newly constructed, knowledge-based scoring function developed on distance-dependent pair-potentials. The atom-by-atom pairwise potential is computed in the case of ligand and protein environments. These potential values are calculated by means of an appropriate probe at the intersection at each grid point constructed around the binding pocket.
2. *Interaction field calculations*: A potential field map generated for complexes of ligand and receptor is employed as an interaction field to calculate atom type and distance-dependent interaction for each atom at each grid point.
3. *Correlation between interaction field value calculations and binding affinity prediction*: Theoretically calculated interaction field values are correlated with experimentally determined biological affinity for ligands using PLS analysis.
4. *Interpretation*: The results are displayed graphically by using contribution maps.

The distinguishing characteristics of this method are:

- A fitting scoring function is combined with a protein-based CoMFA approach, thus conquering the prerequisite to involve entire ligand training sets.
- The steady shift from commonly valid knowledge-based potentials to protein-specific pair-potentials reflects the amount and the degree of structural diversity existing in the ligand training data.
- Atom-type specific interaction fields are employed that are jointly orthogonal in nature, making the interpretation of the PLS result easy.
- In addition to the enthalpic involvement, the process is anticipated to include the entropic effects resulting from desolvation, since structural knowledge from experimentally determined complexes is transformed into statistical pair potentials.

Recently, the formalism has been modified to account for the multiple ligand conformations in an ensemble of protein configurations. The superior method has been defined as consensus AFMoC (AFMoCcon) [19].

8.6.1.5 Genetically evolved receptor modeling

Genetically evolved receptor modeling (GERM) is a 3D-QSAR approach for constructing useful 3D models of macromolecular binding sites in the absence of experimental structures, like X-ray crystallography and NMR spectroscopy- or homology-modeled structures of the target receptor [20]. The primary requirement for GERM is a structure–activity series for which a sensible alignment of realistic and sensible bioactive conformers has been determined. All the aligned conformers are enclosed in the receptor active site, allocating them as a shell of atoms (analogous to the first layer of atoms in the active site). The allocated shells of atoms are considered an explicit set atom (aliphatic H, aliphatic C, polar H, etc.) and matched at the receptor active site analogous to those originate in the receptor active site. Hence, the shell of aliphatic carbon is disseminated by a uniform sphere of an aligned training set ligands, and the positions of model aliphatic carbon atom and aligned ligand training set are adjusted so that maximum van der Waals interactions are obtained. Once the position of aliphatic carbon has been recognized, their position can be occupied by any of the atom types, including no atom at all. One practical problem arises when the number of shell atoms and their atom types increase: the number of possible combinations rises to a huge value, thereby rendering it impracticable to systematically get the best possible model. To deal with this dilemma and to generate a number of probable conformers into the active site of receptor, the method uses genetic algorithms (GAs). Thereafter, the ligands of the training set are docked into the GA-generated receptor active-site model, one at a time, and intermolecular nonbonded interaction energies like van der Waals and electrostatic terms are calculated employing a chemistry at HARvard Macromolecular

Mechanics (CHARMM) molecular mechanics force field. Finally, the computed interaction energies are correlated with the biological activities of the molecules.

The positive prospect of this method is that the model is accessible as a 3D display of the receptor properties in space. The restriction of the GERM methodology is that it considers only a single conformation of each ligand in the training set, as well as its single orientation in the binding site. Not only that, as this method is oriented on the computation of interaction energies with the hypothetical receptor, it is prone to all the limitations of such methods, including the alignment problem. However, if all the compounds of the set do bind in a manner that does not vary the binding site too much, GERM could be a fine approach.

8.6.1.6 Hint interaction field analysis

Hint interaction field analysis (HIFA) is a newly developed, alignment-dependent 3D-QSAR method employed to calculate empirical hydrophobic interaction [21]. It is important to mention that the method is an extension of the CoMFA approach. As a result of the introduction of hydrophobicity calculation in CoMFA, the predicative capability of this type of QSAR model has enhanced. It calculates key hydrophobic features that are atom-based analogs of the fragment constant. The methodology of HIFA includes two steps:

1. Calculating the hydrophobic field interaction by aligning the ligands (in the same manner as with CoMFA).
2. Placing the aligned ligands into a grid, followed by interpreting the net sum of hydrophobic interaction

8.6.2 Alignment-independent 3D-QSAR models

8.6.2.1 Comparative molecular moment analysis

The comparative molecular moment analysis (CoMMA) technique [22] uses second-order moments of the shape, mass distribution, and charge distributions. These moments relate to center of the mass and center of the dipole. The CoMMA descriptors include principal moments of inertia, magnitudes of dipole moment, and principal quadrupole moment. Descriptors relating charge to mass distributions are defined; that is, magnitudes of projections of dipole upon principal moments of inertia and displacement between center of mass and center of dipole. Finally these molecular moment descriptors are correlated with the biological activities of molecules using the PLS tool.

It is important to mention that CoMMA descriptors are sensitive to molecular conformations, but less sensitive than CoMFA field parameters. The CoMMA descriptors play a potential role in virtual screening and molecular diversity. A web version of the CoMMA program is provided by the IBM informatics group [23]. A slight variant of this approach, termed as CoMMA2, has also been developed recently [24].

8.6.2.2 Weighted holistic invariant molecular descriptor analysis

Weighted holistic invariant molecular (WHIM) [25] descriptors provide invariant information by employing the PCA on the constructed coordinates (Cartesian coordinates around the *x*-, *y*-, *z*-axes) of the atoms constituting the molecule. This transforms the molecule into the space that captures the most variance. In this space, several statistics are calculated, including variance, proportions, symmetry, and kurtosis, and serve as directional descriptors. By combining the directional descriptors, nondirectional descriptors are also defined. The WHIM descriptors are calculated from the Cartesian coordinates of a molecule within different weighting schemes, such as atomic mass, van der Waals volume and Mulliken atomic electronegativity, atomic electronegativity, atomic polarizability, the electrotopological index of Kier and Hall, and molecular electrostatic potential. These descriptors contain information about the 3D structure of a molecule, such as size, shape, symmetry, and atomic distribution. The molecular surface (MS)–WHIM indices are computed from MS points weighted by their molecular electrostatic potential values by applying a WHIM-based mathematical approach. The grid-weighted holistic invariant molecular (G-WHIM) is a modification of the WHIM method where G-WHIM descriptors are calculated using Grid [26].

8.6.2.3 VolSurf

The VolSurf [27] approach is based on probing the grid around the molecule with specific probes. The resulting lattice boxes are used to compute the descriptors relying on volumes or surfaces of 3D contours, defined by the same value of the probe molecule interaction energy. By using various probes and cutoff values of the energy, various molecular properties can be quantified. Derivative quantities (e.g., molecular globularity or factors relating the surface of hydrophobic or hydrophilic regions to surface of the whole molecule) can also be computed. VolSurf is employed as a computational procedure for predicting the absorption, distribution, metabolism, and excretion (ADME) properties of a molecule.

8.6.2.4 Compass

Compass, developed by Jain et al. [28], is a method that automatically chooses the conformations and alignments of molecules. In Compass, each molecule is represented by a different set of feature values. Three types of features (steric, hydrogen bond donor, and acceptor) are used in this approach. Donor and acceptor feature values are measured as the distance from the sampling points scattered near the surface of the molecules to the nearest hydrogen bond donor and acceptor groups, respectively. Steric distances are computed from the sampling points to the nearest atom. The probable methodology to execute the Compass is as follows:

a. Conformational analysis is carried out to determine the probable bioactive conformation of each ligand.

b. Descriptors measuring surface shape or polar functionality of each ligand's pose in a specific alignment in the vicinity of a particular point in space are computed.
c. A neural network is constructed and models built, and realignment of molecules is continuously carried out to achieve the best fit to the binding site with improvements in the neural network model.
d. The final model is developed from these improved and realigned molecular poses.

8.6.2.5 GRID

The GRID program is a computational procedure similar to CoMFA [29]. It is used in order to predict specific noncovalent interactions between a molecule of known 3D structure and a small chemical group (the probe) whose properties are defined by the user. Probes are placed on the grid points, and interaction energies with a molecule are calculated. Therefore, GRID calculates not only steric and electrostatic potential, but also the hydrogen-bonding potential using a hydrogen bond donor and acceptor, and the hydrophobic potential using a "DRY probe." The energies calculated with the water probe using GRID contain the steric and hydrogen bonding interaction energies. Since the water probe is not only electrically neutral, but can also donate and accept a hydrogen bond, the energies determined using this probe are supposed to grip steric and hydrogen-bonding interactions as well, while also representing the hydrophobic interaction energy like logP due to its molecular surface area. Along with the water and DRY probes, other probes that are regularly used singly include the methyl group, the amine (NH_2) group, the carboxylate group, and the hydroxyl group. Contour surfaces are calculated at various energy levels for each probe for every point on the grid and are displayed graphically along with the protein structure. While negative energy levels of the contours describe regions at which ligand binding should be favored, positive energy levels normally characterize the shape of the target.

Although this approach is comparable to CoMFA, as it too computes explicit nonbonded interactions between a molecule of known 3D structure and a probe located at the sample positions on a lattice throughout and around the macromolecule, it offers two distinct advantages:

- The use of a 6–4 potential function for calculating the interaction energies, which is smoother than the 6–12 form of the Lennard–Jones type in CoMFA
- The availability of different types of probes to make the calculation more diverse and wide open

The aim of this method is to calculate the interaction energy fields in MFA and to determine the energetically favorable binding sites on molecules with a known structure. The GRID software, supplied by Molecular Discovery Ltd [30], generates a novel class of molecular descriptors that we are calling *grid-independent descriptors (GRIND)*.

8.6.2.6 Comparative spectral analysis

The comparative spectral analysis (CoSA) method has employed molecular spectroscopy techniques to determine the 3D molecular descriptors of chemical compounds [31]. The molecular spectra are utilized to predict biological activity of the 3D structures. The spectroscopic method generally comprises proton (^{1}H)-NMR, carbon (^{13}C)-NMR, IR, and mass spectrometry. The basic steps of this method are as follows:

a. The data computed through spectroscopic studies are converted into matrices with the assistance of an appropriate tool.

b. The developed data matrix is correlated with the experimental biological activity by using PLS analysis.

c. The mathematical equation is interpreted, and the important structural fragments for the activity of the studied compounds are identified.

8.6.2.7 Quantum chemical parameters in QSAR analysis

In QSAR analysis, quantum chemical parameters provide information regarding the electronic effects of compounds, considering atom-by-atom as well as cumulative electronic profiles of the chemical structure. The application of quantum chemical procedures and the indices was restricted to the Hückel molecular orbital (HMO) and extended HMO (EHMO) methods for a long time due to limited computational resources, although descriptors computed at higher levels of theory have been used recently. The Hartree–Fock self-consistent field (SCF) method is the most common approach used for solving the electronic Schrödinger equation [32]. The molecular Schrödinger equations have undergone a significant amount of implementation with the discovery and use of a wide variety of *ab initio* and semiempirical quantum-chemical methods [33]. Atomic charges (qX), molecular orbital energies (such as EHOMO, ELUMO, and ELUMO–EHOMO), superdelocalizabilities (Sr), molecular polarizability (α), dipole moments (μ), and energies (ET) are some of the descriptors used for semiempirical analysis.

8.7 OVERVIEW AND CONCLUSIONS

There is no doubt about the usefulness of the 3D-QSAR approaches compared to 2D-QSAR, as the former can handle more diverse structures. However, the 3D approaches still have some shortcomings; for example, a very large number of compounds cannot be handled at a time and just for this reason, one still has to employ the high-throughput virtual screening method. Exploration of the active conformation of flexible compounds in the study set is critical, followed by the specification for the molecular alignment in constructing a 3D-QSAR model. The intermolecular interactions with receptors also need to be studied because different types of interaction may take place at different sites. Despite all the pitfalls, the usefulness of the mentioned 3D-QSAR approaches have been globally established and recognized in the drug design and discovery process. The ever-increasing information from structural biology will present valuable feedback to the assumptions that form the basis of 3D-QSAR methods. Before applying the predictive models to real-life situations, one must look at the technicalities of the underlying QSAR methodologies in order to avoid their improper use and misapprehension. More specifically, the problems associated with alignment dependency and conformational sensitivity must be considered carefully to reduce the chance of error. A comprehensive understanding and error-free practice of these strategies in QSAR modeling should assist medicinal chemists in prioritizing their experimental endeavors and significantly intensify the experimental hits.

REFERENCES

[1] Akamatsu M. Current state and perspectives of 3D-QSAR. Curr Top Med Chem 2002; 2:1381–94.

[2] Hopfinger AJ, Tokarski JS. Three-dimensional quantitative structure–activity relationship analysis. In: Charifson PS, editor. Practical application of computer-aided drug design. New York, NY: Marcel Dekker, Inc.; 1997. pp. 105–64.

[3] Oprea TI. 3D QSAR modeling in drug design. In: Bultinck P, Winter HD, Langenaeker W, Tollenaere JP, editors. Computational medicinal chemistry for drug discovery. New York, NY: Marcel Dekker, Inc.; 2004. pp. 571–616.

[4] Bolton EE, Kim S, Bryant SH. PubChem3D: conformer generation. J Cheminform 2011;3:4.

[5] Cramer III RD, Patterson DE, Bunce JD. Comparative molecular field analysis (CoMFA). i. Effect of shape on binding of steroids to carrier proteins. J Am Chem Soc 1988;110(18):5959–67.

[6] Kim KH. Comparative molecular field analysis (CoMFA). In: Dean PM, editor. Molecular similarity in drug design. Glasgow, UK: Blackie Academic & Professional; 1995. pp. 291–331.

[7] Allen F. The Cambridge structural database: a quarter of a million crystal structures and rising. Acta Crystallogr B 2002;58:380–8.

[8] Berman HM, Westbrook J, Feng Z, Gilliland G, Bhat TN, Weissig H, et al. The protein data bank. Nucleic Acids Res 2000;28(1):235–42.

[9] Norinder U. Recent progress in CoMFA methodology and related techniques. In: Kubinyi H, Folkers G, Martin YC, editors. 3D QSAR in drug design—recent advances, vol. 3. New York, NY: Kluwer Academic Publishers; 1998. pp. 24–39.

[10] Richard D, Cramer III RD, Bunce JD, Patterson DE, Frank IE. Crossvalidation, bootstrapping, and partial least squares compared with multiple regression in conventional QSAR studies. Quant Struct-Act Relat 1988;7:18–25.

[11] Klebe G, Abraham U, Mietzner T. Molecular similarity indices in a comparative analysis (CoMSIA) of drug molecules to correlate and predict their biological activity. J Med Chem 1994;37(24): 4130–46.

[12] Cerius2, version 4.8; Accelrys Inc.: San Diego, CA; 1998.

[13] Hahn M. Receptor surface models. 1. Definition and construction. J Med Chem 1995;38(12):2080–90.

[14] Robinson DD, Winn PJ, Lyne PD, Richards WG. Self-organizing molecular field analysis: a tool for structure–activity studies. J Med Chem 1999;42(4):573–83.

[15] Doweyko A. The hypothetic al active site lattice. An approach to modelling active sites from data on inhibitor molecules. J Med Chem 1988;31(7):1396–406.

[16] Chuman H, Karasawa M, Fujita T. A novel three-dimensional QSAR procedure: Voronoi field analysis. Quant Struct-Act Relat 1998;17(4):313–26.

[17] Amat L, Robert D, Besalu E, Carbo-Dorca R. Molecular quantum similarity measures tuned 3D QSAR: an antitumoral family validation study. J Chem Inf Comput Sci 1998;38:624–31.
[18] Silber K, Heidler P, Kurz T, Klebe G. AFMoC enhances predictivity of 3D QSAR: a case study with DOXP-reductoisomerase. J Med Chem 2005;48(10):3547–63.
[19] Breu B, Silber K, Gohlke H. Consensus adaptation of fields for molecular comparison (AFMoC) models incorporate ligand and receptor conformational variability into tailor-made scoring functions. J Chem Inf Model 2007;47:2383–400.
[20] Walters DE, Hinds RM. Genetically evolved receptor models: a computational approach to construction of receptor models. J Med Chem 1994;37:2527–36.
[21] Semus SF. A novel hydropathic intermolecular field analysis (HIFA) for the prediction of ligand–receptor binding affinities. Med Chem Res 1999;9(7–8):535–47.
[22] Silverman BD, Platt DE. Comparative molecular moment analysis (CoMMA): 3D-QSAR without molecular superposition. J Med Chem 1996;39(11):2129–40.
[23] CoMMA. IBM Bioinformatics Group, <http://cbcsrv.watson.ibm.com/Tco.html> [accessed 16.10.14].
[24] Silverman BD. Three-dimensional moments of molecular property fields. J Chem Inf Comput Sci 2000;40:1470–6.
[25] Todeschini R, Lasagni M, Marengo E. New molecular descriptors for 2D- and 3D-structures. J Chemom 1994;8:263–73.
[26] Bravi G, Gancia E, Mascagni P, Pegna M, Todeschini R, Zaliani A. MS-WHIM, new 3D theoretical descriptors derived from molecular surface properties: a comparative 3D-QSAR study in a series of steroids. J Comput Aided Mol Des 1997;11:79–92.
[27] Crivori P, Cruciani G, Carrupt PA, Testa B. Predicting blood–brain barrier permeation from three-dimensional molecular structure. J Med Chem 2000;43(11):2204–16.
[28] Jain AN, Koile K, Chapman D. Compass: predicting biological activities from molecular surface properties. Performance comparisons on a steroid benchmark. J Med Chem 1994;37(15):2315–27.
[29] Goodford PJ. A computational procedure for determining energetically favorable binding sites on biologically important macromolecules. J Med Chem 1985;28(7):849–57.
[30] GRID. Molecular Discovery Ltd., <http://www.moldiscovery.com/soft_grid.php> [accessed 19.10.14].
[31] Asikainen A, Ruuskanen J, Tuppurainen K. Spectroscopic QSAR methods and self-organizing molecular field analysis for relating molecular structure and estrogenic activity. J Chem Inf Comput Sci 2003;43(6):1974–81.
[32] Roothaan CC, Sachs J, Lester M, Weiss AW. Analytical self-consistent field functions for the atomic configurations 1s2, 1s22s, and 1s22s2. Rev Mod Phys 1960;32:186.
[33] Karelson M, Lobanov VS, Katritzky AR. Quantum-chemical descriptors in QSAR/QSPR studies. Chem Rev 1996;96(3):1027.

CHAPTER 9

Newer QSAR Techniques

Contents

Understanding the Basics of QSAR for Applications in Pharmaceutical Sciences and Risk Assessment.
ISBN: 978-0-12-801505-6, DOI: http://dx.doi.org/10.1016/B978-0-12-801505-6.00009-0

9.1 INTRODUCTION

Drug design is driven by innovation and technological advancement involving a combination of sophisticated experimental and computational approaches. Innovation in medicinal chemistry and biology has generated an imperative foundation in the search for new drug candidates. With the advances in scientific knowledge, high-performance hardware, and sophisticated software, a new wave of drug discovery has emerged in pharmaceutical research and development (R&D) through computational chemistry [1]. Quantitative structure–activity relationship (QSAR) methods are among the most important computational strategies that have been applied for the identification of hits, generation of leads, and finally optimization of these leads into drug candidates over the past 10 years [2].

Among the newer QSAR techniques, hologram-based QSAR (HQSAR) has emerged as one of the powerful new two-dimensional (2D) fragment-based QSAR (FB-QSAR) techniques where specialized molecular fragments are employed. HQSAR is fast and easy to use, and it can accurately predict activity for lead identification, facilitating future synthesis programs. A number of recent publications have shown that HQSAR can give results comparable to complicated and exhaustive 3D-QSAR techniques, but the former is much easier to use [3,4]. A new method called *group-based QSAR (G-QSAR)* uses descriptors evaluated for the fragments of the molecules generated using specific fragmentation rules [5]. Another simple QSAR method based on 2D image analysis for congeneric series of compounds is known as *multivariate image analysis QSAR (MIA-QSAR)* developed by Freitas et al. [6]. MIA has been used in chemical problems by using spectral data and widely used in the fields of scientific imaging for a long time. With the advancement of computation tools, new methods like *Laboratório de QuimiometriaTeórica e Aplicada* QSAR (LQTA-QSAR) [7], *ensemble* QSAR (*e*QSAR) [8], and other novel approaches like FB-QSAR, fragment-similarity-based QSAR (FS-QSAR), self-organizing map QSAR (SOM-QSAR), QUASAR (5D-QSAR), 6D-QSAR, and 7D-QSAR have been introduced by QSAR researchers with the intention of making the study of QSAR more useful, productive, and interpretable for designing new drug candidates with enhancement of the general acceptability of QSARs to the scientific community [9,10].

9.2 HQSAR

9.2.1 Concept of HQSAR

HQSAR is a modern technique based on the concept of using molecular substructures expressed in a binary pattern (i.e., fingerprints) as descriptors in QSAR models. HQSAR is a 2D FB-QSAR method that employs specialized molecular 2D fingerprints. HQSAR [11] does not require any physicochemical descriptors or three-dimensional (3D) structures to generate the structure–activity model. In this method, 2D structures and biological activity are used as inputs and the structures are converted to all possible linear, branched, and overlapping fragments. These fragments are assigned to integer values using a cyclic redundancy check algorithm, and these integer values are used to make a fixed-length integer array. These arrays are known as *molecular holograms*, and space occupancies of the molecular holograms are used as descriptors. The fundamental difference from other fragment-based techniques is that it encodes all possible fragments, including overlapping fragments. Partial least squares (PLS) regression is used to build the model, which is validated by the leave-one-out (LOO) method. The final model (as represented in the following equation) is obtained using PLS:

$$A_i = C + \sum_{i=1}^{L} X_{il} C_{il} \tag{9.1}$$

In Eq. (9.1), A_i is the activity of compound i, X_{il} is the hologram occupancy value at position i or bin l, C is a constant, C_{il} is the coefficient for the corresponding bin from the PLS run, and L is the hologram length.

9.2.2 How to develop an HQSAR model

The HQSAR technique involves three main steps [12]: (i) generation of substructural fragments for each of the training set molecules, (ii) representation of the fragments in the form of holograms, and (iii) correlation of the molecular holograms with the activity data of the training set compounds using the PLS technique to generate an HQSAR model. The bin occupancies of the molecular holograms are the structural descriptors encoding the specific compositional and topological molecular information. A graphical illustration of the generation of molecular holograms and the HQSAR model is demonstrated in Figure 9.1.

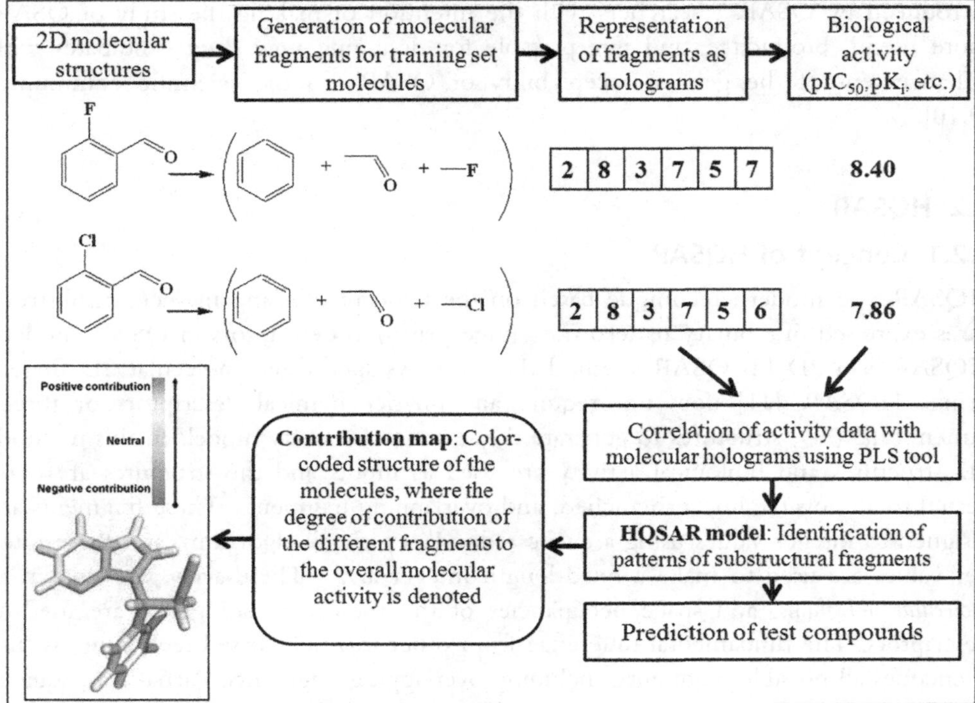

Figure 9.1 A flowchart for HQSAR model development.

The number and nature of fragments denoting the molecular fingerprint are specified based on the minimum (*M*) and maximum (*N*) number of atoms in a fragment. The substructure fingerprints are then hashed into hologram bins of varying lengths (*L*), such as 53, 59, 61, 71, and 97. A *hologram bin* is an integer array with a fixed length ranging from 50 to 500. The molecular fingerprint maintains a count of the frequency of the various molecular fragment types occupying each bin of the fixed-length array. The array refers to the molecular hologram, while the bin occupancies represent the descriptor variables.

The various type of fragments thus obtained are placed into different bins, with similar ones occupying the same bin. The molecular holograms are then correlated with the activity data based on PLS analysis, and the number of components yielding optimally predictive models is determined using the LOO cross-validation (LOO-CV) technique. The graphical display of the HQSAR analysis provides a color-coded structure of the molecules, where the degree of contribution of the different fragments to the overall molecular activity is denoted by a specific color. As an example, we can cite that in the case of SYBYL software [13], the colors at the red end of the spectrum reflect poor contributions, while those at the green end show favorable contributions; and white atoms signify intermediate contributions and cyan ones refer to the common skeleton shared by all training set compounds. It is interesting to point out that the color codes may vary from software to software. The chance of overfitting the developed model should be reduced by limiting the maximum number of components to $R/5$ (with R being the number of training set compounds). Followed by the selection of the component number, the QSAR analysis should be redone and the final PLS model obtained with the optimum component number based on the specific fragment distinction parameters, fragment size, and bin length. A statistically significant HQSAR model with an optimum number of components should be selected based on the maximum value of Q^2 and the minimum value of cross-validated standard error (SE_{cv}). The HQSAR model should be validated using the test set compounds, and the accuracy of prediction of the test set activity data is judged based on the value of the R^2_{pred} (Q^2_{ext}) parameter.

9.2.3 HQSAR parameters

HQSAR models can be affected by a number of parameters considering hologram generation [11,12]. All the parameters are demonstrated through a graphical illustration in Figure 9.2. The parameters are discussed in detail in the next sections of this chapter.

9.2.3.1 Hologram length

Hologram length is a user-defined parameter that controls the number of bins in the hologram fingerprint. As the hologram length (L) is considerably less than the number of fragments in most of the compounds, modifying it will cause the pattern of bin

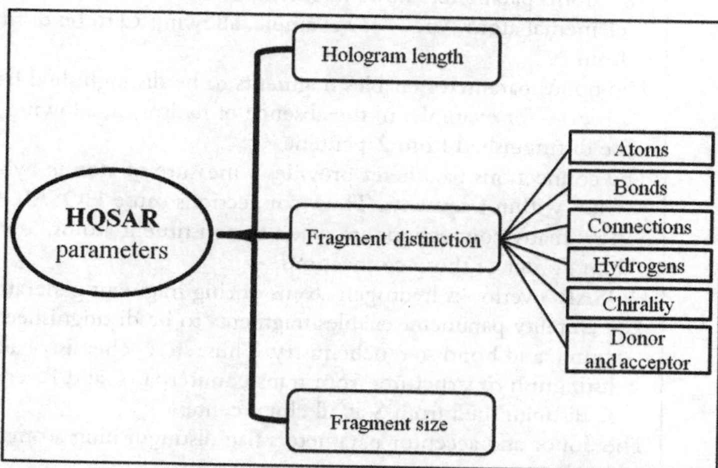

Figure 9.2 HQSAR parameters.

occupancies in data-set holograms to change. Certain patterns of fragment disposition in the molecular holograms enable PLS to more readily detect the relationship between fragments present in the data set and the variance in the biological activity.

9.2.3.2 Fragment size

Fragment size controls the minimum and maximum lengths of fragments to be included in the hologram fingerprint. Molecular holograms are produced by the generation of all linear and branched fragments between *M* and *N* atoms in size. The parameters *M* and *N* can be changed to include smaller or larger fragments in the holograms.

9.2.3.3 Fragment distinction

HQSAR allows fragments to be distinguished based on various parameters, which are defined in Table 9.1.

9.2.4 Why use HQSAR over other techniques?

A key dissimilarity between HQSAR fingerprints and traditional 2D fingerprints is that 2D fingerprints are binary strings that record the presence or absence of substructures, while molecular holograms contain all possible molecular fragments within a molecule and maintain a count of the number of times each unique fragment occurs. HQSAR encodes all possible fragments within a molecule, as well as each of the constituent subfragments. This feature allows HQSAR to encode imperative regiospecific information about fragments [11,12].

Table 9.1 Fragment distinction parameters

Atoms	The atoms parameter allows fragments to be determined based on elemental atom types—for example, allowing *O* to be distinguished from *N*.
Bonds	The bonds parameter enables fragments to be distinguished based on bond orders—for example, in the absence of hydrogen, allowing pentane to be distinguished from 2-pentene.
Connections	The connections parameter provides a measure of atomic hybridization states within fragments. Thus, connections cause HQSAR to identify how many connections are made to constituent atoms, as well as the bond order of those connections.
Hydrogens	HQSAR overlooks hydrogen atoms during fragment generation.
Chirality	The chirality parameter enables fragments to be distinguished based on atomic and bond stereochemistry. Thus, stereochemistry allows to distinguish *cis* structures from trans counterparts, and R-enantiomers to be distinguished from S at all chiral centers.
Donor and acceptor	The donor and acceptor parameters flag distinguishing atoms matching the donor and acceptor properties.

Activity variation with the shift of a substituent around a ring system can be readily identified by the HQSAR approach. In addition, HQSAR can distinguish fragments using stereochemical and hybridization state information features that have not been incorporated in other fragment-based methods. HQSAR typically produces correlations that are comparable to 3D-QSAR techniques, such as comparative molecular field analysis (CoMFA), but avoids the time-consuming step of 3D model generation and mutual alignment in 3D space [12]. The technique offers the following advantages over complex 3D techniques:

- HQSAR builds quantitative models that correlate the biological activity or property to the chemical structure and provides a precise prediction of the activity of untested molecules.
- It eliminates the need for generation of 3D structures, putative binding conformations, and molecular alignments.
- It provides a visual display of the active centers in compounds that indicates the fragments contributing maximally to the activity profile of the compounds. Color coding of atoms in molecular fragments indicates a positive or negative contribution to the property of interest.
- It is applicable to large data sets as well as traditional-size sets.
- It allows rapid identification of the structure–activity relationship profile of a data set.
- It searches databases to make predictions for collections of structures.

The advantages of HQSAR over the traditional 2D fingerprints and 3D-QSAR techniques are graphically illustrated in Figure 9.3.

9.2.5 Application of HQSAR models

The main purpose of studying HQSAR is to explore individual atomic contribution to molecular bioactivity with a visual display of active centers in the compounds. Thus, the drug design process can be very fruitfully facilitated by studying QSAR. HQSAR has been successfully applied in different stages of drug discovery by various groups of researchers.

9.2.5.1 A flexible tool in drug design

Many HQSAR models have been generated for a variety of ligands of important molecular targets, including cases where the crystal structure of the target protein is not yet available [14–17]. One has to recognize that along with the prediction of potency and affinity of untested compounds, HQSAR models can provide useful insight into the relationships between structural fragments and biological activity. These fragments can be simply visualized through the generation of contribution maps that replicate the individual contribution of each atom or structural fragment for a query compound. This information, combined with synthetic and medicinal

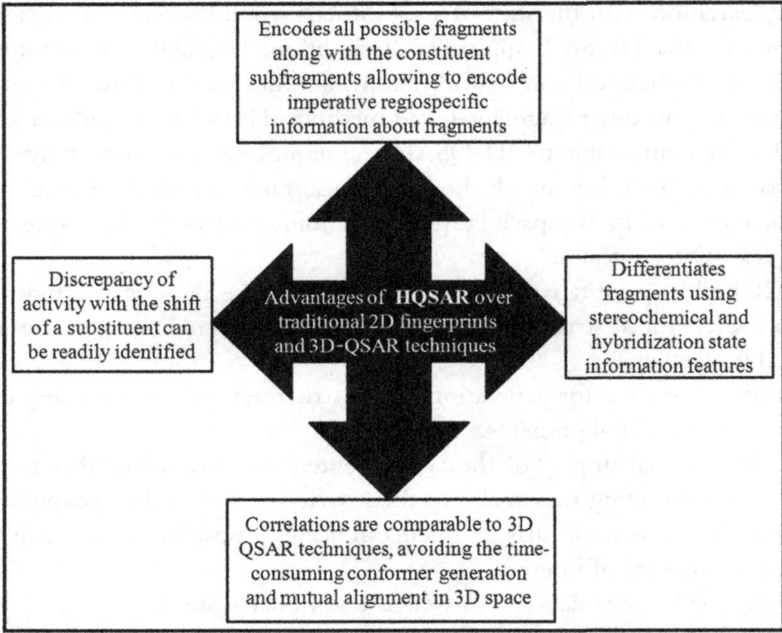

Figure 9.3 The advantages of HQSAR over traditional 2D fingerprints and 3D-QSAR techniques.

chemistry knowledge, could lead to the synthesis of new drug molecules with improved potency. Thus, HQSAR can be considered a flexible tool in drug design.

As an example, we can cite that the most potent compound of a large collection of 9-substituted-9-deazaguanine analogs that inhibit human purine nucleoside phosphorylase (PNP) enzyme has been identified by Castilho et al. [3] with the application of the 2D-HQSAR contribution map. The contribution map allowed the recognition of key structural components essential for intermolecular interactions in the protein active site. Analyzing the contribution map of the most potent inhibitor, the authors concluded that the molecular fragments for the purine ring and cyanil moieties are strongly involved in the inhibitory profile of the compound. Thus, it is possible to identify responsible atomic contributions of a query molecule of increased potency in the absence of the 3D crystal structure of PNP or any other 3D structural information. On the other hand, when 3D structural information is present, this allows a comparison of the HQSAR results to determine if they are in agreement with the 3D chemical environment of the target protein.

HQSAR models have been used in combination with both classical 2D-QSAR and 3D-QSAR methods, suggesting that this method is a valuable tool for lead optimization and drug design process [15–18]. These complementary methods have effectively allowed the integration of additional features in the interpretation of HQSAR models in terms of their chemical and biological significance [19]. As a descriptive example of the amalgamation of QSAR strategies, a study of a large series of flavanoids, dihydrobenzoxathiins, and dihydrobenzodithiins as estrogen receptor (ER) modulators demonstrated that HQSAR and CoMFA can be carried out concurrently to search for a potent drug molecule [4]. The molecular fragments identified by the HQSAR model are strongly correlated to the binding affinity of this series of ligands, which is in accordance with the CoMFA results shown in the steric and electrostatic contour maps. In another study, Avery et al. [20] reported 3D-QSAR (CoMFA) and HQSAR models for a series of 211 artemisinin analogs to develop more potent and less neurotoxic agents for the oral treatment of drug-resistant malaria. The authors found that predictions made with CoMFA and HQSAR models on the test set compounds were in reasonable agreement with the experimentally determined values.

The role of HQSAR in the drug design is evident, and it is enormously vital to realize that the information collected from the patterns of substructural fragments is associated with essential ligand–receptor interactions. We can cite here that in the absence of tubulin-bound discodermolide crystal structures, Salum et al. [21] recently utilized HQSAR to generate molecular recognition patterns that were then combined with molecular modeling studies as a step for the understanding of crucial discodermolide–tubulin interactions associated with the high antiproliferative activity of discodermolide analogs.

9.2.5.2 Mathematical correlation to activity/property prediction

HQSAR has been employed to construct models with internal and external robustness, as well as predictivity. The basic approach of HQSAR can be tactically applied in virtual screening (VS) strategies for the identification of hits [22–24]. The analysis of large data sets generated by combinatorial chemistry and high-throughput screening (HTS) techniques has demonstrated the versatility and range of applications of HQSAR. HQSAR includes several desirable characteristics, such as versatility and reliability. The method is suitable for the identification of important structural fragments and for the rapid evaluation and prediction of large chemical libraries, as well as for database mining.

The originality of this method is that it can distinguish the most important structural fragments related to activity and associate them with unique 2D structural characteristics, which can be found in data sets of chemically diverse compounds. Importantly, HQSAR models carry a set of 2D chemical and structural features that can be quantitatively translated into specific 3D ligand–protein interactions. Furthermore, the attribution of diverse weights to differentiate the relative contribution of molecular fragments is directed by experimental values. Statistically robust HQSAR models have been generated for a set of indole derivatives consisting potent anticancer activity for accurate prediction of the activity [25,26].

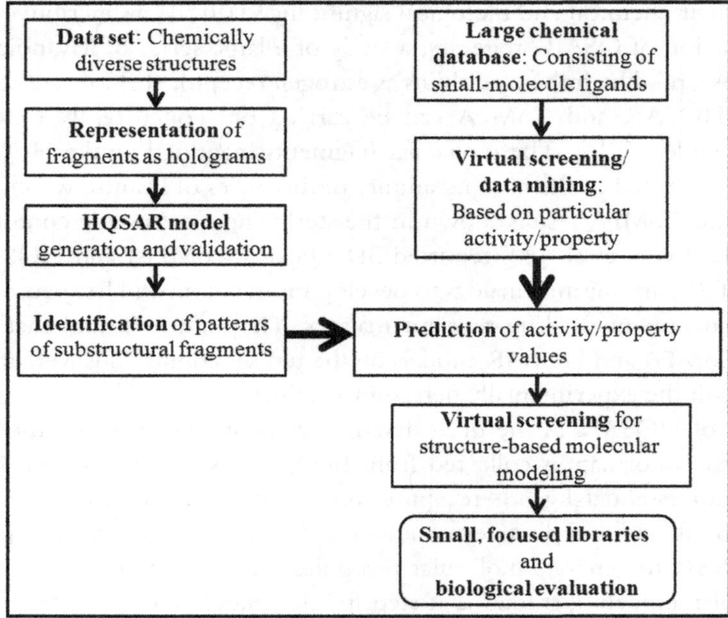

Figure 9.4 Integration of HQSAR models and virtual screening in drug design.

The computational approach can be employed to search large chemical databases to identify probable hits for a given biological target. Identified molecular recognition patterns from HQSAR models can be combined with the structure-based VS, which is graphically illustrated in Figure 9.4. The integration of fragment-based methods and structure-based VS strategies can be utilized successfully in the coming years.

9.2.5.3 Pharmacokinetic studies and ADME prediction

Along with properties like efficacy, potency, and selectivity, a drug should possess desirable pharmacokinetic/dynamic characteristics and safety. Properties such as absorption, distribution, metabolism, and excretion (ADME) have been recently considered in early phases of drug discovery, as undesirable pharmacokinetic properties can negatively affect the clinical development of new drug molecules [27,28]. In terms of resources, reagents, and detection techniques, in vitro and in vivo ADME assays are quite lengthy, complex, and relatively expensive. In this perspective, a variety of useful *in silico* ADME models have been developed for the screening of large data sets of compounds, which can be used as faster, simpler, and cheaper tools than the experimental ones [28].

More recently, it has been observed that reliable HQSAR models have been successfully developed and validated for data sets of highly diverse compounds belonging to various therapeutic classes [29,30]. It is interesting to point out that the HQSAR patterns of substructural fragments could also be useful in pharmacokinetic studies comparing traditional mechanism-based pharmacodynamic modeling. The identified substructural patterns for a particular class of chemicals can be employed as ADME filters in the process of chemical library design and VS. The high chemical diversity and the conformation-independent characteristics signify distinctive advantages in the application of the HQSAR method for ADME property prediction.

9.3 G-QSAR

9.3.1 Concept of G-QSAR

G-QSAR [5] is a novel extrapolation of the FB-QSAR technique that allows establishing a correlation of chemical group variation at different molecular sites of interest with the corresponding biological activity. The technique aims at deriving a quantitative relationship between the activity and descriptors calculated for various molecular fragments of interest using specific fragmentation rules. It provides an ease of interpretation of the essential requisites of the different substituents by not only suggesting the important descriptors, but also reflecting the site where they have to be optimized for the design of new molecules. G-QSAR uses the known 2D/3D descriptors for the different fragments and also includes interaction of fragments using cross-terms that are evaluated as products of vectors of fragment descriptors and used as descriptors.

The advantage of the G-QSAR technique is that it considers the substituent interactions as fragment-specific descriptors to account for the fragment interactions in QSAR model. The 2D-QSAR approaches could only suggest important descriptors, whereas the G-QSAR approach not only reflects the descriptors, but also the site where they have to be optimized for the design of new molecules [5]. Thus, it may be inferred that the G-QSAR approach is a modification of the classical QSAR concept of Hansch, which deals with the calculation of physicochemical and structural parameters specific for the position and type of substitution.

9.3.2 Background of evaluation of G-QSAR method

In the classical Hansch method, substituent properties like Hammett and Taft constants, which are related to chemical environment and steric properties of groups, are used as descriptors for QSAR [31]. The interesting point here is that the substituent constants are completely independent of each other and interactions among them are completely ignored. Again, usually QSAR models are developed from several molecular descriptors such as topological, electronic, structural, and spatial, but the major problem is that these descriptors represent the properties of the whole molecule, ignoring corresponding group contributions. Whole-molecular descriptors have played a significant role in developing quantitative relationship with the activity, but the true interpretation of these traditional QSAR models has always been a challenge to QSAR researchers. The major drawback of these models is that they do not specify the site at which modification is required for the future design of the drug entity.

Consequently, one of the 3D-QSAR techniques, CoMFA, considered descriptors like steric and electrostatic fields calculated at the grid points generated from aligned molecules [32]. As the descriptor space is huge, to reduce dimensionality, models are developed by using regression methods such as PLS. The major advantage of this method is that the model can provide good clues for designing new drug entities by specifying a position along with its steric and electrostatic requirements. However, the major limitations of this method are its dependency on molecular alignment and selection of conformers for the alignment. This feature becomes critical in two cases: first, when the information of bioactive conformation is absent; and second, when the molecule framework is not rigid.

Thus, a QSAR method that allows flexibility to study molecular sites of interest and capture interactions among them is needed. Again, unlike 3D-QSAR methods, this method should not rely on conformational analysis and molecular alignment to identify the sites and way of interactions liable for the activity difference. With this as the background, Ajmani et al. [5] have developed G-QSAR, which allows easy interpretation, unlike any conventional QSAR method. The foremost advantage of this method is that it reflects the site where it has to be optimized for the design of new molecules. The advantage of G-QSAR over HQSAR is that G-QSAR considers the substituent interactions as fragment-specific descriptors when accounting for the fragment interactions in the QSAR model.

9.3.3 G-QSAR methodology

Existing methods like the Free—Wilson approach and HQSAR (as discussed earlier) use fragment descriptors for the generation of QSAR models [5,33—35]. However, the relatively new method G-QSAR differs from them in two ways:

1. In G-QSAR, fragmentation of each molecule is done adhering to a set of predefined rules before their respective fragment descriptors are calculated. This is totally different from the existing methods, which search a predefined group in the molecule and then use traditional 2D/3D descriptors for the different fragments of the molecules for a series of compounds.
2. G-QSAR considers cross-interaction terms as descriptors to explain the fragment interactions in the QSAR model, whereas there is no reflection of these descriptors in the existing methods.

G-QSAR methodology can be precisely explained in three steps, which are detailed in the next sections.

9.3.3.1 Molecular fragmentation

The G-QSAR technique begins with the fragmentation of the molecules under study [5]. The fragmentation of a molecule becomes simple while working with a set of congeneric molecules. The number of sites at which the substituents are present form the different fragments for a given molecule. For example, we can demonstrate that R_1 and R_2 are the substitution sites of a congeneric series of chromone derivatives for antioxidant activity (Figure 9.5). For the G-QSAR study of this set of compounds, the molecules can be divided into two fragments composed of various substitutions at two sites R_1 and R_2.

On the other hand, for a noncongeneric set of molecules (chemically diverse structures or different templates), breaking up of a set of molecules is performed with a predefined set of chemical rules. Here, molecules are considered to consist of different fragments, as presented in Figure 9.6 with a simple example of 3-arylsydonyl and aryl-substituted hydrazine thiazoles with three fragments. To consider the environment of the neighboring fragments, the attachment point atoms are incorporated in the fragments. With respect to steric and electrostatic environments, fragment *B* will be different from fragments *A* and *C*, as it will include the attachment atoms of both *A* and *C*. On the other hand, fragments *A* and *C* have the attachment atom from the *B* fragment only.

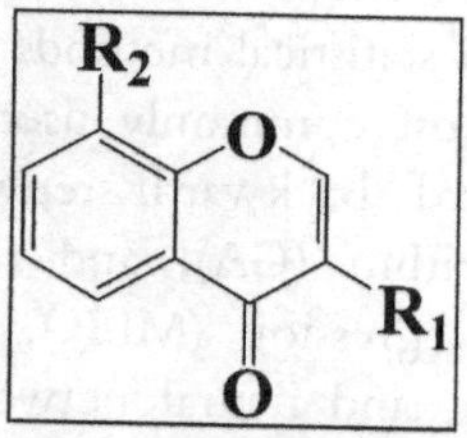

Figure 9.5 A chromone derivative with two substitutions at R_1 and R_2.

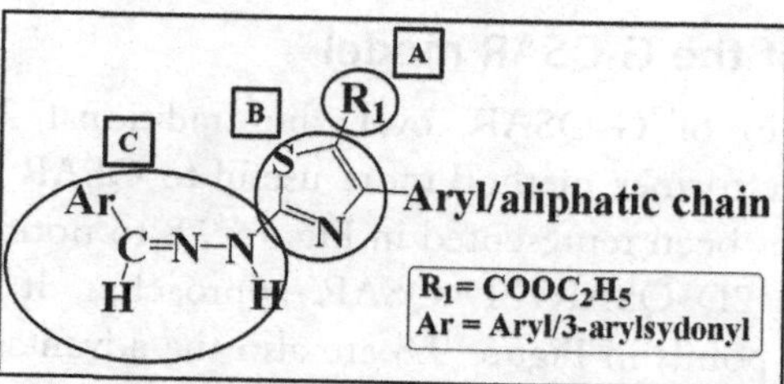

Figure 9.6 A simple example of 3-arylsydonyl and aryl-substituted hydrazine thiazole with three fragments.

9.3.3.2 Calculation of fragment descriptors

The molecular fragments are generated for each molecule in the data set, as demonstrated in Figures 9.5 and 9.6. Descriptors would then be calculated for each fragment (e.g., R_1 and R_2) of a given molecule in two ways:

1. 2D descriptors like topological indices, electrotopological indices, other alignment-independent topological descriptors, 3D alignment-independent descriptors like dipole moment, radius of gyration, volume, and polar surface area (PSA) are calculated for fragments present in each molecule in the data set.
2. Besides various 2D/3D descriptors calculated for various fragments present in each molecule, cross-interaction terms between various fragments are also calculated and used as descriptors for the generation of the QSAR model.

For instance, if two descriptors (D1 and D2) are calculated for the fragments R_1 and R_2, the following descriptors will be generated: D1R_1, D1R_2, D2R_1, D2* R_2, D1R_1*D1R_2, D1R_1*D2R_2, D1R_2*D2R_1, D2R_1*D2R_2, D1R_1*D2R_1, and D1R_2*D2R_2, where D1R_1, D1R_2 are the calculated descriptor D1 for the group(s) at R_1 and R_2 sites and D2R_1, D2R_2 are the calculated descriptor D2 for the group(s) at R_1 and R_2 sites. The remaining descriptors are cross-interaction descriptors.

9.3.3.3 G-QSAR model development

The third and final step is the selection of the ideal set of descriptors from the large pool of descriptors to build a quantitative model. To pick an optimal subset of descriptors, various variable selection methods may be applied, and there is the option of combining a variety of statistical methods for constructing the quantitative model. For this purpose, the most commonly used variable selection methods are stepwise forward, stepwise forward–backward, stepwise backward, simulated annealing method, and genetic algorithm (GA), and the quantitative model building approaches are multiple linear regression (MLR), principal component regression (PCR), PLS, *k*-nearest neighbor, and neural networks. As per the requirement of the data set and the G-QSAR model developer, one can use any method from the abovementioned pool. Figure 9.7 represents a complete schematic diagram of the G-QSAR methodology.

9.3.4 Application of the G-QSAR model

The notable advantages of G-QSAR over the traditional 2D-QSAR/3D-QSAR methods have made the former method more useful to QSAR researchers recently. A graphical illustration has been represented in Figure 9.8 to notify the major advantages of G-QSAR over the 2D-QSAR/3D-QSAR approaches. It is interesting to point out that the first three points in Figure 9.8 are also the advantages of 2D-QSAR over 3D-QSAR. The G-QSAR methodology provides a better understanding of the structure–activity relationship, considering the identification of vital chemical variations at

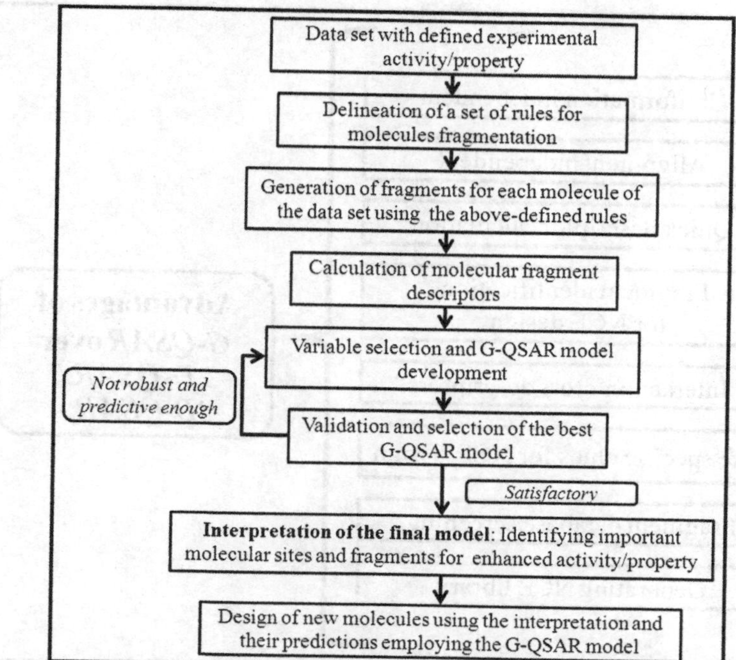

Figure 9.7 A flowchart of G-QSAR methodology.

specific substitution sites and also by providing a predictive mathematical model for the future prediction of new chemical entities (NCEs). The site-specific clarity, along with the interpretation of fragments generated by G-QSAR models, will help chemists to design better drug candidates.

9.3.4.1 NCE design based on fragments

G-QSAR models can generate information based on the employed descriptors on the fragments that contribute maximally to the variation in activity. The relative contribution of each descriptor can provide quantitative information about the importance of the corresponding descriptors. Analysis of the fragments within the reference chemical structure can provide vital information that can be used in the design of new molecules. For example, Goyal et al. [36] constructed G-QSAR models employing pyrazole-derived compounds exhibiting inhibitory activity against *Leishmania* CRK3. Taking into consideration the result of the G-QSAR study, the authors generated a combinatorial library and reported top two compounds after predicting their activity. The study provides a substantial basis for consideration of the designed pyrazole-based leads as potent anti-*Leishmania* CRK3 drugs.

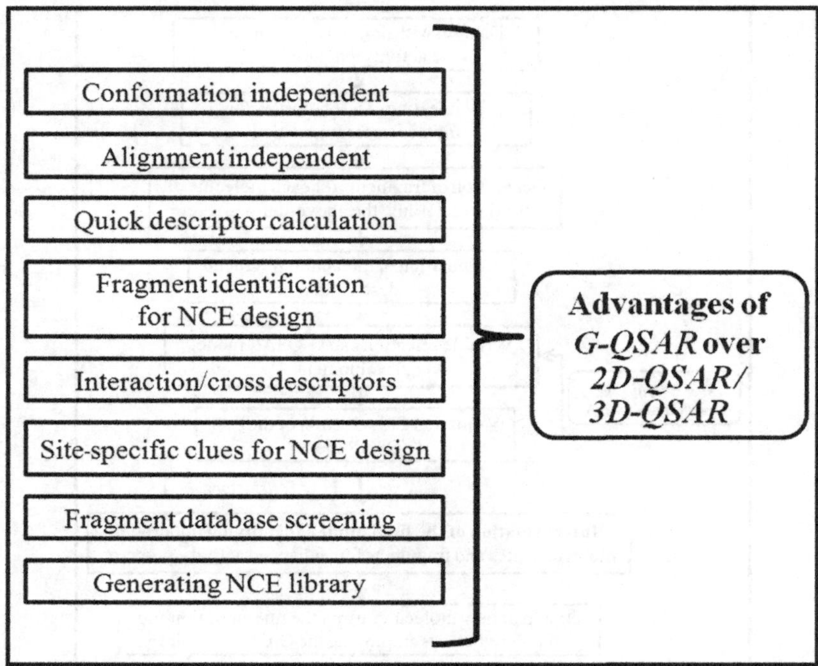

Figure 9.8 Major advantages of G-QSAR over 2D-QSAR/3D-QSAR approaches.

9.3.4.2 Scaffold hopping and lead optimization

G-QSAR is independent of 3D conformations and alignment of the molecules and provides significant information concerning sites and properties responsible for activity disparity. The G-QSAR models can be employed tactically for scaffold hopping and lead optimization by employing descriptor ranges of selected fragments of active molecules for searching the fragment database in order to identify fragments that can replace the original data set fragments. For example, Ajmani and Kulkarni [37] demonstrated the application of G-QSAR in lead optimization of multikinase (PDGFR-beta, FGFR-1, and SRC) and scaffold hopping of multiserotonin target inhibitors. They have developed multiresponse regression G-QSAR models that were useful for scaffold hopping and lead optimization of multitarget inhibitors. In addition, the models provide imperative fragment-based features that can form the building blocks to guide combinatorial library design in the search for optimally potent multitarget inhibitors.

9.3.4.3 Addressing the inverse QSAR problem

G-QSAR addresses the "inverse QSAR" problem, which offers a systematic method to design molecules that satisfy QSAR requirements and thereby design active

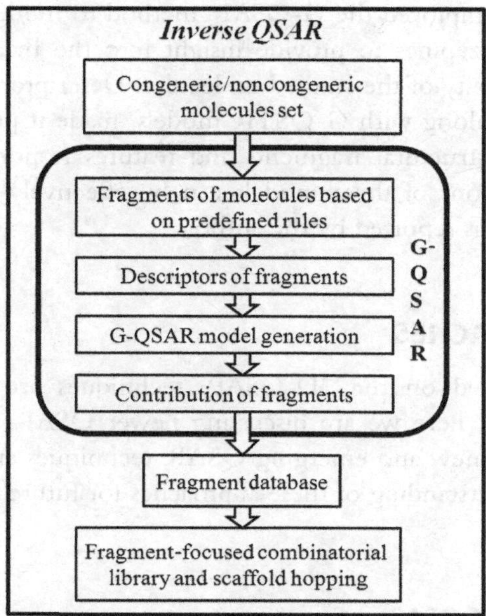

Figure 9.9 The inverse QSAR methodology.

molecules. Interestingly, G-QSAR works systematically to solve the inverse QSAR problem in the following steps:

a. Identifying essential molecular sites and their respective properties
b. Computing descriptors that are found to be important in the G-QSAR model
c. Searching for fragments that correspond to these ranges within fragment databases
d. Generating NCE by combining such fragments and site information

A graphical illustration is provided to promote better understanding of the inverse QSAR problem in Figure 9.9.

9.3.4.4 Mathematical correlation to activity prediction

G-QSAR can be tactically applied for the identification of significant structural fragments and for the rapid evaluation and prediction of databases from different classes of activities. As illustrative examples, two case studies are discussed next.

Ambure and Roy [38] examined a congeneric series of cyclin-dependent kinase 5/p25 (CDK5/p25) inhibitors to understand the structural requirements for improving activity against CDK5/p25 and selectivity over CDK2 by the development of 2D-QSAR, G-QSAR, and quantitative activity–activity relationship (QAAR) models. The 2D-QSAR and G-QSAR models explore the probable structural requirements for improving activity, while the QAAR model assists the improved understanding of the features required for selectivity of the inhibitors.

Kar and Roy [39] employed the G-QSAR method to model the toxicity response of a series of benzodiazepines to provide insight into the main structural fragments responsible for the toxicity of the studied molecules. Descriptor-based QSTR and 3D toxicophore mapping, along with G-QSTR models, made it possible to reach a conclusion regarding the structural fragments and features responsible for the toxicity. The consensus predictions of these models can be effectively utilized to design less toxic benzodiazepines, as reported by the authors.

9.4 OTHER APPROACHES

Newer approaches based on the 3D-QSAR techniques are broadly explained in Section 8.5. Therefore, here we are discussing newer QSAR techniques other than 3D-QSAR. Relatively new and emerging QSAR techniques are outlined in this section for the better understanding of these approaches for future use.

9.4.1 MIA-QSAR

9.4.1.1 Concept of MIA-QSAR

One of the most common and successfully applied methodologies in 3D-QSAR is CoMFA [32]. In CoMFA, the descriptors are mostly generated in a 3D space in order to replicate noncovalent interactions between the active sites and ligands. But the success of this methodology is hugely dependent on the exhaustive conformer generation and the complexity in the alignments of ligands. Working from this background, Freitas et al. [6] have developed a simple and easily accessible QSAR method based on 2D images of congeneric series of compounds.

MIA has been applied successfully in different fields of science for a long time. One of the most common practical applications in the fields of scientific imaging [40], it is a multivariate regression method that is based on data sets obtained from 2D images. In MIA-QSAR, 2D images are employed for the generation of pixels (a *pixel* is the smallest uniform element of an image displayed on the screen) for individual compounds in a particular data set. Then, the pixels of each image are considered as descriptors that are correlated with the respective activities for the development of QSAR models. MIA-QSAR is a very accessible and fast method of QSAR analysis where one can test a large number of compounds with different substituents to check the variation of activity for the specific class of compounds. This is a visual and direct method to predict biological responses in a quantitative way to a series of molecules with congenericity. This method can be successfully applied in various areas like remote sensing and clinical analysis, as suggested by the developer groups [6].

9.4.1.2 Methodology of MIA-QSAR

9.4.1.2.1 Descriptor calculation

Like other QSAR models, the first step in the development of MIA-QSAR is the calculation of descriptors. As images of any chemical structure are considered as rich sources of information, MIA-QSAR tactically applies the image-generated information as descriptors. Images can be divided into univariate and multivariate types. Univariate or grayscale images are expressed as a 2D matrix with height × width dimensions. In the case of multivariate images, each image is a 3D array with height × width × wavelength dimensions. The most common type of multivariate images is a color image where wavelengths corresponding to red, green, and blue lights, respectively, are measured. Thus, dimensions of the 3D array of these types of images are expressed as height × width × 3 (where 3 represents red, green, and blue wavelengths). After constructing binaries of each image, they are superimposed to generate a tensor. The generated tensor is unfolded in order to use two-way analysis methods. Therefore, the generated 2D matrix for the whole data set can be utilized as the total pool of descriptors [6].

In order to make the process easily understandable, we have provided a hypothetical example of the calculation of descriptors for MIA-QSAR. The 2D structures of each compound of a data set are systematically built using any drawing software module and saved in bitmaps. Thereafter, the bitmap of molecules are set to $A \times B$ pixels windows, with resolution of $Z \times Z$ points per inch. Since the bitmaps of molecules should be superimposed as a 2D alignment, a common pixel is chosen among the total set of molecular structures (80 compounds in this example), and then the molecules are totally fixed in that given coordinate (e.g., the $M \times N$ coordinate, common to the whole series). Each 2D image is read and converted into binaries, and the predictor block is assembled by grouping the 80 treated images, giving an $80 \times A \times B$ array. The 3D array is unfolded into a two-way array ($80 \times AB$). This generated X-descriptor matrix is applied in order to be correlated with the dependent variable, which is the vector of activities of the studied molecules. The building of a 3D array to a 2D array of molecules and generation of a descriptor matrix is illustrated in Figure 9.10.

9.4.1.2.2 Model development

In the X-matrix, each row contains the variables (the pixels) describing each molecule, and it is consequently decomposed into a score vector s_1 and a weight vector w_1. The score vector is determined to have the property of maximum covariance with the dependent variable y. The score vectors then replace the original variables as regressors. As the descriptors used in this QSAR model building are pixels of the images of the molecules, the problem of collinearity and noisy descriptors is a very

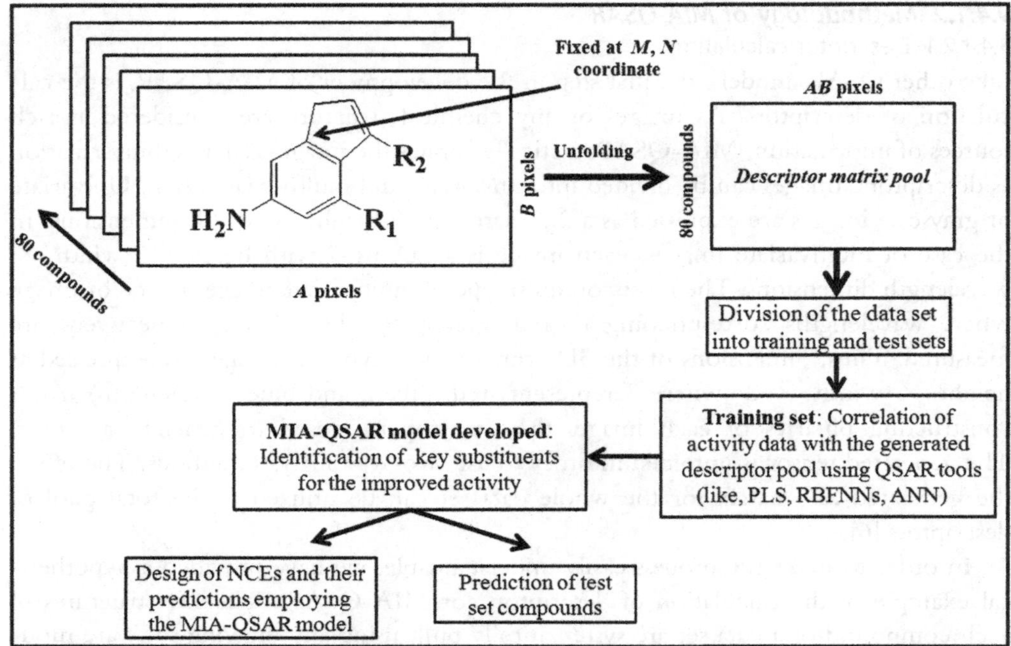

Figure 9.10 The principal steps of MIA-QSAR.

serious issue for MIA-QSAR. Generally, methods such as principal component analysis (PCA) and PLS regression can be used for collinear descriptors, as these methods generate new orthogonal descriptors (principal components for PCA and latent variables for PLS), resulting in better robust and predictive models [6,41]. Again, other chemometric tools can be used successfully for the development of MIA-QSAR based on the requirement of the data set and practices of QSAR researchers. Newer techniques like principal component–radial basis function neural networks (PC-RBFNNs) [41], principal component analysis-adaptive neurofuzzy inference systems (PCA-ANFIS) [42], least squares support-vector machines (LS-SVMs) [43], and N-way PLS squares (N-PLS) [42,44] have successfully been applied in MIA-QSAR model development by different groups of researchers. The developed MIA-QSAR models are then employed for the prediction of test set compounds and, consequently, for the identification of key substituents for the improved activity.

9.4.1.3 Pros and cons of MIA-QSAR

MIA-QSAR is a simple method because neither specific tools nor high-level computations are needed. One can test molecules that have diverse substituents or have scaffolds with some level of similarity. Employing MIA-QSAR, one can rapidly predict any modeled response in a direct or visual way, especially for a congeneric series of molecules depending only on the availability of biological data for some compounds. This approach is free of tridimensional alignment, as well as conformational analysis methods like 3D approaches, but it can give results as good as those obtained from the 3D approaches.

On the other hand, one should be very much concerned about a few characteristics that may be drawbacks of MIA-QSAR. Basically, MIA-QSAR is totally dependent on the 2D images of molecules. Therefore, the drawing and representation of individual structure play a crucial role in the development of the models in terms not only of statistical background, but also interpretability. We have explained this issue in this chapter with the following examples:

- Structure of the molecules can be saved in different font type and size.
- Substituents can be presented in different ways. For example, CN can be represented with $-C{\equiv}N$, and OMe can be presented with O-CH_3.
- Instead of the bitmap format, images can be saved in different standard formats, like joint photographic experts group (JPEG), tagged image file format (TIFF), and portable network graphics (PNG).

Thus, with the various font types and sizes, representations of substituents, and image-saving formats, pixel numbers vary for not only each substituent, but also for the whole molecule. In our point of view, the abovementioned issues may largely affect the reliability of MIA-QSAR. Although Goodarzi et al. [45] revealed that the results of prediction is independent of the way in which molecules are drawn, but to increase the trustworthiness of MIA-QSAR among QSAR researchers, further studies are needed.

9.4.1.4 Application of MIA-QSAR

MIA-QSAR can be successfully applied not only in activity prediction, but also in NCE design, scaffold hopping, and lead optimization. Identification of the key features for the activity profile of a particular class of compounds is one of the important applications of MIA-QSAR, which leads to further NCE design and formation of database for future use. These databases can be used for future scaffold hopping and lead optimization without applying conformational analysis or any alignment studies. For example, we will cite the following case studies for successful application of MIA-QSAR.

A data set of (*S*)-*N*-[(1-ethyl-2-pyrrolidinyl)methyl]-6-methoxybenzamides with affinity to the dopamine D2 receptor subtype was used by Freitas et al. [6] to build MIA-QSAR models employing bilinear PLS and the nonlinear iterative partial least squares (NIPALS) algorithm. The MIA-QSAR method coupled with PCA-ANFIS, which accounts for nonlinearities, was applied on a series of HIV reverse transcriptase inhibitor tetrahydroimidazo [4,5,1-jk][1,4] benzodiazepine (TIBO) derivatives by Goodarzi and Freitas [42]. A set of drug-like compounds derived from Sildenafil, Vardenafil, and Tadalafil analogs was modeled through MIA-QSAR by

Antunes et al. [46]. A highly predictive model was developed and novel phosphodiesterase type-5 (PDE-5) inhibitors were predicted. The promising activities of eight compounds were supported by the docking study, and the calculated absorption, distribution, metabolism, excretion, and toxicity (ADMET) profiles for these compounds suggest advantages over the drugs that are commonly used for the treatment of erectile dysfunction.

9.4.2 Binary QSAR

9.4.2.1 Concept of binary QSAR

The introduction of combinatorial chemistry for designing large libraries compelled researchers to discover rapid robotic methods for assaying millions of compounds in a short period of time. This rapid method is referred to as *high-throughput screening (HTS)*. Often, the results generated by this method are prone to error, and the current QSAR methodologies require fewer heterogeneous compounds having continuous activity data with lower error margins in order to have good predictive values. To overcome the methodological problems in conventional QSAR techniques and to handle a huge amount of binary data from HTS, the *binary QSAR* method was introduced, which can handle data from HTS [47]. The method accepts binary activity measurements (e.g., active or inactive) and molecular descriptor vectors as input. A Bayesian inference technique is used to predict whether a new compound will be active or inactive.

9.4.2.2 Methodology of binary QSAR

The methodology of the binary QSAR is as follows:

a. Binary QSAR makes an estimate, from a training set, of the probability density $Pr(Y=1/X=x)$, where Y is a Bernoulli random variable (i.e., Y takes on values of 0 or 1) representing "active" or "inactive," and X is a random n-vector of real numbers (a random collection of molecular descriptors).

b. A PCA is carried out on the training set to compute an n by p linear transform, Q, and an n-vector, u, such that the random p-vector $Z=Q(X-u)$ has a mean and variance equal to the p by p identity matrix. The quantity p is referred to as the number of *principal components*.

c. The original molecular descriptors are transformed by Q and u to obtain a decorrelated and normalized set of descriptors. The desired probability density is then approximated by applying Bayes' theorem, assuming that the transformed descriptors are mutually independent:

$$Pr(Y=1/X=x) \approx \left[1+\frac{Pr(Y=0)}{Pr(Y=1)}\prod\frac{Pr(Z_i=z_i/Y=0)}{Pr(Z_i=z_i/Y=1)}\right]^{-1} \tag{9.2}$$

$$Z=Q(X-u)=(Z_1,\ldots,Z_p)$$

d. Individual probability density $Pr(Z_i = z_i)$ is estimated by creating a histogram. The usual actions for histogram creation are sensitive to bin boundaries as each observation (no matter how close it is to a bin boundary) is treated as though it fell in the center of the bin. To diminish this sensitivity, each observation is replaced with a Gaussian density with variance σ^2. This variance can be interpreted as an observation error or as a *smoothing parameter.* Once all of the $2p + 2$ probability densities have been estimated from the training set, the desired density $Pr(Y = 1/X = x)$ is constructed using Eq. (9.2).

Remember that binary QSAR assigns a probability to a compound that it would be active in a particular test setting, but it cannot predict specific modifications of lead compounds to enhance their activity. Thus, binary QSAR is not a substitute for the usual QSAR analysis. In a drug discovery setting, these approaches should be complementary. After binary QSAR-guided selection of active compounds, conventional QSAR can be used to optimize their biological activity.

9.4.3 Fragment-based QSAR

Du et al. [48] introduced a molecular FB-QSAR method in conjunction with fragment-based drug design. FB-QSAR is a development and extension of both the Free–Wilson QSAR and traditional 2D-QSAR. The essence of the new method is that the molecule is divided into several fragments according to their substitutions. The response of the molecules is correlated with the physicochemical properties of the molecular fragments through two sets of coefficients in the linear free-energy equations. One coefficient set is for the physicochemical properties, and the other is for the weight factors of the molecular fragments. Meanwhile, an iterative double least squares (IDLS) technique is developed to solve the two sets of coefficients in a training data set alternately and iteratively. The IDLS technique is a feedback procedure with machine-learning capability. The FB-QSAR approach can remarkably enhance the predictive power and provide more structural insights into rational drug design.

Compared with the traditional 2D-QSAR, FB-QSAR can introduce one more type of parameters, structural parameters, which replicate the molecular fragments and their weight factor coefficients $\{b_\alpha\}$. The fragments are not really physicochemical parameters, but rather virtual structural parameters with a clear chemical concept. FB-QSAR uses much less adjustable variables than the Free–Wilson QSAR does. Consequently, the overcorrelation problem can be avoided in FB-QSAR. It is anticipated that FB-QSAR has a better external predictive ability because it can characterize structural features under a fragment basis. In the FB-QSAR approach, IDLS is an iterative and feedback procedure in which the two sets of coefficients $\{a_l\}$ and $\{b_\alpha\}$ are adjusted iteratively and alternately, minimizing the fitted error step by step. Therefore, the FB-QSAR approach possesses the machine learning ability. In this regard, it is quite similar to the artificial neural network (ANN).

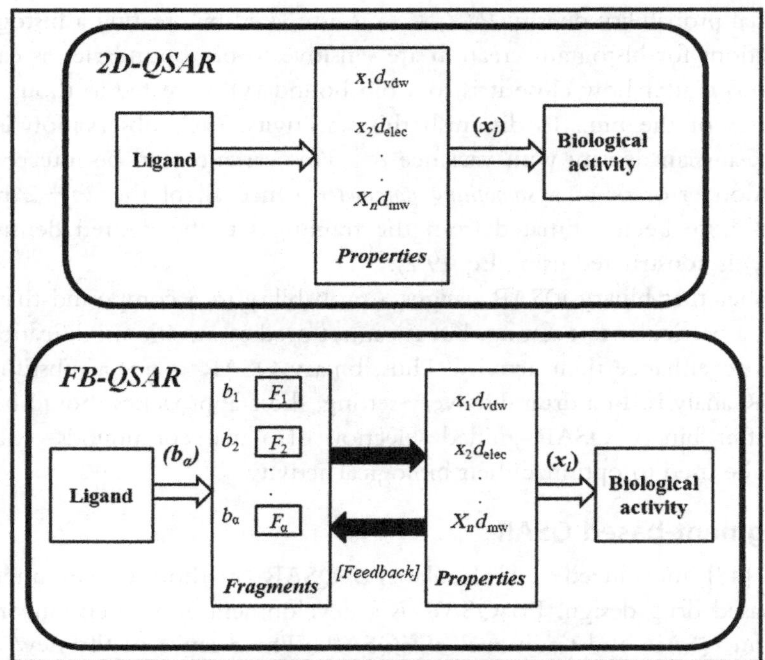

Figure 9.11 The difference between the 2D-QSAR and FB-QSAR methodologies.

The principal thought behind FB-QSAR and its comparison with standard 2D-QSAR is presented in Figure 9.11. In typical 2D-QSAR, the ligand physicochemical properties are directly correlated with the biological activity through a coefficient set $\{x_l\}$ in the linear free-energy equation. On the other hand, in the case of FB-QSAR, the molecular structure is divided into numerous fragments, and the bioactivity is correlated with the physicochemical properties of fragments through two coefficient sets, $\{x_l\}$ and $\{b_\alpha\}$. In this instance, x_l defines the physicochemical properties, and b_α signifies the weight factors of fragments. The two sets of coefficients are solved using the IDLS technique.

9.4.4 Fragment-similarity-based QSAR

FS-QSAR [49] was developed to resolve the major restriction of the original Free–Wilson method by introducing the fragment-similarity concept in the linear regression equation. Such a similarity concept was applied for the first time to improve the traditional Free–Wilson equation instead of using physicochemical properties, which often produce nonunique solutions. In this approach, the fragment-similarity calculation was carried out by the similarity. It used the lowest or highest eigenvalues calculated from Burden CAS University of Texas, BCUT) matrices, which contained partial charges of individual atoms and their atomic connection information in each individual fragments. The equation of the FS-QSAR is as follows:

$$\log(\mathrm{BA}) = \mathrm{const} + \sum_{j=1}^{N}\left[\max\left\{\mathrm{Sim}\left(\overset{P_j}{\underset{k=1}{F_{jk}}}, F_{jg}\right)\right\}\right] \times A_j^{\mathrm{MSF}} \tag{9.3}$$

In Eq. (9.3), BA is biological activity, N is the total number of substituent positions, P_j is the total number of possible substituents at the jth substituent position; max is the max function picks the maximum score among similarity scores; F_{jk} is the kth fragment (a known fragment in the training set) at the jth substituent position; F_{jg} *is* a given fragment (the fragment from a testing/unknown compound) at the jth substituent position; $\mathrm{Sim}[F_{jk}, F_{jg}]$ is the fragment-similarity function comparing F_{jg} to F_{jk}, which calculates a similarity score; and A_j^{MSF} is the coefficient of the most similar fragment (MSF) at the jth substituent position.

The similarity function is defined as

$$\mathrm{Sim}(F_{jk}, F_{jg}) = \mathrm{e}^{-|\mathrm{EV}(F_{jk})-\mathrm{EV}(F_{jg})|} \tag{9.4}$$

where $\mathrm{EV}(F_{jk})$ is the lowest or highest eigenvalue of the BCUT matrix of a fragment (F_{jk}).

The FS-QSAR method was proved to have an effective predictive power compared to the traditional 2D-QSAR method due to the introduction of the similarity concept into the regression equation. However, the predictive accuracy of FS-QSAR may not be as high as other, higher-dimensional QSAR methods, but the method is a unique and reproducible 2D-QSAR model.

9.4.5 *Ensemble* QSAR

9.4.5.1 Concept of eQSAR

eQSAR is a novel dynamic QSAR technique that addresses the significance of low-energy conformers in QSAR studies. The method was developed by Pissurlenkar et al. [8]. The term *ensemble* is employed to depict the efforts at imitating the conformational space of the inhibitor by using a finite set of low-energy conformations. The novelty of this approach is that the biological activity is modeled as a function of physicochemical description initiating from an ensemble of low-energy (active) conformers, rather than as a property generated from the lowest-energy gas phase conformer. The approach first generates an ensemble of low-energy conformations for the ligand through a molecular dynamics (MD) approach that accounts for the diversity of bound conformations accessible in solution. Eigenvalues generated from the "physicochemical property integrated distance matrices" (PD matrices) that encompass both 3D structure and physicochemical properties have been employed as descriptors for model development. The *e*QSAR models possess the ability to select the most biologically pertinent conformations with the relevant physicochemical attributes that can describe the biological activity in the best way. The methodology has the ability to predict whether a particular structural modification would enhance or hamper drug binding.

9.4.5.2 Importance and application of eQSAR

Usually in QSAR studies, the lowest-energy conformer is used for the calculation of descriptors, while all other conformations are ignored. On the other hand, a large number of studies examined the concept that the dynamics influence the number and variety of thermally available conformations. Consequently, these conformers have a significant impact on the biological activity and binding affinity. Therefore, information generated from a single conformer may be inadequate for the whole structural description of a molecule and over time, may lead to the development of an incorrect QSAR model. In *e*QSAR, the biological response for the compounds is modeled as a function of molecular properties originating from specifically selected active conformers, rather than selecting the lowest-energy gas phase conformer, and this has the prospect of improving the quality and predictability of QSAR. The crucial step of this method lies in the selection of suitable active conformers of the ligands as the values of the calculated molecular descriptors can differ drastically for diverse conformers of the identical molecule. These descriptors are distinctive, as they encompass both connectivity information of structure and atomic properties.

9.4.6 LQTA-QSAR

9.4.6.1 Concept of LQTA-QSAR

Martins et al. [7] introduced a novel 4D-QSAR formalism known as *LQTA-QSAR* (LQTA, *Laboratório de Quimiometria Teórica e Aplicada*). This methodology investigates the main features of CoMFA and 4D-QSAR paradigms where conformational flexibility is mostly studied. This approach generates a conformational ensemble profile (CEP) for each compound instead of only one conformation. Thereafter, the MD trajectories and topology information retrieved from the GROMACS free package is used for the calculation of 3D descriptors for a set of compounds. The MD simulations can be executed considering explicit solvent molecules, and the result is a superior approximation of the biological environment. It calculates the intermolecular interaction energies at each grid point, considering probes and all the aligned conformations resulting from MD simulations. These interaction energies are the independent variables or descriptors that are employed in QSAR analysis.

The visualization and interpretation of the descriptors in 3D space support the applicability of this new method in rational drug design. This paradigm is a user-friendly computational method with minimal computation time.

LQTA-QSAR is an open-source tool freely available for the scientific community at http://lqta.iqm.unicamp.br.

9.4.6.2 Methodology of LQTA-QSAR

The basic methodology of LQTA-QSAR is divided into four steps [7]:

a. *Design and recovery of ligands*: The structures of ligands are drawn and their energy is minimized and converted to 3D conformations using suitable force fields. The MD programs like GROMACS are helpful in generating topology and coordinates for ligands.

b. *Generation of ensembles*: The output of the GROMACS file is used as input for calculating the 3D interaction energy descriptors in the grid cell. For the calculation of the interaction energy uniformly, the grid is defined where all the conformations are present. The interaction at each point in the grid is calculated by placing a probe at specific junctions of the grid.

c. *Computation of 3D properties*: To compute energy at regular spaces in 3D grid cells, probes like ions, cations, or a functional group of positive or negative charge are used around 3D grids. Energy in the form of Coulombic and van der Waals interactions is calculated for each atom of the CEP using various force fields. Both energies are calculated for *n* number of atoms and the average of this energy value is useful to calculate the properties for all ligands in each grid point.

d. *Model development with correlation between descriptors and biological activity*: Interaction energies at each grid point are the independent variables or descriptors which are employed in the QSAR analysis. The ordered predictor selection (OPS) algorithm can be applied in the variable selection method and the multivariate regression approaches (PLS/PCR) are used to construct the QSAR model.

Figure 9.12 illustrates the steps involved in the LQTA-QSAR formalism.

9.4.7 SOM 4D-QSAR

The major intention to develop a 4D-QSAR is to model the 3D properties of chemical compounds and to construct and analyze conformational profile of receptor ligands. The self-organizing map (SOM) is a machine-learning approach that is generally used to classify the data according to the similarity between the data. It is a basic type of ANN that is frequently used in QSAR due to its transparency and easy interpretation. It is mostly used for classification and to test the toxicity of chemical compounds. Multiple conformations of ligands are developed in the 4D-QSAR model. The method is suited for experiments where an active bound conformation is searched, taking into account conformation flexibility. The basic methodology of SOM 4D-QSAR can be divided into six basic steps [50,51]:

a. *3D model building and ensemble searching*: SOM 4D-QSAR begins with the generation of 3D conformation of selected ligands in the training set. Consequently, 3D

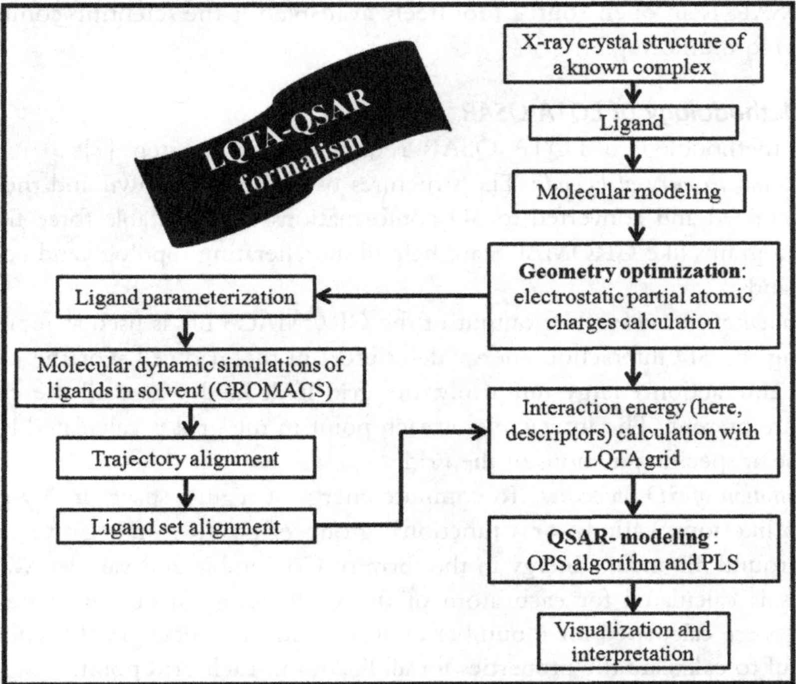

Figure 9.12 The LQTA-QSAR formalism.

structures of the ligands are minimized and active conformations are searched in ensemble sampling.

b. *Trial alignment or superposition*: The selected active conformations of ligands are subjected to trail alignment or superimposition. This work is done on the basis of an active conformer and selecting at least three atoms for superposition in the alignment.

c. *Finding of interaction pharmacophore elements (IPEs)*: In this step, IPEs are identified and selected that play an important role in interaction by placing a selected conformer into the grid cell. The choice of interaction groups like aliphatic, aromatic, hydrogen bond donor, hydrogen bond acceptor, and polar and nonpolar charge groups is done by placing a probe at regular spaces of 3D grid cell.

d. *Creation of CEP*: The training set selected in step *a* after energy minimization is subjected to MD studies, and molecular ensemble created for each ligand molecule is used for the CEP. The MD study also helps in the comparative analysis of ligand conformations. A semiempirical method such as AM1 is used to calculate partial charge of compounds.

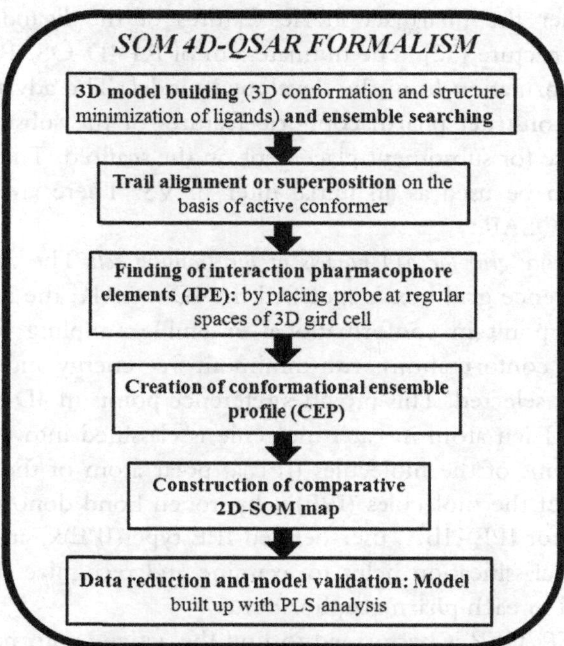

Figure 9.13 The basic steps of SOM 4D-QSAR.

e. *Construction of comparative 2D SOM map*: In this step, 2D self-organization maps are built based on CEP for each ligand after calculating Cartesian coordinates and partial charges. At the training stage, values of each ligand are provided as input data by means of a grid cell occupancy profile (GCOP). Again, the partial charges are supplied to neurons to get occupancy profile maps or partial charge maps.

f. *Data reduction and model validation*: In the final step, specific occupancy and partial charge groups are selected for PLS analysis. In 4D-QSAR, relationships are built up based on the LOO-CV procedure associated with iterative variable elimination (IVE)−PLS. Model validation is done by cross-validating the QSAR model with an external test set data by measuring predictability. To do this, a variety of training and test sets are sampled and monitored by the stochastic model validation (SMV) scheme. A simple graphical illustration of the basic steps of SOM 4D-QSAR is presented in Figure 9.13.

9.4.8 Receptor-independent 4D-QSAR

The study of receptor-independent (RI) 4D-QSAR has a considerable impact in rational drug design. The application of RI 4D-QSAR comes when the researcher wants to find either the pharmacophoric features of the ligand or the projected changes in ligand structure [52]. The ultimate aim of RI 4D-QSAR is to obtain maximum structural information from the developed model. The advantage of RI is that it will design and construct pharmacophoric features of the substituents, design and map the rational base for substituent placement on the scaffold. The designed pharmacophoric model can be used as an initial filter in VS. There are 10 principal steps involved in RI 4D-QSAR:

a. *Initiation of reference grid for 3D models of the training set*: The 3D structure of the training set reference grid box is specified. In 4D-QSAR, the initial 3D structures are the starting point in conformational ensemble sampling of the training set. The training set conformations with minimum free energy and having a common torsion angle are selected. This provides reference points in 4D-QSAR analysis.

b. *Selection of IPE*: Each atom in each molecule is classified into different categories, including all atoms of the molecules (IPE)a, polar atom of the molecules (IPE)p, nonpolar atom of the molecules (IPE)n, hydrogen bond donor(IPE)HBD, hydrogen bond acceptor(IPE)HBA, user-defined IPE types(IPE)x, aromatic carbon, and hydrogen. This classification helps to examine and recognize the diverse interactions concerned in each pharmacophoric site.

c. *Formation of CEP*: CEP is performed to find the active conformation in the training set. A molecular dynamics simulation (MDS) is usually done to generate an ensemble for training molecules. CEP uses Boltzmann sampling techniques. This step is achieved by a systematic conformational search technique or stochastic conformational search technique. Finally, a huge number of conformers are explored and the correct conformation state is selected.

d. *Selection of the trail alignment*: The molecular alignment of 4D-QSAR study can be achieved via rapidly evaluating the trail alignment by searching and sampling operation analogs to CEP. In general, this is achieved by designing RI 4D-QSAR algorithms that help in alignment analysis by the decoupling of conformational analysis and further rapid analysis of conformation to investigate the molecular descriptor on molecular alignment. The CEP for each compound from the training data set is assessed for molecular alignment, which produces unique models of every compound in the grid box.

e. *Construction of GCOP and calculation of GCOD*: Each conformation is placed in the reference cubic lattice reference grid cell, and spacing of cell is fixed as per the trail alignment. The GCOP is calculated for each molecule based on five to six different classes of IPE. These IPEs are used to do trail alignment of 4D-QSAR descriptors. The cell occupancy for each grid cell is taken into consideration after the alignment of each IPE's atom in a grid cell. This step results in the generation of a unique set of IPEs. This set of IPEs for each atom is called a grid cell occupancy descriptor (GCOD).

f. *PLS analysis to reduce the number of GCODs against the biological activity measures*: The data reduction step in 4D-QSAR is similar to CoMFA with a minor difference that the total set of GCODs is incorporated into this study. The PLS is employed to execute regression analysis to remove unnecessary GCODs by establishing the relationship between experiential biological activity and the occupancy value of GCODs. The values obtained from PLS regression are related quantitatively with the 4D-QSAR model, by giving a specific weightage for each GCOD, and the quantitative relationship between small groups of selected GCOD is represented by a graphical mode. In general, a small group (<15) of GCODs is chosen for the 4D-QSAR studies.

g. *4D-QSAR model building, optimization, comparison, and evaluation*: The highly weighted GCODs are selected and employed for RI 4D-QSAR model building by GA and genetic function approximation (GFA), followed by optimization, comparison, and evaluation.

h. *Retrial of trail alignment, construction of IPE and CEPs, and choosing GCODs unless they are included for GA analysis*: Based on the trail alignment, a model is constructed and evaluated with the composite set of 4D-QSAR models constructed on reiteration of steps *d* to *g*. Once the appropriate set of trail alignments is incorporated into building the 4D-QSAR model, proper optimization, comparison, and evaluation of all models are done.

i. *Identification of the best 4D-QSAR model with respect to trail alignment*: The fundamental purpose of this step is to find the best optimized 4D-QSAR model. The best trail alignment is chosen on the basis of highest goodness of fit of regression coefficient and Q^2.

j. *Proposing the hypothesis about active ligand conformations*: The objective of this step is to recognize the active state of conformers generated for each compound and sampled for a conformational search belonging to the lowest energy level ΔE (global minima) of CEP. These selected lowest-energy conformers are evaluated using Q^2 for the best 4D-QSAR model. Also the conformation with maximum grid cell occupancy or consistent with the lowest-energy conformation or after an MD simulation ensemble sampling of GCOD is used to evaluate the activity of the 4D-QSAR model. The hypothesis is completed about prediction of conformation with the lowest energy that is high at activity. The principal steps of RI 4D-QSAR are demonstrated in Figure 9.14.

9.4.9 Receptor-dependent 4D-QSAR

Receptor-dependent (RD) 4D-QSAR is a newly developed approach in QSAR where experimental techniques like X-ray crystallography, nuclear magnetic resonance (NMR) spectroscopy, and comparative modeling/homology modeling are

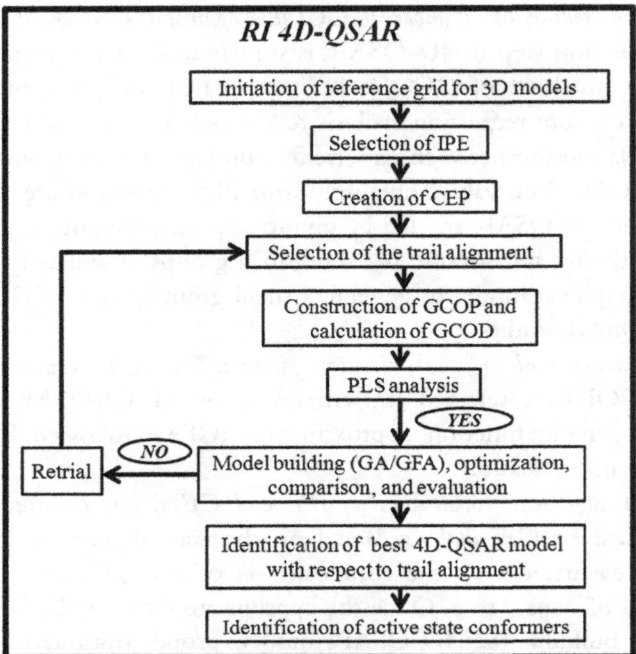

Figure 9.14 Complete methodology of RI 4D-QSAR.

used to determine 3D structures of macromolecules [53]. The 3D structure is determined and the binding site for the ligand is predicted, which allows us to know the binding and alignment modes of ligands. The basic aim of studying RD 4D-QSAR is to map the ligand–receptor interaction mode. The binding mode information from such series of ligands allows one to create site occupancy–weighted 3D pharmacophore models. According to the binding, the interaction weight of the pharmacophore is assigned. The relative occupancy of a pharmacophore is evaluated thermodynamically by accessing the conformational state of the receptor ligand complex. The complex of receptor–ligand is examined as stated previously for binding mode and alignment.

Structure-based drug design (SBDD) has four common limitations when finding novel hits:

a. The conformational flexibility of ligands is not taken into consideration, as only single conformation is used, and this might create indistinctness. The problem is due to the free ligand conformations, which are dissimilar from the actual bound conformation in the active site. The multiple conformations in the form of ensembles may be considered as a single conformation in order to address conformational flexibility.

b. The bonded and nonbonded interactions between the receptor and ligand may vary the conformation of the active site. It can be called the *induced-fit effect*, which may play a role in the recognition of the novel ligand. This has been ignored in most of the SBDD studies and known as the *rigid-fit effect*. In recent studies, multiple protein structures have been taken in the form of ensemble docking to find the induced-fit effect in the binding mode.

c. A number of scoring functions are used, which calculate the free energy of binding between the receptor and the ligand. To do this, a number of force fields are used. Force fields are typically considered for nonbonded interactions between receptor and ligand, but until now, no scoring function has been designed that can calculate the correct binding affinity.

d. Solvation terms like *desolvation* and *resolvation* are not considered generally, and it might affect the ligand–receptor binding interactions.

The specially designed RD 4D-QSAR will concentrate on the faults that arise in SBDD that can be rectified, and the proper quantitative relation can be developed between features of the ligand molecule and biological activity [53]. The basic methodology of RD 4D-QSAR is shown in Figure 9.15.

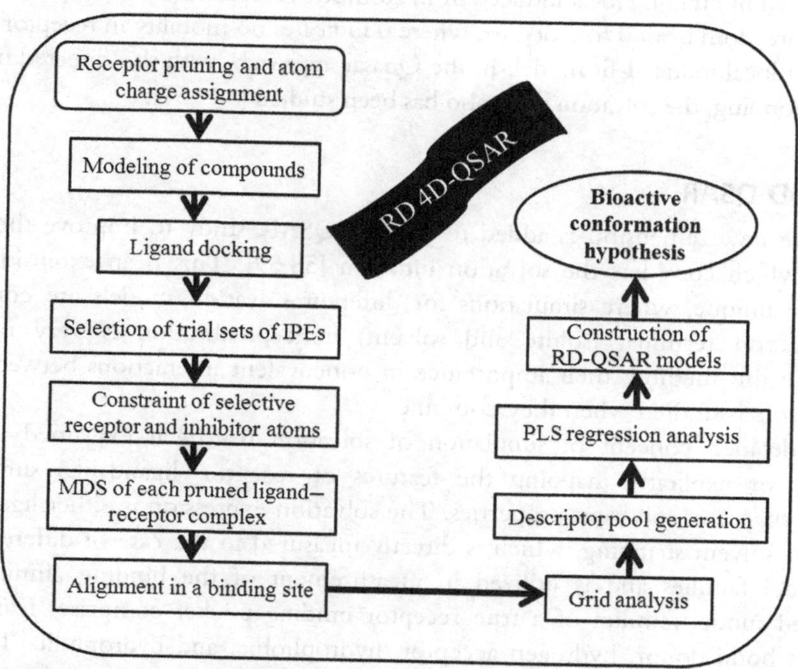

Figure 9.15 Basic methodology of RD 4D-QSAR.

9.4.10 5D-QSAR (QUASAR)

The multiple demonstration of ligand topology to study conformation, isosteriomer, protonation, and orientation is generally called the new dimension to 4D-QSAR, as it can be represented in multiple induced fit, and referred as the new revolution in QSAR called *5D-QSAR* [54,55]. The multiple representations are used as ensembles in studying 5D-QSAR, where molecular simulation and the Boltzmann-weighted selection criterion for bioactive conformation are chosen as genetically evolved from a reservoir of conformations. In the Quasar concept, local induced fit in an atomistic receptor is simulated by initiating "pharmacophore equilibration" mapping ligand in the training set as "inner" and "mean" envelopes. The inner envelope is formed by mapping all training ligand sets at a van der Waals distance, whereas the inner core of the envelope is created by tightly accumulating and accommodating each ligand molecule. The mapping of "inner" and "mean" envelope design on basic approaches is first executed isotropically (linearly), second anisotropically (steric, electric, H-bond, or lipophilicity-potential scaled), and third through energy minimization.

The fifth dimension induced-fit model cannot be constructed without considering a factual receptor. Thus, a number of simulations and induced fit hypothesis are considered to create a factual receptor. To construct a 5D-QSAR model, several techniques have been used like building it on the modus operandi of the mean envelope. The Quasar concept used in building local induced fit in atomistic receptor is created by a changeable degree of freedom from 0 to 1 degree, where 0 indicates no mobility in receptor and 1 as the perfect local induced-fit model. In the Quasar approach, with site-directed hydrogen flip-flop bonding, the solvation term also has been studied [54—57].

9.4.11 6D-QSAR

One more new dimension is added to the 5D-QSAR study to improve the QSAR analysis, which considers the solvation function [58,59]. This is an extension of the Quasar technique, where simulations for different solvation models are considered. The solvation terminal (solute and solvent) conceptualization is very important because in this method, their importance in noncovalent interactions between ligand and receptor is studied when they combine.

The detailed concept of simulation of solvation has been explained by either implicitly or explicitly mapping the features of receptor—ligand-like surface area (size and shape) or solvation properties. The solvation expression is either ligand desolvation or solvent stripping, which is directly measured in the case of different surrogate model families and is utilized in measurement of the binding affinity. These surrogated model families of a true receptor-binding pocket comprises features like hydrogen bond donor, hydrogen acceptor, hydrophobic, and hydrophilic. The result of measuring the binding affinity of a surrogated model family gives us an idea about the solvent's accessible area. The principles used in 4D-QSAR and 5D-QSAR are 3D structures that are generated and simulated using moderate evolutionary pressure. In the 6D-QSAR approach, the inherent characteristics of ligand molecules are screened using receptor properties like hydrophobicity and characteristics of the binding pocket.

9.4.12 7D-QSAR

The most recently introduced higher-dimensional QSAR is 7D-QSAR, where one more dimension is added to the 6D-QSAR study. The 7D-QSAR analysis comprises real receptor or target-based receptor model data [60].

Extensive research is going on for the further development of the 7D-QSAR approach. Polanski [60] cited that the 7D-QSAR protocol should also include virtual target-based receptor models (e.g., obtained by protein homology modeling).

9.5 OVERVIEW AND CONCLUSIONS

Computational techniques play a crucial role in modern medicinal chemistry and biology, presenting unique potential in the early phases of drug research, particularly in terms of time and cost savings. QSAR has evolved into one of the most reliable computational tools, and it has been used for decades to achieve better insight into the relationship between structural features or physicochemical properties and biological activity. A number of possibilities have been explored to make the study of QSAR more acceptable and reliable among biologists and chemists. In the initial days of QSAR development, some classical and milestone studies were done in the field of chemistry by the pioneers of the QSAR field employing 0D-QSAR to 2D-QSAR. After the introduction of 3D-QSAR, a huge amount of research has been performed to establish the correlation between structure and biological activity. More advanced QSAR approaches like 4D-QSAR, 5D-QSAR, 6D-QSAR, and 7D-QSAR have been developed in the last decade to overcome the limitations of 3D-QSAR. Considering some recent findings, multidimensional QSAR might serve as a significant tool in drug discovery in the upcoming years. In this chapter, we have provided an overview of relatively new QSAR methods and recent developments in higher-dimensional QSAR approaches. Since each QSAR method has its own pros and cons, researchers should choose the most appropriate method for modeling as their requirements dictate. However, given the wide range of options, it is challenging to pick the appropriate model for a particular end point being modeled.

REFERENCES

[1] Rester U. From virtuality to reality–virtual screening in lead discovery and lead optimization: a medicinal chemistry perspective. Curr Opin Drug Discov Dev 2008;11:559–68.

[2] Zhao H. Scaffold selection and scaffold hopping in lead generation: a medicinal chemistry perspective. Drug Discov Today 2007;12(3-4):149–55.

[3] Castilho MS, Postigo MP, de Paula CB, Montanari CA, Oliva G, Andricopulo AD. Two- and three-dimensional quantitative structure–activity relationships for a series of purine nucleoside phosphorylase inhibitors. Bioorg Med Chem 2006;14(2):516–27.

[4] Salum LB, Polikarpov I, Andricopulo AD. Structural and chemical basis for enhanced affinity and potency for a series of estrogen receptor ligands: 2D and 3D QSAR studies. J Mol Graph Model 2007;26(2):434–42.

[5] Ajmani S, Jadhav K, Kulkarni SA. Group-based QSAR (G-QSAR): mitigating interpretation challenges in QSAR. QSAR Comb Sci 2009;28(1):36–51.

[6] Freitas MP, Brown SD, Martins JA. MIA-QSAR: a simple 2D image-based approach for quantitative structure–activity relationship analysis. J Mol Struct 2005;738:149–54.

[7] Martins JPA, Barbosa EG, Pasqualoto KFM, Ferreira MMC. LQTA-QSAR: a new 4D-QSAR methodology. J Chem Inf Model 2009;49(6):1428–36.

[8] Pissurlenkar RRS, Khedkar VM, Iyer RP, Coutinho EC. Ensemble QSAR: a QSAR method based on conformational ensembles and metric descriptors. J Comput Chem 2011;32(10):2204–18.

[9] Myint KZ, Xie X-Q. Recent advances in fragment-based QSAR and multi-dimensional QSAR methods. Int J Mol Sci 2010;11:3846–66.

[10] Damale MG, Harke SN, Khan FAK, Shinde DB, Sangshetti JN. Recent advances in multidimensional QSAR (4D-6D): a critical review. Mini Rev Med Chem 2014;14:35–55.

[11] Lowis DR. HQSAR a new, highly predictive QSAR technique, tripos technical notes, vol. 1; 1997.

[12] Doddareddy MR, Lee YJ, Cho YS, Choi KI, Koh HY, Pae AN. Hologram quantitative structure activity relationship studies on 5-HT6 antagonists. Bioorg Med Chem 2004;12(14):3815–24.

[13] Salum LB, Andricopulo AD. Fragment-based QSAR: perspectives in drug design. Mol Divers 2009;13:277–85.

[14] Tong W, Lowis DR, Perkins R, Chen Y, Welsh WJ, Goddette DW, et al. Evaluation of quantitative structure–activity relationship methods for large-scale prediction of chemicals binding to the estrogen receptor. J Chem Inf Comput Sci 1998;38:669–77.

[15] Waller CL. A comparative QSAR study using CoMFA, HQSAR, and FRED/SKEYS paradigms for estrogen receptor binding affinities of structurally diverse compounds. J Chem Inf Comput Sci 2004;44(2):758–65.

[16] So SS, Karplus M. A comparative study of ligand–receptor complex binding affinity prediction methods based on glycogen phosphorylase inhibitors. J Comput Aided Mol Des 1999;13:243–58.

[17] Park Choo HY, Lim JS, Kam Y, Kim SY, Lee J. A comparative study of quantitative structure–activity relationship methods based on antitumor diarylsulfonylureas. Eur J Med Chem 2001; 36:829–36.

[18] Pungpo P, Hannongbua S, Wolschann P. Hologram quantitative structure–activity relationships investigations of non-nucleoside reverse transcriptase inhibitors. Curr Med Chem 2003;10: 1661–77.

[19] Guido RVC, Oliva G, Andricopulo AD. Virtual screening and its integration with modern drug design technologies. Curr Med Chem 2008;15:37–46.

[20] Avery MA, Alvim-Gaston M, Rodrigues CR, Barreiro EJ, Cohen FE, Sabnis YA, et al. Structure–activity relationships of the antimalarial agent artemisinin. 6. The development of predictive *in vitro* potency models using CoMFA and HQSAR methodologies. J Med Chem 2002; 45:292.

[21] Salum LB, Dias LC, Andricopulo AD. Fragment-based QSAR and molecular modeling studies on a series of discodermolide analogs as microtubule-stabilizing anticancer agents. QSAR Comb Sci 2009;2:325–37.

[22] Kaiser D, Smiesko M, Kopp S, Chiba P, Ecker GF. Interaction field based and hologram based QSAR analysis of propafenone-type modulators of multidrug resistance. Med Chem 2005;1: 431–44.
[23] Prakash O, Ghosh I. Developing an antituberculosis compounds database and data mining in the search of a motif responsible for the activity of a diverse class of antituberculosis agents. J Chem Inf Model 2006;46(1):17–23.
[24] Lo Piparo E, Koehler K, Chana A, Benfenati E. Virtual screening for aryl hydrocarbon receptor binding prediction. J Med Chem 2006;49(19):5702–9.
[25] La Regina G, Edler MC, Brancale A, Kandil S, Coluccia A, Piscitelli F, et al. Arylthioindole inhibitors of tubulin polymerization. 3. Biological evaluation, structure–activity relationships and molecular modeling studies. J Med Chem 2007;50(12):2865–74.
[26] Kaufmann D, Pojarová M, Vogel S, Liebl R, Gastpar R, Gross D, et al. Antimitotic activities of 2-phenylindole-3-carbaldehydes in human breast cancer cells. Bioorg Med Chem 2007; 15(15):5122–36.
[27] van deWaterbeemd H, Gifford E. ADMET *in silico* modelling: towards prediction paradise. Nat Rev Drug Discov 2003;2(23):192–204.
[28] Lombardo F, Gifford E, Shalaeva MY. *In silico* ADME prediction: data, models, facts and myths. Mini Rev Med Chem 2003;3(8):861–75.
[29] Moda TL, Montanari CA, Andricopulo AD. *In silico* prediction of human plasma protein binding using hologram QSAR. Lett Drug Des Discov 2007;4(7):502–9.
[30] Moda TL, Torres LG, Carrara AE, Andricopulo AD. PK/DB: database for pharmacokinetic properties and predictive *in silico* ADME models. Bioinformatics 2008;24(19):2270–1.
[31] Kubinyi H. QSAR: Hansch analysis and related approaches. Weinheim, Germany: VCH; 1993.
[32] Cramer RD, Patterson DE, Bunce JD. Comparative molecular field analysis (CoMFA). 1. Effect of shape on binding of steroids to carrier proteins. J Am Chem Soc 1988;110(18):5959–67.
[33] Free Jr. SM, Wilson JW. A mathematical contribution to structure–activity studies. J Med Chem 1964;7:395–9.
[34] Kier LB, Hall LH. Molecular connectivity in chemistry and drug research. New York, NY: Academic Press; 1976.
[35] Winkler DA, Burden FR. Holographic QSAR of benzodiazepines. Quant Struct-Act Relat 1998;17(3):224–31.
[36] Goyal S, Dhanjal JK, Tyagi C, Goyal M, Grover A. Novel fragment-based QSAR modeling and combinatorial design of pyrazole-derived CRK3 inhibitors as potent antileishmanials. Chem Biol Drug Des 2014;84(1):54–62.
[37] Ajmani S, Kulkarni SA. Application of GQSAR for scaffold hopping and lead optimization in multitarget inhibitors. Mol Inf 2012;31(6–7):473–90.
[38] Ambure P, Roy K. Exploring structural requirements of leads for improving activity and selectivity against CDK5/p25 in Alzheimer's disease: an *in silico* approach. RSC Adv 2014;4(13):6702–9.
[39] Kar S, Roy K. Predictive toxicity modelling of benzodiazepine drugs using multiple *in silico* approaches: descriptor-based QSTR, group-based QSTR and 3D-toxicophore mapping. Mol Simul 2014. http://dx.doi.org/10.1080/08927022.2014.888718 [In press]
[40] Geladi P, Wold S, Esbensen K. Image analysis and chemical information in images. Anal Chim Acta 1986;191:473–80.
[41] Saghaie L, Shahlaei M, Madadkar-Sobhani A, Fassihi A. Application of partial least squares and radial basis function neural networks in multivariate imaging analysis—quantitative structure activity relationship: study of cyclin dependent kinase 4 inhibitors. J Mol Graph Model 2010;29(4): 518–28.
[42] Goodarzi M, Freitas MP. MIA-QSAR coupled to principal component analysis—adaptive neuro-fuzzy inference systems (PCA–ANFIS) for the modeling of the anti-HIV reverse transcriptase activities of TIBO derivatives. Eur J Med Chem 2010;45(4):1352–8.
[43] Goodarzi M, Freitas MP. MIA-QSAR, PCA-ranking and least-squares support-vector machines in the accurate prediction of the activities of phosphodiesterase type 5 (PDE-5) inhibitors. Mol Simul 2010;36(11):871–7.

[44] Goodarzi M, Freitas MP. MIA-QSAR modelling of activities of a series of AZT analogues: bi- and multilinear PLS regression. Mol Simul 2010;36(4):267–72.
[45] Goodarzi M, Freitas MP, Ferreira EB. Influence of changes in 2-D chemical structure drawings and image formats on the prediction of biological properties using MIA-QSAR. QSAR Comb Sci 2009; 28(4):458–64.
[46] Antunes JE, Freitas MP, da Cunha EFF, Ramalho TC, Rittner R. *In silico* prediction of novel phosphodiesterase type-5 inhibitors derived from Sildenafil, Vardenafil and Tadalafil. Bioorg Med Chem 2008;16(16):7599–606.
[47] Gao H, Williams C, Labute P, Bajorath J. Binary quantitative structure–activity relationship (QSAR) analysis of estrogen receptor ligands. J Chem Inf Comput Sci 1999;39:164–8.
[48] Du Q-S, Huang R-B, Wei YT, Pang Z-W, Du L-Q, Chou K-C. Fragment-based quantitative structure–activity relationship (FB-QSAR) for fragment-based drug design. J Comput Chem 2009; 30:295–304.
[49] Myint K-Z, Ma C, Wang L, Xie XQ. The fragment-similarity-based QSAR (FS-QSAR): a novel 2D-QSAR method to predict biological activities of triaryl bis-sulfone and COX2 analogs. SAR QSAR Environ Res 2011;22:385–410.
[50] Andrzej B, Jaroslaw PA. 4D-QSAR study on anti-HIV HEPT analogs. Bio Med Chem 2006;14(1): 273–9.
[51] Andrzej B, Jaroslaw P. Modeling robust QSAR 3: SOM-4DQSAR with iterative variable elimination IVE-PLS: application to steroid, azo dye and benzoic acid series. J Chem Inf Model 2007;47(4): 1469–80.
[52] Carolina HA, Kerly FM, Pasqualoto E, Ferreira I, Hopfinger AJ. 3D-pharmacophore mapping of thymidine-based inhibitors of TMPK as potential antituberculosis agents. J Comput Aided Mol Des 2010;24(2):157–72.
[53] Dahua P, Jianzhong L, Craig S, Hopfinger AJ, Yufeng T. Characterization of a ligand–receptor binding event using receptor dependent four-dimensional quantitative structure–activity relationship analysis. J Med Chem 2004;47(12):3075–88.
[54] Christoph O, Thomas JS, Bernhard W. 5D-QSAR for spirocyclic S1 receptor ligands by Quasar receptor surface modeling. Eur J Med Chem 2010;45(7):3116–24.
[55] Angelo V, Max D. 5D-QSAR: the key for simulating induced fit. J Med Chem 2002;45(11): 2139–49.
[56] Angelo V, Max D, Horst D, Kai-Malte H, Franz B, Markus AL. Novel ligands for the chemokine receptor-3 (CCR3): a receptor-modeling study based on 5D-QSAR. J Med Chem 2005;48(5): 1515–27.
[57] Sylvie D, Grant M, Nicholas JL, James PS. Quantitative structure–activity relationship (5D-QSAR) study of combretastatin like analogs as inhibitors of tubulin assembly. J Med Chem 2005;48(2): 457–65.
[58] Angelo V, Anne-Verene D, Morena S, Beat E. Predicting the toxic potential of drugs and chemicals *in silico*: a model for the peroxisome proliferator-activated receptor γ (PPAR γ). Toxicol Lett 2007; 173(1):17–23.
[59] Angelo V, Max D, Markus AL. Combining protein modeling and 6D-QSAR simulating the binding of structurally diverse ligands to the estrogen receptor. J Med Chem 2005;48(11):3700–3.
[60] Polanski J. Receptor dependent multidimensional QSAR for modeling drug–receptor interactions. Curr Med Chem 2009;16(25):3243–57.

CHAPTER 10

Other Related Techniques

Contents

Understanding the Basics of QSAR for Applications in Pharmaceutical Sciences and Risk Assessment.
ISBN: 978-0-12-801505-6, DOI: http://dx.doi.org/10.1016/B978-0-12-801505-6.00010-7

10.1 INTRODUCTION

Computer-assisted tools in drug design and discovery, with an incredible modernization of computational resources, are very much appreciated throughout the world. Both ligand- and structure-based approaches are increasingly being used for the design of small lead and druglike molecules with anticipated multitarget activities [1]. Various ligand-based methods have been developed for effective and comprehensive application in virtual screening (VS), *de novo* design, and lead optimization. Pharmacophore has become one of the major ligand-based tools in computational chemistry for the drug research and development process [2]. Again, molecular recognitions, including enzyme–substrate, drug–protein, drug–nucleic acid, protein–nucleic acid, and protein–protein interactions, play significant roles in many biological responses. As a consequence, identification of the binding mode and affinity of the drug molecule is crucial to understanding the underlying mechanism of action in the respective therapeutic response. In this perspective, structure-based drug design is always a front-runner among all the available drug design approaches. Molecular docking is one of the largely acclaimed structure-based approaches, widely used for the study of molecular recognition, which aims to predict the binding mode and binding affinity of a complex formed by two or more constituent molecules with known structures [3].

There are a handful of novel techniques invented in the last decade employing the combined information computed from receptors and ligands. These tools can be defined as a combination of structure- and ligand-based design tools in the evolution of drug discovery techniques. Undoubtedly, methods like comparative binding energy analysis (COMBINE) [4] and comparative residue interaction analysis (CoRIA) [5] are the front-runners in the abovementioned approach with encouraging successful applications in drug discovery.

In silico screening is generally defined as VS, which is used rationally to select compounds for biological in vitro/in vivo testing from chemical libraries and databases of hundreds of thousands of compounds [6]. The VS approach is used for computationally prioritizing drug candidate molecules for future synthesis by using certain filters. The filters may be created by employing knowledge about the protein target (in structure-based VS) or known bioactive ligands (in ligand-based VS). These computational methods are powerful tools, as they supply a straightforward way to estimate the properties of the molecules and establish them as probable drug candidates from a huge number of compounds in no time in a cost-effective way. A combination of bioinformatics and chemoinformatics is crucial to the success of VS of chemical libraries, which is an alternative and complementary approach to high-throughput screening (HTS) in the lead discovery process [7]. Simply stated, the VS attempts to improve the probability of identifying bioactive molecules by maximizing the true positive rate—that is, by ranking the truly active molecules as high as possible.

10.2 PHARMACOPHORE

10.2.1 Concept and definition

One of the most promising *in silico* concepts of computer-aided drug design (CADD) is that of the pharmacophore. The term *pharmacophore* was first coined by Paul Ehrlich in the early 1900s, but it was Monty Kier [8,9] who introduced the physical chemical concept of pharmacophore in a series of papers published between 1967 and 1971. The pharmacophore technique in modern drug discovery is extremely useful as an interface between the medicinal chemistry and computational chemistry, both in VS and library design for efficient hit discovery, as well as in the optimization of lead compounds to final drug candidates. Recent research has focused on the practice of parallel screening using pharmacophore models for bioactivity profiling and early-stage risk assessment of probable adverse effects and toxicity due to interaction of drug candidates with antitargets.

The hypothesis of pharmacophore is based on that the molecular recognition of a biological target by a class of compounds can be explained by a set of common features that interact with a set of complementary sites on the biological target [10]. Along with the features, their three-dimensional (3D) relationship with each of the features is another crucial component of the pharmacophore concept. It is closely linked to the widely used principle of bioisosterism, which can be adopted by medicinal chemists while designing bioactive compound series.

The pharmacophore can be simply defined by the following, as stated in the International Union of Pure and Applied Chemistry (IUPAC) definition of the term given in Wermuth et al. [11]:

> *A pharmacophore is the ensemble of steric and electronic features that is necessary to ensure the optimal supramolecular interactions with a specific biological target structure and to trigger (or to block) its biological response.*
>
> *A pharmacophore does not represent a real molecule or a real association of functional groups, but a purely abstract concept that accounts for the common molecular interaction capacities of a group of compounds toward their target structure.*
>
> *A pharmacophore can be considered as the largest common denominator shared by a set of active molecules. This definition discards a misuse often found in the medicinal chemistry literature, which consists of naming as pharmacophores simple chemical functionalities such as guanidines, sulfonamides, or dihydroimidazoles (formerly imidazolines), or typical structural skeletons such as flavones, phenothiazines, prostaglandins, or steroids.*
>
> *A pharmacophore is defined by pharmacophoric descriptors, including H-bonding, hydrophobic, and electrostatic interaction sites, defined by atoms, ring centers, and virtual points.*

The pharmacophore describes the essential steric and electronic, function-determining points necessary for an optimal interaction with a relevant pharmacological target. It can also be thought of as a template, a partial description of a molecule where certain blanks need to be filled. The types of ligand molecules and the size and diversity of the data set have a great impact on the resulting pharmacophore model. Although a pharmacophore model signifies the key interactions between a ligand and its biological target, neither the structure of the target nor its identity is required to construct a handy pharmacophore model. As a consequence, pharmacophore approaches are often considered to be vital when the accessible information is very restricted. For example, when one knows nothing more than the structures of active ligands, a pharmacophore is the answer.

A simple hypothetical example is illustrated to define the common pharmacophores of three well-known compounds (namely, epinephrine, norepinephrine, and isoprenaline) in Figure 10.1.

10.2.2 Background and early days of pharmacophore

Introducing the term *pharmacophore* in the year 1909, Ehrlich [12], nicknamed the "father of drug discovery," defined it as "a molecular framework that carries (*phoros*) the essential features responsible for a drug's (*pharmacon*) biological activity." Although the first definition of the term was credited to Ehrlich, it was Kier who introduced the physical chemical concept in the late 1960s and early 1970s when describing common molecular features of ligands of important central nervous system receptors. This was labeled as "muscarinic pharmacophore" by Kier [8,9].

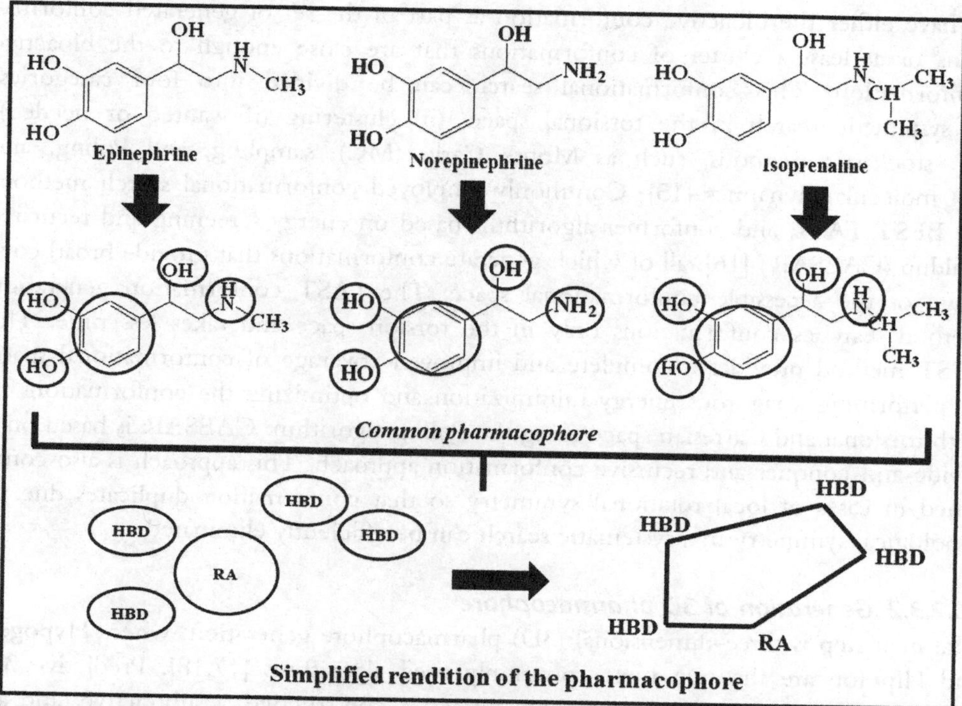

Figure 10.1 Depiction of common pharmacophoric features of three well-known compounds: epinephrine, norepinephrine, and isoprenaline.

In the past, pharmacophore models were mainly worked out manually, assisted through the use of simple interactive molecular graphics visualization programs. Later, the growing complexities of molecular structures required refined computer programs for the determination and use of pharmacophore models. In the evolution of computational chemistry, the fundamental perception of a pharmacophore model as a simple geometric depiction of the key molecular interactions remains unchanged. With the advances in computational chemistry in the past 20 years, a variety of automated tools for pharmacophore modeling and applications emerged. A considerable number of studies have been carried out since the development of the pharmacophore approach [13]. Pharmacophore approaches have been used comprehensively in VS, *de novo* design, as well as in lead optimization and multitarget drug design [14].

10.2.3 Methodology of pharmacophore mapping

10.2.3.1 Diverse conformation generation

Conformational expansion is the most critical step, since the goal is not only to have the most representative coverage of the conformational space of a molecule, but also to have either the bioactive conformation as part of the set of generated conformations or at least a cluster of conformations that are close enough to the bioactive conformation. This conformational search can be divided into four categories: (i) systematic search in the torsional space, (ii) clustering (if wanted or needed), (iii) stochastic methods, such as Monte Carlo (MC), sampling, and Poling, and (iv) molecular dynamics [15]. Commonly employed conformational search methods are BEST, FAST, and conformer algorithms based on energy screening and recursive buildup (CAESAR) [16], all of which generate conformations that provide broad coverage of the accessible conformational space. The FAST conformation generation method searches conformations only in the torsion space and takes less time. The BEST method provides a complete and improved coverage of conformational space by performing a rigorous energy minimization and optimizing the conformations in both torsional and Cartesian space using the Poling algorithm. CAESAR is based on a divide-and-conquer and recursive conformation approach. This approach is also combined in cases of local rotational symmetry so that conformation duplicates due to topological symmetry in a systematic search can be efficiently eliminated.

10.2.3.2 Generation of 3D pharmacophore

The next step is three-dimensional (3D) pharmacophore generation, where Hypogen and HipHop are the two most commonly used algorithms [17,18]. Predictive 3D pharmacophores are generated in three phases: a constructive, a subtractive, and an optimization phase, as follows:

Constructive phase: HipHop is intended to derive common feature hypothesis-based pharmacophore models using information from a set of active compounds. HipHop does not require the selection of a template; rather, each molecule is treated as a template in turn. Different configurations of chemical features are identified in the template molecule using a pruned exhaustive search, which starts with small sets of features and then extends until no larger configuration is found. Next, each configuration is compared with the remaining molecules to identify configurations that are common to all molecules. The resulting pharmacophores are ranked using a combination of how well the molecules in the training set map onto the pharmacophore model. In HipHop, the user can define how many molecules must map completely or partially to a pharmacophore configuration. Again, HypoGen [18] is an algorithm that uses the activity values of the small compounds in the training set to generate hypotheses to build 3D pharmacophore models. HypoGen identifies all allowable pharmacophores consisting of up to five features among the two most active compounds and investigates the remaining active compounds in the list.

Subtractive phase: This phase deals with pharmacophores that were created in the constructive phase and removes pharmacophores from the data structure that are not likely to be useful.

Optimization phase: The optimization phase is performed using the simulated annealing algorithm. A maximum of 10 hypotheses are generated for each run. HypoGen develops models with different pharmacophore features: (i) hydrogen-bond acceptor (HBA); (ii) hydrogen-bond donor (HBD); (iii) hydrophobic (HYD), HYDROPHOBIC (aliphatic) and HYDROPHOBIC (aromatic); (iv) negative charge (NEG CHARGE); (v) negative ionizable (NI); (vi) positive charge (POS CHARGE); (vii) positive ionizable (PI); and (viii) ring aromatic (RA). The hypotheses generated are analyzed in terms of their correlation coefficients and the cost function values.

The basic pharmacophore features are illustrated in Figure 10.2. Pharmacophore models are usually labeled based on the number of features. For example, pharmacophore models consisting of three and four features are termed as three-point pharmacophore and four-point pharmacophore, respectively. A simple graphical representation is shown in Figure 10.3.

10.2.3.3 Assessment of the quality of pharmacophore hypotheses

The *HypoGen* module performs a fixed cost calculation that represents the simple model that fits all the data, and a null cost calculation that assumes that there is no

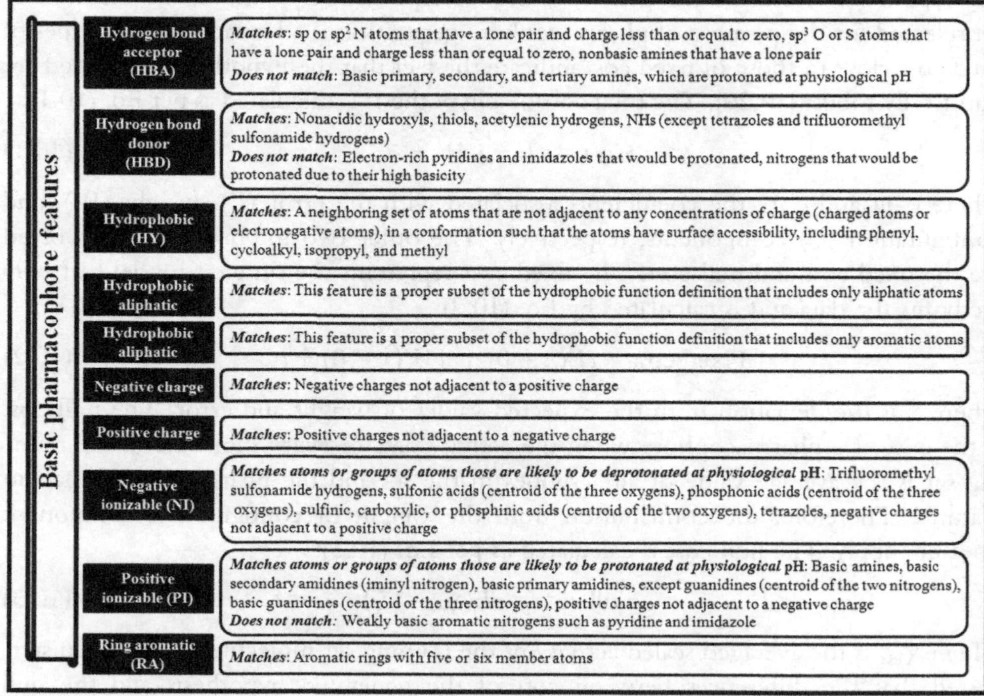

Figure 10.2 Basic pharmacophore features and their definitions.

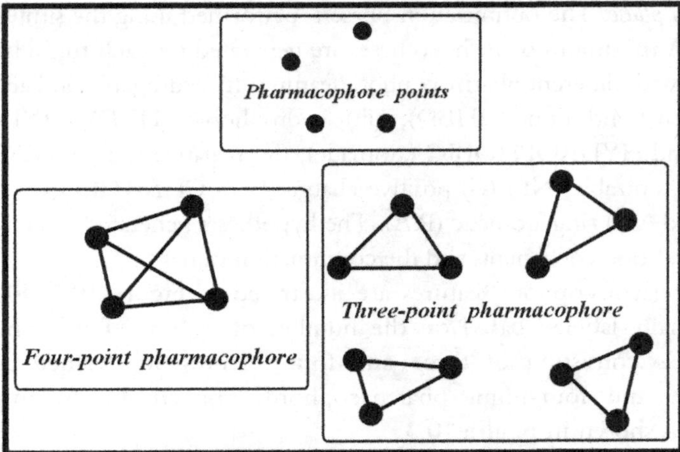

Figure 10.3 Point-based pharmacophore concepts.

relationship in the data set and that the experimental activities are normally distributed about their average value. A small range of the total hypothesis cost obtained for each of the hypotheses indicates homogeneity of the corresponding hypothesis, and the training set selected for the purpose of pharmacophore generation is adequate. Again, values of total cost close to those of fixed cost indicate the fact that the hypotheses generated are statistically robust [19,20]. The total cost of a hypothesis is calculated as per Eq. (10.1):

$$\text{Cost} = eE + wW + cC \tag{10.1}$$

where e, w, and c are the coefficients associated with the error (E), weight (W), and configuration (C) components, respectively. The other two important costs involved are the fixed cost and null cost. The fixed cost represents the simplest model that perfectly fits the data and is calculated by Eq. (10.2):

$$\text{Fixed cost} = eE(x = 0) + wW(x = 0) + cC \tag{10.2}$$

where x is the deviation from the expected values of weight and error. The null cost is the cost of a pharmacophore when the activity data of every molecule in the training set is the average value of all activities in the set and the pharmacophore has no features. Therefore, the contribution from the weight or configuration component does not apply. The null cost is calculated as per Eq. (10.3):

$$\text{Null cost} = eE(\chi_{est} = \overline{\chi}) \tag{10.3}$$

where χ_{est} is the averaged scaled activity of the training set molecules. It has been suggested that the differences between cost of the generated hypothesis and the null hypothesis should be as large as possible; a value of 40–60 bits difference may indicate that it has a 75–90% chance of representing a true correlation in the data set used. The total cost of any hypothesis should be toward the value of fixed cost to represent any meaningful model. Two other very important output parameters are the configuration cost and the error cost. Any value of configuration cost higher than 17 may indicate that the correlation from any generated pharmacophore is most likely due to chance. The error cost increases as the value of the root mean square (RMS) increases. The RMS deviations (RMSDs) represent the quality of the correlation between the estimated and the actual activity data.

10.2.3.4 Validation of the pharmacophore model

The pharmacophore models selected based on the acceptable correlation coefficient (R) and cost analysis, should be validated in three subsequent steps: (i) Fischer's randomization test, (ii) test set prediction, and (iii) Güner–Henry (GH) scoring method.

Fischer's randomization test: First, cross-validation is performed and statistical significance of the structure–activity correlation is estimated by randomizing the data using the Fischer's randomization test [20]. This is done by scrambling the activity data of the training set molecules and assigning them new values, followed by the generation of pharmacophore hypotheses using the same features and parameters as those used to develop the original pharmacophore hypothesis. The original hypothesis is considered to be generated by mere chance if the randomized data set results in the generation of a pharmacophore with better or nearly equal correlation compared to the original one.

Test set prediction: The purpose of the pharmacophore hypothesis generation is not only to predict the activity of the training set compounds [21], but also to predict the activities of external molecules. With the objective of verifying whether the pharmacophore is able to predict the activity of test set molecules in agreement with the experimentally determined value, the activities of the test set molecules are estimated based on the mapping of the test set molecules to the developed pharmacophore model. The conformers are generated for the test set molecules based on the method that is used during the conformer generation of the training set, and they are mapped using the corresponding pharmacophore models. Thus, the predictive capacity of the models is judged based on the predictive R^2 values (R^2_{pred} with a threshold value of 0.5) or classification-based methods (such as sensitivity, specificity, precision, and accuracy). The test set should cover similar structural diversity as the training set in order to establish the broadness of the pharmacophore predictability.

GH scoring: The GH scoring method is employed following test set validation to evaluate the quality of the pharmacophore models [22–24]. The GH score can be successfully applied to quantify model selectivity precision of hits and the recall of actives from a directory of useful decoys (DUD) data set [25] consisting of known actives and inactives. The DUD is a publicly available database for free use, generated based on the observation that physical characteristics of the decoy background can be used for the classification of different compounds. The DUD can be downloaded from http://dud.docking.org.

The method involves evaluation of the following: the percent yield of actives in a database (%*Y*, recall), the percent ratio of actives in the hit list (%*A*, precision), the enrichment factor *E*, and the GH score. The GH score ranges from 0 to 1, where a value of 1 signifies the ideal model. The following are the metrics used for analyzing hit lists by a pharmacophore model–based database search:

$$\%A = \frac{\mathrm{Ha}}{A} \times 100 \tag{10.4}$$

$$\%Y = \frac{\mathrm{Ha}}{\mathrm{Ht}} \times 100 \tag{10.5}$$

$$E = \frac{\mathrm{Ha}/\mathrm{Ht}}{A/D} \tag{10.6}$$

$$\mathrm{GH} = \left[\frac{\mathrm{Ha}(3A + \mathrm{Ht})}{4\mathrm{Ht}A}\right]\left(1 - \frac{\mathrm{Ht} - \mathrm{Ha}}{D - A}\right) \tag{10.7}$$

In these equations, %*A* is the percentage of known active compounds retrieved from the database (precision); Ha is the number of actives in the hit list (true positives); *A* is the number of active compounds in the database; %*Y* is the percentage of known actives in the hit list (recall); Ht is the number of hits retrieved; *D* is the number of compounds in the database; and *E* is the enrichment of the concentration of actives by the model relative to random screening without any pharmacophoric approach.

The basic steps of pharmacophore formalism are represented in Figure 10.4.

10.2.4 Types of pharmacophore

A pharmacophore model can be generated in two ways. The first method is ligand-based modeling, where a set of active molecules are superimposed and common chemical features are extracted that are necessary for their bioactivity; the second is structure-based modeling performed by probing possible interaction points between the macromolecular target and ligands.

10.2.4.1 Ligand-based pharmacophore modeling

Ligand-based pharmacophore (LBP) modeling has become an important computational tool for assisting drug discovery in the case of nonavailability of a

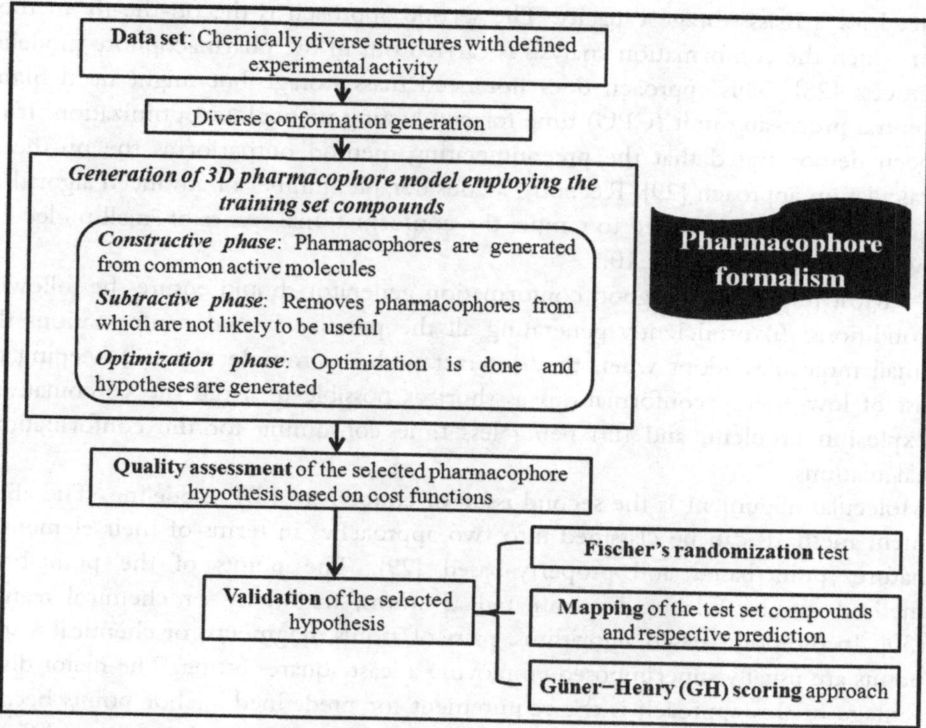

Figure 10.4 Fundamental steps of pharmacophore formalism.

macromolecular target structure [26,27]. The LBP is usually carried out by extracting common chemical features from the 3D structures of a known set of ligands representative of fundamental interactions between the ligands and a specific macromolecular target. In the case of LBP modeling, pharmacophore generation from multiple ligands involves two major steps: First, creation of the conformational space for each ligand in the training set to represent conformational flexibility of the ligands and to align the multiple ligands in the training set, and second, determination of the essential common chemical features to build the pharmacophore model. The conformational analysis of ligands and performing molecular alignment are the key techniques as well as the main complexities in any LBP modeling.

A few challenges still exist in spite of the great advances of LBP modeling:

a. The first problem, and one of the most serious, is the modeling of ligand flexibility. Presently, two strategies are utilized to deal with this problem. The first is the preenumerating method, in which multiple conformations for each ligand are precomputed and saved in a database [28]. The advantage of this approach is lower computing cost for conducting molecular alignment at the expense of a possible need for a mass storage capacity. The second approach is the on-the-fly method, in which the conformation analysis is carried out in the pharmacophore modeling process [28]. This approach does not need mass storage but might need higher central processing unit (CPU) time for conducting meticulous optimization. It has been demonstrated that the preenumerating method outperforms the on-the-fly calculation approach [29]. Recently, a considerable number of advanced algorithms [14] have been established to sample the conformational spaces of small molecules, which are listed in Table 10.1.

Most importantly, a good conformation generator should ensure the following conditions: (i) proficiently generating all the putative bound conformations that small molecules adopt when they interact with macromolecules, (ii) keeping the list of low-energy conformations as short as possible to avoid the combinational explosion problem, and (iii) being less time consuming for the conformational calculations.

b. Molecular alignment is the second issue of concern in LBP modeling. The alignment methods can be classified into two approaches in terms of their elementary nature: point-based and property-based [29]. The points of the point-based method can be further discriminated as atoms, fragments, or chemical features [30]. In the point-based algorithms, pairs of atoms, fragments, or chemical feature points are usually superimposed employing a least-squares fitting. The major disadvantage of this approach is the requirement for predefined anchor points because the generation of these points can become problematic in the case of different ligands. Consequently, the property-based algorithms utilize molecular field descriptors, generally represented by sets of Gaussian functions, to generate alignments. Recently, new alignment methods have been developed, including stochastic proximity embedding [31], atomic property fields [32], fuzzy pattern recognition [33], and grid-based interaction energies [34].

c. The third challenge lies in the appropriate selection of training set compounds. Although this problem is simple and nontechnical, but it often puzzles researchers nonetheless. The type of ligand molecules, the size of the data set, and its chemical diversity largely affect considerably the final generated pharmacophore model [28].

10.2.4.2 Structure-based pharmacophore modeling

Structure-based pharmacophore (SBP) modeling is directly dependent on the 3D structures of macromolecular targets or macromolecule–ligand complexes. As the number of experimentally determined 3D structure of targets has grown to a very large number, SBP methods have attracted significant interest in the last decade. The approach is considered as the complementary one to the docking procedures, providing the same level of information as well as less demanding with respect to required computational resources. The protocol of SBP modeling involves analyzing the

Table 10.1 Various conformational sampling methods

Conformational sampling method	Characteristics
3DGEN	1. An algorithm for exhaustive generation of 3D isomers proceeding from molecular topology 2. A systematic approach 3. Based on a combinatorial process
Balloon	1. A stochastic algorithm 2. A multiobjective GA is employed 3. Removing conformational duplicates 4. Can effectively produce low-energy conformers, which are geometrically distinct from each other
CAESAR	1. A systematic search method 2. Based on a divide-and-conquer and recursive conformer buildup approach 3. Avoids conformer duplicates due to topological symmetry 4. Capable of reproducing the receptor-bound conformation
CONAN	1. A fragment-based, buildup approach combined with the rule-based method 2. Intersection strategy is used for conformational analysis
ConfGen	1. A systematic approach based on divide-and-conquer strategy 2. A rule-based approach is incorporated 3. Intended for the high-throughput generation of 3D databases
Conformation import workflow in the molecular operating environment (MOE)	1. A systematic approach with the use of divide-and-conquer strategy and combined with rule-based method 2. Each fragment is subject to a stochastic search algorithm, expected to locate most its low-energy conformers 3. A high-throughput conformer generator for library preparation
Corina	1. Fast approach 2. Straightforward performance, reasonable execution time, simplicity, and applicability to building large, 3D chemical inventories 3. Often gives a larger average RMSD to the bioactive conformation
Cyndi	1. Nondeterministic method 2. Based on a multiobjective genetic algorithm (MOGA) 3. Efficient, particularly when reproducing a bioactive conformation

(Continued)

Table 10.1 (Continued)

Conformational sampling method	**Characteristics**
Directed tweak	1. Originally for 3D query searches 2. A torsional space minimizer 3. Involving the use of analytical derivatives, and is fast as a result 4. Allowing 3D flexible searching on an interactive time scale
Genetic algorithm	1. Nondeterministic method 2. Suitable for the superimposition of sets of flexible molecules
MED-3DMC	1. Nondeterministic method 2. A Metropolis MC algorithm based on a SMARTS mapping of the rotational bonds and the MMFF94 VDW energy term is used 3. Capable of sampling the conformational space with a small average RMSD to the bioactive conformation.
MIMUMBA	1. A rule-based method 2. The revised version is in conjunction with the OMEGA approach 3. The rules can be extracted from statistical observations from a training portion of the CSD
Molecular dynamics simulation method	1. Can create reasonable conformers 2. Time consuming 3. Depends on temperature and simulation time 4. Is of special interest when dealing with molecular conformations in solution
Monte Carlo	1. A stochastic method 2. Solvation effects can be studied in an explicit solvent 3. Do not guarantee that the conformational space has been explored exhaustively; in particular, the output of a search may depend on the starting conformation 4. Efficient at the beginning of a search, but efficiency degrades as the search proceeds
OMEGA	1. A rule-based method (heuristic) combined with divide-and-conquer strategy 2. A high-throughput conformer generator for library preparation
Poling restraints	1. A stochastic method 2. Promoting conformational variation 3. Avoiding analogous conformers 4. Covering most of the pharmacophore space with significantly fewer conformers

(*Continued*)

Table 10.1 (Continued)

Conformational sampling method	Characteristics
Self-organization method	1. A distance geometry (DG) approach 2. Conformations generated are consistent with a set of geometric constraints, which include interatomic distance bounds and chiral volumes derived from the molecular connectivity table 3. Tending to produce relatively compact conformers
Systematic torsional grid method	1. A systematic search method 2. Uses a recursive tree search algorithm 3. Can generate all conformations of polypeptides which satisfy experimental NMR restraints 4. Time consuming
WIZARD	1. A rule-based method (heuristic) 2. Expert system techniques are adopted

complementary chemical features of the active site and their spatial relationships, and developing a pharmacophore model assembly with selected features [2].

SBP modeling can be further classified into two subclasses: macromolecule–ligand–complex based and macromolecule (without ligand) based. The macromolecule–ligand–complex-based approach is suitable in identifying the ligand binding site of the macromolecular target and determining the key interaction points between ligands and the target protein. LigandScout [35] is an excellent software program that incorporates the macromolecule–ligand–complex-based scheme. Programs like Pocket v.2 [36] and GBPM [37] are based on the same approach. The major limitation of this process is the requirement for the 3D structure of the macromolecule–ligand complex. As a consequence, it cannot be applied to cases when no ligands targeting the binding site of interest are known. This can be solved by the macromolecule-based approach. The SBP method implemented in the Discovery Studio software [18] is a typical example of a macromolecule-based approach [38].

The most commonly encountered difficulty for SBP modeling is the identification of too many chemical features for a specific binding site of the macromolecular target. A pharmacophore model consisting of too many chemical features (e.g., more than seven) is not appropriate for practical applications (e.g., 3D database screening). Therefore, it is always important to pick a restricted number of chemical features (usually three to seven) to create a reliable pharmacophore hypothesis. One more significant drawback is that the obtained pharmacophore hypothesis cannot replicate the quantitative structure–activity relationship (QSAR) because the model is generated based just on a single macromolecule–ligand complex or a single macromolecule.

10.2.5 Application of pharmacophore models

Enrichment in the pharmacophore techniques in the last two decades has made the approach one of the most significant tools in drug discovery. In spite of the advances in key techniques of pharmacophore modeling, there is space for additional improvement to derive more precise and best possible pharmacophore models, which include better handling of ligand flexibility, proficient molecular alignment algorithms, and more precise model optimization. Along with the pharmacophore-based VS and *de novo* design, the applications of pharmacophore have been extended to lead optimization [39], multitarget drug design [40], activity profiling [41], and target identification [42]. Application of the pharmacophore technique is demonstrated in a schematic way in Figure 10.5.

10.2.5.1 Pharmacophore model–based VS

Pharmacophore models can be used for querying the 3D chemical database to search for potential ligands; this process is termed *pharmacophore-based VS*. In the case of the pharmacophore-based VS approach, a pharmacophore hypothesis is taken as a

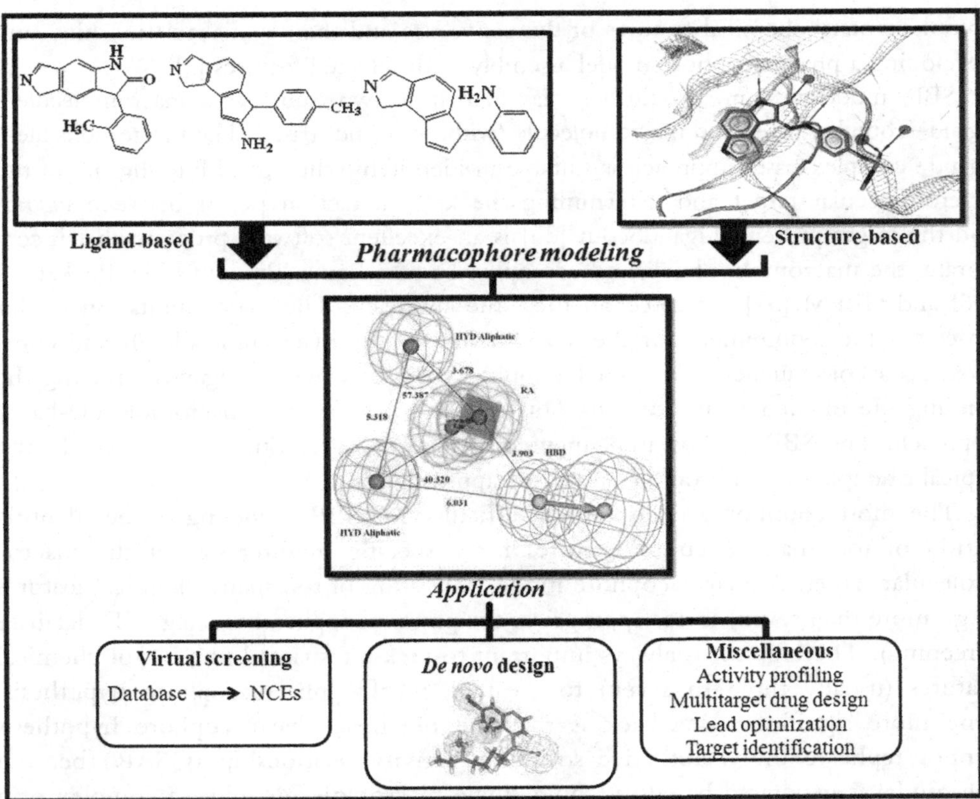

Figure 10.5 Diverse applications of the pharmacophore technique.

template. The intention behind the screening is actually to discover such hits that have chemical features similar to those of the template. Sometimes these hits might be related to known active compounds, but few have completely novel scaffolds. The screening process involves two major difficulties: handling the conformational flexibility of small molecules and pharmacophore pattern identification.

The flexibility of small molecules is handled either by preenumerating multiple conformations for each molecule or conformational sampling at search time. Pharmacophore pattern identification, usually known as *substructure searching*, is performed to check whether a query pharmacophore is present in a given conformer of a molecule. The commonly used approaches for substructure searching are Ullmann [43], the backtracking algorithm [44], and the Generic Match Algorithm (GMA) [45].

The most challenging problem for pharmacophore-based VS is that few percentages of the virtual hits are really bioactive. In simpler words, the screening results produce a higher false-positive rate, a higher false-negative rate, or both. Many factors like the quality and composition of the pharmacophore model and the macromolecular target information can contribute to this problem. The most probable factors are as follows:

a. The most critical one is the development of a robust and reliable pharmacophore hypothesis. Addressing this issue requires an inclusive validation and optimization of the pharmacophore model.

b. Different molecules can be retrieved in VS from different hypotheses of a single pharmacophore model, which is probably an important reason for the higher false-positive/false-negative rates in some studies.

c. The flexibility of target macromolecule in pharmacophore approaches is handled by introducing a tolerance radius for each pharmacophoric feature, which is unlikely to entirely account for macromolecular flexibility in some cases. Recent attempts [46] to integrate molecular dynamics simulation (MDS) into pharmacophore modeling have recommended that the pharmacophore models generated from MDS trajectories explain the considerably enhanced representation of the flexibility of pharmacophores.

d. The steric restriction by the macromolecular target which is not adequately considered in pharmacophore models, although it is partially accounted for by the consideration of excluded volumes. In most of the cases, interactions between a ligand and a protein are distance-sensitive, particularly the short-range interactions, such as the electrostatic interaction, which a pharmacophore model is tricky to account for. As a consequence, the combination of pharmacophore-based and docking-based VS can be considered as an efficient approach for VS.

10.2.5.2 Pharmacophore-based de novo *design*

Another vital application of pharmacophore is *de novo* design of ligands. In the case of pharmacophore-based VS, the obtained compounds are generally existing chemicals that might be patent protected. On the contrary, the *de novo* design approach can be used to generate entirely novel candidate structures that match to the requirements of a given pharmacophore. The first pharmacophore-based *de novo* design program is NEWLEAD [47]. It uses a set of disconnected molecular fragments that are consistent with a pharmacophore model as input. The selected sets of disconnected pharmacophore fragments are subsequently connected by using various linkers (such as atoms, chains, or ring moieties).

The limitation with NEWLEAD is that it can only handle cases in which the pharmacophore features are functional groups (not typical chemical features). The additional inadequacy of the NEWLEAD program is that the sterically illicit region of the binding site is not considered. As a result, the compounds created by the NEWLEAD program might be tricky to chemically synthesize. There are programs like LUDI [10] and BUILDER [48] that can also be used to amalgamate identification of SBP with *de novo* design. Both programs require knowledge of the 3D structures of the macromolecular targets.

More recently, a program called PhDD (a pharmacophore-based *de novo* design method of druglike molecules) has been designed by Huang et al. [49], to overcome the limitations of the present pharmacophore-based, *de novo* design software tools. PhDD can involuntarily create druglike compounds that satisfy the necessities of an input pharmacophore hypothesis. The pharmacophore used in PhDD can be consisted of a set of abstract chemical features and excluded volumes which are the sterically forbidden region of the binding site. In the case of PhDD, it first generates a set of new molecules that entirely conform to the requirements of the given pharmacophore model. Thereafter, a series of evaluation to the generated molecules are carried out, including the assessments of drug-likeness, bioactivity, and synthetic convenience.

10.2.6 Advantages and limitations of pharmacophore

Like any other approach, pharmacophore has both advantages and disadvantages. The major advantages and limitations are as follows:

Advantages

- Pharmacophore models can be used for VS on a large database.
- There is no need to know the binding site of the ligands in the macromolecular target protein, although this is true only for LBP modeling.
- It can be used for the design, optimization of drugs, and scaffolds hopping.
- It can conceptually be obtained even for 2D structural representation.
- This approach is comprehensive and editable. By adding or omitting chemical feature constraints, information can be easily traced to its source.

Limitations

- 2D pharmacophore is faster but less accurate than 3D pharmacophore.

- A pharmacophore is based only on the ligand structure and conformation. No interactions with the proteins are integrated. It is interesting to point out that in this case, SBP modeling can be used to solve the problem.
- It is sensitive to physicochemical features.

10.2.7 Software tools for pharmacophore analysis

Pharmacophore modeling is extensively used because of its immense accessibility through commercial software packages. Also, there is a freely available web server called PharmaGist (http://bioinfo3d.cs.tau.ac.il/PharmaGist/) for detecting a pharmacophore from a group of ligands known to bind to a particular target. A complete list of different commercialized and freely available software and program modules [19,35–38]) used for pharmacophore modeling is given in Table 10.2.

10.3 STRUCTURE-BASED DESIGN–DOCKING

10.3.1 Concept and definition of docking

Molecular docking is the study of how two or more molecular structures (e.g., drug and enzyme or protein) fit together [50]. In a simple definition, docking is a molecular modeling technique that is used to predict how a protein (enzyme) interacts with small molecules (ligands). The ability of a protein (enzyme) and nucleic acid to interact with small molecules to form a supramolecular complex plays a major role in the dynamics of the protein, which may enhance or inhibit its biological function. The behavior of small molecules in the binding pockets of target proteins can be described by molecular docking. The method aims to identify correct poses of ligands in the binding pocket of a protein and to predict the affinity between the ligand and the protein. Based on the types of ligand, docking can be classified as

- Protein–small molecule (ligand) docking
- Protein–nucleic acid docking
- Protein–protein docking

Protein–small molecule (ligand) docking represents a simpler end of the complexity spectrum, and there are many available programs that perform particularly well in predicting molecules that may potentially inhibit proteins. Protein–protein docking is typically much more complex. The reason is that proteins are flexible and their conformational space is quite vast.

Docking can be performed by placing the rigid molecules or fragments into the protein's active site using different approaches like clique-searching, geometric hashing, or pose clustering. The performance of docking depends on the search algorithm [e.g., MC methods, genetic algorithms (GAs), fragment-based methods, Tabu searches, distance geometry methods, and the scoring functions like force field (FF)

Table 10.2 Software and programs for pharmacophore modeling

Ligand-based methods				
Software	**Conformational analysis algorithm**	**Molecular alignment**	**Significant characteristics**	**Remarks**
ALADDIN	N/A*	N/A*	Design and pharmacophore generation from geometric, steric, and substructure searching of 3D structures	Not commercialized
Apex-3D	Preenumerating method	Feature-based method	An expert system developed to represent, elucidate, and utilize knowledge on structure–activity relationships	Catalyst (Biovia, http://accelrys.com/)
APOLLO	Preenumerating method	Feature-based method	Identifying from a set of ligands their interaction points belonging to the receptor site and creating a pseudoreceptor	Not commercialized
CLEW	N/A*	Feature-based method	Utilizing the machine-learning method and geometrical fitting to develop the pharmacophore	Not commercialized
DANTE	N/A*	N/A*	Inferring pharmacophores automatically from structure–activity data, which include information about the shape of the binding cavity	Not commercialized
DISCO	Preenumerating method by Concord and Confort via the Sybyl interface	Bron–Kerbosh clique-detection algorithm	Considering 3D conformations of compounds as sets of interpoint distances	Integrated into the Sybyl interface, which is available from Tripos Inc. (www.tripos.com)
GALAHAD	Both preenumerating method and on-the-fly	Atom-based method	A more sophisticated GA is used for pharmacophore modeling	Integrated into the Sybyl interface, which is available from Tripos Inc. (www.tripos.com)

(*Continued*)

Table 10.2 (Continued)

Ligand-based methods				
Software	**Conformational analysis algorithm**	**Molecular alignment**	**Significant characteristics**	**Remarks**
GAMMA	On-the-fly	Atom-based method	The conformational search and the pattern identification are performed simultaneously by utilizing the GA technique	Not commercialized
GASP	On-the-fly	Atom-based method	A flexible GA is used for pharmacophore identification	Integrated into the Sybyl interface, which is available from Tripos Inc. (www.tripos.com)
HipHop	Preenumerating method by the Poling algorithm	Feature-based method	Identifying common features by a pruned exhaustive search (qualitative model)	Discovery Studio (Biovia, http://accelrys.com/)
HypoGen	Preenumerating method by the Poling algorithm	Feature-based method	Designed to correlate structure and activity (quantitative model)	Discovery Studio (Biovia, http://accelrys.com/)
HypoRefine	Preenumerating method by the Poling algorithm	Feature-based method	An extension to the HypoGen Exclusion volumes are involved	Discovery Studio (Biovia, http://accelrys.com/)
MOE	Preenumerating method ranging from molecular dynamics to stochastic methods and systematic search	Property-based algorithm	A pharmacophore is defined manually by applying schemes using a Pharmacophore Query Editor	Chemical Computing Group, Inc. (www.chemcomp.com)
MPHIL	On-the-fly	Atom-based method (rigid)	Based on clique detection and GA	Not commercialized
PharmaGist	On-the-fly	Feature-based method	A webserver for LBP detection	http://bioinfo3d.cs.tau.ac.il/PharmaGist
PHASE	Preenumerating method by Schrödinger's ConfGen technology	Feature-based method (called *sites*)	Very flexible and user friendly. SMARTS pattern matching is used for feature location. Excluded volumes are included.	Schrödinger Inc. (www.schrodinger.com)

(*Continued*)

Table 10.2 (Continued)

Ligand-based methods

Software	Conformational analysis algorithm	Molecular alignment	Significant characteristics	Remarks
RAPID	Preenumerating method	Atom-based method	A rigid alignment based on mapping triangles of 3D atom coordinates	Not commercialized
SCAMPI	On the fly	Feature-based method	Can handle large heterogeneous data sets	Not commercialized
XED	Preenumerating method	Molecular field-based method	Using field points to describe the VDW and electrostatic potential that surround molecules	Marketed by Cresset Biomolecular (http://www.cresset-group.com/)

Structure-based methods

Software	Molecular alignment	Significant characteristics	Remarks
GBPM	Complex-based	Based on logical and clustering operations with 3D maps computed by the GRID program on structurally known molecular complexes. Particularly suitable for identifying protein–protein interaction areas.	Not commercialized
LigandScout	Complex-based	Incorporating a complete definition of 3D chemical features. Pharmacophoric feature points-based pattern-matching alignment algorithm is used. Intuitive and easy to use.	Marketed by Inte:Ligand (www.inteligand.com/ligandscout/)
Pocket v.2	Complex-based	Capable to generate a pharmacophore model with a rational number of features when one complex structure is available.	Not commercialized
SBP	Apoprotein-based	Directly converting LUDI interaction maps within the protein binding site into Catalyst pharmacophoric features.	Discovery Studio (Biovia, http://accelrys.com/)

N/A*: Not applicable or the exact information is not available.

methods and empirical free energy scoring functions]. The first step of docking is the generation of composition of all possible conformations and orientations of the protein paired with the ligand. The second step is that the scoring function takes input and returns a number indicating favorable interaction [51].

To identify the active site of the protein, first, selection of the required X-ray cocrystallized structure from the protein data bank (PDB) is performed, and then extracting the bound ligand, one can optimize the protein active site of interest. But the process of identification of the active site in a protein is critical when the bound ligand is absent in the crystal structure. In that case, one has to do the following procedures:

a. One can perform comprehensive literature review of the source papers (from which the X-ray crystal structure has been included in PDB) to identify the active site of residues.

b. If any established drug giving the same pharmacological action of interest is available for the protein, then the active sites for this drug should be identified. In the initial phase of analysis, one can try these residues as active binding sites for the test ligands.

c. Every docking software program usually has a particular algorithm to identify the active site of the protein by allowing binding of the ligand in different parts of the protein and exploring the best possible binding position of the ligands with the protein.

10.3.2 Definition of fundamental terms of docking

To understand the docking study better, one needs to know the basic terms related with the docking study. The most commonly used terms connected with docking studies are defined next. All the discussed terms are graphically represented in Figure 10.6:

Receptor: A *receptor* is a protein molecule or a polymeric structure in or on a cell that distinctively recognizes and binds a molecule (ligand) acting as a molecular messenger. When such ligands bind to a receptor, they cause some kind of cellular response.

Ligand: A *ligand* is the complementary partner molecule that binds to the receptor for effective bimolecular response. Ligands are most often small drug molecules, neurotransmitters, hormones, lymphokines, lectins, and antigens, but they could also be another biopolymer or macromolecule (in the case of protein–protein docking).

Docking: *Docking* is a molecular modeling technique designed to find the proper fit between a ligand and its binding site (receptor).

Dock pose: A ligand molecule can bind with a receptor in a multiple positions, conformations, and orientations. Each such docking mode is called a *dock pose*.

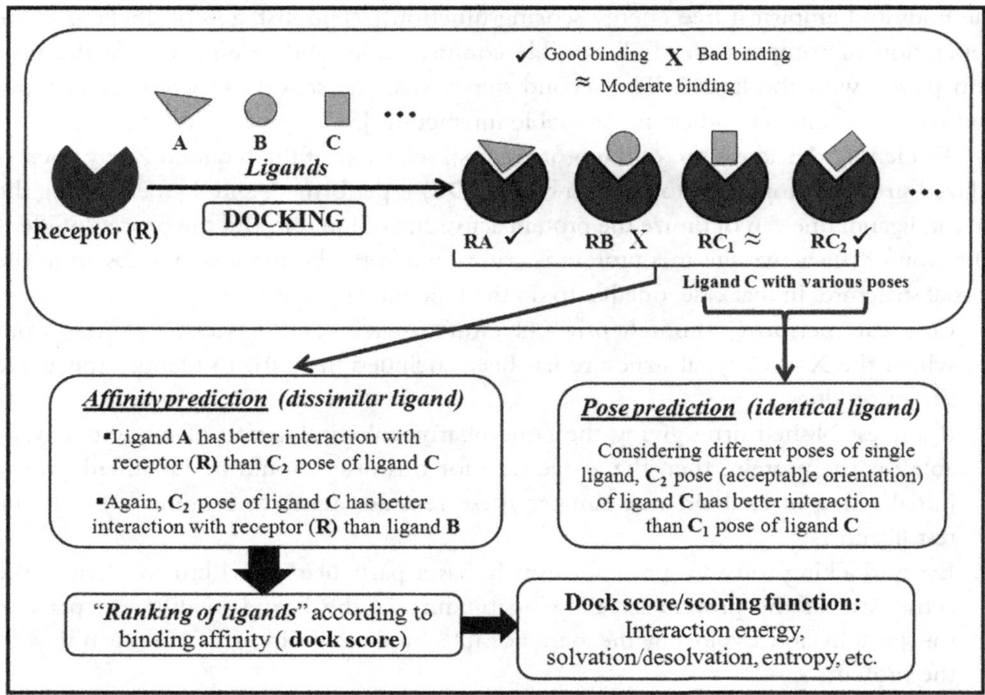

Figure 10.6 Graphical representation of commonly used terms in docking studies.

Binding mode: *Binding mode* is the orientation of the ligand relative to the receptor, as well as the conformation of the ligand and receptor when they are bound to each other.

Dock score: The process of evaluating a particular pose by counting the number of favorable intermolecular interactions such as hydrogen bonds and hydrophobic contacts. In order to recognize the energetically most favorable pose, each pose is evaluated based on its compatibility to the target in terms of shape and properties such as electrostatics and generate corresponding dock score. A good dock score for a given ligand signifies that it is potentially a good binder.

Ranking: *Ranking* is the process of classifying which ligands are most likely to interact favorably to a particular receptor based on the predicted free energy of binding. After completion of docking, all ligands are consequently ranked by their respective dock scores (i.e., their predicted affinities). This rank-ordered list is then employed for further synthesis and biological investigation only for those compounds that are predicted to be most active.

Pose prediction: *Pose prediction* can be defined as searching for the accurate binding mode of a ligand, which is typically carried out by performing a number of trials and keeping those poses that are energetically best. It involves finding the correct orientation and the correct conformation of the docked ligand due to their flexible nature.

Scoring or affinity prediction: Affinity prediction or scoring functions are applied to the energetically best pose or *n* number of best poses found for each ligand, and comparing the affinity scores for different ligands give their relative rank ordering. [52].

Scoring functions are generally divided into two main groups. One main group comprises knowledge-based scoring functions that are derived using statistics for the observed interatomic contact frequencies, distances, or both in a large database of crystal structures of protein–ligand complexes. The other group contains scoring schemes based on physical interaction terms [53]. These so-called energy component methods are based on the assumption that the change in free energy upon binding of a ligand to its target can be decomposed into a sum of individual contributions:

$$\Delta G_{\text{bind}} = \Delta G_{\text{int}} + \Delta G_{\text{solv}} + \Delta G_{\text{conf}} + \Delta G_{\text{motion}} \tag{10.8}$$

The terms defined for the main energetic contributions to the binding event are as follows: specific ligand–receptor interactions (ΔG_{int}), the interactions of ligand and receptor with solvent (ΔG_{solv}), the conformational changes in the ligand and the receptor (ΔG_{conf}), and the motions in the protein and the ligand during the complex formation (ΔG_{motion}).

10.3.3 Essential requirements of docking

1. *Receptor crystal structures*: To execute the docking study, it is essential to have the receptor structures of interest. The structure of the receptor can be determined by experimental techniques such as X-ray crystallography or nuclear magnetic resonance (NMR), and can be easily downloaded from the PDB (http://www.rcsb.org/pdb/home/home.do). The quality of the receptor structure plays a crucial role in the success of docking studies. In general, the higher the resolution (preferably <2 Å) of the employed crystal structure, the better the observed docking results are. Another important criterion for examining the quality of a receptor structure is Debye–Waller factor (DWF), or *B*-factor; or the temperature factor, which is used to describe the attenuation of X-ray scattering or coherent neutron scattering caused by thermal motion. It signifies the relative vibrational motion of different parts of the protein. Atoms with low *B*-factors belong to a part of the structure that is well ordered, and atoms with large *B*-factors generally belong to part of the structure that is very flexible. As a consequence, it is important to ensure that the *B*-factors of the atoms in the binding site region are logical, as high values imply that their coordinates are less reliable. Identification of the bound-ligand in the cocrystal structure and the knowledge about its interaction

with the corresponding protein's amino acid residues are very important before starting a docking study.

2. *Receptor homology modeling and threading techniques*: On the contrary, if the X-ray crystal structure of the protein is not available, one can opt for the protein structure prediction techniques. In that case, most commonly applied techniques are "threading" and "homology modeling" [54,55]. In the case of threading or the fold recognition technique, an estimation is made whether a given amino acid sequence is compatible with one of the ligands in a database. On the other hand, homology or comparative modeling relies on a correlation or homology between the sequence of the target protein and at least one known structure. Correct homology models can be generated, provided that the sequence identity of a given target sequence is >50% to a known structure template. Modest homology model building efforts could potentially create receptor structures for entire target families. Importantly, homology modeling is a comparatively economical method for generating a diversity of receptor conformations using either single-template or multiple-template structures enhancing the understanding of selectivity.
3. *A set of ligands of interest*: Once the 3D structure of the protein of interest has been attained from either experiments (X-ray crystal structure) or predictions (receptor from homology modeling), the docking study can be performed using ligands of interest employing a multiplicity of docking techniques. If the function of the protein is unknown, it may be vital to search its structure for hypothetical binding sites. These binding sites can be explored for the binding of selected ligands or they can be compared with known binding sites. An analysis of the binding site characteristics and the interactions with a given ligand can lead to important insights for the design of novel ligands or the docking of assumed ligand molecules [56].

10.3.4 Categorization of docking

As discussed earlier in Section 10.3.1, docking can be categorized into three main classes: (i) protein–ligand docking, (ii) protein–nucleic acid docking, and (iii) protein–protein docking. Among these, protein–ligand docking is a common research area because of its importance to structure-based drug design [3]. Again, the protein–ligand docking can be classified in the following manner: (a) rigid-body docking, where both the receptor and ligand are treated as rigid; (b) flexible ligand docking, where the receptor is held rigid, but the ligand is treated as flexible; and (c) flexible docking, where both receptor and ligand flexibility is considered. Thus far, the most commonly used docking algorithms use the rigid receptor/flexible ligand model. Here, we have categorized the protein–ligand docking in terms of the three most important aspects: (i) protein flexibility, (ii) ligand sampling, and (iii) scoring function, as illustrated in Figure 10.7.

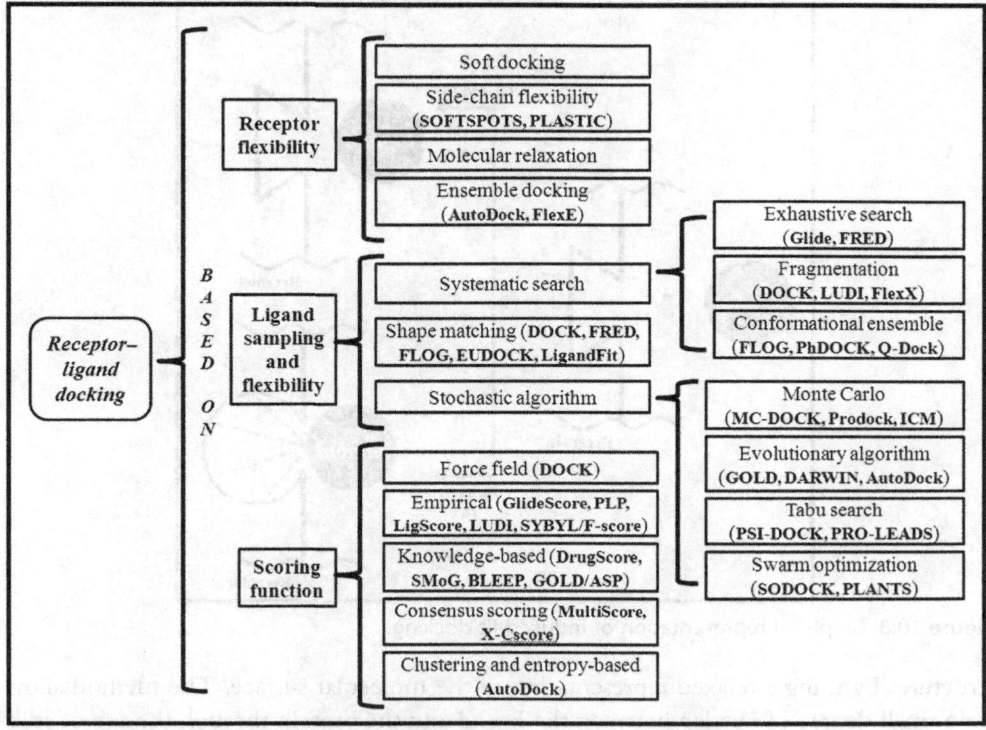

Figure 10.7 Categorization of protein–ligand docking.

10.3.4.1 Receptor/protein flexibility

Ligand binding usually induces protein conformational changes (ranging from local rearrangements of side-chains to large domain motions) or induced fit (Figure 10.8) upon ligand binding in order to maximize energetically favorable interactions with the ligand [57]. The algorithm behind the most induced-fit mechanisms is hydrophobic interaction or hydrophobic collapse of the receptor around the bound ligand [58]. Due to the large size and many degrees of freedom of proteins, their flexibility is one of the most challenging issues in molecular docking. There are varying degrees of receptor flexibility. The degree of flexibility that one could incorporate in a given experiment is directly proportional to computational complexity and cost. The protein flexibility can be grouped into four major categories: (i) soft docking, (ii) side-chain flexibility, (iii) molecular relaxation, and (iv) protein ensemble docking [59].

10.3.4.1.1 Soft docking

Soft docking is the simplest approach, which considers protein flexibility in absolute terms. Soft docking algorithms attempt to allow flexibility of the receptor and ligand

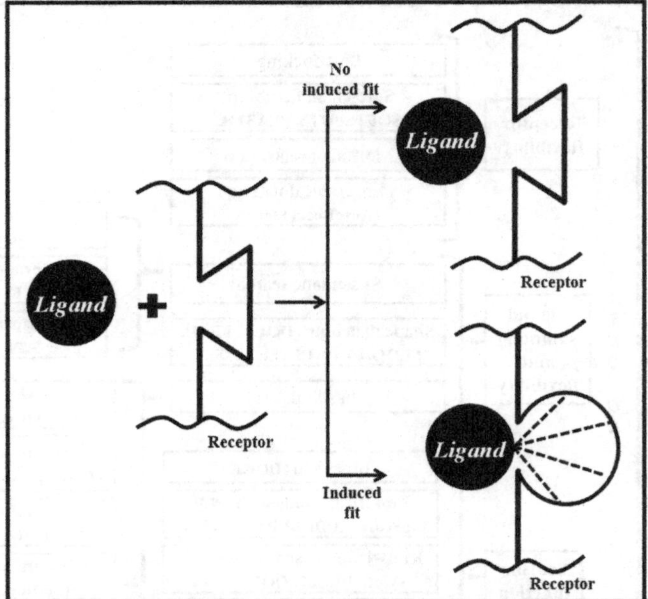

Figure 10.8 Graphical representation of induced-fit docking.

structures by using a relaxed representation of the molecular surface. The method allows for a small degree of overlap between the ligand and the protein through the use of additional energy terms—usually interatomic van der Waals (VDW)—in the empirical scoring function [60]. The advantages of soft docking are its computational competence and easiness for implementation. It is important to remember that soft docking can account for only minute conformational changes. The soft docking concept proposed by Jiang and Kim describes the molecular surface and volume as a "cube representation" [61]. This cube representation implies implicit conformational changes by way of size/shape complementarity, close packing, and, most important, liberal steric overlap.

10.3.4.1.2 Side-chain flexibility

Allowing active site side-chain flexibility is another way to provide receptor flexibility, in which backbones are kept fixed and side-chain conformations are sampled. The method originally proposed by Leach [62] uses pregenerated side-chain rotamer libraries that subsequently are subjected to optimization during a ligand docking procedure via the dead-end elimination algorithm. The optimized ligand/side-chain orientations are then scored in order to rank the lowest energy combination of side-chain and ligand conformers. Since the invention of this approach, researchers have proposed many improved techniques to incorporate continuous or discrete side-chain flexibility in ligand docking [63,64].

10.3.4.1.3 Molecular relaxation

The molecular relaxation method accounts for protein flexibility by first using rigid-body docking to place the ligand into the binding site and then relaxing the protein backbone and side-chain atoms nearby. Initially, the rigid-body docking allows atomic clashes between the protein and the placed ligand conformations in order to consider the protein conformational changes. Thereafter, the formed complexes are relaxed or minimized by MC, MDS, or other methods [65]. The MDS calculate the time-dependent behavior of a molecular system, which provides detailed information on the fluctuations and conformational changes of proteins and nucleic acids. These methods are now regularly used to examine the structure, dynamics, and thermodynamics of biological molecules and their complexes.

The advantage of the molecular relaxation method is the addition of certain backbone flexibility in addition to the side-chain conformational changes. However, compared to the side-chain flexibility methods, the relaxation method is more demanding on the scoring function because it involves not only the side-chain movement, but also the more challenging task of backbone sampling. One of the significant drawbacks of this approach is that it is time consuming.

10.3.4.1.4 Docking of multiple protein structures/ensemble docking

Ensemble docking, which has gained considerable attention as a method of incorporating protein flexibility, utilizes an ensemble of protein structures to represent different possible conformational changes [66]. Commonly, the full receptor ensembles are generated by MDS, MC simulation, or homology modeling approaches. The ensembles can be generated experimentally from NMR solution structure determination or multiple X-ray crystal structures. Strict comparisons have revealed that there is a considerable overlap of dynamic information between theoretically derived molecular dynamics ensembles and experimentally derived NMR ensembles [67]. The first ensemble study was done by Knegtel et al. [68], in which an averaged energy grid was constructed by combining the energy grids generated from each experimentally determined protein structures using a weighting scheme, followed by standard ligand docking. Generally, the ensemble docking algorithm is not used for generating new protein structures; instead, it is used for selecting the induced-fit structure from a given protein ensemble.

10.3.4.2 Ligand sampling and flexibility

Ligand sampling is one of the most basic components in protein–ligand docking. Given a protein target, the sampling algorithm generates possible ligand orientations or conformations (poses) around the selected binding site of the protein. It is interesting to point out that the binding site can be the experimentally determined active site, a dimer interface, or another site of interest. Without any doubt, ligand sampling and its flexibility are the significant areas in protein–ligand docking research. There are three types of ligand-sampling algorithms: shape matching, systematic search, and stochastic algorithms, all of which are discussed in the next sections.

10.3.4.2.1 Shape matching

The shape matching approach is one of the common sampling algorithms that is employed in the initial stages of the docking or in the earlier step of other, more advanced ligand sampling methods. The ligand is placed using the criterion that the molecular surface of the placed ligand must harmonize the molecular surface of the binding site on the protein. Generally, three translational and three rotational degrees of freedom of the ligand are allocated for many possible ligand-binding orientations. Therefore, how the placed ligand gets bound in the protein site with a good shape complementarity is the major goal of the shape matching algorithm. It is important to remember that the conformation of the ligand is normally fixed during shape matching [69]. The major advantage of shape matching is its computational efficiency.

10.3.4.2.2 Systematic search

Systematic search algorithms are usually employed for flexible ligand docking, which create all the probable ligand binding conformations by exploring all degrees of freedom of the ligand. The systematic search method can be divided into three subclasses:

a. *Exhaustive search*: The most uncomplicated systematic algorithms are exhaustive search methods, in which flexible ligand docking is performed by systematically rotating all possible rotatable bonds of the ligand at a given interval. In spite of its sampling totality for ligand conformations, the number of the choices can be huge due to an increase in the number of rotatable bonds. As a consequence, to make the docking process realistic, geometric and chemical constraints are normally applied to the initial screening of ligand poses, and the filtered ligand conformations are further subject to the more precise refinement and optimization measures.

b. *Fragmentation approach*: The basic idea behind this approach is that the ligand is first divided into a number of fragments. Then, the ligand-binding conformation is grown by placing one fragment at a time in the binding site or by docking all the fragments into the binding site and linking them covalently.

c. *Conformational ensemble*: In the conformational ensemble methods [69], ligand flexibility is achieved by rigidly docking an ensemble of pregenerated ligand conformations with other programs (e.g., OMEGA). Then, ligand-binding modes from different docking runs are collected and ranked according to their binding energy scores.

10.3.4.2.3 Stochastic algorithms

The fundamental algorithm behind the stochastic approach is that ligand-binding orientations and conformations are sampled by making random changes to the ligand at each step in the conformational space and the translational and rotational space of the ligand, respectively. The random change will be accepted or rejected according to a probabilistic criterion. The stochastic algorithms can be classified into four different categories [70]:

a. *MC methods*: The probability to allow a random change is determined by employing the Boltzmann probability function.

b. *Evolutionary algorithms*: These involve a search for the right ligand-binding mode based on the idea from the evolutionary process in biological systems.

c. *Tabu search methods*: The probability of approval relies on the explored areas in the conformational space of the ligand. The random change will be rejected if the RMSD between the present ligand-binding conformation and any of the formerly recorded solutions is less than a cutoff; otherwise, the random change will be accepted.

d. *Swarm optimization method*: This particular algorithm tries to determine the best possible solution in a search space by modeling swarm intelligence. Movements of a ligand mode through the search space are directed by the information of the best positions of its neighbors.

10.3.4.3 Docking scoring functions

The fundamental element behind determining the accuracy of a protein–ligand docking algorithm is the generated scoring function during the docking study [71]. Swiftness and precision are the two essential aspects of any scoring function. An ideal scoring function would be both computationally proficient and consistent. Numerous scoring functions have been developed since the introduction of docking studies. The scoring functions are broadly grouped into five basic categories according to their methods of derivation.

10.3.4.3.1 FF scoring functions

FF scoring functions [72] rely on the partitioning of the ligand-binding energy into individual interaction terms such as VDW energies, electrostatic energies, and bond stretching/bending/torsional energies, employing a set of derived FF parameters such as the AMBER [73] or CHARMM [74] FFs. The major challenges in FF scoring functions are accounting for the solvent effect and accounting for the entropic effect.

10.3.4.3.2 Empirical scoring functions

The binding energy score of a complex is calculated by adding up a set of weighted empirical energy terms (such as VDW energy, electrostatic energy, hydrogen-bonding energy, desolvation term, entropy term, and hydrophobicity term) in empirical scoring functions.

Compared to the FF scoring functions, the empirical scoring functions are usually much more computationally proficient due to their simple energy terms. It is interesting to point out here that the general applicability of an empirical scoring function relies on the training set due to the fact that it fits known binding affinities of its training set.

10.3.4.3.3 Knowledge-based scoring functions

Knowledge-based scoring functions result from the structural information in experimentally determined protein–ligand complexes [75]. The theory beneath the knowledge-based scoring functions is the potential of mean force, which is defined by the inverse Boltzmann relation. This scoring function maintains a good balance between accuracy and speed. The difficulty for this scoring function is the calculation for the aforementioned reference state. It can be classified into three categories based on the methods of computation: (a) traditional atom-randomized reference state, (b) corrected reference state, and (c) circumventing the reference state.

10.3.4.3.4 Consensus scoring

Consensus scoring is not a typical scoring function; rather, it is a technique involved in protein–ligand docking [76]. It advances the probability of finding an accurate solution by amalgamating the scoring information from multiple scoring functions in anticipation of eliminating the inaccuracies of the individual scoring functions. As a consequence, the main difficulty in consensus scoring is how to create the combination rule for each score so that the true binders can be discriminated from others according to the consensus rule.

10.3.4.3.5 Clustering- and entropy-based scoring methods

To enhance the performances of scoring functions, there is another new technique called the *clustering-based scoring method*, which includes the entropic effects by dividing generated ligand-binding modes into different clusters [77]. The entropic contribution in each cluster is calculated by the configurational space covered by the ligand poses or the number of ligand poses in the cluster. One disadvantage of clustering-based scoring methods is that its performance relies on the ligand sampling protocol, which is highly dependent on the docking program.

10.3.5 Basic steps of docking

Fundamentally, docking is a three-step process irrespective of software and docking algorithms [78]. The steps are as follows:

a. *Ligand preparation*: The first step is to prepare the ligands. In this process, all the duplicate structures should be removed, and options for ionization change, tautomer, isomer generation, and 3D generator must be set in the working software platform for the respective ligands.

b. *Protein preparation*: Hydrogen atoms should be added and the protein must be minimized using software-specific FF, followed by the removal of water molecules except in the active site. The protein should be adjusted by fixing any serious errors like incomplete residues near the active site. The charges and atom types for any metal atoms should be set properly, if needed. If there are bonds to metal ions, the bonds should be deleted, followed by adjusting the formal charges of the atoms that were attached to the metal, as well as the metal itself. The protein molecule, thus prepared, is the total receptor ready for docking.

c. *Ligand–protein docking*: After ensuring that protein and ligands are in the correct form for docking, in a few cases the receptor grid files are generated using a grid–receptor generation program for grid-based docking. The grid box is generally generated at the centroid of the ligand bound to the active site of the receptor. In other cases, active pockets of the protein are identified to dock the prepared ligand in those identified pockets. Initially, all the molecules of the data set should be docked into the active site of the protein and the interaction energies between each ligand and the receptor can be calculated. The obtained results are then needed to be compared with those of the bound ligand of the crystallized protein structure in order to assess whether the molecules fit into the specified active site of the receptor or not. A set number of ligand poses should be saved for each conformation of the ligand. A predefined number of docking poses thus saved for each conformation of the compound can be ranked according to their dock score function, and then their interaction with the receptor can be analyzed. From the docking studies, the receptor–ligand interactions are correlated with the biological activity of the data set compounds. The structural validation of the docking procedure is done by extracting the cocrystallized ligand from the active site of the receptor and redocking it to the receptor to ensure that it binds to the same active site and interacts with the same amino acid residues as before. The basic steps are schematically illustrated in Figure 10.9.

10.3.6 Challenges and required improvements in docking studies

A significant amount of work has been performed to devise superior docking programs and scoring functions over the past years. However, there is still room for improvement. This section presents some of the primary challenges and the required improvements that will advance the performance of docking and scoring [79].

Challenges:

a. *Water molecules in protein*: Water molecules often play a significant role in protein–ligand interaction. If water-mediated interactions during docking is ignored, the estimated interaction energy of a given ligand conformation may be too low. On the contrary, if one holds water molecules present in the crystal

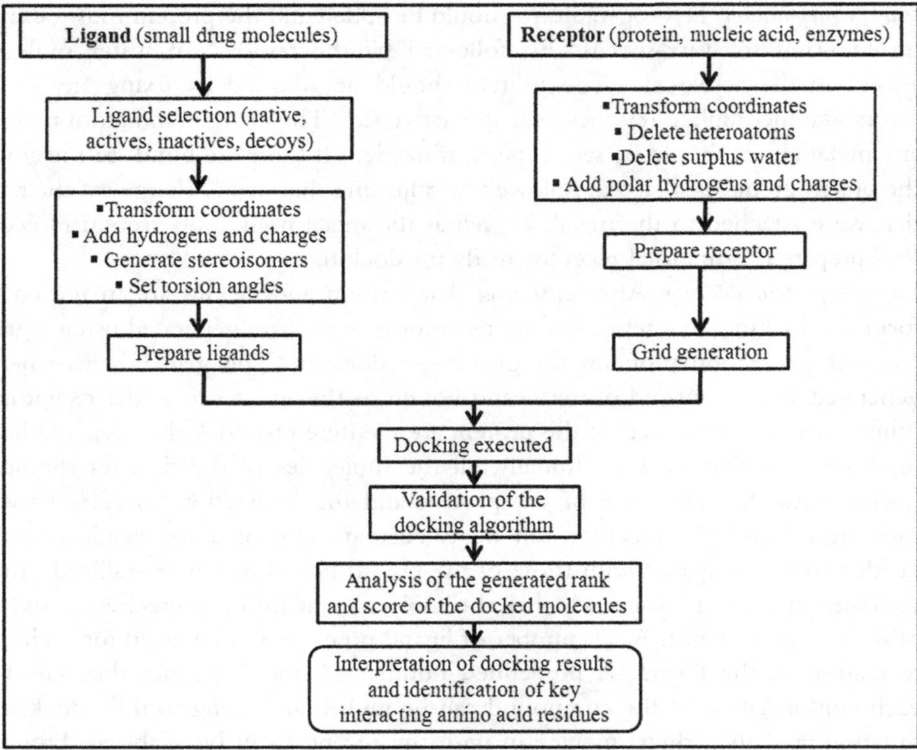

Figure 10.9 Basic steps of the docking formalism.

protein structure, then the binding pose and affinity of a ligand will not be reliable. Thus, it is very difficult to treat the water molecules effectively. To perform reliable and acceptable docking, one first need to recognize probable positions for water molecules where they could interact with the protein and ligand, and subsequently, one must be capable to predict whether a water molecule is indeed present at that position.

b. *Tautomers and protomers*: Another significant challenge with docking is consideration for the various tautomeric and protomeric states that the molecules can adopt. Most of the time, molecules such as acids or amines are stored in their neutral forms. As they are ionized under physiological conditions, it is essential to ionize them prior to docking. Although ionization is easy to attain, but the problem of tautomer generation is already much more difficult, as other questions will arise, such as: Which tautomer should one use? Should one use more than one or all possible tautomers for a given molecule? Not only tautomers, but also different ionization states of ligands provide real challenges in docking.

c. *Docking into flexible receptors*: One of the most challenging problems in docking is dealing with flexible receptors. Numerous examples have become known where the same protein adopts different conformations depending on which ligand it binds to [80]. In order to deal with the trouble of flexible receptors in docking, several approaches have been proposed: (1) letting the receptor or parts of it move during docking; (2) docking the compounds into numerous different conformations of the same receptor and aggregating the results; and (3) docking into averaged receptor representations. In a few cases, more than one of these methods are used based on the requirements in question.

Required improvements:

d. *Multiple active-site corrections (MASC)*: A possible way of improving docking results is the application of MASC, a simple statistical correction [81]. The scoring functions prefer certain ligand types or characteristics, such as large or hydrophobic ligands. As a consequence, some ligands are predicted to be good binders regardless of whether these ligands will bind to specific active sites. Therefore, MASC has been introduced, which can be interpreted either as a statistical measure of ligand specificity or as a correction for ligand-related bias in the scoring function. In order to calculate the MASC scores, each ligand is docked into a number of unrelated binding sites of different binding site characteristics. The corrected score (or MASC score) S'_{ij} for ligand molecule i in binding site j is calculated as follows:

$$S'_{ij} = \frac{(S_{ij} - \mu_i)}{\sigma_i} \tag{10.9}$$

where S_{ij} is the uncorrected score for the ligand, and μ_i and σ_i represent the mean and standard deviation of the scores for the ligand molecule i across the different binding sites. Thus, the MASC score S'_{ij} represents a measure of specificity of molecule i for binding site j compared to the other binding sites.

e. *Docking with constraints*: By introducing a constraint during docking, it is feasible to control the way the poses are generated and the ones that are preferentially set aside. For example, in the case of the DockIt program [82], one can apply distance constraints between the ligand and protein that are consequently utilized during pose generation via a distance geometry approach.

f. *Postprocessing*: There are two approaches of postprocessing that can be employed in the case of a docking study: (i) applying postdock filters and (ii) using tailor-made rescoring functions. The postdock filters are theoretically simple and may correspond to certain geometric criteria, like the existence of certain interactions (e.g., a hydrogen bond with a selected residue or a polar interaction) or the filling of a specified pocket in the active site. Again, all scoring functions may exhibit biased behavior with certain compound classes or functional groups. To diminish the impact of this difficulty and to decrease the statistical noise, composite scoring, or rescoring methods have been introduced [83]. Rather than using a single scoring function, several scoring functions are merged such that in order to be classified as a potential binder, a molecule has to be scored well by a number of different scoring functions. Another way of postprocessing is to use the docking results as input to develop a Bayesian model with the aim of reducing the numbers of false positives and false negatives [84].

10.3.7 Applications of docking

The docking technology is successfully applied at multiple stages of the drug design and discovery process for three main purposes: (1) predicting the binding mode of a known active ligand, (2) identifying new ligands using VS, and (3) predicting the binding affinities of allied compounds from a known active series. The prediction of a ligand-binding mode in a protein active site has been the most successful area. In the broader perspective, the major specific applications of docking are listed here to get a proper dimension of the use of docking studies in the drug discovery process:

- The determination of the lowest free-energy structures for the receptor–ligand complex
- Calculation of the differential binding of a ligand to two different macromolecular receptors
- Study of the geometry of a particular ligand–receptor complex.
- Searching of a database and ranking of hits for lead generation and optimization for future drug candidate.
- To propose the modification of lead molecules to optimize potency or other properties.
- Library design and data bank generation.
- Screening for the side effects that can be caused by interactions with proteins, like proteases and cytochrome P450, can be done.
- It is also possible to check the specificity of a potential drug against homologous proteins through docking.
- Docking is also a widely used tool in predicting protein–protein interactions.
- Docking can create knowledge of the molecular association, which aids in understanding a variety of pathways taking place in the living system.
- To reveal possible potential pharmacological targets.
- Docking-based virtual HTS is less expensive than normal HTS and faster than conventional screening.

The docking study has a huge role not only in lead drug identification process, but also in search of potential target identification for different diseases [79]. A representative list of marketed or clinical trial drugs employing structure-based drug design–docking study is given in Table 10.3. For a more elaborate illustration, please see Chapter 11.

Table 10.3 Representative examples of marketed drugs employing the structure-based drug design–docking study

Generic name	Manufacturer	Inhibit/Target
AG85, ag337, ag331	Agouron	Thymidylate synthase
Aliskiren	Novartis	Renin inhibitors
Amprenavir	GlaxoSmithKline	HIV protease
Boceprevir	Schering–Plough	Protease inhibitor used for treating hepatitis caused by hepatitis C virus (HCV)
Captopril	Bristol Myers–Squibb	Reversible inhibitor of angiotensin-converting enzyme (ACE)
Dorzolamid	Merck Sharp and Dohme	Carbonic anhydrase (hypercapnic ventilatory failure)
ERα and ERβ	Information not available	Estradiol (E2) analogs
Indinavir	Merck	HIV protease
Inverase	Hoffman La Roche	HIV protease
LY-517717	Lilly/Protherics	Inhibitors of factor Xa serine protease
Nelfinavir	Hoffman La Roche	HIV protease
Nolatrexed dihydrochloride	Agouron	Thymidylate synthase (TS)
Norvir	Abbot	HIV protease
NVP-AUY922	Novartis	Heat shock protein 90 (HSP90)
Raltitrexed	AstraZeneca	Thymidalate
Raltegravir	Merck	HIV integrase
Rupintrivir	Agouron	Irreversible inhibitors of human rhinovirus (HRV) 3C protease
Saquinavir	Hoffman La Roche	HIV protease
TMI-005	–	Dual inhibitor of tumor necrosis factor-α (TNFα) converting enzyme (TACE) and matrix metalloproteinases (MMPs)
Zanamivir	Gilead Sciences	Neuraminidase inhibitor

10.3.8 Docking software tools

A large number of docking programs and search algorithms have been reported since the invention of docking [79]. Although the basic steps of docking processes are more or less identical, these docking programs vary fundamentally with respect to the docking algorithm, ligand search strategy, and scoring function techniques. A list of popular docking software programs is given in Table 10.4.

Table 10.4 Available software tools for the docking study

Software	Algorithm and remarks
AutoDock	AutoDock is a suite of automated docking tools capable of predicting how small molecules, such as substrates or drug candidates, bind to a receptor of a known 3D structure. The Lamarckian GA is used as the algorithm. Website: http://autodock.scripps.edu/
Discovery Studio	The conformational search of the ligand poses is performed by the MC trial method. Preprocessing of ligands is performed using the ligand fit program with selecting one of the energy grid out of three energy grids (PLP1, Dreiding, and CFF) available in Discovery Studio. The docking poses saved for each conformation of the compound are ranked according to their dock scores based on LigScore1, LigScore2, PLP1, PLP2, Jain, and PMF function. Website: http://accelrys.com/
DOCK	DOCK is a program that can examine possible binding orientations of protein–protein and protein–DNA complexes. It can be used to search databases of molecular structures for compounds that act as enzyme inhibitors or bind to target receptors. The shape matching (sphere images) algorithm is employed here. Website: http://www.cmpharm.ucsf.edu/kuntz/dock.html
DOT	Daughter Of Turnip (DOT) is a program for docking macromolecules to other molecules of any size. It can predict binding modes of small molecule–protein complexes. The intermolecular energies for all configurations generated by this search are calculated as the sum of electrostatic and VDW energies. Website: http://www.sdsc.edu/CCMS/DOT/
FADE and PADRE	Fast Atomic Density Evaluator (FADE) and Pairwise Atomic Density Reverse Engineering (PADRE) programs are designed to aid in the molecular modeling of proteins. In particular, the programs can rapidly elucidate features of interest such as crevices, grooves, and protrusions. The topographical information produced by FADE and PADRE can help researchers easily pinpoint the most prominent features of a protein, regions that are likely to participate in interactions with other molecules. In addition, it provides shape descriptors to aid in analyzing single molecules.
FlexiDock	FlexiDock is a commercial software performs flexible docking of ligands into receptor binding sites. Website: http://www.tripos.com/software/fdock.html
FlexX	Incremental construction algorithm is employed in FlexX. The FlexX predicts the geometry of the protein–ligand complex and estimates the binding affinity. The two main applications of FlexX are complex prediction and VS. Complex prediction is used, when one have a protein and a small molecule binding to it but no structure of the protein–ligand complex is available. Website: http://www.biosolveit.de/flexx/

(*Continued*)

Table 10.4 (Continued)

Software	Algorithm and remarks
FRED	The shape matching (Gaussian functions) algorithm is employed in the Fast Rigid Exhaustive Docking (FRED) software.
FTDock	Fourier Transform Docking (FTDock) is a free program that performs rigid-body docking on two biomolecules in order to predict their correct binding geometry.
Glide	Glide is a fast and accurate docking program that addresses a number of problems, ranging from fast database screening to highly accurate docking. The descriptor matching/MC is the principal algorithm of Glide. The hierarchical filters in Glide ensure a fast and efficient reduction of large data sets to the few drug candidates that bind best with the target. Website: http://www.schrodinger.com/Glide/
GOLD	GOLD is a GA-based method for ligand protein docking. GOLD accounts for receptor flexibility through side-chain flexibility and, most important, ensemble docking. Website: http://www.ccdc.cam.ac.uk/Solutions/GoldSuite/Pages/GOLD.aspx
GRAMM	Global Range Molecular Matching (GRAMM) is a free program for protein docking. To predict the structure of a complex, it requires only the atomic coordinates of the two molecules (no information of the binding sites is needed). The molecular pairs may be two proteins, a protein and a smaller compound, two transmembrane helices, etc. The program performs an exhaustive 6D search through the relative translations and rotations of the molecules. Website: http://vakser.bioinformatics.ku.edu/resources/gramm/grammx/
Hammerhead	Hammerhead is suitable for screening large databases of flexible molecules by binding to a protein of known structure. The approach is completely automated, from the elucidation of protein binding sites, through the docking of molecules, to the final selection of compounds.
HINT	HINT is a software package that utilizes experimental solvent partitioning data as a basis for an empirical molecular interaction model. The program calculates empirical atom-based hydropathic parameters that, in a sense, encode all significant intermolecular and intramolecular noncovalent interactions implicated in drug binding or protein folding.
Liaison	Liaison is a commercial program for fast estimation of free energy of binding between a receptor and a ligand. The free energy of binding can be approximated by an equation in which only the free and bound states of the ligand are calculated. The method combines high-level molecular mechanics calculations with experimental data to build a scoring function for the evaluation of ligand–receptor binding free energies.
LigandFit	The shape matching (moments of inertia) algorithm is employed.

(*Continued*)

Table 10.4 (Continued)

Software	Algorithm and remarks
MOE	MOE is a fast and accurate docking program. The dock poses were ranked according to the GBVI/WSA binding free-energy calculation and minimized using MMFF94x within a rigid receptor.
Molegro Virtual Docker	Molegro Virtual Docker is an integrated platform for predicting protein–ligand interactions. Molegro Virtual Docker handles all aspects of the docking process, from preparation of the molecules to determination of the potential binding sites of the target protein, and prediction of the binding modes of the ligands.
QSite	QSite is a mixed-mode QM/MM program for highly accurate energy calculations of protein–ligand interactions in the active site. The program is specifically designed for proteins and allows a number of different QM/MM boundaries for residues in the active site. QSite uses the power and speed of Jaguar to perform the quantum mechanical part of the calculations and OPLS-AA to perform the molecular mechanical part of the calculations.
Situs	Situs is a program package for the docking of protein crystal structures to single-molecule, low-resolution maps from electron microscopy or small-angle X-ray scattering.
SLIDE	Descriptor matching algorithm is employed in SLIDE.
SuperStar	SuperStar is a program for generating maps of interaction sites in proteins using experimental information about intermolecular interactions. The generated interaction maps are therefore fully knowledge-based. SuperStar retrieves its data from IsoStar, CCDC interaction database. IsoStar contains information about nonbonded interactions from both the Cambridge Structural Database (CSD) and the Protein Data Bank (PDB).

10.4 COMBINATION OF STRUCTURE- AND LIGAND-BASED DESIGN TOOLS

In recent years, there has been increasing attention paid to developing new methods employing the combined information generated from receptors and ligands. Most of the common present-day and potential future approaches are discussed in this section.

10.4.1 Comparative binding energy analysis

10.4.1.1 The concept of comparative binding energy

Comparative binding energy (COMBINE) analysis is a method of developing a system-specific expression to compute binding free energy using the 3D structures of receptor–ligand complexes [4]. This technique is based upon the hypothesis that the free energy of binding can be correlated with a subset of energy components calculated from the structures of receptors and ligands in bound and unbound forms [4,85]. Computation of binding free energies is very challenging due to the need to sample conformational space effectively in order to compute entropic contributions. Empirical scoring functions, which are fast to calculate, have been derived to approximate binding free energy using a single structure of a receptor–ligand complex [86]. If some experimental binding data are accessible for a set of related complexes, then this information can be used to derive a target-specific scoring function. This algorithm is taken in the COMBINE analysis in which the binding free energy (ΔG) or inhibition constant (K_i) or other related properties are correlated with a subset of weighted interaction energy components determined from the structures of energy minimized receptor–ligand complexes. The receptor binding free energy (ΔG) of a ligand can be expressed as

$$\Delta G = \sum_{i=1}^{n} \omega_i \, \Delta u_i^{\text{rep}} + C \tag{10.10}$$

The n terms Δu_i^{rep} of the ligand–receptor binding energy ΔU are selected, and the coefficients ω_i and constant C are determined by the statistical analysis. ΔU is calculated for representative conformations of the ligand–receptor complexes and the unbound ligands and the receptor using a molecular mechanics FF. The ligands are divided into n_l fragments, and the receptor into n_r regions (e.g., amino acid residues), and thus

$$\begin{aligned} \Delta U = & \sum_{i=1}^{n_l}\sum_{j=1}^{n_r} u_{ij}^{\text{VDW}} + \sum_{i=1}^{n_l}\sum_{j=1}^{n_r} u_{ij}^{\text{ELE}} + \\ & \sum_{i=1}^{n_l} \Delta u_i^{B,L} + \sum_{i=1}^{n_l} \Delta u_i^{A,L} + \sum_{i=1}^{n_l} \Delta u_i^{T,L} + \sum_{i<i'}^{n_l} \Delta u_{ii'}^{\text{NB},L} + \\ & \sum_{j=1}^{n_r} \Delta u_j^{B,R} + \sum_{j=1}^{n_r} \Delta u_j^{A,R} + \sum_{j=1}^{n_r} \Delta u_j^{T,R} + \sum_{j<j'}^{n_r} \Delta u_j^{\text{NB},R} \end{aligned} \tag{11.10}$$

The first two terms on the right side of the equation describe the intermolecular interaction energies between each fragment i of the ligand and each region j of the receptor. The next four terms describe changes in the bonded (bond, angle, and torsion) and the nonbonded (a combination of Lennard–Jones and electrostatic) energies of the ligand fragments upon binding to the receptor, and the last four terms account for changes in the bonded and nonbonded energies of the receptor regions upon binding of the ligand.

10.4.1.2 The methodology of COMBINE

To derive the COMBINE model, fundamentally three steps are to be followed: namely, modeling the molecules and their complexes, measuring the interaction energies between ligands and the receptor, and finally, performing chemometric analysis to derive the regression equation [4]. The methodology for the COMBINE analysis is outlined schematically in Figure 10.10.

a. *Molecular modeling*: To develop the COMBINE models, the ligands should be divided into fragments, and then the same number of fragments must be allocated to all the compounds, adding dummy fragments to the ligands lacking the correct number. The 3D models of the ligand–receptor complexes and the unbound receptor and ligands can be derived with a standard molecular mechanics program. Different regression equations can be produced by using the following factors:
   - Different starting conformations of the receptor
   - The inclusion of positional restraints on parts of the receptor
   - Different convergence criteria during energy minimization
   - Different ways of treating the solute–solvent interface
   - The dielectric environment

b. *Measurement of the interaction energies*: The objective of this step is the computation of the nonbonded (VDW and electrostatic) interaction energies between each residue of the receptor and every fragment of the ligand, using a molecular mechanics FF. Along with the interaction energies, the energies between all pairs of residues/fragments for the complexes and for the free ligands and receptor on the basis of the distance-based dielectric constant should be computed as well. Finally, a matrix will be formed, with columns representing the energy components and rows

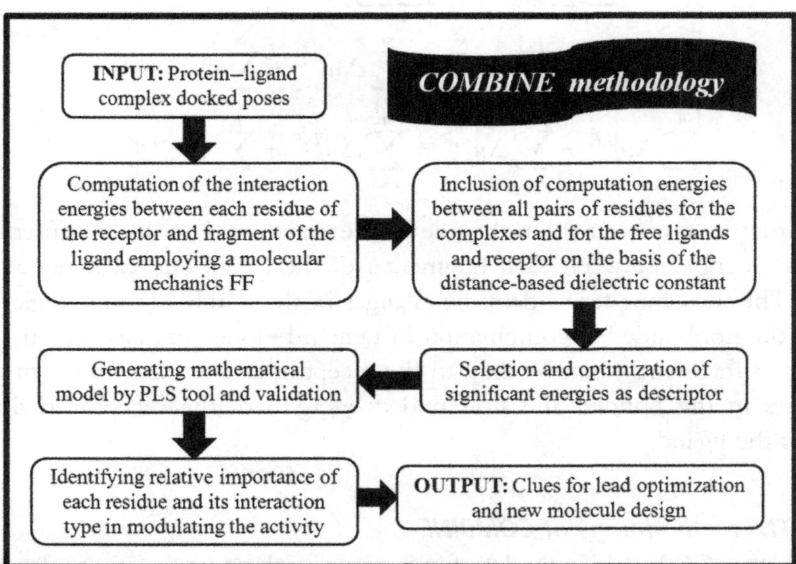

Figure 10.10 The methodology of the COMBINE analysis.

representing each compound in the set. A final column containing experimental activities or inhibitory activities or binding affinities is then added to the matrix as the dependent variable for model development.

c. *Chemometric analysis*: After the completion of steps 1 and 2, significant descriptors should be retained and others must be eliminated from the study matrix. Due to the large number of variables and their intercorrelation nature, partial least squares (PLS) is the technique of choice for deriving the QSAR model that can quantify the most important energy interactions in terms of activity prediction [87,88].

10.4.1.3 Importance and advantages of COMBINE

Comparing the COMBINE method with the calculation of binding energies via classical molecular mechanics, the advantages of ligand–receptor interaction energies to statistical analysis are as follows [4]:

a. The noise due to inaccuracy in the potential energy functions and molecular models can be reduced.
b. Mechanistically important interaction terms can be identified.
c. Compared to more traditional QSAR analysis, this approach can be anticipated to be more predictive, as it incorporates more physically relevant information about the energies of the ligand–receptor interaction.
d. It helps in the screening of lead compounds based on the required properties that interact favorably with the key residues.

10.4.1.4 Drawbacks and required improvements

COMBINE experiences the intrinsic errors implicated in the computation of the interaction energies between ligand and macromolecular complexes like all other interaction energy-based 3D-QSAR methods. The predictability of the method can be improved by making advances in several aspects, like the description of the electrostatic term, the addition of appropriate descriptors for solvation and entropic effects, and the optimization of the methodology, such as the choice of ligand fragment definitions and the details of the variable selection protocol [4].

10.4.1.5 Applications of COMBINE

COMBINE analysis was originally developed to study the interactions of one target protein with a set of related ligands. It has been established in recent times that the approach can be applied tactfully to a wide range of complexes, including enzyme–substrate and inhibitor complexes [89], protein–protein/peptide complexes [90], and protein–DNA complexes [91]. It has also been employed to examine binding to more than one target protein receptor.

10.4.1.6 Software for COMBINE

SCOPE: To make the COMBINE method more user friendly, the method has been implemented in the structure-based compound optimization, prioritization, and evolution (SCOPE) module of VLifeMDS, which uses this approach to derive a 3D-QSAR between the experimental biological activities and the calculated ligand interaction energy terms [92]. First, to execute COMBINE analysis, each of the ligands against a particular target has to be docked into its target. It requires a training set of docked and optimized ligand–receptor complexes, and the unbound ligands and receptor for which intermolecular and intramolecular interaction energies are calculated. The calculated descriptors are then correlated with the experimental activity of the studied compounds to develop a QSAR model. Finally, the interpretation of the developed mathematical equation can enlighten the important ligand–receptor interactions for future drug designing and development process.

gCOMBINE: gCOMBINE is an user-friendly tool for performing COMBINE analysis in drug design research programs. It is a graphical user interface (GUI) written in Java with the purpose of performing COMBINE analysis on a set of ligand–receptor complexes with the intention of deriving highly informative QSAR models [93]. The objective of this method is to generate the ligand–receptor interaction energies into a series of variables, explore the origins of the variance within the set employing principal component analysis (PCA), and then allocate weights to the chosen ligand–residue interactions by using PLS analysis to correlate with the experimental activities or binding affinities. The major advantages of using a GUI are that it allows plenty of interactivity and provides multiple plots representing the energy descriptors entering the analysis, scores, loadings, experimental versus predicted regression lines, and the evolution of classical validation parameters. Using the GUI, one can carry out numerous added tasks, such as possible truncation of positive interaction energy values and generation of ready-made PDB files containing information related to the importance of the activity of individual protein residues. This information can be aptly displayed and color-coded using a molecular graphics program like PyMOL.

10.4.2 Comparative residue interaction analysis

10.4.2.1 Concept of CoRIA

The CoRIA analysis is a relatively recent innovation in the field of QSAR studies. It is a 3D-QSAR approach, which uses the descriptors that describe the thermodynamic events involved in ligand binding to the receptor to explore both the qualitative and quantitative facets of the ligand–receptor recognition process. The main emphasis of CoRIA is to calculate and analyze the receptor–ligand complex and thereafter predict the binding affinity of the complex [5]. The binding free-energy difference (ΔG_{bind})

between the free and bound states of the receptor and ligand ($\Delta G_{complex} - \Delta G_{uncomplexed}$) is related to the binding constant (K_d) of the ligand to the receptor and can be expressed as an additive interaction of different events using the classical binding free energy equation [94]:

$$\Delta G_{bind} = \Delta G_{solv} + \Delta G_{conf} + \Delta G_{inter} + \Delta G_{motion} \tag{10.12}$$

That is, the total free energy of binding (ΔG_{bind}) is an additive interaction of solvation of ligand (ΔG_{solv}), which is the difference between the unbound (e.g., cellular) and bound states, conformational changes that occur in the receptor and ligand (ΔG_{conf}), specific interactions between the ligand and receptor as a consequence of their proximity (ΔG_{inter}), and the motion in the receptor and ligand once they are close to each other (ΔG_{motion}).

10.4.2.2 Methodology of CoRIA

The first step of CoRIA is the calculation of the binding energies in the form of non-bonded interaction energies (like VDW and Coulombic), which describe thermodynamic events involved in ligand binding to the active site of the receptor. Thereafter, employing a genetic version of the PLS technique (namely, G/PLS), these calculated energies should be correlated with the biological activities of molecules, along with the other physiochemical variables like molar refractivity, surface area, molecular volume, Jurs descriptors, and strain energy [5,95,96]. Further, validation has to be performed for the developed CoRIA models based on various validation metrics to ensure the acceptability of the developed models. The methodology of the CoRIA is schematically presented in Figure 10.11.

10.4.2.3 Variants of CoRIA

In recent years, to deal with the problems of peptide QSAR, CoRIA methodology has gone through several advanced modifications. Two newly developed variants of CoRIA are [5,95]:

a. *reverse*-CoRIA (*r*CoRIA): When the peptide (ligand) is fragmented into individual amino acids, and the interaction energies (VDW, Coulombic, and hydrophobic interactions) of each amino acid in the peptide with *the total receptor* is calculated, the technique is known as *rCoRIA*.

b. *mixed*-CoRIA (*m*CoRIA): When the interaction energies of each amino acid in the peptide with the *individual active site residues in the receptor* is calculated, the approach is defined as *mCoRIA*.

For both approaches, along with the interaction energies, other thermodynamic descriptors (like free energy of solvation, entropy loss on binding, strain energy, and solvent assessable surface area) are also included as independent variables, which are correlated to the biological activity using a G/PLS technique like general CoRIA.

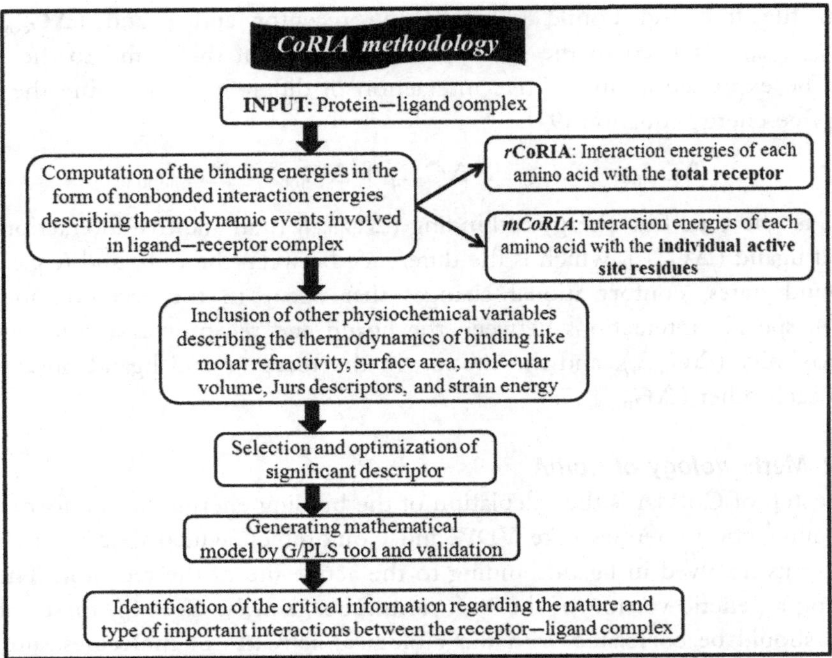

Figure 10.11 The methodology of the CoRIA analysis.

10.4.2.4 Importance and application of CoRIA

The most significant importance of the CoRIA methodology is that it is capable of extracting critical information regarding the nature and type of important interactions at the level of both the receptor and the ligand. The generated rich source of information can be directly employed in the design of new molecules and drug targets [87]. The approaches have the ability to forecast modifications in both the ligand and the receptor, provided that structures of some ligand—receptor complexes are available. The CoRIA approach can be used to identify crucial interactions of the inhibitors with the enzyme at the residue level, which can be profitably exploited in optimizing the inhibitory activity of ligands. Furthermore, it can be used to guide point mutation studies—yet another advantage.

10.4.2.5 Drawback of CoRIA

The major drawback of CoRIA is that it cannot be applied with small organic molecules. This is because unlike peptides, there is no rational or unanimously established protocol for fragmenting small molecules [87].

10.4.2.6 Future perspective of CoRIA

The algorithm of this methodology can be further improved in the near future by considering the following points:

- Solvation of the entire ligand–protein complexes
- Extensive conformational sampling by molecular dynamics
- Inclusion of other important interactions like hydrogen bonding

10.5 *IN SILICO* SCREENING OF CHEMICAL LIBRARIES: VS

10.5.1 Concept

VS is a technique to identify novel hits (i.e., bioactive molecules) from large chemical libraries through computational means by applying knowledge about the protein target (structure-based VS) or known bioactive ligands (ligand-based VS) [97]. The ligand-based approaches utilize structure–activity data from a set of known actives in order to identify drug candidates for experimental evaluation. The ligand-based methods include approaches like similarity and substructure searching, QSAR, pharmacophore-based search, and 3D shape matching [98,99]. Apparently, structure-based VS mainly employ the docking approach, where the 3D structure of the biological target protein or receptor is used to dock the candidate molecules and rank them based on their predicted binding affinity (docking score). These techniques, like ePharmacophore and protein–ligand fingerprints, also can be used under structure-based VS. It is important to mention that based on the requirements of the researchers, one can use ligand- and structure-based approaches one by one, as a layered screening technique, or both approaches concurrently.

The VS technology has emerged as a response to the pressure from the combinatorial/HTS community. VS can be considered as the mining of chemical spaces with the aim to identify molecules that possess a desired property [100]. The VS approach is highly dependent on the quantity and quality of available data and the predictability of the underlying algorithm. As a consequence, there is no universal guideline or workflow for the VS approaches, and the researcher has to apply his computational knowledge and experience to find the active drug candidate from the sea of drug databases and chemical libraries applying the best possible source of tools as per his requirements.

10.5.2 Workflow and types of VS

The experimental efforts to carry out the biological screening of billions of compounds are still considerably high, and therefore, CADD approaches have become attractive alternatives. One has to remember that the workflows employed in the VS are not universal. The workflow is solely dependent on the researchers' needs, the diversity of chemical library, and available sources for sensible and practical VS. Here, we have tried to describe a general, commonly employed workflow.

10.5.2.1 Selection of chemical libraries/databases

The first criterion of any VS approach is the selection of the required chemical library. Taking the requirements into consideration, the researcher has to select the chemical library from the available large pool of public and commercial databases. The database may cover a particular class of compounds (structural or pharmacological) or diverse classes of molecules. A significant amount of information regarding various types of chemical libraries has been provided in Section 10.5.6.

10.5.2.2 Preprocessing of chemical libraries

After selection of the required database, one has to perform the preprocessing of the chemical library by removing the duplicate structures, tautomers, counter ions, and protonated ones.

10.5.2.3 Filtering of druglike molecules

In the next step, to filter the druglike molecules from the preprocessed chemical library, different druglike filters need to be employed:

a. *Lipinski's rule of five*: It is a well-known rule of thumb of encoding a simple profile for the permeability of orally available drugs. The filter demonstrates that poor absorption or permeation are more likely to occur when (i) molecular weight (MW) is over 500, (ii) calculated octanol/water partition coefficient (logP) is over 5, (iii) presence of more than 5 HBDs, and (iv) presence of more than 10 HBAs [101]. With the exception of logP, all other criteria are additive and can be accurately computed for screening of virtual libraries. However, Lipinski's rule of five fails to distinguish between drugs and nondrugs, rather serves as a method to predict compounds with poor absorption or permeability. One has to remember that antibiotics fall outside the scope of this rule.

b. *ADMET filter*: In addition to the Lipinski's filter, ADMET filters [102] can be employed for filtering. To get the early information regarding absorption, distribution, metabolism, excretion (ADME), and toxicity data (ADMET data), the ADMET filter screen is very useful. The late stage failure of the molecules in the clinical trials is primarily attributed to their inability to meet the necessary pharmacokinetic profile. Accurate prediction of ADMET properties enables to eliminate unwanted molecules and aids the lead optimization process.

10.5.2.4 Screening

The ultimate screening step of the VS of the filtered druglike compounds is based on two fundamental approaches; namely, a ligand-based approach and a receptor-based approach [103].

a. *Ligand-based approach*: In this approach, molecules with physical and chemical properties similar to those of the known ligands are identified using QSAR models, pharmacophore-based search, substructure search, and 2D and 3D atomic property-based search approaches. The ligand-based approach is possible without protein information and can be employed for scaffold hopping. Again, since this technique is biased by the properties of known ligands, it limits the diversity of the hits generated.

b. *Receptor-based approach*: The approach uses techniques like protein—ligand docking, different scoring functions, and active-site-directed SBPs for the molecular recognition between a ligand and a target protein to select chemical entities that bind to the active sites of biologically relevant targets with known 3D structures. The major advantages of this approach are the following: It is possible to carry out this process without ligand information, the entire capability of the protein pocket is taken into account, prediction of binding modes is possible, scaffold hopping and profiling without any bias toward existing ligands can be done.

c. *Combination of ligand- and receptor-based approach*: As there is no universal method for the VS, one can use ligand- and structure-based methods separately (e.g., pharmacophore and docking one by one as a two-layer technique), or can employ the combined ligand- and structure-based methods like COMBINE and CoRIA. The COMBINE and CoRIA approaches are reliable. as they consider the ligand and receptor information as well as information regarding their binding complexes.

d. *Machine learning techniques*: Apart from the ligand- and receptor-based approaches, machine learning techniques like support vector machine (SVM) and binary kernel discrimination (BKD) can be tactfully applied in a few cases of VS. The SVM predicts the bioactivity by representing the lead in *n*-dimensional real space using molecular descriptors and fingerprint technology, where *n* represents the number of features or attributes. The SVM approach is based on the fuzzy logic fingerprint. The BKD is a recently developed computational approach. In BKD, the molecule is represented as 2D fragment bit-string. It consists of three components. First, the structural representation section; second, the similarity searching section using different coefficients; and third, the section with different weighting schemes for lead compounds.

10.5.2.5 Hit selection to new chemical entity generation

Once hits are selected from the final screening process, one has to synthesize or purchase the hits for further study. The selected hits have to go through different in vitro/in vivo bioassays for final confirmation of their pharmacological actions. Compounds showing encouraging pharmacological activity are considered as the leading ones for further preclinical and clinical studies to establish them as the final drug candidates. A schematic illustration of various steps of the VS is presented in Figure 10.12.

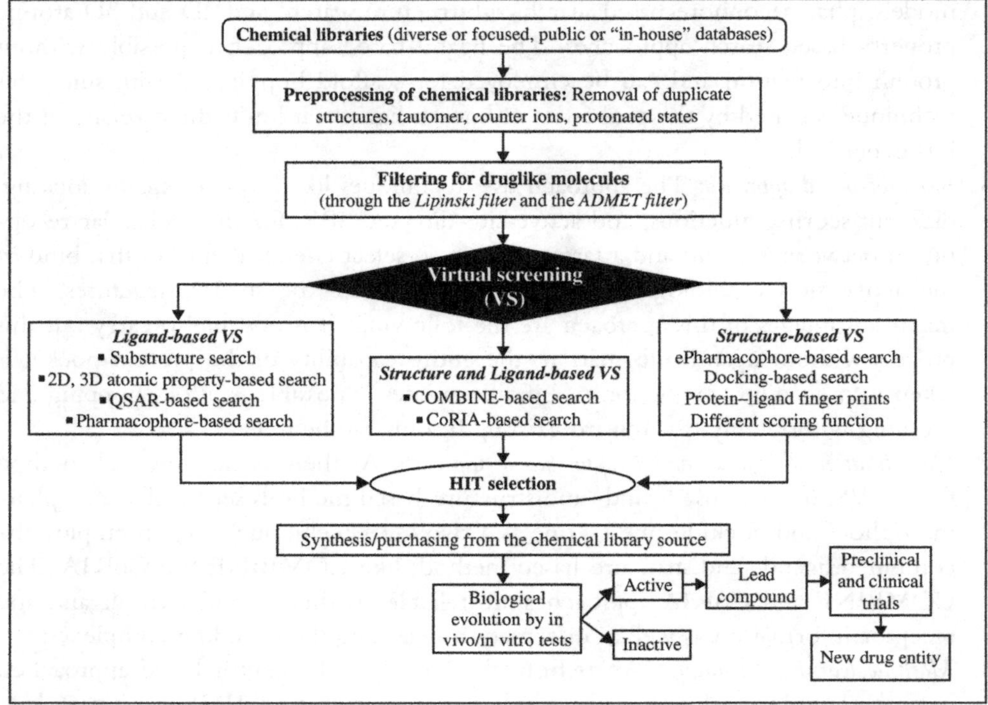

Figure 10.12 Fundamental steps of the VS approach.

10.5.3 Successful application of VS: A few case studies

Employing VS approaches, many drugs have been obtained that are already on the market, and a few others are in the different stages of clinical trials. Liebeschuetz et al. [104] used library design- and structure-based VS to develop inhibitors of factor Xa serine protease, an important target in the blood coagulation cascade. Sharma et al. [105] carried out VS to find the neuraminidase inhibitors (potential targets for swine flu), and two of the metabolites (Hesperidin and Narirutin) were predicted to be more potent than the existing drugs (Oseltamivir). Dahlgren et al. [106] developed salicylidene acylhydrazides as inhibitors of type III secretion (T3S) in the gram-negative pathogen *Yersinia pseudotuberculosis* from a set of 4416 virtual compounds employing three QSAR models. As the studies are so numerous, we have made a representative list of successful applications of VS-based [107] drug discovery in Table 10.5.

10.5.4 Advantages of VS

Application of the VS techniques increases the chance of successful drug discovery by many times. Without any hesitation, we can say that the VS has emerged as a reliable,

Table 10.5 Representative case studies of successful application of VS

Target			Database	Methods employed	Structure of the most active hit
Receptor	G protein –coupled	*α_{1A} adrenergic*	Aventis in-house compound and MDDR	Pharmacophore and docking	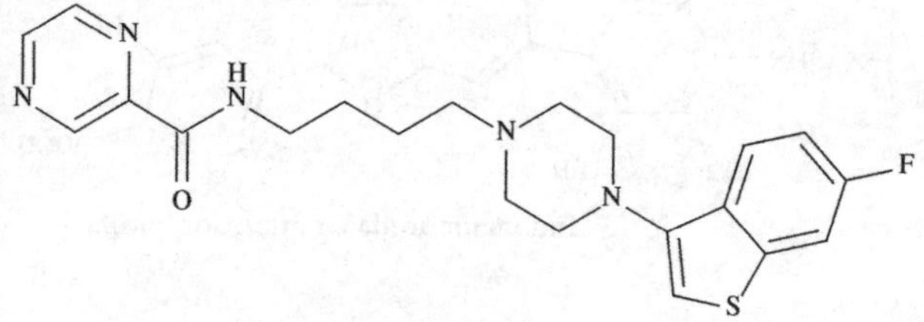 α_{1A} adrenergic receptor antagonist
		Dopamine D3	NCI	Pharmacophore and docking	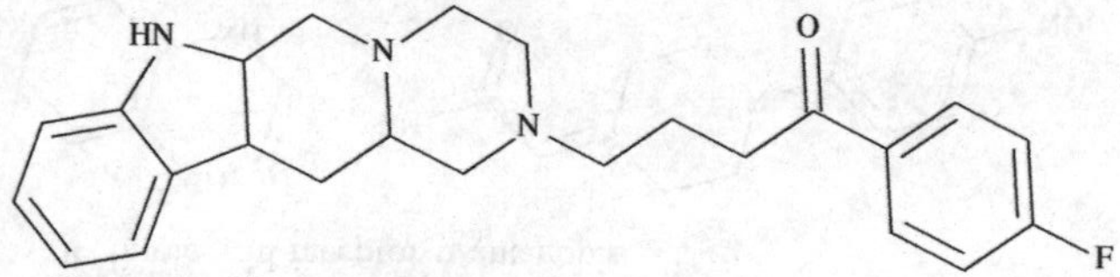 Dopamine D3 receptor antagonist
		Endothelin A	Maybridge database	Pharmacophore	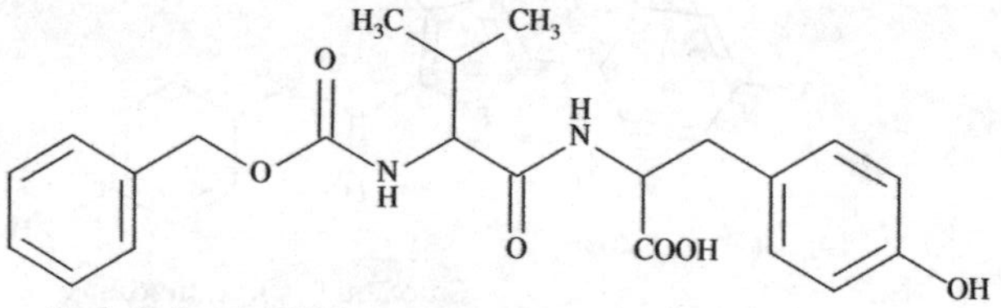 Endothelin A (ET_A) receptor antagonist
		Muscarinic M3	Astra Charnwood in-house compound repository	Pharmacophore	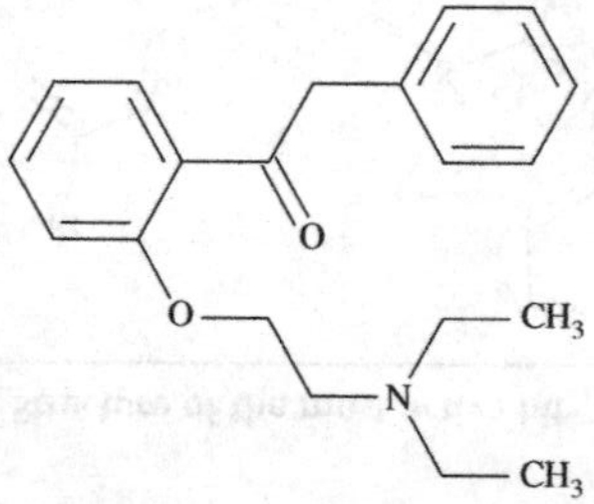 Muscarinic M3 receptor antagonist

(*Continued*)

Table 10.5 (Continued)

Target			Database	Methods employed	Structure of the most active hit
		Neurokinin-1 (NK_1)	826,952 compounds Merging various databases	Pharmacophore and docking	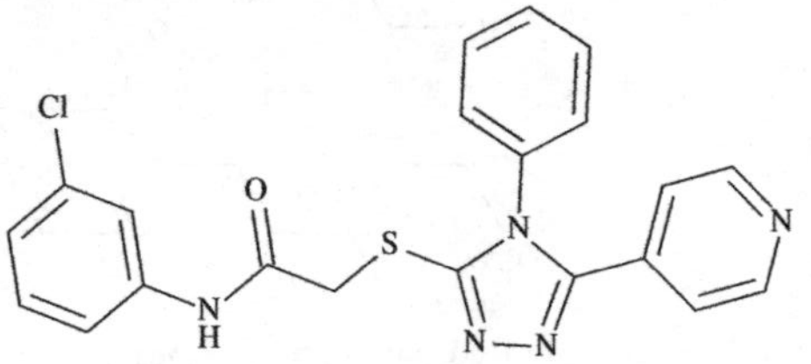 Cl; O; N H; S; N; N—N; N Neurokinin NK_1 antagonist
	Nuclear receptors	*Retinoic acid receptor*	ACD	Docked into the retinoic acid receptor (RAR) binding site	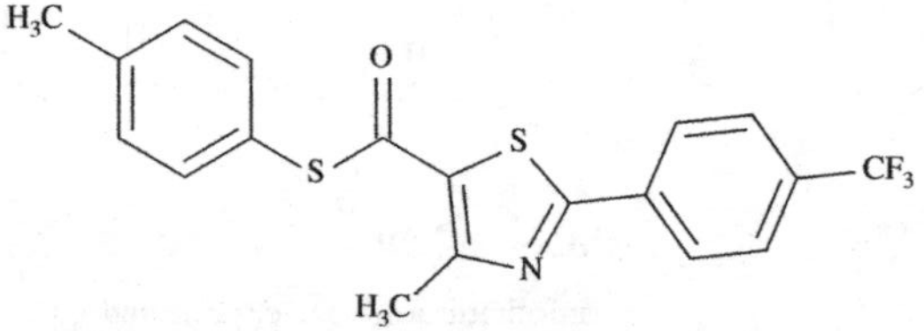 H_3C; O; S; S; N; H_3C; CF_3 Retinoic acid receptor α antagonist
		Thyroid hormone receptor	ACD	Docking	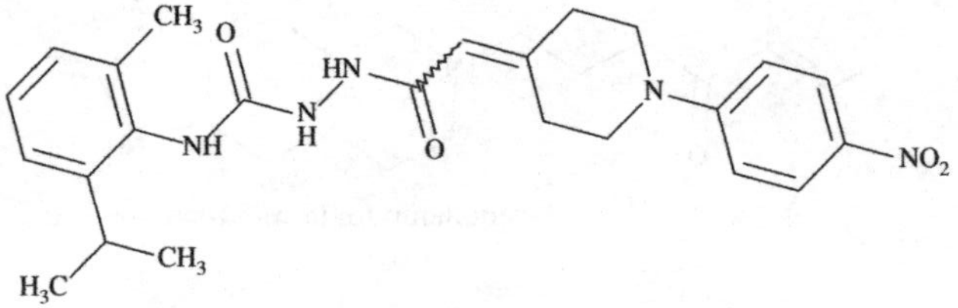 CH_3; O; NH; N H; HN; O; N; NO_2; H_3C; CH_3 Thyroid hormone receptor antagonist
Enzymes	Kinase	*Akt 1 (protein kinase Bα, PKBα)*	ChemBridge	Flexible docking and employing different scoring functions	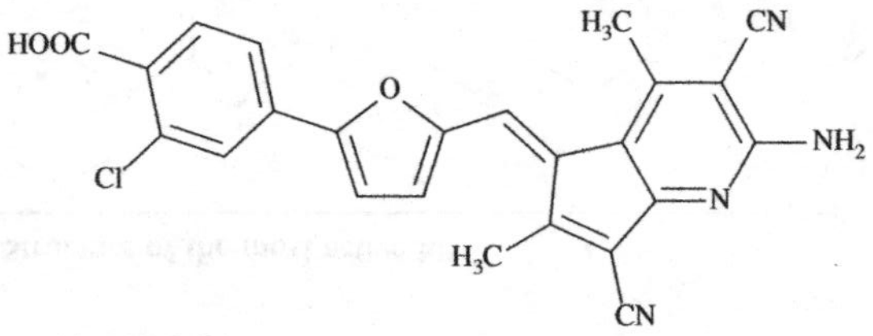 HOOC; Cl; O; H_3C; CN; NH_2; N; H_3C; CN Akt 1 inhibitor

		Bcr-Abl tyrosine kinase	ChemDiv	Lipinski filter and docking	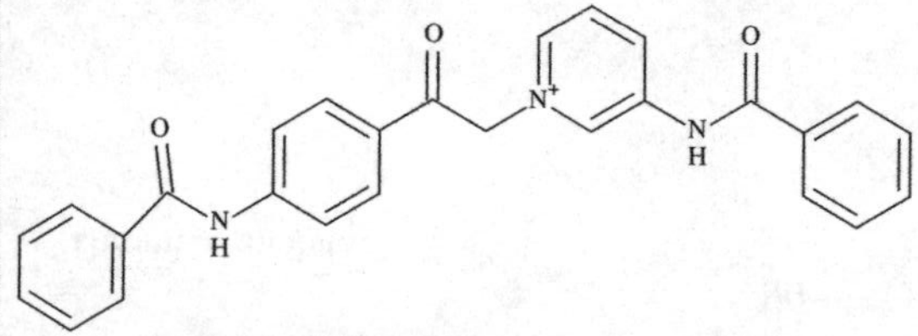 Bcr-Abl Tyrosine kinase inhibitor
		Checkpoint kinase 1 (Chk-1)	AstraZeneca in-house compound	Pharmacophore and flexible docking	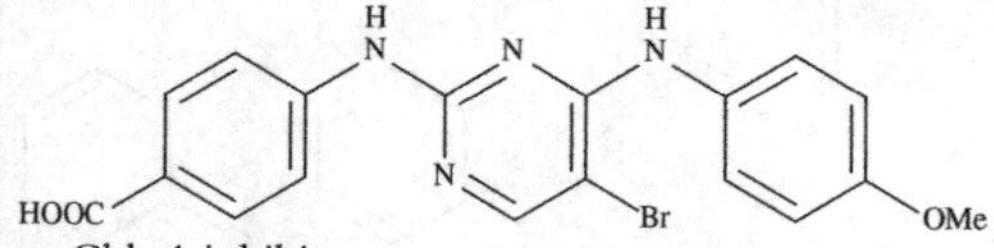 Chk-1 inhibitor
		Cyclin-dependent kinase 4 (Cdk4)	ACD	*De novo* design program LEGEND was combined with the program SEEDS to extract relevant scaffolds	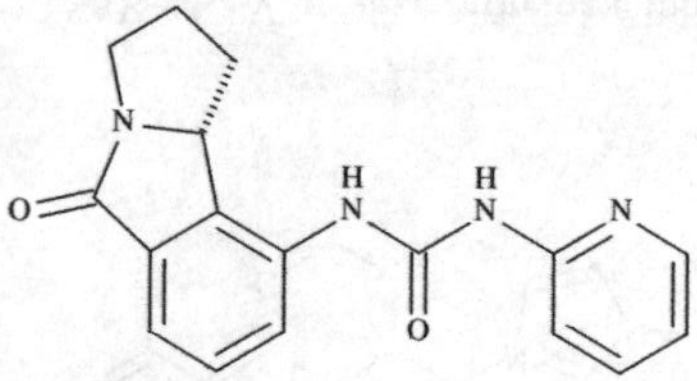 Cdk4 inhibitor
		p56 Lymphoid T cell tyrosine kinase (Lck)	3D database of 2 million commercial compounds	Docking	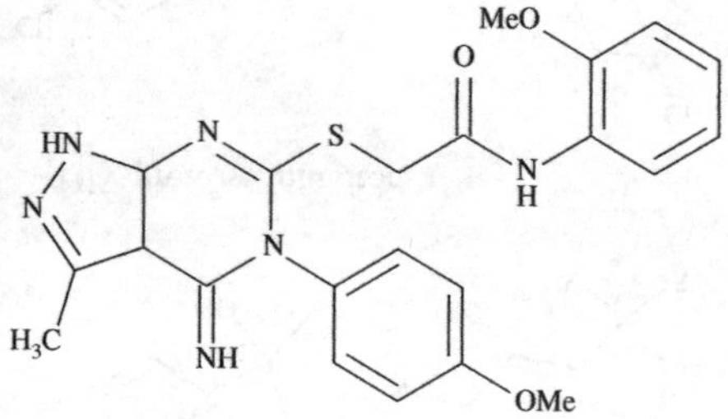 Lck inhibitor
	Proteases	*Falcipain-2*	ChemBridge	Lipinski and ADMET filters, homology modeling along with docking	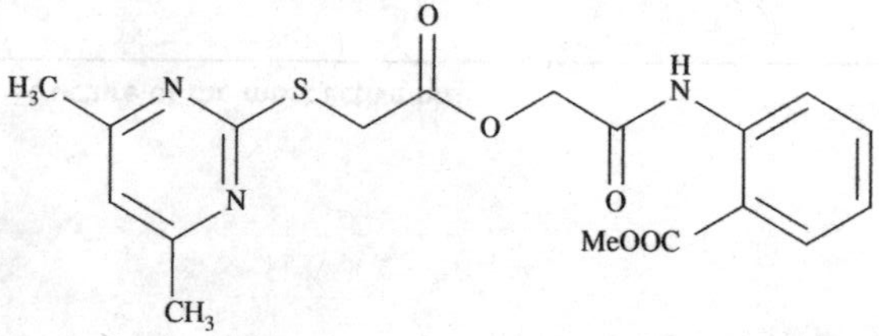 Falcipain inhibitor

(*Continued*)

Table 10.5 (Continued)

Target			Database	Methods employed	Structure of the most active hit
		HIV protease	Cambridge	Docking	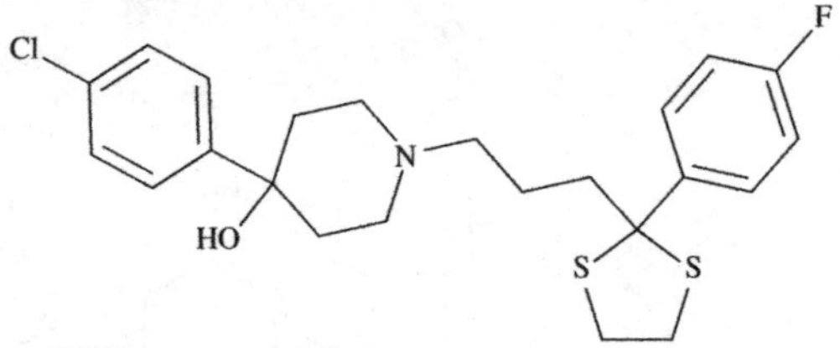 HIV protease inhibitor
		SARS CoV 3C-Like proteinase	ACD, MDDR, and NCI	Homology modeling, docking and molecular dynamics,	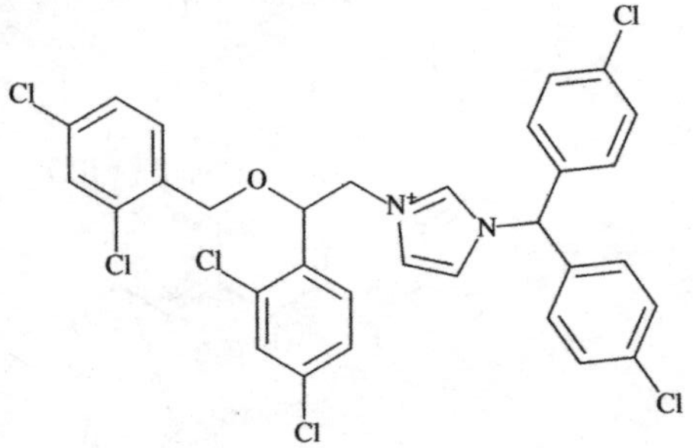 SARS CoV 3C-like proteinase inhibitor
		Thrombin	5300 commercial compounds	Docking and *de novo* design	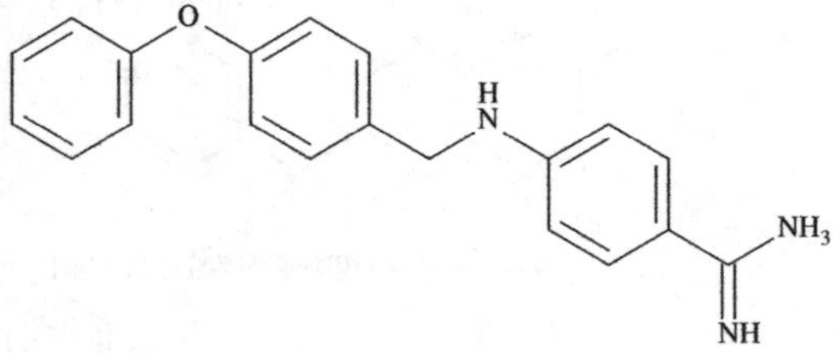 Thrombin inhibitor

Hydrolases	*Adenylyl cyclase (edema factor and CyaA)*	ACD	Docking	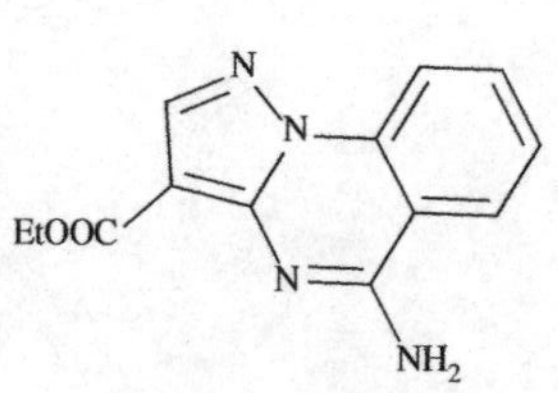 Edema factor (EF) adenylyl cyclase inhibitor
	AmpC β-lactamase	ACD	Docking	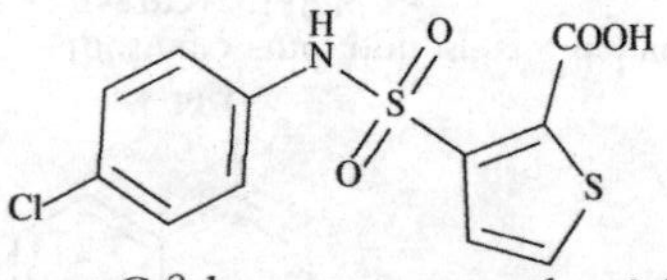 mpC β-lactamase noncovalent inhibitor
	Protein tyrosine phosphatase 1B	Pharmacia, the in-house compound	Docking	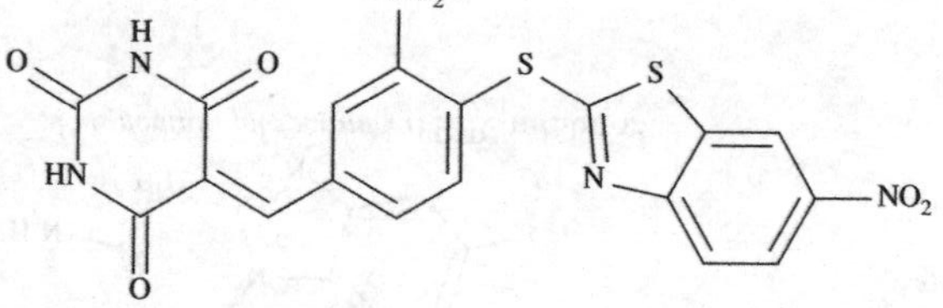 Protein tyrosine phosphatase 1B (PTP1B) inhibitor
Oxidases/ reductases	*Aldose reductase*	ADAM and EVE docking program	Docking	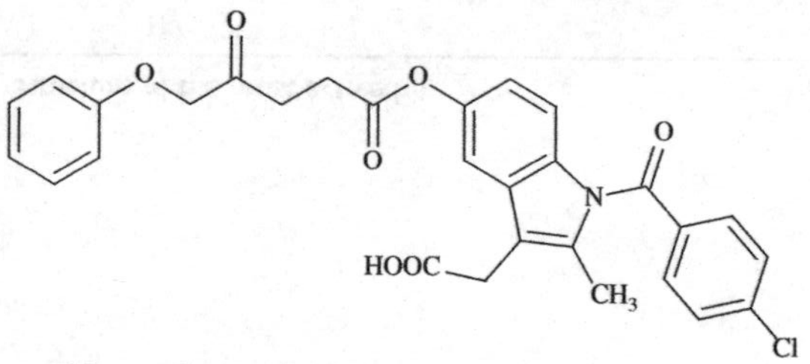 Aldose reductase inhibitor

(*Continued*)

Table 10.5 (Continued)

Target			Database	Methods employed	Structure of the most active hit
		Dihydrofolate reductase	ACD	Docking	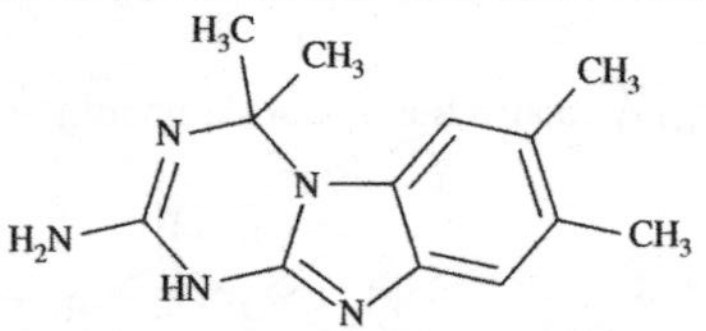 H_3C, CH_3, N, N, H_2N, HN, N, CH_3, CH_3 *Plasmodium falciparum* DHFR inhibitor
		Inosine 5′-monophosphate dehydrogenase Inhibitors (IMPDH)	In-house reagent inventory system	Docking and different scoring functions	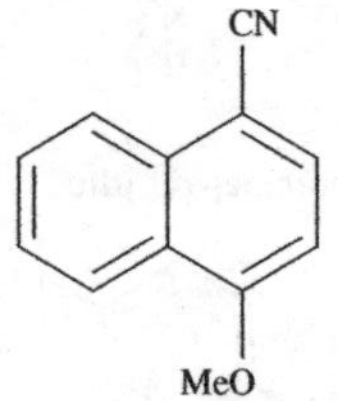 CN, MeO Inosine 5′-monophosphate dehydrogenase (IMPDH) inhibitor

cost-effective, and time-saving technique for the discovery of lead compounds [108]. The main advantages of this method compared to laboratory experiments are described in the next sections.

10.5.4.1 Cost-effective

As no compounds have to be purchased externally or synthesized by a chemist at the initial stages, VS is one of the most cost effective of the drug discovery processes.

10.5.4.2 Time-saving

Synthesis can take an extremely long time, especially in the case of large databases with millions of chemical compounds. But employing computational tools, the VS approach is always efficient in drug discovery.

10.5.4.3 Labor-efficient

Synthesis and bioassays always involve a great amount of human strength, and the chance of getting false positives is always present, even after spending a lot of physical and mental labor. Although undeniably VS also has a chance of resulting in false positives, but it is always labor-efficient in drug development.

10.5.4.4 Sensible alternative

It is possible to investigate compounds that have not been synthesized yet; and conducting HTS experiments is costly, time-consuming, and laborious for large numbers of chemicals. As a result, VS is always a rational option to minimize the initial number of compounds before using HTS methods.

10.5.5 Pitfalls

While applying the VS technique, the researcher must face many difficulties, such as finding the best possible balance between efficiency and precision when evaluating a particular algorithm, determining which method achieves better results and in what situations, and defining whether there is any universal method or workflow for VS. Considering the altitude of settings, parameters, and data sets, researchers have to explore a large number of *ifs* and *buts* during execution of VS. There are many known limitations (as well as still-unreported ones) of VS techniques. The probable pitfalls are discussed in the following section, along with possible ways to resolve them [109]. The pitfalls can be classified into four categories: (a) erroneous assumptions and expectations, (b) data design and content, (c) choice of software, and (d) conformational sampling, as well as ligand and target flexibility. A schematic representation has been shown in Figure 10.13.

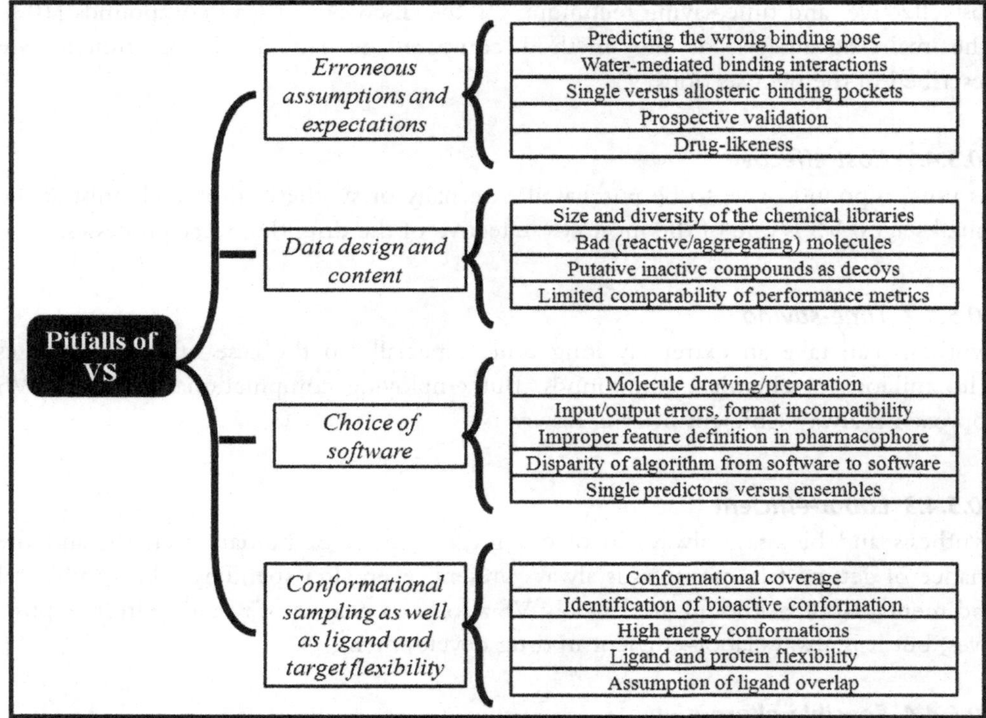

Figure 10.13 Major pitfalls of the VS approach.

a. *Erroneous assumptions and expectations*:

- *Predicting the wrong binding pose*: There are a few cases where even though the predicted docking binding poses are wrong, docking screening can accidentally generate high scores to many hits.
- *Water-mediated binding interactions*: In many docking studies, hydrogen bonds between ligand and protein are formed by water, which is often visible in the crystal structure of the complex. Those water-mediated hydrogen bonds can be taken into account in a structure-based VS study, but it is very difficult to predict the exact number, position, and orientation of these interactions.
- *Single- versus allosteric-binding pockets*: Both structure- and ligand-based VS approaches have intrinsic limitations, in that they are incapable of identifying bioactive ligands for the binding pockets, which are not explicitly docked against or implicitly represented in the training set. Again, the unknown binding site of a ligand complicates the problem of properly assessing hit rates in the VS experiments.
- *Prospective validation*: The VS is habitually performed on data sets with known actives, but often only putatively inactive molecules. As a result, in many cases,

a good number of inactive molecules are absent to identify the true inactives after the VS approach.

- *Druglikeness*: The majority of the VS approaches are based on the screening of druglike compounds by employing Lipinski's rule of five as the preliminary screening steps of the VS. One should remember that the rule applies only to oral bioavailability, and that many bioactivity classes such as antibiotics fall outside the scope of this rule. Hence, VS protocols are generally applied and validated on a relatively small fraction of chemical space, and their performance may change drastically from one database to another.

b. *Data design and content*:

- *Size and diversity of the chemical libraries*: In many cases, the employed libraries in the VS are either too small or contain too many closely related analogs, or often both. A data set that lacks sufficient chemical diversity is never an ideal choice for VS.
- *Experimental errors and inappropriate bioassays*: A large pool of data sets is often assembled from different sources, where different bioassay procedures and detection techniques have been used. As a consequence, there is a huge risk of experimental errors and inappropriate assays from molecule to molecule.
- *Bad (reactive/aggregating) molecules*: The data set provided for VS often includes molecules that contain chemically reactive groups or other undesirable functionalities that may interfere with the HTS detection techniques.
- *Putative inactive compounds as decoys*: Experimentally confirmed inactive compounds are helpful as negative controls because only few of them should appear in the hit list when a reliable VS protocol is employed. However, many of the decoys used in VS benchmark studies are only putatively inactive; hence, some assumed true negatives may actually be positives.

c. *Choice of software*:

- *Molecule drawing/preparation*: Adding implicit hydrogen atoms, handling the ionization states of the molecule, and assigning the correct charges at the initial stages of VS screening can easily be forgotten in many cases, where the final result will totally mislead the scientific community.
- *Input/output errors, format incompatibility*: Various errors are introduced when interconverting different molecular formats from one software to another. There is a high possibility of getting distorted information, like changes in atomic coordinates, chirality, hybridization, and protonation states of the employed compounds.
- *Improper feature definitions in the pharmacophore*: Incorrect feature definitions can be detrimental to the outcome of VS. In pharmacophore queries, the definition of pharmacophore features needs to be applied with caution. For example, it is known that nitrogen and oxygen atoms in the same heterocycle (such as

an oxazole) do not both behave as HBAs simultaneously. In the majority of cases, the acceptor in the oxazole ring is the nitrogen.

- *Disparity of algorithm from software to software*: Various software tools apply different algorithms for a particular job. For example, in the case of docking for energy minimization, different forms of FFs are applied from one software to another. Therefore, there is a high probability of getting different hits and making the VS process highly dependent on the use of particular software.
- *Single predictors versus ensembles*: Multiple statistical tools (both free and commercial software and descriptors) are available to perform VS studies. Each module captures different characteristics of molecular similarity. As a consequence, it is always difficult to identify a preferred tool/software/descriptor; therefore, it is often necessary to account for several approaches rather than one.

d. *Conformational sampling as well as ligand and target flexibility*:

- *Conformational coverage*: One of the main challenges in 3D-VS is generating a convenient set of conformations to cover the molecule's conformational space effectively.
- *High-energy conformations*: One has to remember that good conformational coverage is very important, and on the contrary, high-energy or physically unrealistic conformations can be detrimental to VS. Few conformational sampling approaches do not utilize energy minimization to refine and properly rank the resulting geometries. Therefore, the resulting list could contain many false positives.
- *Ligand and protein flexibility*: A common practice in many 3D database search systems is to set a limit on the number of conformations stored for each molecule. The number of conformations accessible to a molecule depends greatly on its size and flexibility. Of course, it is not only the ligands that are flexible; it is the biological targets as well. Protein flexibility is probably the most unexploited aspect of VS.
- *Assumption of ligand overlap*: In 3D shape-based VS, most programs attempt to maximize the overlap between the query and the database molecules. Indeed, different ligands may occupy different regions in the same protein, even in the same binding site, and the overlap between them in 3D space can be much less than assumed by a shape-based VS tool, resulting in more false negatives.

10.5.6 Databases for the VS

Chemically diverse libraries are particularly attractive for identifying novel scaffolds for new or relatively unexplored targets, such as those resulting from diversity-oriented synthesis. One needs to remember that the database library must fit the purpose of the experiment before its selection for screening. A large number of databases are publicly available and the number is increasing day by day. Recent initiatives requiring greater use of *in silico* technologies have called for transparency and development of strong database information that is available to the public at no cost. Electronic information on chemical structure, pharmacological activity, and specificity against known molecular targets can serve a wide variety of purposes in the field of VS. Table 10.6 summarizes a list of most current public and commercial chemical databases that are commonly screened in practice. The scientific community should take initiatives to develop more databases for public and administration use in the near future.

10.6 OVERVIEW AND CONCLUSIONS

The LBP approach and structure-based molecular docking play promising roles in the identification and optimization of leads in modern drug discovery. Pharmacophore and docking-based approaches, employed both alone or concurrently in VS, lead to a much higher hit rate than traditional screening methods (e.g., HTS). In a complete, structurally diverse data set, pharmacophore gives immense confidence about the best probable features that are solely responsible for particular pharmacological activity. On the contrary, the docking method provides an opportunity for the designing of active compounds considering the binding aspects of the ligand with the amino acid residues in the respective receptors. Methods like CoRIA and COMBINE provide a blend of ligand- and structure-based drug design at once, where the best possible interactions of the ligand–receptor complex can be identified. These methods are capable of extracting critical information regarding the nature and type of important interactions at the level of both the receptor and the ligand.

VS approaches have been vigorously implemented by pharmaceutical industries with the intent to obtain as many potential compounds as possible, and with the hope of a greater chance of finding hits from the available large pool of chemical libraries. Many successful examples have been demonstrated recently in the field of computer-aided VS for lead identification. There appears to be no universal method to execute these studies, as each biological target system is unique. Although one cannot ignore the intrinsic restrictions of VS, it remains one of the best possible options to explore a large chemical space, in terms of cost effectiveness and commitment of time and material needed. With the development of new docking methodologies, ligand-based screening techniques and machine-learning tools, the VS techniques are capable of giving better hit prediction rates, and undoubtedly, these will play the front-runner role in drug design in the near future either as a complementary approach to HTS or as a stand-alone approach. One has to remember that technologies are available that need to be employed in the right way and in the right direction to identify novel chemical substances with the scientific use of VS techniques. However, it must be emphasized that VS is not intended to replace the actual experimental approaches. As a matter of fact, the VS and experimental methods are highly complementary to each other.

Table 10.6 Commonly used chemical databases for the VS approach

Compound database	Availability	No. of compounds[a]	Website
ACD	Commercial	3,870,000	http://accelrys.com/products/databases/sourcing/available-chemicals-directory.html
Asinex	Commercial	550,000	http://www.asinex.com
Binding DB	Public	284,206 small ligands with 648 915 binding data, for 5662 protein targets	http://www.bindingdb.org
Chem ID	Public	3,88,000	http://chem.sis.nlm.nih.gov/chemidplus/
ChemBank	Public	800,000	http://chembank.broadinstitute.org
ChEMBL db	Public	658,075 differing bioactive compounds and 8091 targets	https://www.ebi.ac.uk/chembldb/
ChemBridge	Commercial	700,000	http://www.chembridge.com
ChemDiv	Commercial	1.5 million	http://www.chemdiv.com
Chemical Entities of Biological Interest (ChEBI)	Public	584,456	http://www.ebi.ac.uk/chebi/init.do
ChemMine	Public	6,200,000	http://bioweb.ucr.edu/ChemMineV2/
ChemNavigator	Commercial	55.3 million	http://www.chemnavigator.com
ChemSpider	Public	26 million	http://www.chemspider.com
Chimiotheque nationale	Public	44,817 compounds	http://chimiotheque-nationale.enscm.fr/index.php
CoCoCo	Public	6,957,134 molecules	http://cococo.unimore.it/tiki-index.php
Desmond Absolute Solvation Free Energies Set	Public	239	http://www.schrodinger.com/Desmond/Absolute-Solvation-Free-Energies-Set
Developmental Therapeutics Program (DTP)	Public	4,73,965	http://dtp.nci.nih.gov/
DNP	Public	40,000	http://dnp.chemnetbase.com/intro/index.jsp
DUD	Commercial	2950	http://dud.docking.org/
DUD.E	Commercial	22,886	http://dude.docking.org/

DrugBank	Public	7739 drugs	http://www.drugbank.ca
e-Drug3D	Public	1632	http://chemoinfo.ipmc.cnrs.fr/MOLDB/index.html
Enamine	Commercial	1.7 million	http://www.enamine.net
GLIDA	Public	G protein–coupled receptors (GPCRs) related Chemical Genomics database, Over 200	http://pharminfo.pharm.kyoto-u.ac.jp/services/glida/index.php
Glide Fragment Library	Commercial	441	http://www.schrodinger.com/Glide/Fragment-Library
Glide Ligand Decoys Set	Commercial	1000	http://www.schrodinger.com/Glide/Ligand-Decoys-Set
GLL	Commercial	25,145	http://cavasotto-lab.net/Databases/GDD/
GVK BIO	Commercial	Focused libraries with target inhibitor	http://www.gvkbio.com/informatics.html
HerbMedPro	Commercial	246	http://www.herbmed.org/
i:lib diverse	Commercial	Druglike fragment set for combinatorial library generation	http://www.inteligand.com/
Interbioscreen	Public	440,000 synthetic and 47,000 natural	http://www.ibscreen.com/index.htm
KKB	Public	>1.54M	http://www.eidogen.com/kinasekb.php
Maybridge	Commercial	56,000	http://www.maybridge.com
Mcule	Commercial	–	https://mcule.com/
MDDR	Commercial	150,000	http://accelrys.com/products/databases/bioactivity/mddr.html
MMsINC	Public	–	http://mms.dsfarm.unipd.it/MMsINC/search/
MORE	Commercial	9.7 million	https://itunes.apple.com/us/app/mobile-reagents-universal/id417616789
Mother of All Databases (MOAD)	Public	14,720 ligand–protein complexes, 4782 structures with binding data, 7064 ligands	http://www.bindingmoad.org
NCI	Public	140,000 million	http://dtp.nci.nih.gov/index.html
NRDBSM	Public	17,000	http://www.scfbio-iitd.res.in/software/nrdbsm/index.jsp

(*Continued*)

Table 10.6 (Continued)

Compound database	Availability	No. of compounds[a]	Website
PDB bind	Commercial	3214 ligand − protein complexes	http://www.pdbbind.org/
PubChem	Public	49,875,000	http://pubchem.ncbi.nlm.nih.gov
Specs	Commercial	240,000	http://www.specs.net
SPRESI^{web}	Commercial	5.68 million	http://www.spresi.com/
Super Drug Database (SDD)	Public	2,396 compounds with 1,08,198 conformers	http://bioinf.charite.de/superdrug/
TCM	Public	32,000	http://tcm.cmu.edu.tw
Therapeutic Target Database	Commercial	1906 targets, 5124 drugs	http://bidd.nus.edu.sg/group/cjttd/TTD_HOME.asp
U.S. Food and Drug Administration (FDA) database	Public	Drugs@FDA includes most of the drug products approved since 1939	http://www.fda.gov/Drugs/InformationOnDrugs/ucm135821.htm
WOMBAT	Commercial	331,872 molecules, 1966 targets	http://www.sunsetmolecular.com
ZINC	Public	13 million	http://zinc.docking.org
ZINClick	Public	16 million	http://www.symech.it/index.asp?catID=31&lang=en

[a]These are approximate numbers; -no exact information is available.

REFERENCES

[1] Schneider G. *De novo* design—hop(p)Ing against hope. Drug Discov Today Technol 2013;10: e453–60.

[2] Langer T. Pharmacophores in drug research. Mol Inf 2010;29(6–7):470–5.

[3] Kolb P, Ferreira RS, Irwin JJ, Shoichet BK. Docking and chemoinformatic screens for new ligands and targets. Curr Opin Biotech 2009;20:429–36.

[4] Ortiz AR, Pisabarro MT, Gago F, Wade RC. Prediction of drug binding affinities by comparative binding energy analysis. J Med Chem 1995;38(14):2681–91.

[5] Datar PA, Khedkar SA, Malde AK, Coutinho EC. Comparative residue interaction analysis (CoRIA): a 3D-QSAR approach to explore the binding contributions of active site residues with ligands. J Comput Aided Mol Des 2006;20:343–60.

[6] Tropsha A. Integrated chemo and bioinformatics approaches to virtual screening. In: Tropsha A, Varnek A, editors. Chemoinformatics approaches to virtual screening. London: RSC Publishing; 2008. pp. 295–325.

[7] Oprea TI. Virtual screening in lead discovery: a viewpoint. Molecules 2002;7:51–62.

[8] Kier LB. Molecular orbital calculation of preferred conformations of acetylcholine, muscarine, and muscarone. Mol Pharmacol 1967;3:487–94.

[9] Kier LB. MO Theory in drug research. New York, NY: Academic Press; 1971.

[10] Wermuth CG. Pharmacophores: historical perspective and viewpoint from a medicinal chemist. In: Langer T, Hoffmann RD, editors. Pharmacophores and pharmacophore searches. Weinheim: Wiley-VCH; 2006. pp. 3–13.

[11] Wermuth CG, Ganellin CR, Lindberg P, Mitscher LA. Glossary of terms used in medicinal chemistry (IUPAC Recommendations 1997). Pure Appl Chem 1998;70(5):1129–43.

[12] Ehrlich P. Ueber den jetzigen Stand der Chemotherapie. Ber Dtsch Chem Ges 1909;42:17–47.

[13] Leach AR, Gillet VJ, Lewis RA, Taylor R. Three-dimensional pharmacophore methods in drug discovery. J Med Chem 2010;53(2):539–58.

[14] Yang S-Y. Pharmacophore modeling and applications in drug discovery: challenges and recent advances. Drug Discov Today 2010;15(11–12):444–50.

[15] Smellie A, Teig S, Towbin P. Poling: promoting conformational variation. J Comput Chem 1995; 16:171–87.

[16] Kristam R, Gillet VJ, Lewis RA, Thorner D. Comparison of conformational analysis techniques to generate pharmacophore hypotheses using catalyst. J Chem Inf Model 2005;45(2):461–76.

[17] Sutter J, Guner OF, Hoffman R, Li H, Waldman M. In: Guner OF, editor. Pharmacophore perception, development, and use in drug design. La Jolla, CA: International University Line; 2000.

[18] Accelrys Inc. Discovery studio 2.1. San Diego, CA: Accelrys Inc.; 2010.

[19] Li H, Sutter J, Hoffmann RD. In: Güner OF, editor. Pharmacophore perception, development, and use in drug design. La Jolla, CA: International University Line; 2000.

[20] Debnath AK. Generation of predictive pharmacophore models for CCR5 antagonists: study with piperidine- and piperazine-based compounds as a new class of HIV-1 entry inhibitors. J Med Chem 2003;46(21):4501–15.

[21] Ekins S, Bravi G, Binkley S, Gillespie JS, Ring BJ, Wikel JH, et al. Drug Metab Dispos 2000; 28:994.

[22] Güner OF, Henry DR. Metric for analyzing hit lists and pharmacophores. In: Güner OF, editor. Pharmacophore perception, development, and use in drug design, IUL biotechnology series. La Jolla, CA: International University Line; 2000. pp. 191–212.

[23] Güner OF, Waldman M, Hoffmann RD, Kim JH. Strategies for database mining and pharmacophore development, 1st. In: Güner OF, editor. Pharmacophore perception, development, and use in drug design, IUL biotechnology series. La Jolla, CA: International University Line; 2000. pp. 213–36.

[24] Clement OO, Freeman CM, Hartmann RW, Handratta VD, Vasaitis TS, Brodie AM, et al. Three dimensional pharmacophore modeling of human CYP17 inhibitors. Potential agents for prostate cancer therapy. J Med Chem 2003;46:2345–51.

[25] Huang N, Shoichet BK, Irwin JJ. Benchmarking sets for molecular docking. J Med Chem 2006;49:6789–801.
[26] Willett P, Clark RD. GALAHAD: 1. Pharmacophore identification by hypermolecular alignment of ligands in 3D. J Comput-Aided Mol Des 2006;20(9):567–87.
[27] Jones G, Willett P, Glen RC. A genetic algorithm for flexible molecular overlay and pharmacophore elucidation. J Comput-Aided Mol Des 1995;9(6):532–49.
[28] Poptodorov K, Luu T, Hoffmann RD. In: Langer T, Hoffmann RD, editors. Methods and principles in medicinal chemistry, pharmacophores and pharmacophores searches, vol. 2. Weinheim, Germany: Wiley-VCH; 2006.
[29] Wolber G, Seidel T, Bendix F, Langer T. Molecule-pharmacophore superpositioning and pattern matching in computational drug design. Drug Discov Today 2008;13(1–2):23–9.
[30] Dror O, Shulman-Peleg A, Nussinov R, Wolfson H. Predicting molecular interactions in silico. I. An updated guide to pharmacophore identification and its applications to drug design. Front Med Chem 2006;3:551–84.
[31] Bandyopadhyay D, Agrafiotis DK. A self-organizing algorithm for molecular alignment and pharmacophore development. J Comput Chem 2008;29:965–82.
[32] Totrov M. Atomic property fields: generalized 3D pharmacophoric potential for automated ligand superposition, pharmacophore elucidation and 3D QSAR. Chem Biol Drug Des 2008;71:15–27.
[33] Nettles JH, et al. Flexible 3D pharmacophores as descriptors of dynamic biological space. J Mol Graph Model 2007;26:622–33.
[34] Baroni M, Cruciani G, Sciabola S, Perruccio F, Mason JS. A common reference framework for analyzing/comparing proteins and ligands. Fingerprints for ligands and proteins (FLAP): theory and application. J Chem Inf Model 2007;47:279–94.
[35] Wolber G, Langer T. LigandScout: 3-D pharmacophores derived from protein bound ligands and their use as virtual screening filters. J Chem Inf Model 2005;45(1):160–9.
[36] Chen J, Lai LH. Pocket v.2: further developments on receptor-based pharmacophore modeling. J Chem Inf Model 2006;46:2684–91.
[37] Ortuso F, Langer T, Alcaro S. GBPM: GRID based pharmacophore model. Concept and application studies to protein–protein recognition. Bioinformatics 2006;22(12):1449–55.
[38] SBP is now incorporated into Discovery Studio, available from Accelrys Inc., San Diego, CA.
[39] Brenk R, Klebe G. "Hot spot" analysis of protein-binding sites as a prerequisite for structure-based virtual screening and lead optimization. In: Langer T, Hoffmann RD, editors. Pharmacophores and pharmacophore searches. Weinheim: Wiley-VCH; 2006. pp. 171–92.
[40] Wei D, Jiang X, Zhou L, Chen J, Chen Z, He C, et al. Discovery of multi-target inhibitors by combining molecular docking with common pharmacophore matching. J Med Chem 2008;51(24):7882–8.
[41] Steindl TM, Schuster D, Laggner C, Langer T. Parallel screening: a novel concept in pharmacophore modeling and virtual screening. J Chem Inf Model 2006;46(5):2146–57.
[42] Rollinger JM, Hornick A, Langer T, Stuppner H, Prast H. Acetylcholinesterase inhibitory activity of scopolin and scopoletin discovered by virtual screening of natural products. J Med Chem 2004;47(25):6248–54.
[43] Ullmann JR. An algorithm for subgraph isomorphism. J ACM 1976;23:31–42.
[44] Barnard JM. Substructure searching methods: old and new. J Chem Inf Comput Sci 1993;33:532–8.
[45] Xu J. GMA: a generic match algorithm for structural homomorphism, isomorphism, maximal common substructure match and its applications. J Chem Inf Comput Sci 1996;36:25–34.
[46] Giménez-Oya V, Villacañas O, Fernàndez-Busquets X, Rubio-Martinez J, Imperial S. Mimicking direct protein–protein and solvent mediated interactions in the CDP-methylerythritol kinase homodimer: a pharmacophore-directed virtual screening approach. J Mol Model 2009;15(8):997–1007.
[47] Tschinke V, Cohen N. The NEWLEAD program: a new method for the design of candidate structures from pharmacophoric hypotheses. J Med Chem 1993;36:3863–70.

[48] Roe DC, Kuntz I. BUILDER v.2: improving the chemistry of a *de novo* design strategy. J Comput Aided Mol Des 1995;9:269–82.
[49] Huang Q, et al. PhDD: a new pharmacophore-based *de novo* design method of drug-like molecules combined with assessment of synthetic accessibility. J Mol Graph Model 2010;28(8):775–87.
[50] Kirkpatrick P. Virtual screening: gliding to success. Nat Rev Drug Disc 2004;3:299.
[51] Ewing JAT, Kuntz ID. Critical evaluation of search algorithms for automated molecular docking and database screening. J Comput Chem 1997;18:1175.
[52] Gohlke H, Klebe G. Approaches to the description and prediction of the binding affinity of small-molecule ligands to macromolecular receptors. Angew Chem Int Ed 2002;41(15):2644–76.
[53] Gohlke H, Kleb G. Statistical potentials and scoring functions applied to protein–ligand binding. Curr Opin Struct Biol 2001;11(2):231–5.
[54] Peitsch MC, Schwede T, Diemand A, Guex N. In: Jiang T, Xu Y, Zhang MQ, editors. Current topics in computational molecular biology. Cambridge, MA: MIT Press; 2002. pp. 449–66.
[55] Zimmer R, Lengauer T. In: Lengauer T, editor. Bioinformatics—from genomes to drugs. New York, NY: Wiley-VCH; 2002. pp. 237–313.
[56] Bitetti-Putzer R, Joseph-McCarthy D, Hogle JM, Karplus M. Functional group placement in protein binding sites: a comparison of GRID and MCSS. J Comput Aided Mol Des 2001;15(10): 935–60.
[57] Leulliot N, Varani G. Current topics in RNA–protein recognition: control of specificity and biological function through induced fit and conformational capture. Biochemistry 2001;40:7947–56.
[58] Davis AM, Teague SJ. Hydrogen bonding, hydrophobic interactions and failure of the rigid receptor hypothesis. Angew Chem Int Ed Engl 1999;38:736–49.
[59] Totrov M, Abagyan R. Flexible ligand docking to multiple receptor conformations: a practical alternative. Curr Opin Struct Biol 2008;18:178–84.
[60] Ferrari AM, Wei BQ, Costantino L, Shoichet BK. Soft docking and multiple receptor conformations in virtual screening. J Med Chem 2004;47:5076–84.
[61] Jiang F, Kim SH. Soft docking: matching of molecular surface cubes. J Mol Biol 1991;219:79–102.
[62] Leach AR. Ligand docking to proteins with discrete side-chain flexibility. J Mol Biol 1994;235: 345–56.
[63] Meiler J, Baker D. ROSETTALIGAND: protein-small molecule docking with full side-chain flexibility. Proteins 2006;65:538–84.
[64] Nabuurs SB, Wagener M, de Vlieg J. A flexible approach to induced fit docking. J Med Chem 2007;50:6507–18.
[65] Davis IW, Baker D. ROSETTALIGAND docking with full ligand and receptor flexibility. J Mol Biol 2009;385:381–92.
[66] Cozzini P, Kellogg GE, Spyrakis F, Abraham DJ, Costantino G, Emerson A, et al. Target flexibility: an emerging consideration in drug discovery and design. J Med Chem 2008;51:6237–55.
[67] Abseher R, Horstink L, Hilbers CW, Nilges M. Essential spaces defined by NMR structure ensembles and molecular dynamics simulation show significant overlap. Proteins 1998;31:370–82.
[68] Knegtel RM, Kuntz ID, Oshiro CM. Molecular docking to ensembles of protein structures. J Mol Biol 1997;266:424–40.
[69] Lorber DM, Shoichet BK. Hierarchical docking of databases of multiple ligand conformations. Curr Top Med Chem 2005;5:739–49.
[70] Huang S-Y, Zou X. Advances and challenges in protein–ligand docking. Int J Mol Sci 2010; 11:3016–34.
[71] Jain AN. Scoring functions for protein–ligand docking. Curr Protein Pept Sci 2006;7:407–20.
[72] Huang N, Kalyanaraman C, Irwin JJ, Jacobson MP. Molecular mechanics methods for predicting protein–ligand binding. J Chem Inf Model 2006;46:243–53.
[73] Weiner PK, Kollman PA. AMBER—assisted model building with energy refinement. A general program for modeling molecules and their interactions. J Comput Chem 1981;2:287–303.
[74] Brooks BR, Bruccoleri RE, Olafson BD, States DJ, Swaminathan S, Karplus M. CHARMM—a program for macromolecular energy, minimization, and dynamics calculations. J Comput Chem 1983;4:187–217.

[75] Verkhivker G, Appelt K, Freer ST, Villafranca JE. Empirical free energy calculations of ligand–protein crystallographic complexes. I. Knowledge-based ligand–protein interaction potentials applied to the prediction of human immunodeficiency virus 1 protease binding affinity. Protein Eng 1995;8:677–91.

[76] Charifson PS, Corkery JJ, Murcko MA, Walters WP. Consensus scoring: a method for obtaining improved hit rates from docking databases of three-dimensional structures into proteins. J Med Chem 1999;42:5100–9.

[77] Lee J, Seok C. A statistical rescoring scheme for protein–ligand docking: consideration of entropic effect. Proteins 2008;70:1074–83.

[78] Venkatesan SK, Shukla AK, Dubey VK. Molecular docking studies of selected tricyclic and quinone derivatives on trypanothione reductase of *Leishmania infantum*. J Comput Chem 2010;31(13):2463.

[79] Kroemer RT. Structure-based drug design: docking and scoring. Curr Protein Pept Sci 2007;8:312–28.

[80] Teague SJ. Implications of protein flexibility for drug discovery. Nat Rev Drug Discov 2003;2 (7):527–41.

[81] Vigers GPA, Rizzi JP. Multiple active site corrections for docking and virtual screening. J Med Chem 2004;47(1):80–9.

[82] DockIt: Metaphorics, Aliso Viejo, CA, <http://www.metaphorics.com/products/dockit>.

[83] Terp GE, Johansen BN, Christensen IT, Jørgensen FS. A new concept for multidimensional selection of ligand conformations (MultiSelect) and multidimensional scoring (MultiScore) of protein–ligand binding affinities. J Med Chem 2001;44(14):2333–43.

[84] Klon AE, Glick M, Davies JW. Application of machine learning to improve the results of high-throughput docking against the HIV-1 protease. J Chem Inf Comput Sci 2004;44:2216–24.

[85] Wade RC, Ortiz AR, Gago F. Comparative binding energy analysis. Persp Drug Discov Des 1998; 11:19–34.

[86] Moitessier N, Englebienne P, Lee D, Lawandi J, Corbeil CR. Towards the development of universal, fast and highly accurate docking/scoring methods: a long way to go. Br J Pharmacol 2008;153 (S1):S7–26.

[87] Verma J, Khedkar VM, Coutinho EC. 3D-QSAR in drug design—a review. Curr Top Med Chem 2010;10(1):95–115.

[88] Lushington GH, Guo JX, Wang JL. Whither combine? New opportunities for receptor-based QSAR. Curr Med Chem 2007;14(17):1863–77.

[89] Kmunicek J, Hynkova K, Jedlicka T, Nagata Y, Negri A, Gago F, et al. Quantitative analysis of substrate specificity of haloalkane dehalogenase LinB from *Sphingomonas paucimobilis* UT26. Biochemistry 2005;44:3390–401.

[90] Wang T, Tomic S, Gabdoulline RR, Wade RC. How optimal are the binding energetics of barnase and barstar? Biophys J 2004;87:1618–30.

[91] Tomic S, Nilsson L, Wade RC. Nuclear receptor–DNA binding specificity: a COMBINE and Free-Wilson QSAR analysis. J Med Chem 2000;43:1780–92.

[92] VLife MDS. 3.5 is a software of VLife Sciences Technologies Private Limited, 2007–2008, <http://www.vlifesciences.com>.

[93] Gil-Redondo R, Klett J, Gago F, Morreale A. gCOMBINE: a graphical user interface to perform structure-based comparative binding energy (COMBINE) analysis. Proteins 2010;78(1):162–72.

[94] Vedani A, Briem H, Dobler M, Dollinger K, McMasters DR. Multiple conformation and protonation-state representation in 4D-QSAR. J Med Chem 2000;43:4416–27.

[95] Verma J, Khedkar VM, Prabhu AS, Khedkar SA, Malde AK, Coutinho EC. A comprehensive analysis of the thermodynamic events involved in ligand–receptor binding using CoRIA and its variants. J Comput Aided Mol Des 2008;22(2):91–104.

[96] Dhaked DK, Verma J, Saran A, Coutinho EC. Exploring the binding of HIV-1 integrase inhibitors by comparative residue interaction analysis (CoRIA). J Mol Model 2009;15(3):233–45.

[97] Dror O, Shulman-Peleg A, Nussinov R, Wolfson HJ. Predicting molecular interactions in silico: I. A guide to pharmacophore identification and its applications to drug design. Curr Med Chem 2004; 11:71–90.

[98] Jahn A, Hinselmann G, Fechner N, Zell A. Optimal assignment methods for ligand-based virtual screening. J Cheminform 2009;1:14.
[99] Villoutreix BO, Renault N, Lagorce D, Sperandio O, Montes M, Miteva MA. Free resources to assist structure-based virtual ligand screening experiments. Curr Protein Pept Sci 2007;8:381–411.
[100] Fox S, Farr-Jones S, Yund MA. High throughput screening for drug discovery: continually transitioning into new technology. J Biomol Screen 1999;4:183–6.
[101] Lipinski CA, Lombardo F, Dominy BW, Feeney PJ. Experimental and computational approaches to estimate solubility and permeability in drug discovery and development settings. Adv Drug Deliv Rev 1997;23(1–3):3–25.
[102] QikProp, version 3.4, Schrödinger, LLC, New York, NY; 2011.
[103] Wilson GL, Lill MA. Integrating structure-based and ligand-based approaches for computational drug design. Future Med Chem 2011;3:735–50.
[104] Liebeschuetz JW, Jones SD, Morgan PJ, Murray CW, Rimmer A, Roscoe JM, et al. PRO_SELECT: combining structure-based drug design and array-based chemistry for rapid lead discovery. 2. The development of a series of highly potent and selective factor Xa inhibitors. J Med Chem 2002;45:1221–32.
[105] Sharma A, Tendulkar AV, Wangikar PP. Drug discovery against H1N1 virus (influenza A virus) via computational virtual screening approach. Med Chem Res 2011;20(9):1445–9.
[106] Dahlgren MK, Zetterström CE, Gylfe Å, Linusson A, Elofsson M. Statistical molecular design of a focused salicylidene acylhydrazide library and multivariate QSAR of inhibition of type III secretion in the Gram-negative bacterium Yersinia. Bioorg Med Chem 2010;18(7):2686–703.
[107] Kubinyi H. Success stories of computer-aided design. In: Ekins S, editor. Computer applications in pharmaceutical research and development. New York: John Wiley & Sons; 2006. pp. 377–424.
[108] Schneider G, Böhm H. Virtual screening and fast automated docking methods: combinatorial chemistry. Drug Discov Today 2002;7:64–70.
[109] Scior T, Bender A, Tresadern G, Medina-Franco JL, Martínez-Mayorga K, Langer T, et al. Recognizing pitfalls in virtual screening: a critical review. J Chem Inf Model 2012;52:867–81.

CHAPTER 11

SAR and QSAR in Drug Discovery and Chemical Design—Some Examples

Contents

11.1 INTRODUCTION

The design and development of new chemicals is a challenging task. The challenge becomes tougher while dealing with molecules of biological importance (e.g., drugs and pharmaceuticals). The act of developing new drug molecules, as well as modifying the existing ones, involves a multifaceted objective covering the aspects of desired pharmacological activity, undesirable side reactions, appreciable pharmacokinetic features, and suitable form of administration. Although it may be argued that many useful drugs, like acetylsalicylic acid, quinine, and penicillin, have come through *serendipitous* discovery as well as classical research, it should be considered that many other drug candidates have failed or been withdrawn due to undesirable outcomes. The major objective of the pharmaceutical and other chemical industries is to develop medicines (or other chemicals) that are suitably valued by regulatory authorities, patients, healthcare professionals and providers, and others to improve the quality of life of consumers. However, considering the existing economic conditions, the industry attempts to provide the best product possible at a suitable cost and time frame in order to cope with the market. Therefore, the criteria about adjustments comprise the quality, speed, and time parameters to make a product economically viable. However, it is definitely not possible to compromise with the quality of medicinal agents that we consume; hence, the need for less time-consuming, alternative, accurate, and economic methods becomes inevitable. Considering the huge cost incurred during the discovery of a drug molecule that comprises steps like initial synthesis and preliminary screening of biological activity, preclinical development (studies on

Understanding the Basics of QSAR for Applications in Pharmaceutical Sciences and Risk Assessment.
ISBN: 978-0-12-801505-6, DOI: http://dx.doi.org/10.1016/B978-0-12-801505-6.00011-9

animals for pharmacological effect and short- and long-term toxicities), phase I clinical trials (studies on healthy human volunteers), phase II clinical trials (studies on limited cohort of human volunteers with the specific disease), phase III clinical trials (studies on larger populations of affected human volunteers), phase IV clinical trials (post-marketing surveillance), and post-developmental quality control and quality assurance operations in order to get final approval for release, classical and empirical techniques seem impracticable. Hence, rational drug-design approaches are highly useful in providing a theoretical basis on the features of an investigational molecule addressing almost all possible aspects of its failure. Various *in silico* molecular modeling studies, including the quantitative structure–activity relationship (QSAR) methodology, enable us to gather sufficient information regarding the response of a chemical by comparing it with several other similar and different molecules, thereby allowing us to choose the one with optimized features. Furthermore, the use of different *in silico* methodologies also provides a good option for reducing animal experimentation, which involves ethical obligations. In this chapter, we present several success stories of representative approved and investigational drugs and other chemicals that have been designed and developed employing QSAR and related *in silico* molecular modeling operations.

11.2 SUCCESSFUL APPLICATIONS OF QSAR AND OTHER *IN SILICO* METHODS: REPRESENTATIVE EXAMPLES

The research and development in the realm of QSAR and related molecular modeling techniques have traversed a long journey from which several successful outcomes have been obtained. We have attempted to present here a few success stories of computational methods in deriving some drugs and other chemicals [1–7] in Tables 11.1 and 11.2, respectively.

11.2.1 Examples of some approved drugs

Example 1

a. Name of the drug: Captopril

b. Disease indication: Used for the treatment of hypertension.

c. Mechanism: Reduction of blood pressure by antagonizing the action of angiotensin-converting enzyme (ACE) that controls the pressure of blood using the rennin–angiotensin pathway. Captopril is considered as a reversible and potent inhibitor of ACE.

d. Brief developmental history: Captopril was designed using the approach of structure-based drug design in the late 1970s [8]. The basic concept came from the inhibition of the enzyme carboxypeptidase A. Among the first developments were L-benzylsuccinic acid [9], a potent inhibitor of carboxypeptidase A and the pentapeptide BPP5a [10], an inhibitor of ACE (which is isolated from the

Sl. No.	Name of the drug agent	Chemical structure	Indication	Mechanism	US FDA approval/clinical trial status	Marketed by	Product	Trade name
Approved drugs								
1	Saquinavir		AIDS	Inhibitor of HIV-1 protease enzyme	1995	Hoffmann-La Roche	Saquinavir mesylate	Invirase®
2	Amprenavir		AIDS	Inhibition of HIV protease enzyme	1999	GlaxoSmithKline	Amprenavir	Agenerase
3	Indinavir		AIDS	Inhibition of HIV protease enzyme	1996	Merck Sharp Dohme	Indinavir sulfate	Crixivan®

(*Continued*)

Table 11.1 (Continued)

Sl. No.	Name of the drug agent	Chemical structure	Indication	Mechanism	US FDA approval/ clinical trial status	Marketed by	Product	Trade name
4	Lopinavir	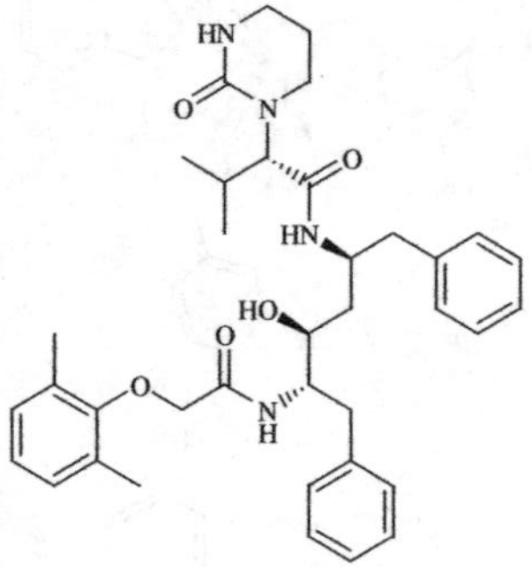	AIDS	Inhibition of HIV protease enzyme	2000	Abott	Lopinavir/ Ritonavir	Kaletra®
5	Nelfinavir	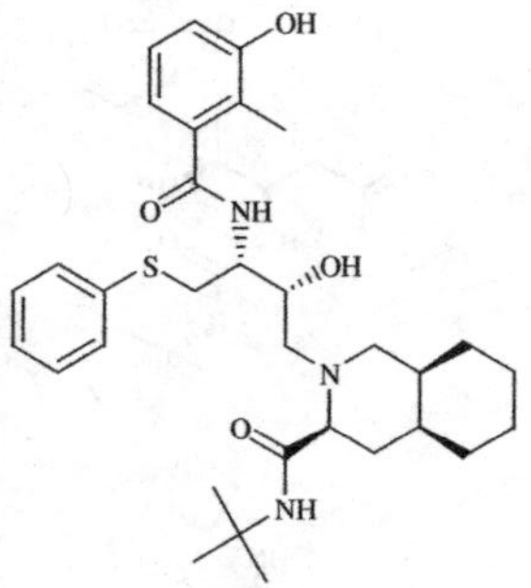	AIDS	Inhibition of HIV protease enzyme	1997	Agouron	Nelfinavir mesylate	Viracept®
6	Raltegravir	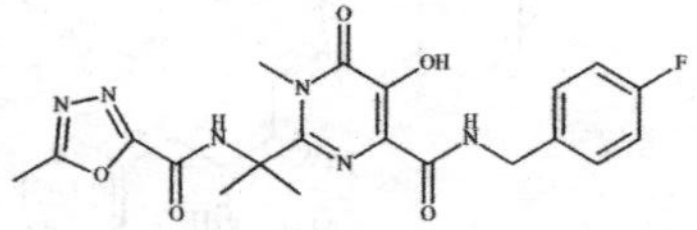	AIDS	Inhibition of HIV-1 integrase enzyme	2007	Merck Sharp Dohme	Raltegravir potassium	Isentress
7	Ritonavir	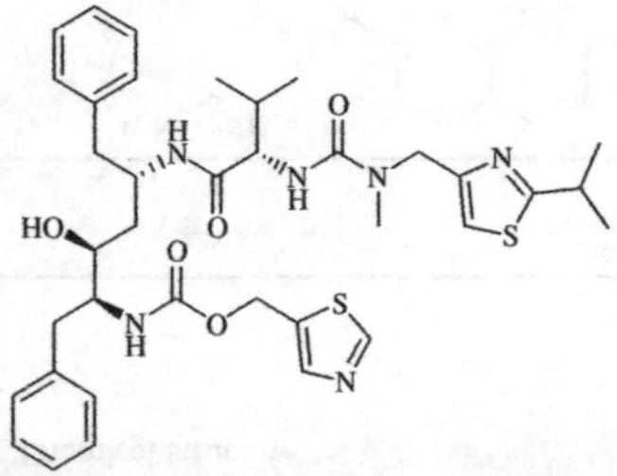	AIDS	Inhibition of HIV protease enzyme	1996	Abott	Ritonavir	Norvir®

		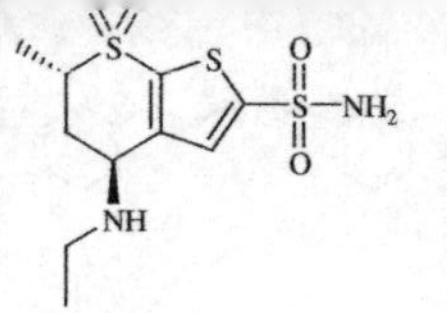	glaucoma and ocular hypertension	carbonic anhydrase II enzyme			hydrochloride	
9	Norfloxacin	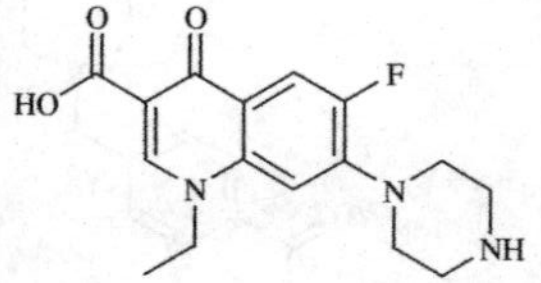	Bacterial infection	Inhibition of bacterial DNA gyrase	1986	Merck	Norfloxacin	Noroxin®
10	Oseltamivir	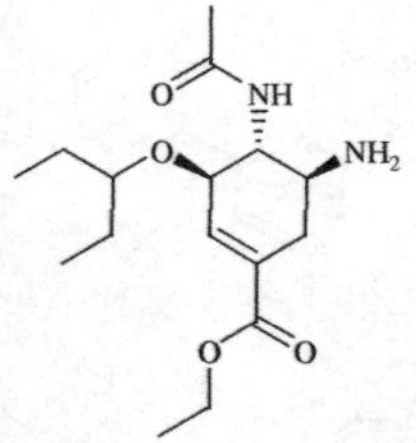	Influenza	Inhibition of NA enzyme	1999	Hoffmann-La Roche	Oseltamivir phosphate	Tamiflu®
11	Zanamivir	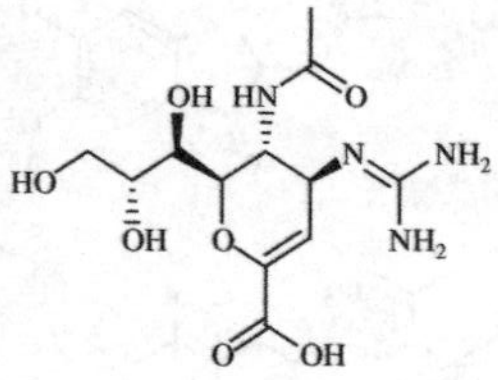	Influenza	Inhibition of NA enzyme	1999	GlaxoSmithKline	Zanamivir	Relenza®
12	Boceprevir	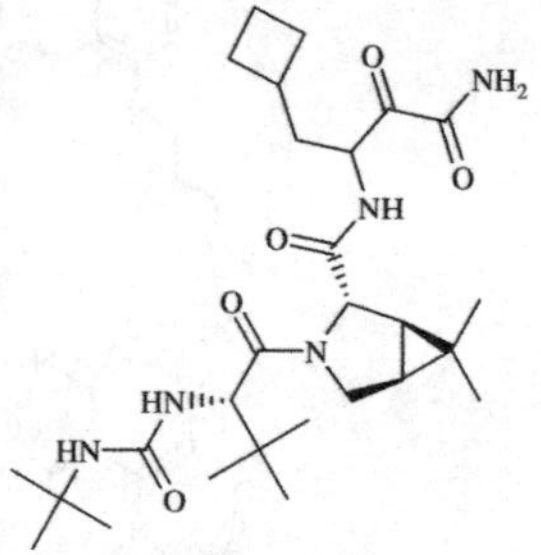	Hepatitis C	Inhibition of NS3-NS4A serine protease of HCV	2011	Merck Sharp Dohme	Boceprevir	Victrelis®

(*Continued*)

Table 11.1 (Continued)

Sl. No.	Name of the drug agent	Chemical structure	Indication	Mechanism	US FDA approval/ clinical trial status	Marketed by	Product	Trade name
13	Captopril	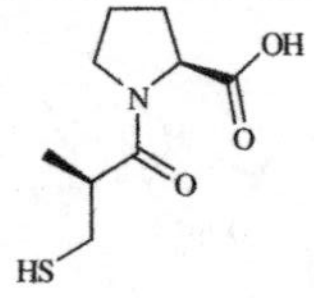	Hypertension	Potent and reversible inhibition of ACE	1981	Bristol Myers-Squibb	Captopril	Capoten®
14	Aliskiren	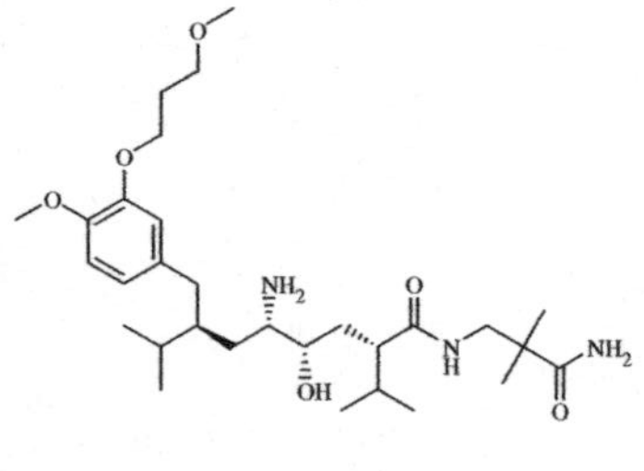	Hypertension	Inhibition of rennin	2007	Novartis	Aliskiren hemifumarate	Tekturna®
15	Donepezil	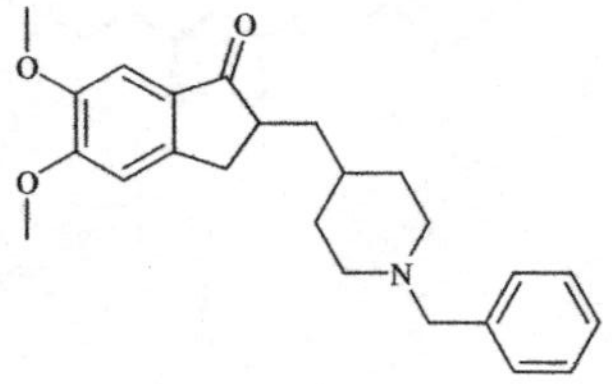	Alzheimer's disease	Inhibition of AChE enzyme	1996	Eisai Inc.	Donepezil hydrochloride	Aricept®
16	Imatinib	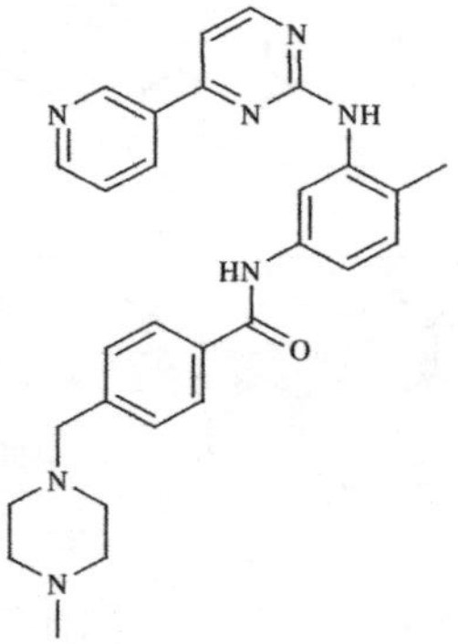	Cancer: Chronic myelogenous leukemia (CML), gastrointestinal stromal tumors (GISTs), etc.	Inhibition of BCR-Abl tyrosine kinase enzyme	2003	Novartis	Imatinib mesylate	Gleevec®
17	Tirofiban	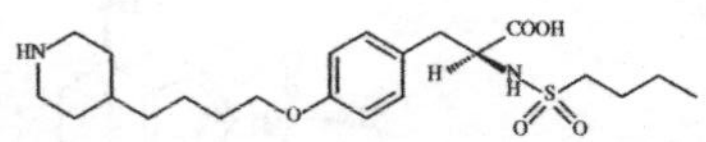	Thrombosis	Inhibition of fibrinogen	2000	Medicure	Tirofiban hydrochloride	Aggrastat®

18	PRX-00023	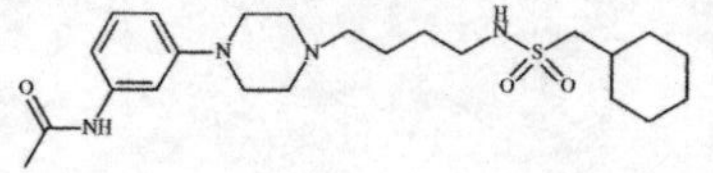	Depression, anxiety	Agonism of $5\text{-}HT_{1A}$	Phase III completed	Epix Pharmaceuticals, Inc.	PRX-00023	–
19	LY-517717	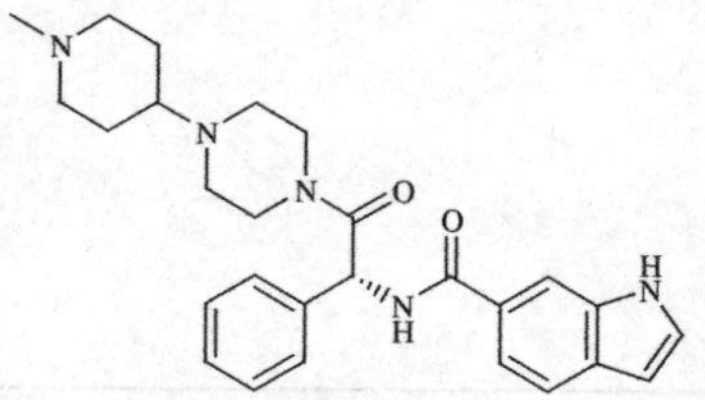	Venous thromboembolism following hip or knee replacement	Inhibition of factor Xa serine protease enzyme	Phase II completed	Eli Lilly/Protherics	LY-517717	–
20	TMI-005	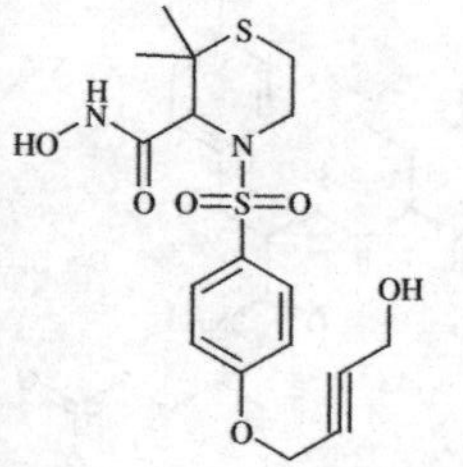	Rheumatoid arthritis	Inhibition of TNF-α convertase enzyme (TACE)	Phase II completed	Wyeth (Pfizer)	TMI-005	–
21	Nolatrexed	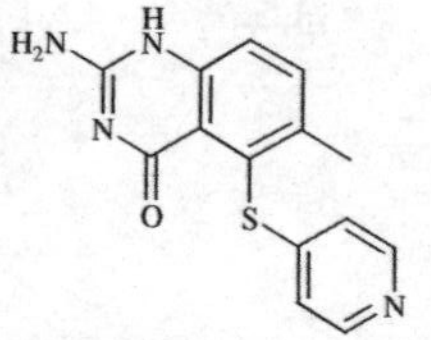	Cancer: Unresectable Hepatocellular Carcinoma (HCC)	Inhibition of thymidylate synthase enzyme	Phase III completed	Agouron	Nolatrexed dihydrochloride	Thymitaq
22	Raltitrexed	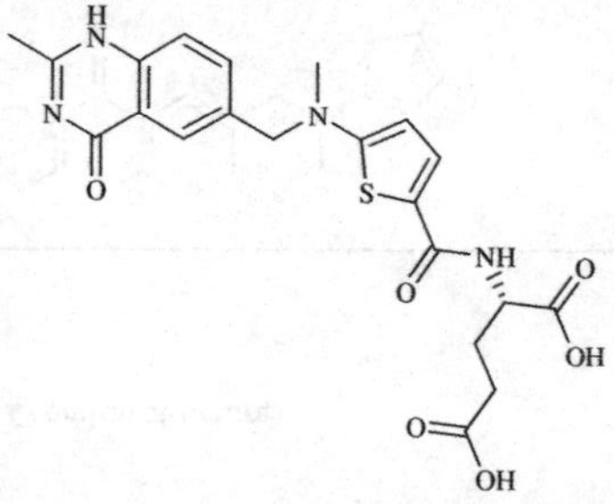	Cancer: malignant neoplasm of colon and rectum	Inhibition of thymidylate synthase enzyme	Phase II completed	Astrazeneca	Raltitrexed	Tomudex

(*Continued*)

Table 11.1 (Continued)

Sl. No.	Name of the drug agent	Chemical structure	Indication	Mechanism	US FDA approval/ clinical trial status	Marketed by	Product	Trade name
23	AUY922 (NVP-AUY922)	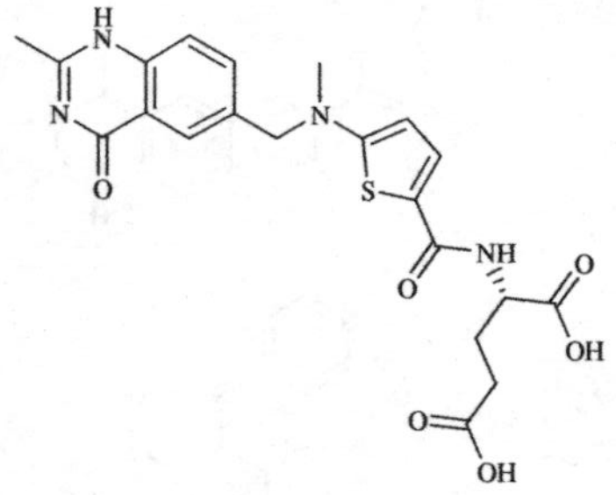 H N N O N S NH O O OH O OH	Cancer	Inhibition of HSP90	Phase II completed	Novartis	AUY922	–
24	Rupintrivir (AG7088)	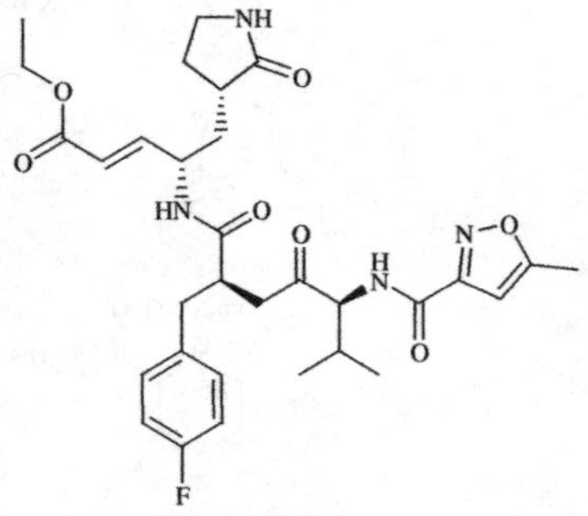 NH O O O HN O O H N N-O O F	Rhinovirus infection	Inhibition of HRV 3C protease enzyme	Phase II completed	Agouron	Rupintrivir	–

Table 11.2 Representative list of registered agrochemicals (pesticides) designed using QSAR techniques

Sl. No.	Name	Chemical structure	Mechanism	EPA registration	Pesticide type
1	Bifenthrin	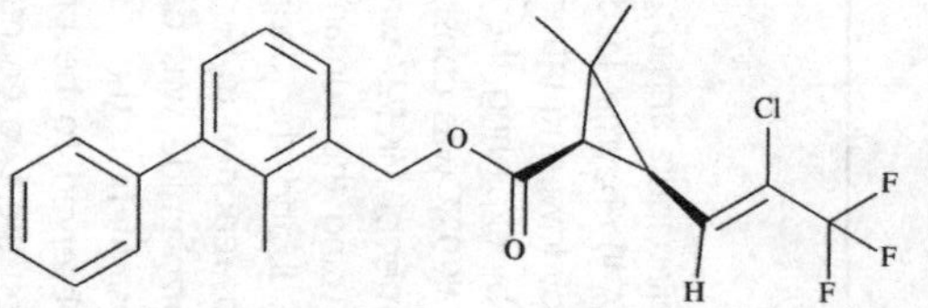	Acts by interfering with the nervous system of insects	1989	Conventional chemical
2	Ipconazole	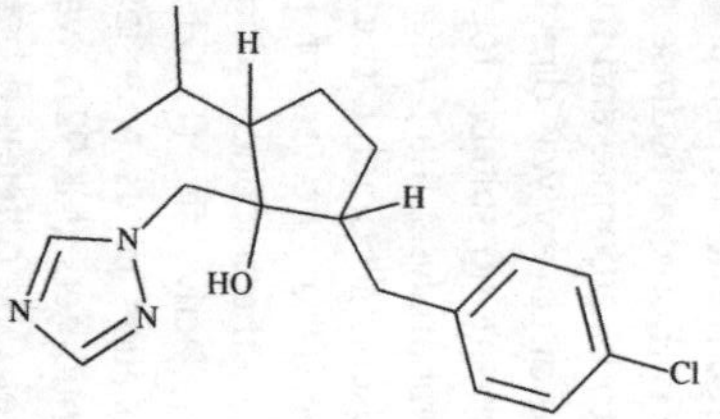	Acts by inhibiting C-14 demethylation during ergosterol biosynthesis	1993	Conventional chemical
3	Metconazole	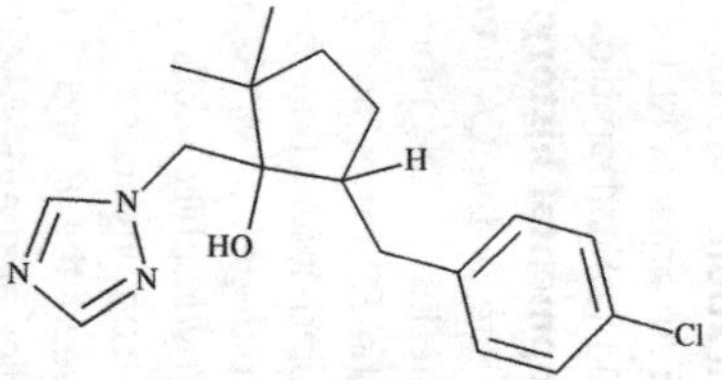	Acts by inhibiting C-14 demethylation during ergosterol biosynthesis	2007	–

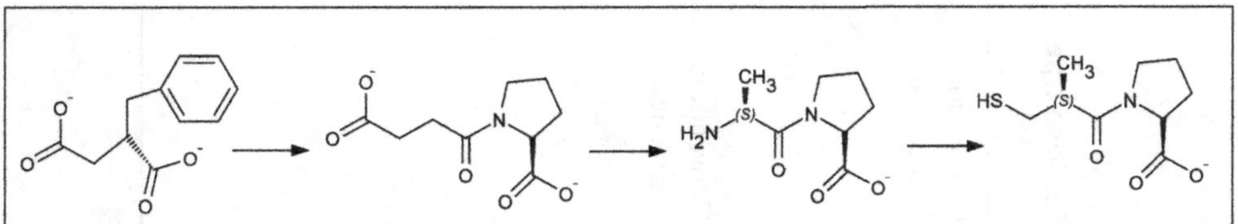

Figure 11.1 The design and development of the captopril molecule.

Brazilian viper, *Bothrops jararaca*). The N-terminal fragment of BPP5a, including dipeptide, tripeptide, and tetrapeptide fragments, possesses the ACE inhibitory activity. Benzylsuccinic acid was considered as a model compound, assuming that succinyl amino acids act as the by-product inhibitors of ACE. Structure—activity relationship (SAR) studies on succinyl-proline moiety led to the design and development of Captopril characterized by an IC_{50} value of 23 nM [8]. Two essential structural modifications were incorporated in succinyl-proline. In order to establish a stronger binding interation with the zinc ion of ACE, the carboxylic acid residue of succinyl-proline was replaced with the mercapto group, and a stereospecific *R*-methyl group was added to the succinyl moiety emulating the methyl group that is similar to that of Ala-Pro (L-Ala residue). Figure 11.1 shows the structural developmental phases of Captopril.

e. Approval status: Approved by the US Food and Drug Administration (FDA) in 1981.

Example 2

a. Name of the drug: Dorzolamide

b. Disease indication: Used for the treatment of open angle glaucoma and ocular hypertension.

c. Mechanism: An antagonist for the carbonic anhydrase II (CA II) enzyme, leading to the blockade of local conversion of carbon dioxide to bicarbonate and thereby lowering intraocular pressure (IOP).

d. Brief developmental history: The discovery was directed by exploring the binding of compounds at the active site of the CA II enzyme using suitable tools. MK-927 was considered as the prototype chemical for reducing IOP. From chiral analysis, the *S*-enantiomer of MK-927 was observed to be more active than the *R* isomer, and X-ray crystallographic studies using the human CA II (HCA II) enzyme showed binding interaction between the zinc ion of HCA II and the deprotonated (presumably) sulfonamide nitrogen of MK-927, while the thiophene ring was reported to be placed between hydrophobic and hydrophilic walls of the active site [11,12]. Dorzolamide was developed from MK-927 through the conformational optimization of its enantiomers. At first, the pseudoequatorial conformation between the *R* and *S* enantiomers (MK-927) was observed to be preferable by employing *ab initio* studies at the 6—31 G* level. One difference between the two enantiomers was in the thiophenesulfonamide N-S-C-S dihedral angle, the ideal being 72°. The *S*-form (150°) showed a preference over the *R* form (170°) since the latter showed an additional twist of the thiophene ring. The second difference was in the geometry of the 4-isobutylamino substituent; an *ab initio* study at the 3—21 G* level showed that the *trans* geometry in the *S*-form is preferable than the *gauche* form in the *R* [12]. Two structural modifications were performed to enhance the inhibitory potency. With the aim of reducing the pseudoaxial energy penalty, a methyl group at the thienothiopyran ring was introduced; and to reduce the lipophilic effect due to the methyl group, ethylamino moiety was used in place of

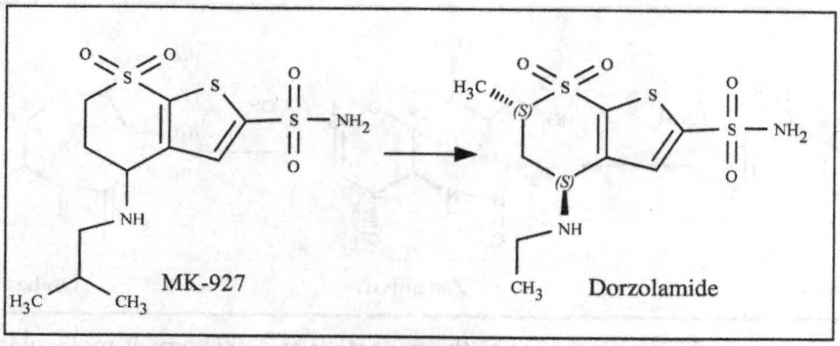

Figure 11.2 The design and development of the dorzolamide molecule.

the 4-isobutylamino group. The final structure was termed *dorzolamide*, and from X-ray crystallographic analysis using HCA II, the *S,S* configuration was observed to be the best characterized by a favorable thiophenesulfonamide N-S-C-S dihedral angle of 140° [12]. Figure 11.2 presents the chemical structures of MK-927 and dorzolamide.

e. Approval status: Approved by the FDA in 1994.

Example 3

a. Name of the drug: Zanamivir

b. Disease indication: Used for the treatment of influenza.

c. Mechanism: Inhibition of the neuraminidase (NA) enzyme for the treatment of influenza A and B viruses.

d. Brief developmental history: The biological target to combat the influenza virus is neuraminidase enzyme (also known as *sialidases*) that comprises two groups: group-1 (N1, N4, N5, N8) and group-2 (N2, N3, N6, N7, N9). The influenza virus envelope comprises NA enzymes that damage the host by the hydrolytic cleavage of glycosidic bonds between the terminal sialic acid residues and adjacent sugars on hemagglutinin or surface cells [13], and the spread of the virus is actually facilitated by the cleavage of sialic acid [14]. The structure-based design and development of drugs against influenza was followed by the establishment of three-dimensional (3D) structural geometry of the group-2 neuraminidase in early 1980s. In 1993, von Itzstein and coworkers [15] used the computational tool GRID while studying the binding site of NA. The design of the NA antagonists was facilitated by the transition-state principle. The binding study of 2-deoxy-2,3-dehydro-*N*-acetylneuraminic acid (DANA) to NA made good progress toward the development of inhibitors, and it concluded with the possibility of further improvement by replacing the 4-hydroxy group with an amino or a larger guanidine moiety [16]. Both substitutions are found to enhance the binding affinity, of which the guanidino moiety showed more effective binding characterized by salt-bridge formation with Glu^{119} residue and charge–charge interaction with Glu^{227} residue, while the amino replacement depicted only salt-bridge interaction with Glu^{119} residue [15]. The guanidino compound was designated as zanamivir, which is the first-in-class NA inhibitor to get approval. The chemical structures of DANA and zanamivir are shown in Figure 11.3. The only problem with zanamivir was its poor bioavailability; hence, inhalation was the route of administration.

e. Approval status: Approved by the FDA in 1999.

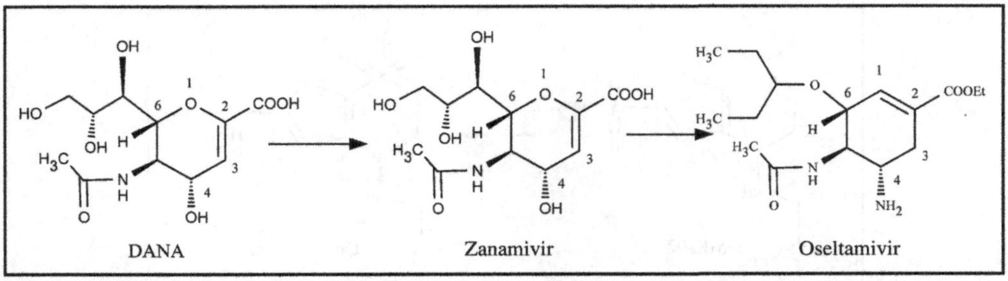

Figure 11.3 The design and development of the zanamivir and oseltamivir molecules.

Example 4

a. Name of the drug: Oseltamivir

b. Disease indication: Used for the treatment of influenza.

c. Mechanism: Inhibition of the NA enzyme for the treatment of influenza A and B viruses.

d. Brief developmental history: The design of oseltamivir followed the success obtained with zanamivir. Considering the oral form as the most convenient and patient-compliant one, especially during epidemics, researchers started developing new analogs with improved oral bioavailability profiles. Scientists at Gilead Sciences (based in Foster City, CA) strategized to develop more stable carbocyclic core moiety in place of the dihydropyran ring and designed transition-state analogs of sialic acid [17]. Further exploration of the binding site depicted the presence of hydrophobic amino acid residues (Ile^{222}, Ala^{246}), and accordingly, SAR modification led to the development of an ester compound called *Oseltamivir*. It is a prodrug that releases the active carboxylic acid form upon hepatic hydrolysis. It was the first orally available medicament to combat influenza types A and B. The chemical structure of oseltamivir (shown in Figure 11.3) is a continuation of anti-influenza drug development, including DANA and Zanamivir.

e. Approval status: Approved by the FDA in 1999.

Example 5

a. Name of the drug: Saquinavir

b. Disease indication: Used for the treatment of acquired immune deficiency syndrome (AIDS).

c. Mechanism: Inhibition of human immunodeficiency virus-1 protease (HIV-1 PR) by incorporating mutation or causing chemical inhibition, leading to the production of immature, noninfectious human immunodeficiency virus (HIV) viral particles [18].

d. Brief developmental history: Following the discovery of the structure of the HIV-protease enzyme, various approaches, including transition-state mimetic [19] and structure-based techniques, have been studied concerning the design and development of successful inhibitors. Saquinavir is the first of these to become an approved drug against AIDS, and there are other similar agents as well. The concept arose from the nonselective nature of mammalian protease toward Phe-Pro substrate, which undergoes cleavage by HIV-1 PR [20]. The design of saquinavir followed the inhibition of HIV-1 PR by the peptide agent Ro 31-8558. Following suitable structure-based optimization operations, this compound was modified into saquinavir (initially identified as Ro 31-8959), a derivative of a pentapeptide

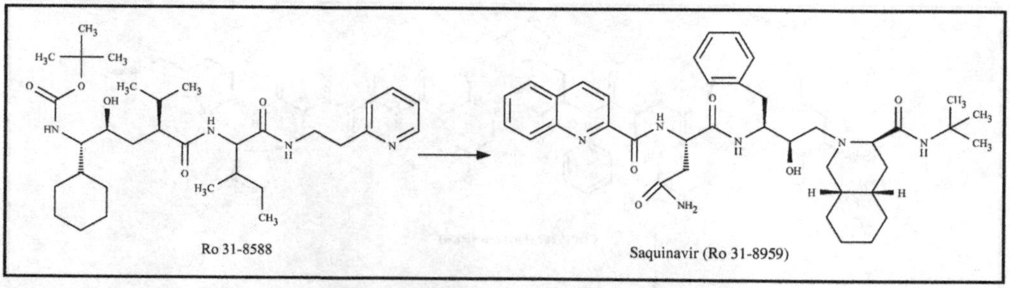

Figure 11.4 The design and development of the saquinavir molecule.

characterized by noncleavable hydroxylethylamine transition state moiety and the bulky (*S,S,S*)-decahydro-isoquinolin-3-carbonyl (DIQ) group. Saquinavir antagonizes the replication of both HIV-1 and HIV-2 virus particles. Figure 11.4 shows the chemical structures of saquinavir with Ro 31-8558.

e. Approval status: Approved by the FDA in 1995.

Example 6

a. Name of the drug: Aliskiren

b. Disease indication: Used for the treatment of hypertension.

c. Mechanism: Antagonism of the action of rennin, thereby inhibiting the pressor action of the rennin–angiotensin system (RAS).

d. Brief developmental history: The RAS system controls blood pressure and body fluid volume. Renin leads to the formation of angiotensin I by peptidic cleavage of angiotensinogen, followed by the action of ACE to give angiotensin II from angiotensin I. Because of the availability of the X-ray crystallographic structure of rennin, a good number of studies involving various *in silico* techniques have been employed toward the design of its potential inhibitors. The compounds developed at the beginning were preferentially peptides. The compound CGP29287 denotes one of the earliest developments in this paradigm employing the "transition state theory," [21] and its chemical structure is related to renin. Then, the next-generation peptidic compound inhibiting the activity of renin was CGP38560, which could not proceed further owing to low oral absorption followed by rapid excretion using the biliary system [22]. After encountering further failures with the peptide analogs, the design paradigm turned into nonpeptidic agents by the use of suitable molecular modeling analyses. Another second-generation lead compound could be identified (Figure 11.5), the structure of which was modified further by the incorporation of methoxy and alkylether substituents on the aromatic ring in place of *tertiary* butyl and methyl acetoxy groups. X-ray crystallographic analysis of this molecule showed a previously undiscovered binding subpocket that previously had not been used by the peptide analogs. Optimization of hydrophobic interaction at this binding subpocket led to the development of Aliskiren. Structure-based drug design analysis depicted that the methoxypropoxy side chain was optimal in terms of length, providing suitable H-bonding interaction with Tyr^{14} in the subpocket [23], while the presence of terminal carboxamide group provided additional H-bonding interaction with Arg^{74} and the geminal methyl groups allowed van der Waals interactions with renin.

e. Approval status: Approved by the FDA in 2007.

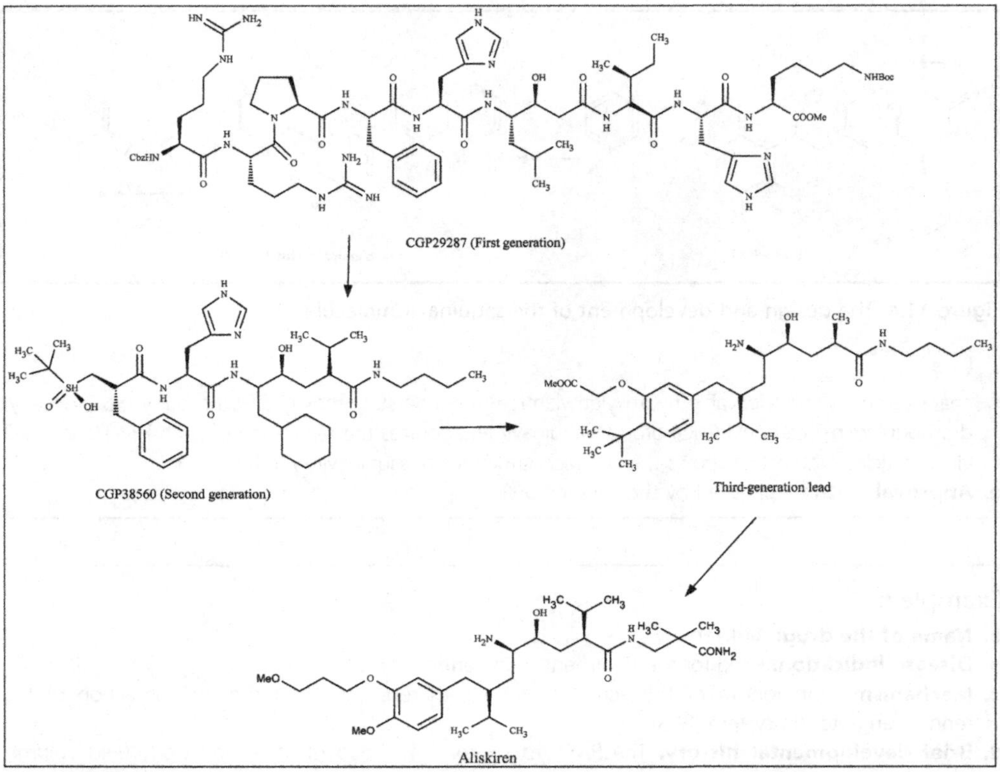

Figure 11.5 The design and development of the aliskiren molecule.

Example 7

a. Name of the drug: Boceprevir

b. Disease indication: Used for the treatment of hepatitis C.

c. Mechanism: Inhibition of NS3-NS4A serine protease in hepatitis C virus (HCV), leading to the prevention of the replication of virus particles.

d. Brief developmental history: The initial attempts of high-throughput screening (HTS) analysis toward the development of successful inhibitors of HCV failed, which led to a structure-based design approach for potential molecules. Initial observations showed that the inhibition of NS3-NS4A protease is facilitated by compounds that release N-terminal peptides. Later, in a study involving serine protease inhibitors, Ser^{139} in the viral protease was observed to be a target for electrophilic reaction with groups like aldehyde and ketones. [24,25]. A series of α-ketoamide inhibitors were designed at the Schering-Plough Research Institute, and these were derivatives of amino acid residues spanning from P6 to P5′ [26]. In Figure 11.6, an early lead has been presented (compound A), which was later optimized to give compound B. Further SAR exploration at the P1, P2, and P3 capping positions of compound B gave rise to boceprevir, in which cyclobutylalanine at P1 position, dimethylcyclopropylproline moiety at the P2 position, and urea type moiety at P3 positions were observed to be optimal [26,27].

e. Approval status: Approved by the FDA in 2011.

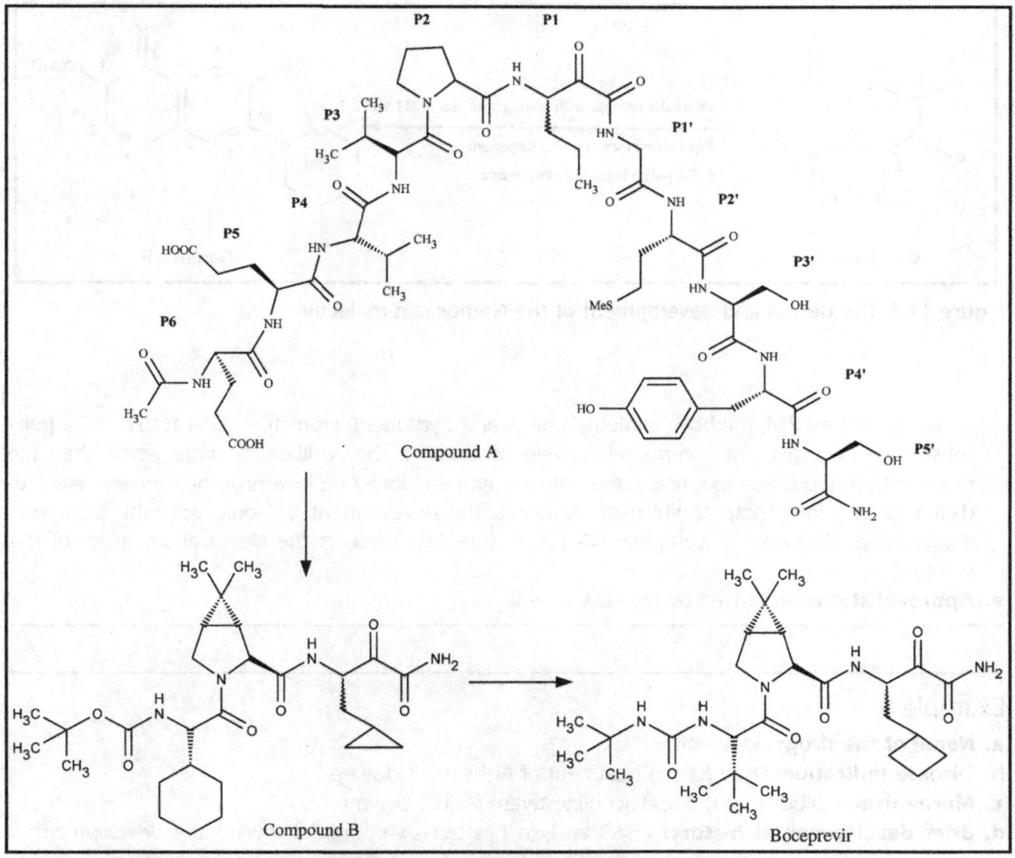

Figure 11.6 The design and development of the boceprevir molecule.

Example 8

a. Name of the drug: Norfloxacin

b. Disease indication: Used for the treatment of bacterial infection.

c. Mechanism: Inhibition of the bacterial DNA gyrase enzyme.

d. Brief developmental history: The study for the development of more potent fluoroquinolone compounds started after nalidixic acid was observed to be active against gram-negative bacteria in the early 1960s. The development was principally achieved using the 2D-QSAR technique employing the famous Hansch equation. A QSAR study on the antibacterial activity of 6-, 7-, or 8-monosubstituted 1-ethyl-1,4-dihydro-4-oxo-quinoline-3-carboxylic acid derivatives (compound A) showed a parabolic correlation between the activity and steric parameters (STERIMOL) for the substituents at positions R_1 and R_3 (compound A). Even though no such correlating relationship between the physicochemical constants values for R_2 substituent with activity was found, the piperazinyl group at this position was observed to be the most promising one among other groups (*viz.*, nitro,

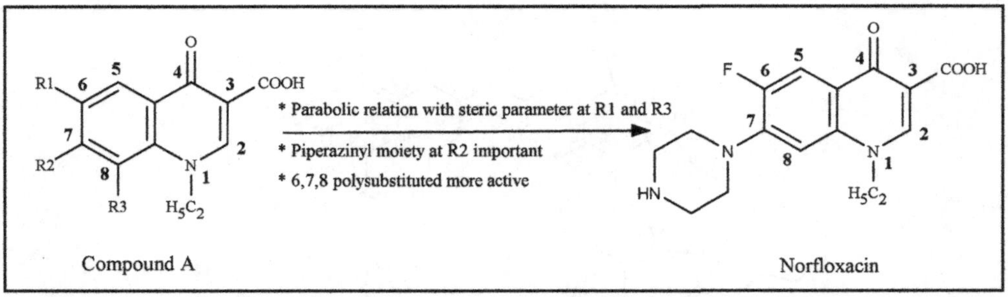

Figure 11.7 The design and development of the Norfloxacin molecule.

acetyl, chloro, methyl, methoxy, dimethylamino, and hydrogen). From the QSAR results, 6,7,8-polysubstituted derivatives of compound A were observed to be additionally more active than the mono-substituted ones. Specifically, the 6-fluoro- and 6-chloro-7-(l-piperazinyl) derivatives were predicted to be highly potent, which finally led to the development of norfloxacin, the 6-fluoro-7-(l-piperazinyl) derivative of compound A [28]. Figure 11.7 presents the chemical structures of this substance.

e. Approval status: Approved by the FDA in 1986.

Example 9

a. Name of the drug: Donepezil

b. Disease indication: Used for the treatment of Alzheimer's disease.

c. Mechanism: Inhibition of the acetylcholinesterase (AChE) enzyme.

d. Brief developmental history: QSAR analysis has been very fruitful toward the development of donepezil [29] from the rational exploration of a series of indanone and benzylpiperidine ring substructures possessing AChE inhibitory activity. At first, the benzylpiperazine analog compound A was obtained as an inhibitor of AChE enzyme following a random screening operation. A second screening was made employing a library of similar chemical structures that identified another chemical that consists of the benzylpiperazine system with a benzamide connector (compound B). During lead optimization, a methyl substitution on the amide nitrogen was observed to be a requirement. Conformational analysis was performed on the *N*-alkyl benzamide analogs considering the potential of the methyl group in amide nitrogen in changing the *cis* and *trans* isomer ratio. Different molecular modeling techniques, including molecular shape comparison, QSAR, and X-ray diffraction analysis, were employed for the enhancement of the lead structure, and the resulting observations depicted that the *cis*-conformation of benzamide was the active form, the activity increased with the presence of bulky substituent at the *para* position of the benzamide, and amide carbonyl oxygen took part in intermolecular hydrogen bond formation. The structural knowledge aided in the development of the molecule donepezil [29,30], which is used as a hydrochloride salt. The chemical structures of the mentioned compounds are demonstrated in Figure 11.8.

e. Approval status: Approved by the FDA in 1996.

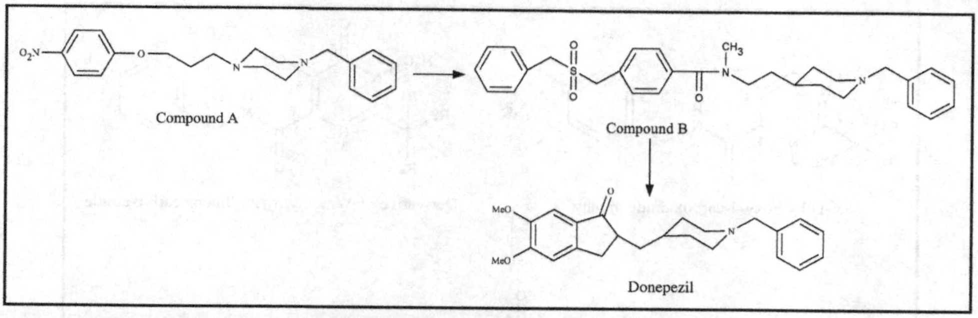

Figure 11.8 The design and development of the Donepezil molecule.

Example 10

a. Name of the drug: Raltegravir

b. Disease indication: Used for the treatment of AIDS.

c. Mechanism: Inhibition of HIV-1 integrase enzyme, thereby interfering with the incorporation of viral DNA into the cellular genome.

d. Brief developmental history: HIV-1 integrase presents an attractive target to combat the virus particles, and it is the first FDA-approved inhibitor of HIV-1 integrase. In addition, 4-aryl-2,4-diketobutanoic acids are recognized as the first class of chemicals with activity against HIV-1 integrase. The binding site of HIV-1 integrase was in the process of exploration using the molecular dynamics trajectory [31]. The AutoDock program, along with the relaxed complex method, was employed for the identification of novel binding modes. The derived information was utilized later, which gave the molecule known as *Raltegravir*. Two classes of chemicals (namely 5,6-dihydroxypyrimidine-4-carboxamides and *N*-methyl-4-hydroxy-pyrimidinone-carboxamides) showing inhibitory potential to HIV-integrase-catalyzed transfer of DNA were the initial molecules. Through a series of structural changes and optimization, raltegravir became prominent [32]. The chemical structures of the mentioned compounds can be seen in Figure 11.9.

e. Approval status: Approved by the FDA in 2007.

Example 11

a. Name of the drug: Tirofiban

b. Disease indication: Used for the treatment of platelet aggregation; that is, formation of the thrombus.

c. Mechanism: Antagonism of the fibrinogen receptor by the prevention of its binding to the GP IIb/IIIa glycoprotein complex.

d. Brief developmental history: It may be interesting to note that arginyl-glycyl-aspartyl (RGD), a tripeptide sequence is considered as the basic required sequence for the binding of fibrinogen to GP IIb/IIIa [33]. Tirofiban presents a nonpeptide inhibitor of fibrinogen by imitating the Arg-Gly-Asp sequence of active peptides. The search for synthetically designed molecule started with compound A bearing comparable potency to Arg-Gly-Asp-Ser through the optimization of N-terminus attributes. By comparing a series of derivatives, several structural modifications were made toward the achievement of a potent molecule, which includes change of secondary hydroxyl group and variation of

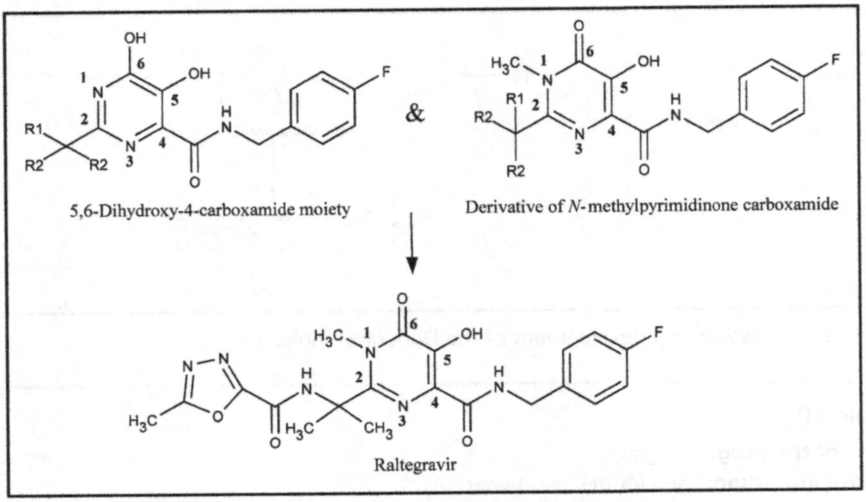

Figure 11.9 **The design and development of the raltegravir molecule.**

the chain-length of the CH_2 group. A seven-methylene linkage was observed to exert potent activity (compound B) by providing a great distance between the tyrosine moiety and the basic center. In order to account for the conformational restriction of the amino terminal chain, compound C was formed containing a piperidine ring at the end, and this molecule showed a significant activity profile. Structural optimizations were also performed in the C-terminal (including removal of the carbobenzyloxy group, elimination of polar α-amino substituent, and replacement of the carbamate oxygen with methylene group), and finally, the presence of a benzylsulfonyl group provided enhanced activity. The C-terminal of compound C was subjected to optimization by introducing a hexanoyl group giving compound D, which was further modified using a benzylsulfonyl replacement, and finally, the use of *n*-butylsulfonyl group resulted in tirofiban. Molecular modeling analysis depicts that the nitrogen atom of piperidine ring imitates the action of basic guanidino moiety of Arg, while the tyrosine carboxyl group functions as a surrogate to the carboxyl group of aspartic acid. The mechanism of tirofiban was termed as an "exosite" inhibitory action since molecular modeling showed that the (*S*)-$NHSO_2$*n*-C_4H_9 group takes part in a favorable noncovalent interaction with GP IIb/IIIa at a site different from that of Arg-Gly-Asp-based antagonists [34]. The chemical structures are presented in Figure 11.10.

e. Approval status: Approved by the FDA in 2000.

11.2.2 Examples of other approved chemicals

Example 1

a. Name of the chemical: Ipconazole

b. Type of application: As a potential fungicide in the field of agriculture.

c. Mechanism: The inhibition of C-14 demethylation during the biosynthesis of ergosterol.

d. Brief developmental history: Different types of azoles have been exploited as fungicides in agrochemistry since the 1960s. An initial *trans* geometry among the azole substituents was identified.

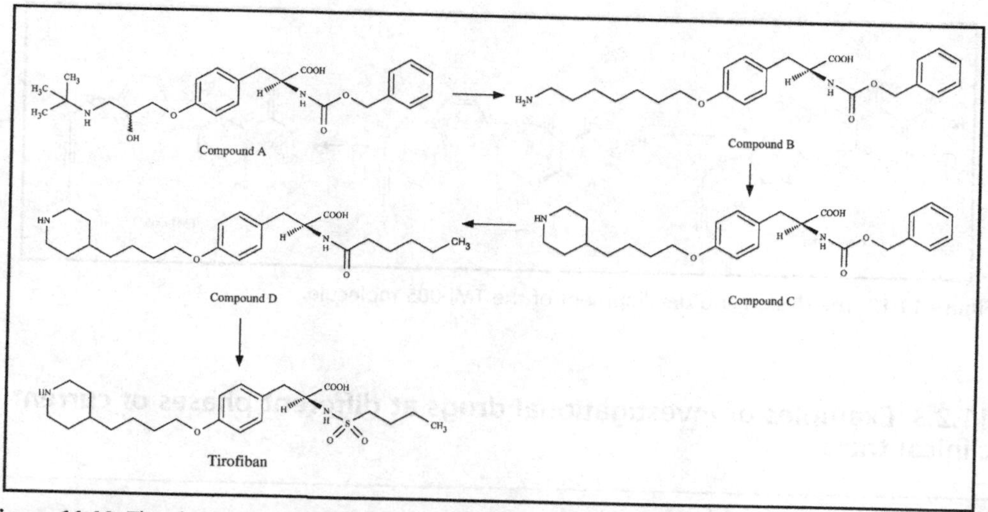

Figure 11.10 The design and development of the tirofiban molecule.

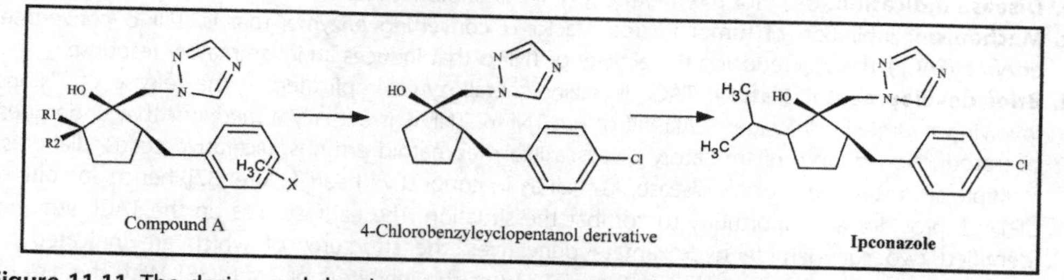

Figure 11.11 The design and development of the ipconazole molecule.

Considering Compound A as the basic skeleton, a series of derivatives were formed by varying substituents at 'X' while keeping $R_1 = R_2 = H$, and linear QSAR equations were developed using 16–18 compounds with the inhibition data of *Botrytis cinerea* and *Gibberella fujikuroi*. The obtained result containing hydrophobic and steric characteristics involving partition coefficient measure (logP) and STERIMOL parameters were exploited for the development of the next potential compound, 4-Cl-benzylcyclopentanol [35]. Further optimizations were implemented considering the steric and hydrophobicity measures, followed by a 3D structural comparison accounting for molecular conformational freedom and semiempirical analysis involving the MNDO formalism. Based on the derived information, another set of molecules were synthesized, tested, and subjected to predictive QSAR model development, from which a member was chosen that showed potent activity against rice diseases, known as *Ipconazole*. The commercial product consists of an equipotent mixture of ipconazole racemic isomers [35,36]. The chemical structures of the compounds are presented in Figure 11.11.

e. Status: First introduced in Japan. It was registered on the pesticide list of the US Environmental Protection Agency (EPA) in 1993 for the treatment of seed on various crops, turf grass, ornamental flowers, and conifers.

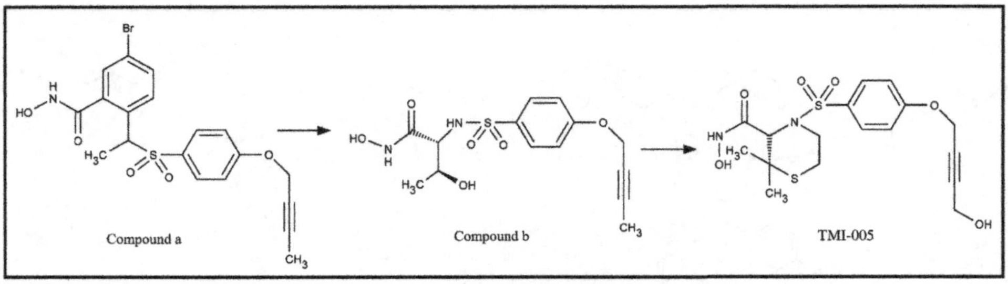

Figure 11.12 The design and development of the TMI-005 molecule.

11.2.3 Examples of investigational drugs at different phases of current clinical trials

Example 1

a. **Name of the drug:** TMI-005
b. **Disease indication:** Used for the treatment of rheumatoid arthritis.
c. **Mechanism:** Inhibition of tumor necrosis factor-α converting enzyme; that is, TNF-α convertase enzyme (TACE), thereby reducing the activity of TNF-α that induces an inflammatory response.
d. **Brief developmental history:** TACE is a zinc metallozyme implicated in the release of TNF-α, involving hydrolytic cleavage of Ala-Val of pro-TNF-α. TNF-α is actually a mediator that undergoes overproduction during inflammatory diseases like rheumatoid arthritis, ulcerative colitis, diabetes, multiple sclerosis, and Crohn's disease, as well as in congestive heart failure [37]; hence, inhibition of TACE provides an opportunity to combat the situation. The early studies on the TACE enzyme identified two sulfonamide hydroxamate derivatives, the structures of which are indicated as "Compound a" and "Compound b" in Figure 11.12 as the inhibitors of TACE [38]. With the aim of enhancing the binding efficacy of the compounds, a library of phenoxyacetylene hydroxamate derivatives was generated employing the solid phase combinatorial synthetic method, followed by optimization of SAR and pharmacokinetic criteria that led to the design of a propargylic hydroxyl-hydroxamic acid compound known as *TMI-005* [39]. The chemical structure of TMI-005 is shown in Figure 11.12.
e. **Clinical trial status:** Phase II clinical trial completed.

Example 2

a. **Name of the drug:** Nolatrexed
b. **Disease indication:** Used for the treatment of unresectable hepatocellular carcinoma (HCC).
c. **Mechanism:** Antagonism of the action of the thymidylate synthase (TS) enzyme, leading to the prevention of the conversion of deoxyuridine monophosphate (dUMP) to deoxythymidylate monophosphate (dTMP).

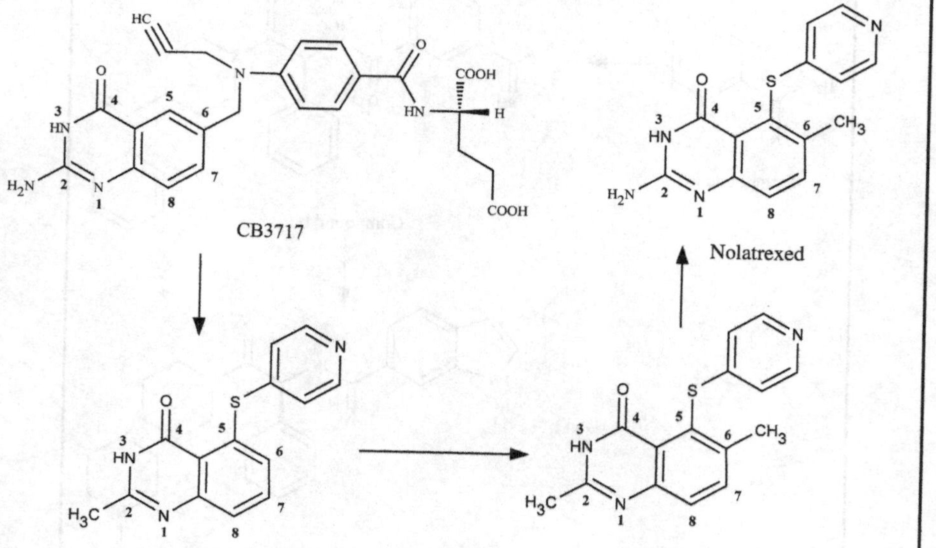

Figure 11.13 The design and development of the Nolatrexed molecule.

d. Brief developmental history: Inhibition of the TS enzyme has emerged as an attractive target for the design of anticancer drugs. Studies involving different structure-based molecular modeling methods and X-ray crystal structure data on TS have led to the design of a potent quinazoline derivative CB3717 [40]. The study employing CB3717 was carried out using TS of *Escherichia coli*, which is highly homologous to human TS [41]. Hence, during further modification of this compound, some basic features were kept constant, such as the 4-ketoquinazoline ring accounting for hydrogen bonding and π–π stacking interaction. Changes were made in the 2, 5, and 6 positions of the ring. The initial modifications include substitution of amino with methyl at position 2 and bringing the *para*-aminobenzoyl moiety to the 5 position with a one-atom linkage, allowing similar interaction with a hydrophobic cavity in the receptor [42]. The next potential molecule observed was a pyridine substituent with better potency (compound b), which was further optimized to compound c with an addition of a methyl group at position 6 that allows hydrophobic interaction with Trp^{80} of TS [42]. Compound c showed an improved docking result, and finally, an amino group was introduced at position 2 that showed better hydrogen bonding interaction with Ala^{263} of TS. The final compound, Nolatrexed, elicited very high inhibitory potential. Figure 11.13 presents the structures of all the compounds mentioned with respect to this series.

e. Clinical trial status: Phase III clinical trial completed.

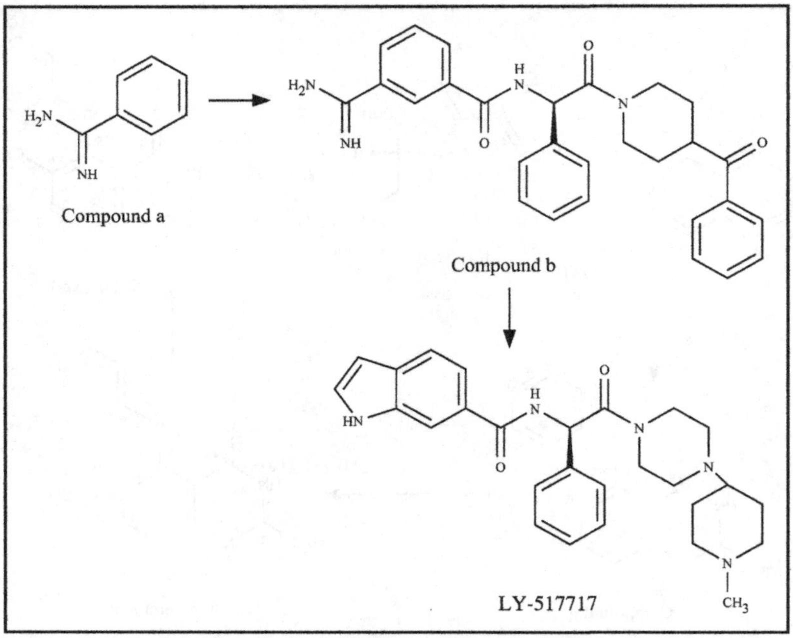

Figure 11.14 The design and development of the LY-517717 molecule.

Example 3

a. Name of the drug: LY-517717

b. Disease indication: Used for the treatment of venous thromboembolism after hip or knee replacement.

c. Mechanism: Inhibition of factor Xa serine protease enzyme, thereby preventing the formation of thrombus.

d. Brief developmental history: A structure-based virtual screening coupled with library design strategy was adopted for the development of factor Xa serine protease inhibitors [43]. The study started using benzamidine fragment (compound a), which followed to the amidine derivative (compound b) through an iterative library design. However, because of the oral bioavailability issue, the benzamidine moiety was replaced with an uncharged indole that allows favorable interaction with aspartate residue, leading to the development of LY-517717. Hence, the final compound was characterized by both anti-thrombotic activity and enhanced oral pharmacokinetic property [44]. The chemical structures are presented in Figure 11.14.

e. Clinical trial status: Phase II clinical trial completed.

Example 4

a. Name of the drug: NVP-AUY922

b. Disease indication: Used for the treatment of cancer.

c. Mechanism: Inhibition of heat shock protein 90 (HSP90), causing interference with the client protein implicated in the progression of tumors.

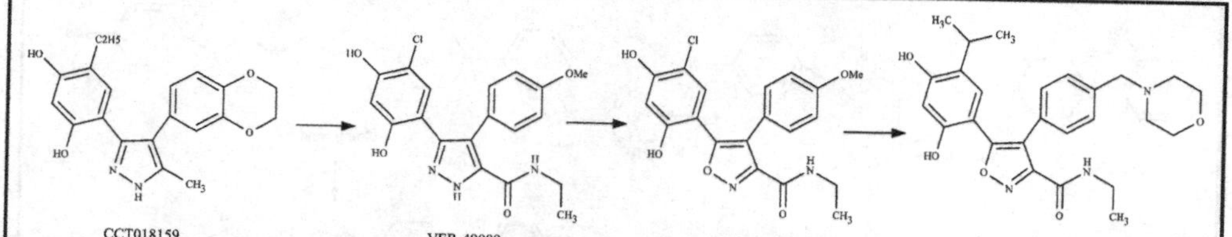

Figure 11.15 The design and development of the NVP-AUY922 molecule.

d. Brief developmental history: HSP90 presents a good target for study because of its high-resolution crystal structure. A pyrazole resorcinol compound CCT018159 was developed using a high-throughput screening (HTS) technique [45], followed by the use of iterative structure-based design formalism for optimization. Structural modifications were made according to the need at the binding site of HSP90, which includes the addition of an amide group, addition of different substituents, and replacement of pyrazole moiety with isoxazole. The next series of compounds includes VER-49009 [46], VER-50589 [47], and finally, NVP-AUY922. Figure 11.15 shows the chemical structures of these compounds.

e. Clinical trial status: Phase I clinical trial completed.

Example 5

a. Name of the drug: PRX-00023

b. Disease indication: Used for the treatment of depression, anxiety, and attention deficit hyperactivity disorder (ADHD).

c. Mechanism: Potentiation of the activity of the 5-HT_{1A} receptor.

d. Brief developmental history: PRX-00023 was developed as a selective amidosulfonamide nonazapirone agonist of the 5-HT_{1A} receptor. Considering the information gap while studying structure-based drug discovery involving G-protein-coupled receptor (GPCR), a nonhomology method called *PREDICT* [48] was used for modeling the 3D structure of the 5-HT_{1A} receptor. Following the validation of the target, virtual screening methodology was employed on Predix's compound library involving the docking and scoring of 40,000 compounds, giving 78 virtual hits that were subjected to experimental testing. The lead compound obtained was compound a, an arylpiperazinylsulfonamide derivative showing appreciable binding affinity to the 5-HT_{1A} receptor. Compound a was subjected to various structure-based *in silico* lead optimization formalisms for enhancing the selectivity over the α_1-adrenergic candidates by introducing alkylamino, arylamino, alkylsulfonylamino, acylamino groups, and the conformationally constrained analog compound b was obtained. However, owing to the *hERG* K^+ channel blockage action of compound b, it was modified by introducing nonaromatic hydrophobic group in place of the existing aromatic *p*-toluene substituent to avoid interaction with the Tyr^{562} amino acid of hERG. A series of molecules were obtained by the incorporation of various alkyl substituents from which one compound with a cyclohexylmethyl group showed desired conformational stability along with improved 5-HT_{1A} agonistic action with minimal effect on the hERG K^+ channel. This molecule was presented as PRX-00023 (Figure 11.16).

e. Clinical trial status: Phase III clinical trial completed.

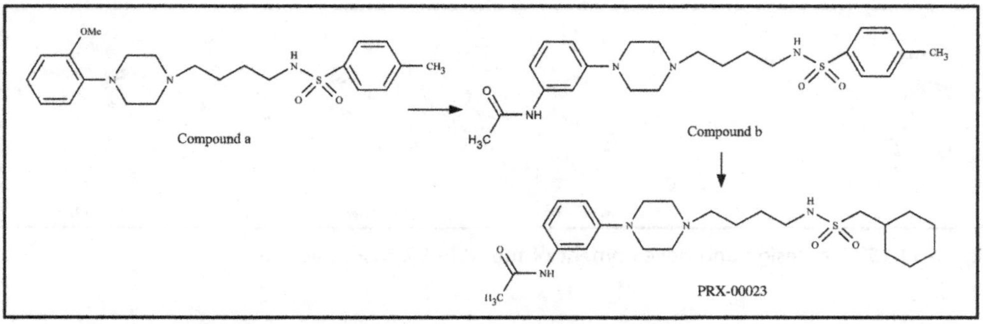

Figure 11.16 The design and development of the PRX-00023 molecule.

11.3 CONCLUSION

Innovation is the backbone and strength of any process. Molecular modeling techniques are useful to rationalize the design and discovery paradigm of chemicals. They aid these processes by providing a suitable alternative means, and they enable success at a shorter time span with limited financial investment while still maintaining the quality of the product. The economic investment of pharmaceutical companies for the research and development (R&D) is very significant, especially in accordance with the generation of revenue. The global revenues for pharmaceutical products in the United States and Europe were $856 billion, accounting for 60% of sales (approximately) in 2010. The developmental cost of pharmaceuticals has risen to $1.2 billion in the early 2000s from $140 million in the 1970s. The investment in R&D is estimated to be about $51.1 billion in 2013, compared to $2 billion in 1980 [49]. The quality of a research protocol is maximized when the possible failure routes are taken care of. QSAR, along with other molecular modeling techniques, provide a rational optimization strategy to the developers that can be extremely fruitful if implemented properly. One more point to be noted is that readers should not think that molecular modeling techniques are applicable to synthetic drugs only; it has good applications in the design of drug molecules from natural sources as well. QSAR and other *in silico* techniques are not meant to replace the experimental techniques, but they present a set of principles that can be used to explore the knowledge of innovation in the discovery of drugs and other chemicals cogently and efficiently.

REFERENCES

[1] Talele TT, Khedkar SA, Rigby AC. Successful applications of computer aided drug discovery: moving drugs from concept to the clinic. Curr Top Med Chem 2010;10:127–41.

[2] Ooms F. Molecular modeling and computer aided drug design. examples of their applications in medicinal chemistry. Curr Med Chem 2000;7:141–58.

[3] Kubinyi H. Success stories of computer-aided design. In: Ekins S, editor. Computer applications in pharmaceutical research and development. USA: John Wiley & Sons Inc.; 2006. pp. 377–424.
[4] Fujita T. Recent success stories leading to commercializable bioactive compounds with the aid of traditional QSAR procedures. Quant Struct-Act Relat 1997;16:107–12.
[5] ClinicalTrials.gov is a Web-based resource maintained by the National Library of Medicine (NLM) at the National Institutes of Health (NIH) and provides easy access to information on publicly and privately supported clinical studies on a wide range of diseases and conditions. 2014. Accessible at <http://clinicaltrials.gov/>. (Nov 8, 2014).
[6] Orange book: approved drug products with therapeutic equivalence evaluations. U.S. Department of Health and Human Services, Food and Drug Administration. 2014. Accessible at <http://www.accessdata.fda.gov/scripts/cder/ob/default.cfm>. (Nov 8, 2014).
[7] Pesticides. Chemical search: conventional, antimicrobial and biopesticide active ingredients. Accessible at <http://iaspub.epa.gov/apex/pesticides/f?p = chemicalsearch:1>. (Nov 8, 2014).
[8] Cushman DW, Cheung HS, Sbo EF, Ondetti MA. Design of potent competitive inhibitors of angiotensin converting enzyme. Carboxyalkanoyl and mercaptoalkanoyl amino acids. Biochemistry 1977;16:5484–91.
[9] Byers LD, Wolfenden R. Binding of the by-product analog benzylsuccinic acid by carboxypeptidase A. Biochemistry 1973;12:2070–8.
[10] Ferreira SH, Bartelt DC, Greene LJ. Isolation of bradykinin-potentiating peptides from *Bothrops jararaca* venom. Biochemistry 1970;9:2583–93.
[11] Erikeson AE, Jones TA, Liljas A. Refined structure of human carbonic anhydrase II at 2.0 Å resolution. Proteins 1988;4:274–82.
[12] Baldwin JJ, Ponticello GS, Anderson PS, Christy ME, Murcko MA, Randall WC, et al. Thienothiopyran-2-sulfonamides: novel topically active carbonic anhydrase inhibitors for the treatment of glaucoma. J Med Chem 1989;32:2510–13.
[13] Seto JT, Rott R. Functional significance of sialidase during influenza virus multiplication. Virology 1966;30:731–7.
[14] Moscona A. Neuraminidase inhibitors for influenza. N Engl J Med 2005;353:1363–73.
[15] von Itzstein M, Wu W-Y, Kok GB, Pegg MS, Dyason JC, Jin B, et al. Rational design of potent sialidase-based inhibitors of influenza virus replication. Nature 1993;363:418–23.
[16] Bossart-Whitaker P, Carson M, Babu YS, Smith CD, Laver WG, Air GM. Three-dimensional structure of influenza A N9 neuraminidase and its complex with the inhibitor 2-deoxy 2,3-dehydro-*N*-acetyl neuraminic acid. J Mol Biol 1993;232:1069–83.
[17] Kim CU, Lew W, Williams MA, Liu H, Zhang L, Swaminathan S, et al. Influenza neuraminidase inhibitors possessing a novel hydrophobic interaction in the enzyme active site: design, synthesis, and structural analysis of carbocyclic sialic acid analogues with potent anti-influenza activity. J Am Chem Soc 1997;119:681–90.
[18] Kohl NE, Emini EA, Schleif WA, Davis LJ, Heimbach JC, Dixon RA, et al. Active human immunodeficiency virus protease is required for viral infectivity. Proc Natl Acad Sci USA 1988;85: 4686–90.
[19] McQuade TJ, Tomasselli AG, Liu L, Karacostas B, Moss B, Sawyer TK, et al. A synthetic HIV protease inhibitor with antiviral activity arrests HIV-like particle maturation. Science 1990;247:454–6.
[20] Roberts NA. Rational design of peptide-based HIV proteinase inhibitors. Science 1990;248: 358–61.
[21] Wolfenden R. Analog approaches to the structure of the transition state in enzyme reactions. Acc Chem Res 1972;5:10–18.
[22] Rahuel J, Priestle JP, Grutter MG. The crystal structures of recombinant glycosylated human renin alone and in complex with a transition state analog inhibitor. J Struct Biol 1991;107:227–36.
[23] Wood JM, Maibaum J, Rahuel J, Grutter MG, Cohen NC, Rasetti V, et al. Structure-based design of Aliskiren, a novel orally effective renin inhibitor. Biochem Biophys Res Commun 2003;308: 698–705.
[24] Turk B. Targeting proteases: successes, failures and future prospects. Nat Rev Drug Discov 2006;5: 785–99.

[25] Yan Y, Li Y, Munshi S, Sardana V, Cole JL, Sardana M, et al. Complex of NS3 protease and NS4A peptide of BK strain hepatitis C virus: A 2.2 Å resolution structure in a hexagonal crystal form. Protein Sci 1998;7:837−47.

[26] Malcolm BA, Liu R, Lahser F, Agrawal S, Belanger B, Butkiewicz N, et al. SCH 503034, a mechanism based inhibitor of hepatitis C virus NS3 protease, suppresses polyprotein maturation and enhances the antiviral activity of alpha interferon in replicon cells. Antimicrob Agents Chemother 2006;50:1013−20.

[27] Njoroge FG, Chen KX, Shih N-Y, Piwinski JP. Challenges in modern drug discovery: a case study of boceprevir, an HCV protease inhibitor for the treatment of hepatitis C virus infection. Acc Chem Res 2008;41:50−9.

[28] Koga H, Itoh A, Murayama S, Suzue S, Irikura T. Structure−activity relationships of antibacterial 6,7- and 7,8-disubstituted 1-a1kyl-1,4-dihydro-4-oxoquinoline-3-carboxylic acids. J Med Chem 1980;23:1358−63.

[29] Cardozo MG, Kawai T, Iimura Y, Sugimoto H, Yamanishi Y, Hopfinger AJ. Conformational analyses and molecular-shape comparisons of a series of indanone-benzylpiperidine inhibitors of acetylcholinesterase. J Med Chem 1992;35:590−601.

[30] Cardozo MG, Iimura Y, Sugimoto H, Yamanishi Y, Hopfinger AJ. Quantitative structure−activity relationship. QSAR, analyses of the substituted indanone and benzylpiperidine rings of a series of indanone-benzylpiperidine inhibitors of acetylcholinesterase. J Med Chem 1992;35:584−9.

[31] Schames JR, Henchman RH, Siegel JS, Sotriffer CA, Ni H, McCammon JA. Discovery of a novel binding trench in HIV integrase. J Med Chem 2004;47:1879−81.

[32] Summa V, Petrocchi A, Bonelli F, Crescenzi B, Donghi M, Ferrara M, et al. Discovery of raltegravir, a potent, selective orally bioavailable HIV-integrase inhibitor for the treatment of HIV-AIDS infection. J Med Chem 2008;51:5843−55.

[33] Phillips DR, Charo IF, Parise LV, Fitzgerald LA. The platelet membrane glycoprotein IIb−IIIa complex. Blood 1988;71:831−43.

[34] Hartman GD, Egbertson MS, Halczenko W, Laswell WL, Duggan ME, Smith RL, et al. Non-peptide fibrinogen receptor antagonists. 1. Discovery and design of exosite inhibitors. J Med Chem 1992;35:4640−2.

[35] Chuman H, Ito A, Saishoji T, Kumazawa S. ACS Symp Ser No 606. In: Hansch C, Fujita T, editors. Classical and three-dimensional QSAR in agrochemistry. Washington, DC: American Chemical Society; 1995. p. 171.

[36] Kumazawa S, Ito A, Saishoji T, Chuman H. Jan Chem Program Exch Newslett 1995;6:3.

[37] Vassalli P. The pathophysiology of tumor necrosis factors. Ann Rev Immunol 1992;10:411−52.

[38] Maskos K, Fernandez-Catalan C, Huber R, Bourenkov GP, Bartunik H, Ellestad GA, et al. Crystal structure of the catalytic domain of human tumor necrosis factor-R converting enzyme. Proc Natl Acad Sci USA 1998;95:3408−12.

[39] Levin JI, Chen JM, Cheung K, Cole D, Crago C, Delos Santos E, et al. Acetylenic TACE inhibitors. Part 1. SAR of the acyclic sulfonamide hydroxamates. Bioorg Med Chem Lett 2003; 13:2798−803.

[40] Jones TR, Calvert AH, Jackman AL, Brown SJ, Jones M, Harrap KR. A potent antitumor quinazoline inhibitor of thymidylate synthetase: synthesis, biological properties and therapeutic results in mice. Eur J Cancer 1981;17:11−19.

[41] Matthews DA, Appelt K, Oatley SJ, Xuong NH. Crystal structure of *Escherichia coli* thymidylate synthase containing bound 5-fluoro-2′-deoxyuridylate and 10-propargyl-5,8-dideazafolate. J Mol Biol 1990;214:923−36.

[42] Webber SE, Bleckman TM, Attard J, Deal JG, Kathardekar V, Welsh KM, et al. Design of thymidylate synthase inhibitors using protein crystal structures: the synthesis and biological evaluation of a novel class of 5-substituted quinazolinones. J Med Chem 1993;36:733−46.

[43] Liebeschuetz JW, Jones SD, Morgan PJ, Murray CW, Rimmer AD, Roscoe JM, et al. PRO_SELECT: combining structure-based drug design and array-based chemistry for rapid lead discovery. 2. The development of a series of highly potent and selective factor Xa inhibitors. J Med Chem 2002;45:1221−32.

[44] Jones SD, Liebeschuetz JW, Morgan PJ, Murray CW, Rimmer AD, Roscoe JM, et al. The design of phenylglycine containing benzamidine carboxamides as potent and selective inhibitors of factor Xa. Bioorg Med Chem Lett 2001;11:733–6.
[45] Cheung KM, Matthews TP, James K, Rowlands MG, Boxall KJ, Sharp SY, et al. The identification, synthesis, protein crystal structure and in vitro biochemical evaluation of a new 3,4-diarylpyrazole class of Hsp90 inhibitors. Bioorg Med Chem Lett 2005;15:3338–43.
[46] Dymock BW, Barril X, Brough PA, Cansfield JE, Massey A, McDonald E, et al. Novel, potent small-molecule inhibitors of the molecular chaperone Hsp90 discovered through structure-based design. J Med Chem 2005;48:4212–15.
[47] Sharp SY, Prodromou C, Boxall K, Powers MV, Holmes JL, Box G, et al. Inhibition of the heat shock protein 90 molecular chaperone *in vitro* and *in vivo* by novel, synthetic, potent resorcinylic pyrazole/isoxazole amide analogues. Mol Cancer Ther 2007;6:1198–211.
[48] Becker OM, Dhanoa DS, Marantz Y, Chen D, Shacham S, Cheruku S, et al. An integrated *in silico* 3D model-driven discovery of a novel, potent, and selective amidosulfonamide 5-HT1A agonist (PRX-00023) for the treatment of anxiety and depression. J Med Chem 2006;49:3116–35.
[49] Pharmaceutical Research and Manufacturers of America (PhRMA). 2014 Profile, Washington, DC. 2014, Accessible at <http://www.phrma.org/sites/default/files/pdf/2014_PhRMA_PROFILE.pdf>. (Nov 8, 2014).

CHAPTER 12

Future Avenues

Contents

12.1 INTRODUCTION

The quantitative structure–activity relationship (QSAR) is originally a ligand-based statistical approach. However, in combination with receptor-based approaches, it has demonstrated useful applications and has had success for the optimization of ligands in the context of drug discovery. It has also been used for pharmacokinetic data modeling of drug substances, which is very useful in the early phases of drug discovery. In view of the Registration, Evaluation, and Authorization of Chemicals (REACH) regulations in the European Union (EU) and increasingly strict rules for use of animals in toxicity studies, QSAR has emerged as an alternative method for risk assessment of chemicals in the context of environmental safety. QSAR has also helped in developing pesticides and insecticides for possible use in agriculture. Apart from these commonly known applications, QSAR has also been used to model and design chemicals with special uses (such as antioxidants [1,2], odorants [3,4], sweetening agents [5,6]). In this chapter, we will list some areas that will find potential applications of QSAR in the coming days. Although some studies in these areas have already been done, it is anticipated that more extensive applications will be observed in the near future [7]. Also note that this is not an exhaustive list; applications of QSAR may be seen in other related areas based on intuitive experimental design and requirements of the particular research fields.

Understanding the Basics of QSAR for Applications in Pharmaceutical Sciences and Risk Assessment.
ISBN: 978-0-12-801505-6, DOI: http://dx.doi.org/10.1016/B978-0-12-801505-6.00012-0

12.2 APPLICATION AREAS

12.2.1 QSAR of mixture toxicity

In the environment, chemicals remain in a mixture form, whereas in traditional QSAR, models are developed usually for isolated compounds. Chemicals in a mixture form may behave in a different way due to the interactions with and effects of other chemicals. The lack of reliable data poses one of the biggest challenges for the development of QSARs for toxicity of chemical mixtures. In addition, proper external validation is less straightforward for QSAR models of mixtures because the same compounds with different ratios may be present in the data set. The QSAR modeling of mixtures requires the use of appropriate descriptors. Some of the approaches already applied [7] include descriptors based on the mixture partition coefficient [8], additive molecular descriptors [9], integral nonadditive descriptors of mixtures [10], and fragment nonadditive descriptors [11]. Modeling of mixture toxicity is a relatively new application field of QSAR; further efforts are to be directed to the development of new methods (including descriptors) and the improvement of existing QSAR approaches for mixtures.

12.2.2 Peptide QSAR

In view of increasing antibiotic resistance by pathogens, antimicrobial peptides have drawn significant attention as an alternative class of antimicrobial therapeutics. Although a broad spectrum of antimicrobial peptides have been reported, their structure–activity relationships (SAR) are not well understood, largely because of substantial diversity in their structures and their nonspecific mechanism of action. There is the possibility that QSAR could be applied in further understanding their SAR. The majority of the previous work in this direction was sequence-based modeling efforts in a qualitative manner. There are some recent reports [12–15] on residue- and atom-based approaches in modeling antimicrobial peptides. It has emerged [7] that the atomic level of consideration combined with machine learning techniques may result in models delivering more active peptides. More extensive studies are needed in this area.

12.2.3 QSAR of nanoparticles

Nanoparticles (NPs) have found a wide range of applications in different fields of human life. They are employed in diverse industrial sectors, such as electronics, biomedical, pharmaceutical, cosmetics, and many others. Interestingly, our understanding regarding the harmful interactions of NPs with biological systems, as well as with the environment, is insufficient, and also the current understanding of the toxicity of NP, including possible mutagenic and carcinogenic effects, is very limited. In this background, theoretical methods like QSAR modeling might be applicable for the comprehensive risk exposure and assessment of NPs at the early stage of their development [16]. Information on the properties and toxicities of NPs is required under multiple regulatory documents, including REACH, the Biocides Directive, the Plant Protection Products Directive, the Water Framework Directive, and the Cosmetics Directive, where information shall be generated whenever possible by means other than vertebrate animal tests, through the use of alternative methods such as in vitro methods or QSAR models. The term *nano-QSAR* has recently been coined to describe this. A few nano-QSAR models have been recently reported for different end points, including cellular uptake of NPs in pancreatic cancer cell (PaCa2) [17–19], toxicity of metal oxide NPs for human bronchial epithelial (BEAS-2B) and murine myeloid (RAW 264.7) [20], and for the nanotoxicity of surface-modified multiwalled carbon nanotubes [21].

The most important encountered problems for developing QSAR models of NPs are the following:

1. Scarcity and inconsistency of the experimental data suitable for modeling and risk assessment of NPs
2. Lack of appropriate descriptors that are capable of expressing the specific characteristics of the "nano" structures
3. Inadequate knowledge of the interactions between NP and biological systems
4. Lack of rational structure–activity modeling procedures to screen large numbers of NPs for toxicity and hazard assessment

Efforts should be made to develop new descriptors and methodologies for developing QSAR models for this special class of chemicals.

12.2.4 QSAR of ionic liquids

Ionic liquids (ILs) have emerged as a class of highly useful chemicals with good thermal and chemical stability, appreciable task specificity, and minimal environmental release, with diverse applications in synthetic chemistry, electrochemistry, analytical chemistry, separation and extraction, and other engineering and biological applications. Theoretically, there are well over 1 million ILs that can be synthesized, although the experimental property and toxicity data have been reported for only a small fraction of them. It is possible to tune the physicochemical properties and toxicities of ILs via the choice of certain anionic and cationic components when designing a specific IL ideally suited for a specific process. This can be easily done by exploring the quantitative structure–property relationship (QSPR)/QSAR of ILs. There are already several reports on the QSPR of ILs for different properties; however, QSAR reports of different toxicity end points of ILs are rather limited in number [22]. Along with toxicity, equal importance has to be given to the chemical degradation and biodegradation parameters of ILs. QSAR may provide an enormous opportunity to the designer and synthetic chemists for searching of new analogs of ILs in search of "greener" solvents.

12.2.5 QSAR of cosmetics

The animal testing ban on cosmetic finished products and ingredients was applied in EU legislation with due regard to the Organisation for Economic Co-operation and Development (OECD) validation process in September 2004 and March 2009, respectively, whether or not an alternative method is available. Thereafter, a second measure introduced by the seventh amendment imposes a marketing ban on cosmetics in Europe if the finished product or its ingredients have been tested using animals. In the marketing ban, the first deadline was scheduled on March 2009 and the final cutoff date was March 2013, for when no cosmetic product containing an ingredient safety-tested using animals for the purposes of the directive could be allowed for sale in Europe, regardless of the availability of alternative, nonanimal tests (http://ec.europa.eu/consumers/archive/sectors/cosmetics/regulatory-framework/index_en.htm). The development of alternative methods is a tremendous scientific challenge. In the present scenario, the QSAR models may emerge as one of the leading alternatives for the testing of cosmetics safety and risk assessment (both for raw materials and the finished products). In the future, the QSAR of cosmetics will be one of the leading research areas to be explored in various dimensions. As an example, see Shen et al. [23], who developed and successfully validated the practical skin absorption model (SAM) for 131 fragrance materials.

The possible toxicological end points for the development of QSAR model relevant to cosmetics are as follows:

- Acute toxicity (oral, dermal, and inhalation)
- Irritation and corrosion of the skin and eyes
- Skin sensitization
- Dermal absorption
- Repeated dose toxicity
- Mutagenicity/genotoxicity
- Carcinogenicity
- Reproductive toxicity
- Toxicokinetics
- Photo-induced toxicities

12.2.6 PKPD-linked QSAR modeling

Computational QSAR and pharmacophore models are used to rapidly screen commercial databases of molecules and identify those likely to bind as substrates or inhibitors of a particular receptor or enzyme. The ultimate goal of the *in silico* modeling approach is the prediction of drug effects in vivo, by extrapolation of models using in vitro data. Successful extrapolation, however, is more likely when multiple models are combined to form a unified framework for the prediction of drug action. Several such fields have emerged, such as pharmacokinetic–pharmacodynamic (PKPD) modeling, population PKPD simulations, and physiologically based pharmacokinetic (PBPK) modeling. By understanding PKPD and related relationships, it is possible to estimate the in vivo doses required for efficacy. Such methods may provide a useful screening tool to rank candidate compounds with minimal use of extensive animal testing. Cooper et al. [24] developed a QSAR model based on calculated physical properties that predicted the partitioning of 34 compounds between lung and plasma. It was possible to use this relationship to predict the lung concentration at a given dose and time point. Exploring QSAR and pharmacophore models to predict drug transporter binding represents a way to anticipate drug–drug interactions of novel molecules from molecular structure [25]. These models may also be utilized on PKPD models to improve predictions of in vivo drug effects.

12.2.7 Material informatics

The theory of QSPR/QSAR modeling is applicable to model different properties of materials. Some useful applications include modeling of rheological and mechanical properties of chloroprene rubber accelerators [26], glass transition temperature (T_g) and mechanical properties of uncross-linked systems [27], solubility of fullerenes [28], modeling of catalysts [29], and biomaterials [30]. The QSPR models have the capacity to make good predictions (at least near their domains of applicability), so they merit being used to design materials with improved properties [31]. Although the application of QSPR in material science is not novel, there may be new response properties and materials that may be subjected to modeling by this approach.

12.2.8 Ecotoxicity modeling of pharmaceuticals

Low levels of pharmaceuticals have been detected in many countries in surface waters, groundwater, and drinking water. Although pharmaceuticals receive extensive pharmacological and clinical testing, information on the ecotoxicity of these biologically active compounds is very limited in general. The major routes of entry of pharmaceuticals into the environment are from the disposal of unwanted or expired drugs by users. Due to the fact that these compounds are intentionally designed to exert an effect on humans, residues of pharmaceuticals could be as important, or even more important, for human health than those of pesticides. A limited number of QSAR models have been constructed to date on the ecotoxicity of pharmaceuticals [32].

12.2.9 Interspecies toxicity modeling

Even though the toxicity data of an industrial chemical to a particular biological species may be available, it may be that the chemical's quantitative toxicity to another biological species is not known. Interspecies toxicity correlations provide a tool for estimating a contaminant's sensitivity with known levels of uncertainty for many different species. This approach can be applied for the reduction of animal testing by gathering and extrapolating information from tested to untested species, as well as from tested to untested chemicals [33].

12.2.10 QSAR of phytochemicals

With the increasing acceptance that chemical diversity of plant products is well suited to provide core scaffolds for future drugs, there is increasing use of novel plant products and chemical libraries based on phytochemicals in drug discovery programs. However, only a limited number of *in silico* models have been reported in the literature so far based on phytochemicals. The world may truly benefit from the wealth of knowledge of traditional plant medicine on successful integration of ethnopharmacology and *in silico* approaches [34].

12.3 CONCLUSION

QSAR has come a long way from its introduction in the form of classical Hansch and Free–Wilson approaches. It has gradually evolved with time though the refinement of approaches, use of newer descriptors, application of diverse chemometric tools, employment of rigorous validation tests, and integration with receptor structure information. QSAR has now emerged as a distinct scientific discipline in its own right. Apart from its use in ligand optimization in the context of drug discovery and predictive risk assessment in ecotoxicology, there are several new emerging fields in which QSAR is finding its application. A good practice of QSAR modeling though usage of OECD-recommended guidelines can develop good predictive models with demonstrated practical applications in diverse chemical biological areas, which may further strengthen its acceptability to the scientific community.

REFERENCES

[1] Pal P, Mitra I, Roy K. Predictive QSPR modeling for olfactory threshold of a series of pyrazine derivatives. Flavour Frag J 2013;28(2):102–17.

[2] Pal P, Mitra I, Roy K. QSPR approach to determine the essential molecular functionalities of potent odorants. Flavour Frag J 2014;29(3):157–65.

[3] Mitra I, Saha A, Roy K. Quantification of contributions of different molecular fragments for antioxidant activity of coumarin derivatives based on QSAR analyses. Can J Chem 2013;91(6):428–41.

[4] Das S, Mitra I, Batuta S, Alam MN, Roy K, Begum NA. Design, synthesis and exploring the quantitative structure–activity relationship of some antioxidant flavonoid analogues. Bioorg Med Chem Lett 2014;24(21):5050–4.
[5] Zhong M, Chong Y, Nie X, Yan A, Yuan Q. Prediction of sweetness by multilinear regression analysis and support vector machine. J Food Sci 2013;78:S1445–50.
[6] Yang X, Chong Y, Yan A, Chen J. In-silico prediction of sweetness of sugars and sweeteners. Food Chem 2011;128(3):653–8.
[7] Cherkasov A, Muratov EN, Fourches D, Varnek A, Baskin II, Cronin M, et al. QSAR modeling: where have you been? Where are you going to? J Med Chem 2014;57(12):4977–5010.
[8] Wei DB, Zhai LH, Hu HY. QSAR-based toxicity classification and prediction for single and mixed aromatic compounds. SAR QSAR Environ Res 2004;15(3):207–16.
[9] Ajmani S, Jadhav K, Kulkarni SA. Three-dimensional QSAR using the k-nearest neighbor method and its interpretation. J Chem Inf Model 2006;46(1):24–31.
[10] Zhang L, Zhou P-J, Yang F, Wang Z-D. Computer-based QSARs for predicting mixture toxicity of benzene and its derivatives. Chemosphere 2007;67(2):396–401.
[11] Muratov EN, Varlamova EV, Artemenko AG, Polishchuk PG, Nikolaeva-Glomb L, Galabov AS, et al. QSAR analysis of poliovirus inhibition by dual combinations of antivirals. Struct Chem 2013; 53:1665–79.
[12] Jenssen H, Gutteberg TJ, Lejon T. Modelling of anti-HSV activity of lactoferricin analogues using amino acid descriptors. J Pept Sci 2005;11(2):97–103.
[13] Sánchez-Gómez S, Japelj B, Jerala R, Moriyón I, Alonso MF, Leiva J, et al. Structural features governing the activity of lactoferricin-derived peptides that act in synergy with antibiotics against *Pseudomonas aeruginosa* in vitro and in vivo. Antimicrob Agents Chemother 2011;55(1):218–28.
[14] Cherkasov A, Hilpert K, Jenssen H, Fjell CD, Waldbrook M, Mullaly SC, et al. Use of artificial intelligence in the design of small peptide antibiotics effective against a broad spectrum of highly antibiotic-resistant superbugs. ACS Chem Biol 2009;4(1):65–74.
[15] Jenssen H, Fjell CD, Cherkasov A, Hancock REW. QSAR modeling and computer-aided design of antimicrobial peptides. J Pept Sci 2008;14(1):110–14.
[16] Puzyn T, Leszczynska D, Leszczynski J. Toward the developement of "Nano-QSARs": advances and challenges. Small 2009;5(22):2494–509.
[17] Fourches D, Pu D, Tassa C, Weissleder R, Shaw SY, Mumper RJ, et al. Quantitative nanostructure–activity relationship modeling. ACS Nano 2010;4(10):5703–12.
[18] Epa VC, Burden FR, Tassa C, Weissleder R, Shaw S, Winkler DA. Modeling biological activities of nanoparticles. Nano Lett 2012;12(11):5808–12.
[19] Kar S, Gajewicz A, Puzyn T, Roy K. Nano-quantitative structure–activity relationship modeling using easily computable and interpretable descriptors for uptake of magnetofluorescent engineered nanoparticles in pancreatic cancer cells. Toxicol In Vitro 2014;28(4):600–6.
[20] Liu R, Zhang HY, Ji ZX, Rallo R, Xia T, Chang CH, et al. Development of structure–activity relationship for metal oxide nanoparticles. Nanoscale 2013;5(12):5644–53.
[21] Shao CY, Chen SZ, Su BH, Tseng YJ, Esposito EX, Hopfinger AJ. Dependence of QSAR models on the selection of trial descriptor sets: a demonstration using nanotoxicity endpoints of decorated nanotubes. J Chem Inf Model 2013;53(1):142–58.
[22] Das RN, Roy K. Advances in QSPR/QSTR models of ionic liquids for the design of greener solvents of the future. Mol Divers 2013;17(1):151–96.
[23] Shen J, Kromidas L, Schultz T, Bhatia S. An in silico skin absorption model for fragrance materials. Food Chem Toxicol 2014;74:164–76.
[24] Cooper A, Potter T, Luker T. Prediction of efficacious inhalation lung doses via the use of in silico lung retention quantitative structure–activity relationship models and in vitro potency screens. Drug Metab Dispos 2010;38(12):2218–25.
[25] Ekins S, Ecker GF, Chiba P, Swaan PW. Future directions for drug transporter modelling. Xenobiotica 2007;37(10–11):1152–70.
[26] Todeschini R, Consonni V, Ballabio D, Mauri A, Cassotti M, Lee S, et al. QSPR study of rheological and mechanical properties of chloroprene rubber accelerators. Rubber Chem Technol 2014; 87:219–38.

[27] Hopfinger AJ, Koehler MG, Pearlstein RA, Tripathy SK. Molecular modeling of polymers. 4. Estimation of glass-transition temperatures. J Polym Sci Polym Phys 1988;26(10):2007–28.
[28] Toropova AP, Toropov AA, Benfenati E, Gini G, Leszczynska D, Leszczynski J. CORAL: QSPR models for solubility of [C60] and [C70] fullerene derivatives. Mol Divers 2011;15(1):249–56.
[29] Yao S, Shoji T, Iwamoto Y, Kamei E. Consideration of an activity of the metallocene catalyst by using molecular mechanics, molecular dynamics and QSAR. Comp Theor Polym Sci 1999;9(1): 41–6.
[30] Gubskaya AV, Kholodovych V, Knight D, Kohn J, Welsh W. Prediction of fibrinogen adsorption for biodegradable polymers: integration of molecular dynamics and surrogate modeling. J Polymer 2007;48(19):5788–801.
[31] Le T, Epa VC, Burden FR, Winkler DA. Quantitative structure–property relationship modeling of diverse materials properties. Chem Rev 2012;112(5):2889–919.
[32] Kar S, Roy K. First report on interspecies quantitative correlation of ecotoxicity of pharmaceuticals. Chemosphere 2010;81:738–47.
[33] Cassani S, Kovarich S, Papa E, Roy PP, van der Wal L, Gramatica P. Daphnia and fish toxicity of (benzo)triazoles: validated QSAR models, and interspecies quantitative activity–activity modeling. J Hazard Mater 2013;258– 259:50–60.
[34] Kar S, Roy K. QSAR of phytochemicals for the design of better drugs. Expert Opin Drug Discov 2012; 7(10):877–902.

INDEX

Note: Page numbers followed by "*f*", "*t*", and "*b*" refer to figures, tables and tables, respectively.

0-9, and Symbols

A

B

D

G

H

N

S

T

U

V

W

X

Y

Z

Printed in the United States
By Bookmasters